INTRODUCTION TO GLOBAL HEALTH PROMOTION

INTRODUCTION TO GLOBAL HEALTH PROMOTION

Rick S. Zimmerman, Ralph J. DiClemente,
Jon K. Andrus, Everold N. Hosein, and
Society for Public Health Education (SOPHE)

JB JOSSEY-BASS™
A Wiley Brand

Published by Jossey-Bass
A Wiley Brand
One Montgomery Street, Suite 1000, San Francisco, CA 94104–4594—www.josseybass.com

Library of Congress Cataloging-in-Publication Data

Names: Zimmerman, Rick S., editor. | DiClemente, Ralph J., editor. | Andrus, Jon Kim, editor. | Hosein, Everold N., editor. | Society for Public Health Education, sponsoring body.
Title: Introduction to global health promotion / [edited by] Rick S. Zimmerman, Ralph J. DiClemente, Jon K. Andrus, Everold N. Hosein and Society for Public Health Education.
Description: San Francisco, CA : Jossey-Bass, 2016. | Includes index.
Identifiers: LCCN 2015051179 (print) | LCCN 2016003678 (ebook) | ISBN 9781118897799 (pbk.) | ISBN 9781118897881 (pdf) | ISBN 9781118897836 (epub)
Subjects: LCSH: Health promotion. | Health education. | World health.
Classification: LCC RA427.8 .I5862 2016 (print) | LCC RA427.8 (ebook) | DDC 362.1—dc23
LC record available at http://lccn.loc.gov/2015051179

Cover design by Wiley
Cover image: Hands Image: © Zurijeta/Shutterstock;
Village Image: © pamuk/Shutterstock;
Child Image: © Lucian Coman/Shutterstock

Printed in the United States of America
FIRST EDITION

PB Printing 10 9 8 7 6 5 4 3 2 1

CONTENTS

The editors dedicate this book to the millions of people around the world who work tirelessly to prevent needless suffering caused by diseases that especially afflict the impoverished.

PREFACE

When my coeditors and I decided to respond to SOPHE's (Society for Public Health Education) request for prospectuses for a book on global health promotion, we were excited to have the opportunity to create the kind of book that we really hadn't seen: one that is focused on the relatively new domain of health promotion and disease prevention globally. With so much of the history of epidemiology presenting largely communicable diseases and mortality related to childbirth and the first few years of life, it has been only in the past 60 or so years that health promotion and disease prevention have become central to public health: first in what used to be called developed nations (and what we now refer to as high-income countries); and, second, in the past 15 or so years, during which life expectancies have increased sufficiently in low- and middle-income countries that the focus of public health in these countries has begun to include health promotion and disease prevention. So it was with great enthusiasm that we submitted a prospectus, and with which we reacted when our prospectus was chosen by SOPHE to become this book.

Organization of the Book

We put the book together wanting to share the best evidence with our readers about the approaches that have been successful in promoting health and reducing morbidity and mortality in a variety of areas. We also decided that health promotion strategies and approaches should be viewed through the lenses of theories and models of behavior change, human rights, and the exploding use of technology. As a result of these decisions, we organized the book as follows:

- introductory chapters,
- foundational chapters,
- strategies and best practices in global health promotion in topical areas,
- concluding chapters.

Three introductory chapters set the stage for the rest of the book. In "The State of Global Health," Richard Skolnik, the author of a major global health text, presents data about trends in causes of morbidity and mortality around the world. In "Global Health Promotion: The State of the Science," David McQueen, an internationally renowned global health promotion (GHP) scholar, talks about a fairly new and increasingly evidence-based approach to global health promotion strategies. Then, in "Global Health Promotion and the Social Determinants of Health," Kumanan Rasanathan and Alyssa Sharkey, both of whom work with UNICEF on children's health in under-resourced parts of the world, present the critical role of social and social structural variables as determinants of global health and health promotion. These introductory chapters present important ideas that are referred to throughout the book: (a) prevalence and incidence of various causes of morbidity (illness and risk factors for illness and various conditions) and mortality (death) patterns over time and across regions of the world, which should drive approaches to health promotion around the world; (b) the current status of the development and use of science- and evidence-based approaches to health promotion around the world; and (c) key underlying causes of health and illness related to social structure, processes, and resources—known as "social determinants."

The next section of the book (Chapters 4 through 7) includes foundational chapters on theory and models, human rights, and the use of technology as they relate to global health promotion. Indeed, these three lenses are used to present examples of best practices in disease and mortality reduction and prevention in the major portion of the book. Rick Zimmerman, one of the co-editors of the book and an expert in HIV prevention and behavior change theory development, and his colleagues Zhiwen Xiao, Purnima Mehrotra, and Charles Roy present "Models of Health Behavior Change: International Applications," in which key health behavior change models are described and international applications of these models are discussed, as Chapter 4. Everold Hosein (co-editor of the book), and his colleagues (senior health communication scholars May Kennedy and Sandra de Castro Buffington) describe two additional communication approaches related to behavior change, in Chapter 5, "Two Health Communication Approaches: Communication for Behavioral Impact (COMBI) and Entertainment Education." Elvira Beracochea, an internationally known advocate for health and for implementation of health systems that see health as a right, and her co-author, Lubna Ahmed, present some definitions of ethical concepts, articulate the overlap between health promotion and human rights, and describe case examples to show how sometimes health is but sometimes how it is not delivered as a right in Chapter 6, "Global Health Promotion in the Context of Human Rights." Sheana Bull, one of the international experts in the use of technology and social media in the delivery of health promotion interventions, and co-authors Gretchen Domek and Deborah Thomas, discuss ways that technology can be used most effectively in "eHealth and Global Health Promotion," Chapter 7.

The next nine chapters (Chapters 8–16) present what is currently known about best practices in global health promotion and disease prevention in nine different domains:

- Chapter 8, "Reducing Maternal and Infant Mortality: Meeting a Global Challenge" by Padmini Murthy, an obstetrician/gynecologist who is an expert on global health;
- Chapter 9, "Malaria Prevention and Control," by Fouzia Farooq and Elke Bergmann-Leitner, scientists in the US Military Malaria Research Program;

- Chapter 10, "Global Immunization Initiatives From a Health Promotion Perspective," by Marilyn Rice, a seasoned international health worker, with extensive experience in Latin America, and her colleagues Jon K. Andrus, Virginia Swezy, and Rick S. Zimmerman;
- Chapter 11, "The Evolving Global HIV Pandemic: Epidemiology, Prevention, and Future Priorities," by Ralph DiClemente, one of the co-editors of the book and an internationally renowned expert in HIV prevention, and his colleagues Puja Seth and Purnima Mehrotra;
- Chapter 12, "Community-Based Risk Communication in Epidemics and Emerging Disease Settings," by Renata Schiavo, well-known researcher and advocate in health equity and health communication, and her colleagues Karen Hilyard and Ewart Skinner;
- Chapter 13, "Noncommunicable Diseases (NCDs): Moving Toward Health Promotion," by C. James Hospedales (emphasis on Latin America) and André Pascal Kengne (emphasis on Africa), both international experts in NCDs, and their colleagues Adriana Blanco Marquizo and Branka Legetic;
- Chapter 14, "Women's Cancers," by Silvana Luciani and Irene Arguto, both of whom have spent years working for PAHO (Pan-American Health Organization, a regional arm of the World Health Organization) in the area of cancer;
- Chapter 15, "Health Promotion in Families and Communities: An Integrated Approach From Latin America and the Caribbean," by Fernando Zacarias and Gina Tambini, both experts in family and community health with experience at PAHO, and their colleagues Adrian Diaz, Manuel Pena, Adela Paez Jimenez, and Leticia Martinez; and
- Chapter 16, "Oral Health Promotion," by Margaret Scarlett, an internationally known leader in global oral health, and Gary Kreps, an internationally known global health communication researcher.

Each chapter in this core section of the text includes text boxes that highlight theories and models, human rights, and the use of technology relevant to their topic. We believe this is an important feature of this book: linking of applications across diseases/conditions/prevention domains to models and theories (the two are often presented separately, not showing the way theories are *used*), human rights (we believe this lens is used too rarely in considering global health promotion efforts), and technology (in ways that might suggest to readers how to use technology within their content areas of greatest interest).

The final three chapters cover issues we thought should be considered as broader concerns in moving forward with global health promotion. In Chapter 17, "Adaptation and Implementation of Public Health Innovations in Developing Countries," Bonita Stanton, Xiaoming Li, and Linda Kaljee, all senior researchers who have adapted and implemented Western-developed interventions in various international settings, discuss that process. In Chapter 18, "Health Promotion in the Global Setting: The Role of International Organizations and Governments," Jack Bryant, a pioneer in global health promotion, and Curtiss Swezy, a longtime global health program administrator, describe the history of the role of international organizations and governments in global health promotion. In the final chapter, "The Future of Global Health Promotion," Rick Zimmerman, Jon Andrus (a co-editor of the book and a long-time public health expert with more than 30 years of experience of working in the field of vaccines, immunization, and primary care in developing countries, including as deputy director of PAHO), and C. James Hospedales (long-time expert on health promotion in Latin America and the Caribbean) first look at progress in disease prevention and health promotion via the status of various diseases, conditions, and causes of morbidity and mortality around the world, and then talk about some of the key work that remains to be done in GHP.

We Knew We Couldn't Cover Everything

In creating this book, of course we have come to realize that we could not cover every important topic in global health promotion. Indeed, some reviewers expressed concerns that mental health, substance use and addiction, and/or adolescent health are not covered in the book. Chapter 19 reviews data about prevalence and incidence of mental illness and substance use disorder. But we acknowledge that it is only fairly recently that health promotion and disease prevention have become ways of thinking about mental health and mental illness. *Prevention* is typically used to describe health promotion efforts related to substance use and abuse, and certainly we might have covered this topic as well. We have also emphasized the state of activities in low- and middle-income countries—under-resourced parts of the world—in this book, and we acknowledge that with very high rates of mortality because of childhood diseases, malaria, HIV, and vaccine-preventable illnesses, mental health and substance use and abuse have been less of a focus in these parts of the world. Luckily they are becoming an increasing focus, though they aren't treated as chapters in this book. Adolescent health, though not the topic of an entire chapter, is a significant focus within several chapters, including HPV vaccination in Chapter 10, HIV and other sexually transmitted infections (STIs) in Chapter 11, and adapting interventions in Chapter 17. Finally, some might wonder why oral health is included as a topic. We simply state here (and encourage you to find out more by reading the chapter!) that there are a variety of strong relationships between oral health and other aspects of health, including heart disease, diabetes, a multitude of infections, and negative outcomes of pregnancy (see, for example, US Dept. of Health and Human Services, 2000, pp. 97–152).

Features and Resources for Students or Instructors

We have organized the book and book chapters, and have developed additional resources, that we believe will benefit students or instructors using this book.

- Each chapter has learning objectives that should help students and instructors easily identify the key goals/focus of the chapter.
- Each chapter has a list of key terms.
- Each chapter includes review questions.

- We have created test questions for instructors that are available on the book's website. Use the following link: www.wiley.com/go/globalhealth promotion
- We have created PowerPoint presentations for instructors that are available on the website. Use the following link: www.wiley.com/go/global healthpromotion

As we discussed earlier in the preface, we believe it is important that chapters be read more or less in the order they are presented. The first three chapters present topics, information, or perspectives that are fundamental for understanding the remainder of the book. Chapters 4–7 present theories and models, a description about the importance of human rights within GHP, and a discussion about the potential role of technology for GHP. Chapters 8–16 form the core of the book and contain text boxes related to theories and models, human rights, and technology. Chapters 17–19 present broader issues to consider in applying or learning about GHP.

Final Thoughts for the Reader

As more countries move from low to middle income (we hope) during the next several years and decades, their epidemiological profiles are likely to show an increase in morbidity and mortality related to chronic illness and a reduction in the prevalence of infant mortality, childhood diseases, and other communicable diseases. During this transitional period, however, the combination of communicable and noncommunicable diseases may introduce some new opportunities for health promotion packaged in different ways. And as the field of global health promotion grows and changes in response to emerging diseases and/or increases in the size of the middle class around the world, you may be the pioneers exploring this new world. We sincerely hope that this book facilitates your discovery of new ways of applying its knowledge to promote health and prevent disease around the world!

REFERENCES

US Department of Health and Human Services. (2000). *Oral health in America: A report of the Surgeon General*. Rockville, MD: US Department of Health and Human Services, National Institute of Dental and Craniofacial Research, National Institutes of Health.

ACKNOWLEDGMENTS

First, I acknowledge the love regularly shared with me by my adult children, Eli and Heidi. It means a lot to me and keeps me going when I have a chapter to finish. I also acknowledge all of the contributors to this volume for their work. I know there have been times when you had many other things on your plates but responded to urgent requests from me to keep things moving on your chapters. Thank you for helping to make this book what I hope will be a significant contribution to the emerging field of global health promotion!

—RSZ

I acknowledge the unwavering support of my family: Gina Maria, Sahara Rae, and Sianna Rose. They are the axis on which my world revolves and the inspiration and motivation for everything I do.

—RJD

I dedicate this book to the millions of people who work from bench to delivery to provide life-saving vaccines to those who need them most.

—JKA

There are hundreds of individuals who have helped shape the communication planning method called "Communication for Behavioral Impact" (COMBI) over the years, and I thank them all. But I take this opportunity to highlight two: first, my wife, Dr. Barbara Hosein, who patiently waited for my return after more than a hundred field missions abroad for COMBI work. Second, Dr. Elil Renganathan of the World Health Organization, who was my supervisor and guide as we introduced COMBI into the work of WHO globally.

—ENH

THE EDITORS

Rick S. Zimmerman, PhD, is currently a professor and associate dean for research in the College of Nursing at the University of Missouri–St. Louis. He received his PhD in sociology with an emphasis in medical sociology at the University of Wisconsin–Madison in 1983. His work focuses on understanding why individuals do or do not engage in risky or protective health behaviors. Much of his work during the past 25 years has focused on HIV, STD, and unwanted pregnancy prevention. He has received 10 National Institutes of Health grants on HIV and/or substance abuse prevention (from National Institute of Mental Health, National Institute on Alcohol Abuse and Alcoholism, National Institute on Drug Abuse, and National Institute of Nursing Research) in the past 25 years, most focusing on prevention in adolescents. His research group has conducted school-based curriculum interventions and adapted school-based interventions from Western to developing country settings; has conducted a successful development, implementation, and rigorous evaluation of a televised public service announcement campaign that increased condom use in young adults; and implemented and evaluated a campaign in two southern US cities to encourage early adolescents to wait to become sexually active. He and his research group have also conducted experimental work to help understand the influence of substance use and sexual arousal on sexual decision making. His international work has included the adaptation of alcohol and HIV prevention curricula for secondary school students in Kwa Zulu Natal, South Africa; the adaptation of a school-based dating prevention program in Capetown, South Africa; and the adaptation of a parent and teen intervention to reduce alcohol use and sexual behavior in Bangkok, Thailand. He is the lead author of the Multiple Domain Model, expanding social psychological models of behavior change to include social structural, personality, situational, and preparatory behavior components. He has also conducted research and written about how to improve the validity of self-reports about sensitive behaviors. His current work explores the impact of news reporting about biomedical advances in HIV on risk behavior; attempts to understand contextual and organizational characteristics that determine success of rural teen pregnancy prevention coalitions; and how to improve the validity of reporting about condom use in high-risk settings.

Ralph J. DiClemente, PhD, is Charles Howard Candler Professor of Public Health and associate director, Emory Center for AIDS Research. He holds concurrent appointments as professor, School of Medicine, Department of Pediatrics (Division of Infectious Diseases, Epidemiology, and Immunology), Department of Medicine (Division of Infectious Diseases), and the Department of Psychiatry. He was most recently chair, Department of Behavioral Sciences and Health Education at the Rollins School of Public Health, Emory University. Dr. DiClemente was trained as a health psychologist at the University of California, San Francisco, where he received his PhD in 1984 after completing a Master of Science in Public Health in behavioral sciences at the Harvard School of Public Health and his undergraduate degree at the City University of New York.

DiClemente is a recognized expert on the development and evaluation of STD/HIV prevention programs tailored to African American adolescents and young adults. He has been the recipient of myriad awards and Centers for Disease Control and National Institutes of Health grants. He has published extensively, authoring more than 500 peer-reviewed publications and editing or authoring 18 books.

Jon K. Andrus, MD, joined the Sabin Vaccine Institute in October 2014, where he serves as executive vice president and director of the Vaccine Advocacy and Education (VAE) program. VAE works to reduce the suffering caused by vaccine-preventable diseases by bringing together key stakeholders to foster collaboration, share best practices, and develop improved vaccine policy and access. Previously, Dr. Andrus served as deputy director of the Pan American Health Organization (PAHO). Prior to that, he was the lead technical advisor for PAHO's immunization program, providing oversight and guidance for technical cooperation to member countries.

Dr. Andrus holds faculty appointments at the University of California, San Francisco, and the Johns Hopkins University Bloomberg School of Public Health. He began his global health career as a Peace Corps volunteer, serving as a district medical officer in Malawi, and has since held positions in the US Centers for Disease Control's (CDC) Global Immunization Division, as head, Vaccinology and Immunization Program at the Institute for Global Health at the Universities of California at San Francisco and Berkeley, and as director of the Global Health MPH Program at George Washington University.

Dr. Andrus has received numerous awards for his leadership in the eradication of polio, measles, rubella, and congenital rubella syndrome, as well as the introduction of new vaccines in developing countries. In 2013, Dr. Andrus received the Transformational Leadership Award of the University of California. In 2011, he received the Global Leadership Award of the Pneumococcal Awareness Committee of Experts. In 2007, he received the Philip R. Horne Award for global leadership in immunization. In 2000, he received the Distinguished Service Medal, the highest award of the US Public Health Service, for his leadership in working to eradicate polio in Southeast Asia. Dr. Andrus holds a Bachelor of Science degree from Stanford University, obtained his medical degree from the University of California, Davis, and completed his residencies in family medicine at the University of California, San Francisco School of Medicine and preventive medicine at the CDC. He has published more than 100 scientific peer-reviewed papers on disease eradication, the introduction of new vaccines, and primary care.

Everold N. Hosein, PhD, a senior communication advisor-consultant for the World Health Organization (WHO), and communication consultant for the United Nations Children's Fund (UNICEF), is an international communication specialist (born in Trinidad and Tobago) with more than 45 years of experience in strategic communication, integrated marketing communication, advocacy and public relations, communication for development (C4D), health education, and IEC (information-education-communication) related to social development issues and behavioral impact and behavior change.

Hosein is also the co-director of the Global Health Communication Center at Indiana University and an adjunct professor and coordinator of the WHO-New York University Summer Institute on Integrated Marketing Communication for Behavioral Impact in Health and Social Development at New York University. He is the founder of the strategic communication planning methodology called COMBI—Communication for Behavioral Impact—initiated at New York University in 1994, adopted and refined at WHO since 2000, and more recently combined with UNICEF's Communication for Development work.

Hosein was the recipient of the prestigious 2010 Mayhew Derryberry Award of the Public Health Education and Health Promotion (PHEHP) section of the American Public Health Association (APHA). Formerly, Dr. Hosein was senior counselor for social development at Burson-Marsteller Public Relations in New York. Prior to that he served as director of Program Support (Public Relations, IEC and Fundraising) at International Planned Parenthood Federation, New York. He was the director of the University of the West Indies Institute of Mass Communication in Jamaica.

Hosein's global professional experience extends from Africa and Asia to the Caribbean, Latin America, Europe, and North America. He has completed more than 300 consulting assignments around the world. His communication work has focused on the following program areas: nutrition, early childhood education, children's welfare and girls' education, children protection, water and sanitation, communicable diseases prevention and control, influenza, environmental education, noncommunicable diseases (including cancer prevention and care), pandemics, general public health, reproductive health (including maternal/child health, family planning, and HIV/AIDS/STD prevention), public sector pharmaceutical policies, gender equality, health promotion, university education, agricultural and rural development, population and development, and banking/monetary policies.

SOPHE

The Society for Public Health Education (SOPHE) is a nonprofit professional organization founded in 1950. SOPHE's mission is to provide global leadership to the profession of health education and health promotion and to promote the health of society through advances in health education theory and research, excellence in professional preparation and practice, advocacy for public policies conducive to health, and the achievement of health equity for all. SOPHE is the only independent professional organization devoted exclusively to health education and health promotion.

SOPHE's membership extends health education principles and practices to many settings, including schools; universities; medical and health care settings; work sites; voluntary health agencies; international organizations; and federal, state, and local governments.

Contact SOPHE at 10 G Street N.W., Suite 605, Washington, DC 20002-4242; telephone: (202) 408-9804; Web site: www.sophe.org.

THE CONTRIBUTORS

Irene Agurto, PhD, is an international health consultant. She received her BS degree from the Universidad Catolica de Chile and her PhD degree as social and political scientist from the Universidad Complutense de Madrid, Spain. She has many years of experience in health promotion and education, having held a position as regional advisor at the Pan American Health Organization/World Health Organization, Regional Office for the Americas, for 5 years, based in Washington, DC and 6 years afterwards as a consultant, based in Chile.

She has conducted extensive qualitative research among underserved populations in Latin American and the Carribean and developed and carried out cervical cancer service improvement projects. She has contributed to chronic disease prevention and control through research, education, and training of health providers. She has several publications in these areas.

Lubna Ahmed, MA, grew up in Sudan and moved to the United States in 2000, where she obtained her bachelor's degree in biology. She has eight years of pharmaceutical research experience as well as project management. She received her master's degree in public health from George Mason University in 2014. Ahmed has a strong passion for helping developing countries through awareness and managing projects.

Elvira Beracochea, MD, MPH, has more than 25 years of experience as a physician and a global health expert and has worked in more than 60 countries. She is the founder and president of "Realizing Global Health" (RGH), a global health consulting company that assists donors, governments, and global health organizations to develop self-reliant sustainable health systems that deliver quality health care to everyone everywhere every day. Dr. Beracochea has developed the "Health for All NOW" model to deliver integrated quality health care, the RGH100, a system for improving health care delivery in 100 days, the Asset-Based Management (ABM) system to strengthen health system performance, and numerous other solutions and training and coaching programs that improve the delivery of quality health services worldwide. She is an active advocate for the right to health through her participation in various professional organizations. She is chair of the Community Based Primary Health Care work group of the International Health Section of the American Public Health Association (APHA) and co-chair of the International Health and Nutrition Work Group at the Society for International Development in Washington, DC (SIDW). Her recent books include *Improving Aid Effectiveness in Global Health* (Springer 2015); *Health for All NOW: How to Transform the Delivery of Health Services in Developing Countries, Medicines for All,* and *Rights-Based Approaches to Public Health* (co-editor). Dr. Beracochea received her MD from the University of the Republic of Uruguay and her MPH from Hadassah Hebrew University in Israel.

Elke S. Bergmann-Leitner, PhD, has been a cellular immunologist in the US Military Malaria Research Program since 2001. She also serves as associate research professor (Department of Medicine) at the Uniformed Services University of the Health Sciences, Bethesda, Maryland. She received her PhD from the University of Salzburg, Austria, characterizing splenic regeneration and immunological competence after auto-transplantation. She trained as post-doctoral fellow at the Laboratory for Tumor Immunology and Biology (LTIB) National Cancer Institute/National Institutes of Health (NIH) characterizing anti-tumor T-cell responses in cancer patients, which completed her training in human immunology. Bergmann-Leitner now heads the Flow Cytometry Center, a core facility substantially involved in the evaluation of vaccine-induced responses as well as in the development of novel readout methods. The goal is the identification of immune correlates of protection against malaria induced either by natural exposure or vaccination.

John (Jack) Bryant, MD, is a pioneer in global health and health promotion. Throughout a very full career he worked with the Rockefeller Foundation on a study of 22 developing countries that resulted in the book *Health and the Developing World* (Cornell University Press, 1969). Among his memorable contributions to the field, he was a delegate at the Tübingen, Germany, conferences, helped establish the Christian Medical Commission, and helped guide the World Health Organization Primary Health Care Conference in Almaty. Among his many professional appointments, he was dean, Columbia University School of Public Health, 1971–1978; deputy assistant secretary of international health, Department of Health and Human Services, 1978–1985; and founding chair, Department of Community Health Science, Aga Khan University, Karachi, 1985–1994. He currently holds faculty appointments at the Johns Hopkins School of Public Health, Great Lakes University (Kisumu, Kenya), and the University of Virginia Department of Health Sciences. In recent years he has traveled regularly to Africa to provide health care in urban slums of Nairobi.

Sheana S. Bull, PhD, MPH, is a professor and chair of the Department of Community and Behavioral Health at the Colorado School of Public Health. Her work is focused on testing and determining the efficacy of interventions for health promotion using mobile and social media technologies in the US and global settings. She was among the first NIH-funded researchers to explore the efficacy of the Internet and cell phones for prevention of chronic illness, and published one of the first investigations showing efficacy for using social media to sustain healthy behavior. Her publications include numerous articles describing ethics, theory based program development, recruitment, engagement with material in the social media environment, the influence peers or "friends" on Facebook have on social norms, and the efficacy of using social media for behavior change. She established and currently directs the mHealth Impact Laboratory at the University of Colorado Denver, intended to shorten the timeline to establish mHealth app efficacy, to curate effective mHealth apps, and facilitate their widespread dissemination and scale.

Sandra de Castro Buffington, MPH, is a global leader in entertainment for social change. As the founding director of the Global Media Center for Social Impact at UCLA's Fielding School of Public Health, de Castro Buffington works closely with Hollywood and other creative capitals worldwide to develop health and justice storylines to affect knowledge and behavior, and new media tools to move audiences to action. Her research measures the impact of storytelling on viewers and maps the pro-social content on top TV shows. Named one of the "100 Most Influential Hispanics" in America by *PODER* magazine in 2012, de Castro Buffington's vasectomy campaign in Brazil earned seven international awards, including a Bronze Lion at the Cannes Film Festival and Gold Medal at the London International Advertising Awards. Formerly director of Hollywood, Health & Society, she created a global network of centers, including India and Nigeria with the hub in Hollywood, to improve the accuracy of health-related storylines in top TV shows and films. Her groundbreaking work resulted in 565 storylines on 91 shows across 35 networks between 2009 and 2012.

Adrián Díaz, MD, received his degree from the University of Buenos Aires and is a pediatrician certified by the Argentina Society of Pediatrics. He completed a postgraduate degree in Tropical Medicine at "Prince Leopold" Institute in Anvers, Belgium, and in Public and Community Health at the University of Nancy II, France. He completed an internship in International Health at the Pan American Health Organization/World Health Organization (PAHO/WHO) in Washington, D.C. He has developed an undergraduate course in nutrition at the University of Belgrano, Argentina, and the Master's in Public Health Program at the University of Buenos Aires and the National University of Rosario, Argentina. He has been consultant in various international organizations (UNICEF, Interamerican Development Bank, PAHO/WHO) and NGOs (MSF, Medecins du Monde, Action Against Hunger). He rejoined PAHO/WHO in 2007 as a consultant in Family and Community Health in Peru, where he held the position until June 2014. He is currently advisor in Family and Community Health, PAHO/WHO in Ecuador.

Gretchen Domek, MD, is an assistant professor in pediatrics at the Colorado School of Medicine, University of Colorado Anschutz Medical Campus. Dr. Domek received her medical degree at Harvard Medical School and trained in pediatrics at the University of Colorado. Prior to medical school, Dr. Domek received a master of philosophy degree in medical anthropology at Oxford University as a Rhodes Scholar. She completed a Global Health Fellowship through the Center for Global Health at the Colorado School of Public Health and is a senior investigator at the Center for Global Health. She is the director of the International Adoption Clinic at Children's Hospital Colorado. Her research focuses on using emerging technology for global health promotion as well as promoting early childhood health and development in low-resource settings.

Fouzia Farooq, MPH, has been the laboratory manager and research scientist within the US Military Malaria Research Program at Walter Reed Army Institute of Research (WRAIR)/Naval Medical Research Center (NMRC) since 2007. She is a crucial team member of the Flow Cytometry Center, characterizing Phase I clinical trials testing malaria vaccines for travelers and the military as well as developing new analysis panels for flow cytometry. Farooq is one of the key expert microscopists for controlled human malaria challenge trials at WRAIR/NMRC. She serves on various consortia and international working groups with the goal of harmonizing and optimizing readout methods for vaccine evaluation. She received her master's degree in public health from George Mason University in 2015. One of her accomplishments has been designing public health policies for hospitals in Swaziland, Africa.

Karen M. Hilyard, PhD, is an assistant professor of health promotion and behavior at the University of Georgia College of Public Health, where she teaches health communication and social marketing. Her research is in health communication and disparities related to vaccine behavior and decision making. Hilyard is currently co-principal investigator on a $1.6 million grant from the National Institutes of Health National Institute of General Medical Sciences to develop new computational methodologies to understand vaccine discourse on social media. She was also a UGA Lilly Teaching Fellow from 2013 to 2015. Prior to her career in academia, Hilyard was a professional communicator. She spent eight years at CNN, where she was an Emmy-winning producer covering breaking news stories, and she worked as a public relations executive for six years at agencies in New York City and central Kentucky, overseeing accounts for major national clients in a variety of industries including health care, technology, financial services, manufacturing, and agriculture.

C. James Hospedales, MD, MS, a citizen of Trinidad & Tobago, is the executive director of the Caribbean Public Health Agency. From 2006 to 2012, Dr. Hospedales was responsible for the PAHO program for prevention and control of chronic noncommunicable diseases (NCDs). He played a key role in increasing priority and resources for NCDs, including helping organize the CARICOM Heads of Government Summit on NCDs. He pioneered the Pan American Forum for Action on NCDs, which brings together governments, civil society, academia, and business. He has also been a champion for civil society involvement in efforts to improve health, and helped catalyze the formation of the Healthy Caribbean Coalition.

From 1998 to 2006, Dr. Hospedales was director of the Caribbean Epidemiology Centre. He was instrumental in developing donor partnerships for HIV/AIDS prevention and a partnership with the Caribbean tourism industry to improve health, safety, and environmental conditions.

He was a member of the Caribbean Commission on Health and Development, which made policy recommendations in 2005 to the Heads of Government and named chronic diseases as a super-priority for the region.

His career has included service as an epidemic intelligence service officer with the US Centers for Disease Control, as an epidemiologist at CAREC, and several years working in public health for the UK National Health Service.

Dr. Hospedales graduated with honors in medicine from the University of the West Indies. He has a master's of science degree in community medicine from the London School of Hygiene and Tropical Medicine, is a fellow of UK Faculty of Public Health, and an accredited partnership broker with the Partnering Institute of the UK. He has published more than 60 papers and reports.

Adela Páez Jiménez, DrPH, joined the Pan American Health Organization as Program Management and Partnerships Specialist in 2011. Since 2014, she is based at the European Center for Disease Control as Scientific Coordinator of the Mediterranean Program for Intervention Epidemiology (MediPIET). Holder of a Doctorate in Clinical Epidemiology by the Medicine Faculty & Public Health School of Paris XI, she has over twelve years of experience as epidemiologist in Europe (Institut de Veille Sanitaire, Institut Pasteur), the Middle-East (Ain Shams University-Faculty of Community Medicine), West and Central Africa (UNAIDS Regional Support Team) and Latin America and the Caribbean (PAHO/AMRO).

Linda Kaljee, PhD, is a senior research investigator at the Henry Ford Health System, Global Health Initiative in Detroit, Michigan. Since 1989, she has been engaged in sexual and reproductive health research and program development with a focus on adolescents and emerging adults. She has been a principal investigator or investigator on reproductive health and HIV prevention program development and evaluation studies in diverse communities within the United States as well as internationally, including work in China, India, the Bahamas, and Vietnam. Through her work in the Bahamas, she has been engaged in implementation research and program dissemination and sustainability. More recently she has been involved with research focused on psychosocial issues for children and adolescents living in low-resource settings, including programs in China and Zambia, as well as development of a Web-based and social media HIV and reproductive health intervention for US youth in an urban juvenile detention center.

May G. Kennedy, PhD, MPH, received her doctorate in community/organizational psychology in 1982 from Georgia State University. She taught psychology at Mercer University, and was awarded an APA Congressional Science Fellowship in 1988. She was assigned to the health staff of the Labor and Human Resources Committee in the Senate and then worked for the Select Committee on Children, Youth and Families of the House of Representatives until she was awarded an NIH HIV/AIDS prevention fellowship at the Centers for Disease Control (CDC) in 1993. Earning her master's of public health degree at Emory University in 1995, she spent the next decade as a behavioral scientist at CDC. Assigned to the Division of HIV/AIDS Prevention, the White House Office on AIDS, and the CDC director's Office of Communication, she specialized in adolescent risk reduction, social marketing and evaluating entertainment education collaborations with Hollywood. From 2005 to 2013, Kennedy taught health communication in the public health program at Virginia Commonwealth University, where she conducted federally funded communication research. She is now an affiliate associate professor at VCU in Richmond, Virginia, and a program design and evaluation consultant.

André Pascal Kengne, MD, PhD, is a medical doctor and internist from the School of Medicine of the Yaounde I University in Cameroon and holds a PhD in medicine from the Sydney University, Australia. He is the current director of the South African Medical Research Council's Non-Communicable Diseases Research Unit and holds conjoint appointments as associate professor in the Department of Medicine of the University of Cape Town, South Africa. He is a fellow of the George Institute for Global Health (Australia) and the Julius Center for Health Sciences and Primary Care (Holland). His areas of research include chronic disease epidemiology and prevention in developing countries and decision making in diabetes and cardiovascular diseases. He has been involved in major research projects in these areas in Africa and around the world. He is co-author of numerous peer-reviewed articles, book chapters, and monographs on chronic diseases in Africa and beyond.

Gary L. Kreps, PhD, University of Southern California (1979), is a University Distinguished Professor and director of the Center for Health and Risk Communication at George Mason University. He studies health and risk communication, health promotion, and social influence, with a focus on reducing health inequities. He publishes widely (more than 400 articles, books, and monographs) concerning the applications of communication knowledge. His research has been funded by numerous federal agencies, foundations, health systems, foreign governments, and corporations. He served as the founding chief of the Health Communication and Informatics Research Branch at the National Cancer Institute, where he planned national research programs for promoting cancer prevention and control. He also served as the founding dean of the School of Communication at Hofstra University, executive director of the Greenspun School of Communication at the University of Nevada Las Vegas, and as a professor at Northern Illinois, Rutgers, Indiana, and Purdue universities. He is the recipient of many honors, including the Lewis Donohew Outstanding Health Communication Scholar Award, the ICA/NCA Outstanding Health Communication Scholar Award, and the 2015 American Academy for Health Behavior Research Laureate Award.

Branka Legetic, MD, PhD, is a citizen of Uruguay. She is currently advisor on tobacco control at the Pan American Health Organization (PAHO), World Health Organization Regional Office for the Americas. She obtained her medical degree from the University of the Republic of Uruguay and a specialization in drug addictions at the University Centro Latinoamericano de Economía Humana (CLAEH). She also has a master's degree from the same university on policies for prevention of drug addictions in children and youth. In her native country she worked in the municipality of Montevideo and was a member of the health division advisor team in the area of tobacco control and drugs. She was in charge of the development of the municipality's smoking cessation clinics.

Since 2000, she has actively worked on the tobacco control process in Uruguay. She was a member of the National Alliance for Tobacco Control, the Advisory Tobacco Control Commission of the Ministry of Health and the Tobacco Control Committee of the Medical Union. In May 2006, Dr. Legetic joined the regional tobacco control team at PAHO.

Xiaoming Li, PhD, received his doctorate in educational psychology from the University of Minnesota, Minneapolis, and is professor and endowed chair of Health Promotion, Education, and Behavior at the University of South Carolina Arnold School of Public Health and director of the South Carolina SmartState Center for HealthCare Quality. He served as professor and founding director of the Wayne State University Pediatric Prevention Research Center for more than 12 years prior to joining the University of South Carolina in 2015. Over the past two decades, Li has been a principal investigator or site principal investigator on 12 research projects (including 7 NIH funded projects) and a co-investigator on 28 research projects (including 22 from NIH and other federal agencies). In addition to his specialties in advanced statistics and research methodology, Li is experienced in research on health risk behaviors and perceptions among minority adolescents and other vulnerable or at-risk populations. He has worked on HIV-related prevention/intervention research in the United States, China, Namibia, Vietnam, the Bahamas, Zambia, and India. Li has published more than 300 peer-reviewed articles, book chapters, and special reports and is the editor-in-chief of *Health Psychology and Behavioral Medicine: An Open Access Journal* (Taylor & Francis).

Silvana Luciani, MHSc, is a public health professional, working at the Pan American Health Organization in the Department of Noncommunicable Diseases (NCDs) and Mental Health, where she is developing programs on NCDs and cancer, in collaboration with Ministries of Health in Latin America and the Caribbean. She has been advocating for and providing evidence on the need for comprehensive NCD and cancer programs, and collaborating with governments in Latin America and the Caribbean to create national plans for NCDs and cancer. She has been developing and evaluating community based cancer programs, with a focus on awareness, prevention and early detection. She is also leading a multi-sector partnership on women's cancers to increase health service capacity and use of evidence-based guidelines for breast and cervical cancer control.

Adriana Blanco Marquizo, PhD, MSc, is regional advisor on prevention and control of noncommunicable diseases in the Department of Noncommunicable Diseases and Mental Health at the Pan American Health Organization. She holds a doctorate in prevention of noncommunicable diseases and a master's degree on integrated cardiovascular health prevention and specialization in community medicine and organization of health services. Her areas of expertise are health planning and evaluation, health promotion, noncommunicable disease (NCD) prevention, capacity building, health economics, and epidemiology of NCDs. She was responsible for development and led the process of consultations on the draft of the Regional Plan for Prevention and Control of NCDs 2013–2019 that serves as reference document for regional policy related to NCDs in the Americas. Currently, her work is focused on economic aspects of NCDs, population-based cardiovascular diseases prevention programs, with special attention to reduction of salt consumption in population and surveillance of NCDs and their risk factors.

Leticia Martínez, MSc, obtained her degree in biochemistry and molecular biology from the University of Oviedo, Spain, and carried out her final project at the University of Turku, Finland. She worked as a researcher at the University Children's Hospital in Zurich, Switzerland, at the Division of Infectious Diseases and Hospital Epidemiology.

Martínez obtained her master's of global health and public policy from the University of Edinburgh, Scotland, which was followed by an internship at the Pan American Health Organization/World Health Organization (PAHO/WHO) in Peru.

She joined the Pan American Alliance for Nutrition and Development in 2012, working as technical advisor for the project "Strengthening the Knowledge Management of Programs and Projects to Combat Malnutrition in Latin America" for two years, in pursuit of the Millennium Development Goals under the approach of determinants of food insecurity and malnutrition.

Since then, Martínez has joined the Regional Tobacco Control Team, from the Department of Non-communicable Diseases and Mental Health at PAHO/WHO, supporting the implementation of the Framework Convention on Tobacco Control to curb the tobacco epidemic as one of the risk factors for NCDs.

David V. McQueen, PhD, is a global consultant in health promotion based in Atlanta. His doctoral work was at the Johns Hopkins University. He is retired from 20 years at the Centers for Disease Control, where he was chief of the behavioral risk factor surveillance system (BRFSS), director of the Division of Adult and Community Health (DACH), and associate director for global health promotion. He held professorships at the University of Edinburgh, directing the Research Unit in Health and Behavioral Change, 1983–1992; and the Johns Hopkins University School of Public Health, 1972–1983. He is a globally elected board member of the International Union of Health Promotion and Education (IUHPE), and served eight years as the vice president for science and four years as president; he is currently the IUHPE vice president for scientific affairs. He has served on numerous consultancies and committees with the World Bank, WHO, PAHO, EURO, NAS, the Canadian government, as well as other public and private agencies. He is widely published in academic journals and is the author/editor of several books, including the comprehensive *Global Handbook on Noncommunicable Diseases and Health Promotion* (Springer, 2013). He is an adjunct professor in the Department of Behavioral Sciences and Health Education at Emory University and an adjunct professor of Social and Preventive Medicine, Universität Bern, Switzerland.

Purnima Mehrotra, PhD, has 12 years of experience conducting research in the areas of HIV and risky sexual behavior, focused on young adolescents in the United States and poor urban married women in India. She also has extensive research experience evaluating reproductive, maternal, neonatal, and child health (RMNCH) among most marginalized communities in India (including in community health program design, implementation, and evaluation) and implementing and evaluating behavior change communication campaigns. She has given numerous presentations at national and international conferences and has published more than 20 reports, book chapters, and peer-reviewed publications, the majority on populations at high risk for HIV.

Padmini Murthy, MD, is a physician (a trained obstetrician and gynecologist) and an activist who did her residency in obstetrics and gynecology. She has practiced medicine and public health for the past 28 years in various countries. Dr. Murthy has been the recipient of several awards and honors. Currently she is associate professor of public health practice and global health director at New York Medical College.

Dr. Murthy has been the recipient of several awards and honors, including induction as an inaugural fellow of the American Medical Women's Association in April 2015 and receiving the Millennium Milestone Maker Award at the Ninth Annual Women's Symposium at Sias University, China, in June 2015.

D. Murthy is widely published and is the author and editor of *Women's Global Health and Human Rights* (Jones & Bartlett), which is used as a textbook worldwide, and she serves as a peer reviewer for several publications. Her poetry book, *Mini's Musings,* was published in 2012. She has made more than 100 presentations on women's and children's health nationally and internationally at scientific conferences and at the United Nations, and in other countries where she has been invited.

Manuel Peña, MD, PhD, obtained his medical degree from the University of Havana and specialized in pediatrics and nutrition. He holds a doctoral degree from the Hungarian Academy of Science and was senior research fellow of the University of Pennsylvania and the University of United Nations.

Peña was a professor in pediatrics and was appointed in 1982 as vice dean of Research and Post-Graduate Education at the Institute of Basic Sciences of the Medical University of Havana.

He joined PAHO/WHO as nutrition adviser in the Andean Region, and in 1992 as the nutrition regional adviser in PAHO headquarters in Washington, D.C. He was the PAHO/WHO representative in Jamaica (1999–2003) and in Peru (1994–1999). From 2010 through 2011 he was the coordinator of the Pan American Alliance of Nutrition, involving 15 agencies of the United Nations, whose main objective was to tackle undernutrition with a comprehensive approach.

He has published more than 70 scientific articles in the field of nutrition, obesity and public policy. Currently, Dr. Peña is the PAHO/WHO representative ad interim in Peru.

Kumanan Rasanathan, MD, is a public health physician currently working as a senior health specialist for UNICEF in New York. He is the UNICEF focal point for health in the post-2015 development agenda and for social determinants of child health. He also works on district health system strengthening to improve the delivery of maternal and child health services in Asia and sub-Saharan

Africa, including links to universal health coverage. Before arriving at UNICEF, Dr. Rasanathan worked at WHO in Geneva on primary health care and social determinants of health. He has worked in a range of roles in a number of countries as a clinician, researcher, policymaker, and program manager in clinical practice, vaccine clinical trials, primary health care, national health policy, and reducing inequities in maternal and child health.

Marilyn E. Rice, MA, MPH, is chief executive officer (CEO) of merci (Marilyn E Rice Consulting International), an international consulting firm specializing in advising on promoting equity in health and development. Until June 2011 she was the senior advisor in health promotion and coordinator of the Urban Health and Determinants of Health Team for the Pan American Health Organization (PAHO/WHO). With more than 40 years of experience working in multicultural, multilingual environments, she is known globally for her work in community development, social mobilization, health promotion and education, participatory research and evaluation, and the emerging field of urban health. Serving on boards of numerous international, nonprofit, and professional organizations, as well as on editorial boards of numerous peer-reviewed journals, she has published extensively in her fields of expertise based upon her experiences in countries throughout the world. She continues to conduct workshops, courses, and conferences in many of those places in any of four languages (English, French, Spanish, and Portuguese). She holds degrees in sociology, English, public health, and health education.

Charles Roy, BSN, graduated with his bachelor of science in nursing from the University of Missouri-St. Louis and is currently at Saint Louis Psychiatric Rehabilitation Center as a behavioral nurse. His interest in neurology and behavior sparked early on during his time at Washington University in St. Louis School of Medicine as part of the Young Scientist Program. Charles assisted in the lab of Dr. David Holtzman with a primary focus on the etiology, manifestations, and progression of Alzheimer's disease both in the lab and clinical settings. In college, he was an undergraduate research assistant to Dr. Rick Zimmerman and collaborated in multiple projects exploring risky behavior and sexually transmitted diseases. He also co-authored a chapter in this book under Dr. Zimmerman's guidance during this time. Roy plans on sharing his passion for community health, education, research, and medicine in the future by pursuing his doctoral degree and empowering men and women in underserved areas through knowledge and compassion.

Margaret Scarlett, DMD, is an internationally recognized public health leader in oral health, focusing on infectious and chronic diseases. Early in her career, she provided dental care in three rural clinics in the southern United States, serving a rural minority population. Leveraging her firsthand experience with disparities in oral health promotion and care, she served in various lead roles in policy, administrative, research, and program activities at the Centers for Disease Control and Prevention (CDC) in oral health, women's, health and HIV/AIDS. A contributor to the US Surgeon General's Report on Oral

Health, she has numerous publications and has served as an advisor to the WHO, PAHO, and to eight ministries of health. Following her retirement from CDC, Scarlett provides international consulting and speaking to academic institutions, medical and dental industry, and the dental profession to improve population-based health outcomes.

Renata Schiavo, PhD, MA, is a global health, health care, and social innovation specialist with more than 20 years of experience in different settings, including the United States and several countries in Europe, Latin America, and Africa. She is founding president of Health Equity Initiative, a nonprofit membership organization dedicated to advancing health equity; senior lecturer at Columbia University Mailman School of Public Health; editor-in-chief of the *Journal of Communication in Healthcare: Strategies, Media, and Engagement in Global Health;* and founder and principal, Strategic Communication Resources, a global expert consultancy. She is the author of the internationally acclaimed book *Health Communication: From Theory to Practice* (Jossey-Bass) and dozens of other publications. Her work has been supported by the Office of Minority Health Resource Center, US HHS Office of Minority Health; UNICEF; and the World Health Organization, among others. Schiavo's professional interests focus on system-changing strategies and lie at the intersection of strategic health communication for behavioral, social, and organizational change; strategic planning for system change; multisectoral partnerships; health equity; community health; risk communication; and global health. She was recognized as one of 300 Women Leaders in Global Health (2015) by an initiative of the Graduate Institute of International and Development Studies in Geneva.

Puja Seth, PhD, has 15 years of experience conducting research in HIV and risky sexual behavior among minority populations. She has specialized experience working with HIV-positive clients in a clinical context for mental health issues and has specifically focused on high-risk populations when evaluating and designing HIV interventions. Seth has worked internationally and domestically on programmatic and research efforts on HIV testing and HIV service delivery, prevention with positives, program evaluation, HIV-related workgroups, national-level data and data quality issues, providing technical assistance and capacity building. She has more than 80 presentations at national and international conferences and has more than 40 reports, book chapters, and peer-reviewed publications, with the majority on populations at high risk for HIV. Seth is currently a lead behavioral scientist and an adjunct assistant professor in the Rollins School of Public Health at Emory University.

Alyssa Sharkey, PhD, is a health specialist for UNICEF in New York. She focuses on monitoring and evaluation of UNICEF's priority health programs that support UNICEF's equity agenda, implementation research and qualitative analysis of health programs (particularly relating to demand generation), and knowledge management. Prior to joining UNICEF, she worked as a policy researcher, policy analyst, and program officer within academic, research, and nongovernmental settings in the field of maternal, newborn, and child health both internationally and in the United States.

Ewart C. Skinner, PhD, is associate professor in the Department of Telecommunications at Bowling Green State University, where he has taught courses in global health communication, global media, and telecommunications, and media effects. He has taught in the Communication Skills for Medical Students program at the University of the West Indies, Eric Williams Medical Sciences Complex in Trinidad. In the realm of global health, he has published articles and presented conference papers on HIV/AIDS, and in 2014 was a participant in the COMBI (Communication for Behavioral Impact) NYU/WHO workshop on global health.

Richard Skolnik, MPA, is a lecturer at the Yale School of Public Health and the Yale School of Management. He teaches introductory and advanced global health courses at Yale College and introductory global health courses at the School of Public Health and the School of Management.

Mr. Skolnik has more than 40 years of experience in development and global health work. He spent 25 years at the World Bank, retiring as the director for Health and Education for the South Asia Region. After leaving the World Bank, he was the vice president for international programs at the Population Research Bureau and the director of the Center for Global Health at the George Washington University, where he taught undergraduate global health courses for nine years. He also served as the executive director of the Harvard PEPFAR program for AIDS treatment in Botswana, Nigeria, and Tanzania.

He received a BA from Yale University and an MPA from the Woodrow Wilson School of Princeton University. He is the author of the widely used textbook, *Global Health 101,* and has served on numerous international technical and advisory bodies.

Bonita Stanton, MD, is professor of pediatrics and vice dean for research at the Wayne State University School of Medicine. A behavioral researcher for the past 30 years, Stanton has devoted a substantial component of her research effort in countries other than the United States. She and her family lived in Bangladesh for five years and in Egypt for six months, during which time she was focused on community-based research, and she has worked extensively in China and India as well as several countries in Africa and in the Caribbean. For the past decade, a major focus of her research has been implementation of behavioral prevention interventions demonstrated to be effective through randomized, controlled longitudinal trials. Her research has been extensively supported by the National Institutes of Health as well as other national and international research foundations and funding agencies. She and her colleagues developed and evaluated the "Focus on Kids," "Focus on Youth With Informed Parents and Children Together," "My Future! My Choice!" and "Caribbean Focus on Youth +Caribbean Informed Parents and Children Together" programs, which have received recognition from numerous agencies, including the Centers for Disease Control and Prevention and UNAIDS.

F. Curtiss Swezy, DrPH, spent a decade as a community development and public health officer with the United States Agency for International Development (USAID). He then worked for three decades as a global health program administrator in more than 30 countries, primarily with nongovernmental organizations. He had residential assignments of two or more years in five countries in Southeast Asia and Africa. Since 2006 he has had an adjunct appointment to teach global health primarily to master's of public health students at George Mason University.

Virginia Swezy, MPH, has been working in polio eradication since 1999, when she first joined the Centers for Disease Control and Prevention (CDC), as part of the team managing the Stop Transmission of Polio Team project. Before joining CDC, she worked in public health–related projects for two years in Togo, West Africa, and for three years in Turkmenistan. She has a bachelor's degree in anthropology from Beloit College in Wisconsin and a master of public health degree from Emory University in Atlanta. In 2007, she spent two years as a CDC assignee in Kenya focusing on HIV/AIDS and returned to polio in India in 2009 as the WHO deputy project manager for the National Polio Surveillance Project, where she was assigned as a WHO staff member until 2013. She recently completed a six-year tour in India, with the past two years as a WHO staff member in the Accelerated Disease Control Branch of the WHO South East Asia Regional Office in New Delhi.

Gina Tambini, MD, MPH, is a professional with 25 years of experience in public health in the Americas. She is an expert in the area of family and community health with extensive experience in vaccines and immunization, and has been a member of the team responsible for the elimination of vaccine-preventable diseases and for the significant reduction in mortality rates for children and mothers in the Americas.

Dr. Tambini, a national of Peru, obtained her medical degree from the Universidad Peruana Cayetano Heredia and a master's in public health from Johns Hopkins University. She began her professional career at the Universidad Peruana Cayetano Heredia as an associate investigator working with the microcomputers in primary health care project. She joined PAHO as an epidemiologist in the Expanded Program on Immunization in El Salvador, Colombia, and Ecuador. She proceeded to higher responsibilities as regional adviser to the Special Program on Vaccines and Immunization, coordinator of the Expanded Program on Immunization, director of the Division of Vaccines and Immunization, manager of the Family and Community Health Area, and director of the Family, Gender and Life Course Department. Currently, she holds the position of PAHO/WHO representative in Ecuador.

Deborah Thomas, PhD, is associate professor in the Department of Geography and Environmental Sciences at the University of Colorado Denver, where she also has secondary appointments in the Department of Environmental & Occupational Health in the Colorado School of Public Health and in the School of Public Affairs. She specializes in hazards and health geography, and has more than 20 years of experience working with geographic information systems (GIS) in a variety of social science application areas, including health and disaster management in domestic and global settings. In 2005, she had the opportunity to expand these collaborative networks internationally when she was a Fulbright Scholar at Middle East Technical University in Ankara, Turkey. For the past eight years, she has worked on educational and research initiatives in Tanzania in partnership with the Catholic University of Health and Allied Sciences, including a current NIH-funded project examining the adoption and appropriateness of technology for HIV Surveillance in a rural health delivery system in Tanzania.

Zhiwen Xiao, PhD, is an associate professor in health communication and a faculty affiliate of women's studies at University of Houston. She received her doctoral degree in communications at the University of Kentucky. Xiao's research focuses on health behavior change and health campaigns. She explores how individual and social factors determine health-related behaviors and how health campaigns influence such factors to promote desired health outcomes and behaviors. Her work has appeared in a number of peer-reviewed journals, including *International Journal of Public Health, AIDS Patient Care and STDs, AIDS Care, AIDS Education and Prevention, Psychology, Health & Medicine,* and *International Journal of Sexual Health.*

Fernando Zacarías, MD, DrPH, obtained his medical degree from the National Autonomous University of Mexico and specialized in family medicine and infectious diseases in the United States. Upon his return to Mexico, Dr. Zacarías worked as a researcher in public health and professor of family medicine and community health.

He later obtained his master and doctor of public health degrees from Harvard University, and after working as a visiting scientist at the Centers for Disease Control and Prevention (CDC) for five years, he joined the Pan American Health Organization (PAHO/WHO) in 1984.

At PAHO/WHO, Dr. Zacarías was chief of the AIDS/STD Program for 16 years and subsequently became senior policy advisor in the family and community health area; acting chief of health analysis and statistics; and coordinator of two editions of *Health in the Americas,* the quinquennial PAHO publication on the health situation in the Western Hemisphere.

Currently, Dr. Zacarías is director of operations of Global Health International Advisors, a not-for-profit organization based in Washington, D.C., that works on community health projects internationally.

CHAPTER 1

THE STATE OF GLOBAL HEALTH

Richard Skolnik

LEARNING OBJECTIVES

By the end of this chapter, the reader should be able to:

- Explain the concepts of "DALYs" and "burden of disease"
- Outline the leading causes of morbidity and mortality globally
- Discuss the main risk factors for the leading causes of morbidity and mortality
- Explain how the leading causes of morbidity and mortality and their risk factors vary by country income group, age, and sex
- Review broadly how health communication relates to the burden of disease and its risk factors

The state of global health has changed dramatically over the past two decades. Life expectancy has increased globally and in all regions (World Bank, 2015a). The number of under-five children dying every year has fallen from about 11.6 million in 1990 to about 6.3 million in 2013 (UNICEF, 2014, p. 4). The number of women dying maternal deaths decreased from 1990 to 2010 from about 359,000 to 255,000 (Lozano et al., 2012, p. 2122). Even in the face of HIV, the share of total deaths due to **communicable diseases** has fallen from 1990 to 2010, and the share from **noncommunicable diseases** has risen. Today, communicable diseases are the predominant cause of death only in sub-Saharan Africa (IHME, 2015).

The most important **risk factors** for death and disability have also shifted. Twenty years ago, childhood underweight, indoor air pollution from cooking in unventilated spaces with biofuels, and the lack of access to safe drinking water or sanitation were the leading risk factors globally for death and disability. These risk factors remain significant to the lives of poor people in low- and middle-income countries. Today, however, the most important risk factors globally relate to "behavioral risks." These include a diet abundant in salt and saturated fats but lacking in fresh fruits and vegetables; sedentary lifestyle; hypertension; diabetes; and tobacco and alcohol use. There are now more people in the world who are obese than who are undernourished (Lim et al., 2012, p. 2246).

There has also been a change in the composition of healthy life years lost. Twenty years ago, the majority of healthy life years lost was due to premature death. In the face of lower child death rates, lower death rates for some diseases, and greater longevity, however, the predominant cause of healthy life years lost has shifted from death to disability. People are living longer. However, they are also spending more years living with disability (Institute for Health Metrics and Evaluation [IHME], 2013, pp. 24–30).

The promotion of better health requires that we understand *what* people get sick and die from and *why* they get sick and die from these causes. It is also essential that we understand *how* these burdens have changed in the past and how they are likely to change in the future. In addition, **morbidity** and **mortality** vary by age, gender, location, income group, and country income level. Efforts to promote better health must take account of these differences.

The objective of this chapter is help the reader understand the most important causes of morbidity and mortality both globally and as they vary across regions, countries, and groups. It also aims to assist readers in understanding the underlying risk factors and determinants of these causes. The chapter seeks to answer the following questions:

- How long do people live and how many of those years are lived in good health?
- What are the most important causes of morbidity?
- What are the most important causes of mortality?
- What are the most important risk factors associated with these leading causes of morbidity and mortality?
- How do morbidity and mortality and their associated risk factors vary across regions, countries, and groups?
- How have the leading causes of morbidity and mortality changed over time?
- How do we project that the leading causes of morbidity and mortality will change in the future?

A Note on Data Sources and Definitions

Before one begins to examine these questions, it is important to understand the sources of the data for this chapter.

Since the early 1990s, an important foundation for work on global health has been studies of the burden of disease. One of the most recent and important such studies was published in 2012: *Global Burden of Disease: Generating Evidence, Guiding Policy* (Institute for Health Metrics and Evaluation [IHME], 2013). A series of related articles was also published in 2012 in the *Lancet*. The Institute of Health Metrics and Evaluation, the lead author of these studies, also has an extensive interactive website on the burden of disease. This chapter will refer to the main IHME *Global Burden of Disease* report, the *Lancet* series, and the interactive website as the "Global Burden of Disease Study, 2010" or "GBD."

The GBD has coherent and consistent information on the global burden of disease, and it is used extensively in this chapter. Additional data, primarily from the World Health Organization (WHO), UNAIDS, UNICEF, and the World Bank, are presented when needed to complement GBD data.

The GBD 2010 study examined 133 causes of death for 187 countries. These are referred to as "causes" and include conditions such as lower respiratory infections, diarrhea, and HIV/AIDS. The study also assessed the extent to which these causes were attributable to 67 risk factors and clusters of risk factors that they also examined. These are referred to here as "risk factors."

They include factors such as unimproved water and sanitation, indoor and outdoor air pollution, and tobacco smoking.

Earlier studies of the burden of disease grouped disease conditions into three categories: "Group 1": communicable, maternal, nutritional, and perinatal causes; "Group 2": noncommunicable causes; and "Group 3": injuries. This chapter does not explicitly use these groupings, but they are occasionally mentioned here.

The chapter generally uses GBD terms exactly as they are laid out in the GBD. However, a few terms are simplified in this chapter. This chapter, for example, will refer to "cerebrovascular disease" as "stroke." It will refer to "neonatal preterm birth" as "preterm birth."

Much of the data used in work on development and global health are organized by World Bank region, and this chapter follows that convention. However, some data that are not readily available by World Bank region are organized by the regions of the World Health Organization.

Life Expectancy

We can start to explore the health status of different populations by examining life expectancy. Life expectancy at birth in 2013 ranged from 58 years in the sub-Saharan Africa region of the World Bank to 79 years in the high-income countries, as shown in Figure 1.1. This figure indicates that life expectancy

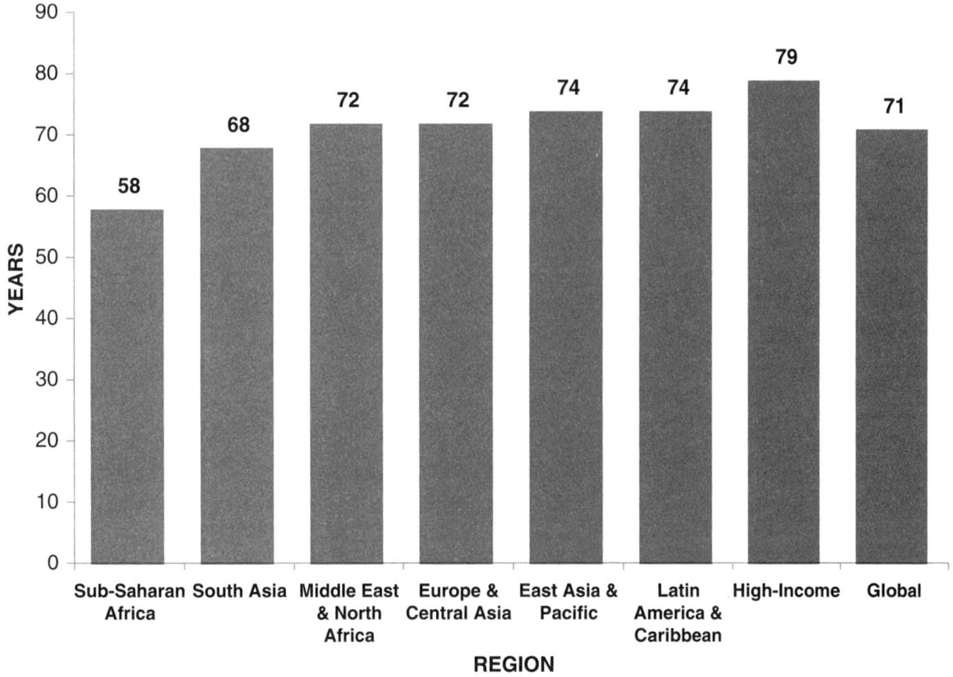

Figure 1.1 Life Expectancy at Birth for World Bank Regions, High-Income Countries, and Globally, 2013
Source: World Bank. World Development Indicators. http://wdi.worldbank.org/table/2.2

at birth in most regions is within 10% of that of the high-income countries, except for South Asia and sub-Saharan Africa. The figure also shows that life expectancy in sub-Saharan Africa substantially lags beyond other regions (World Bank, 2015a).

Figure 1.2 shows the trends in life expectancy by World Bank region from 1960 to 2013.

Figure 1.2 indicates that from 1960 to 2013, life expectancy increased in all World Bank regions. The fastest increase occurred in the East Asia and the Pacific region. However, there were also substantial increases in other low- and middle-income regions, including the Middle East and North Africa, sub-Saharan Africa, and South Asia. Of course, the relatively smaller increases in the high-income countries and in Latin America and the Caribbean largely reflect their already high life expectancies. The relatively small increase in Europe and Central Asia reflects both the high level of life expectancy before the breakup of the former Soviet Union and the social and economic dislocations that occurred after that breakup.

Another valuable data point to use in assessing health status is the share of total deaths in a population that is made up of children under five years of

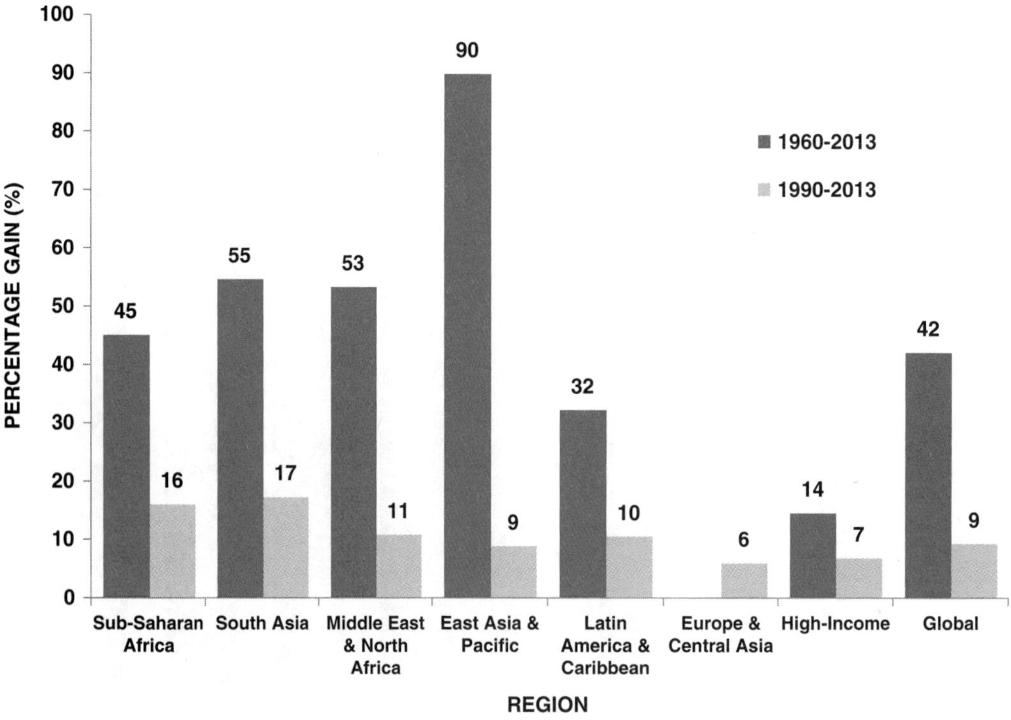

Figure 1.2 Percentage Gain in Life Expectancy for World Bank Regions, High-Income Countries, and Globally, 1960–2013

Note: Data not available for Europe and Central Asia region in 1960.

Source: World Bank. World Development Indicators. http://wdi.worldbank.org/table/2.21; data for 1960 from: Jamison, D. T. (2006). Investing in health. In D. T. Jamison, J. G. Breman, A. R. Measham, et al. (Eds.), *Disease control priorities in developing countries* (2nd ed., p. 6). Washington, DC, and New York, NY: World Bank and Oxford University Press.

age. The world has made important progress in reducing the deaths of children under five as a share of total deaths. Globally, such deaths fell from about 25% of total deaths in 1990 to about 13% in 2010. Nonetheless, under-five child deaths continue to be major shares of total deaths in many low-income countries, as is discussed further in the next section (Wang et al., 2012, pp. 2071, 2075).

Maternal, Neonatal, Infant, and Child Mortality

To understand the "state of global health", we must also understand the maternal mortality ratio and the rates of neonatal, infant, and child mortality and how they vary across country income and other groups.

The maternal mortality ratio is the number of women who die of pregnancy related causes over a given time period, per 100,000 live births over that same period (United Nations Statistical Division, 2015). Figure 1.3 depicts the maternal mortality ratio by World Bank region, for the high-income countries, and globally.

Two main points stand out from this figure. First, two regions, sub-Saharan Africa and South Asia, have substantially higher maternal mortality ratios than any other regions. Second, there is an exceptional variance in maternal mortality ratios by region, with the ratio for sub-Saharan Africa more than 30 times the

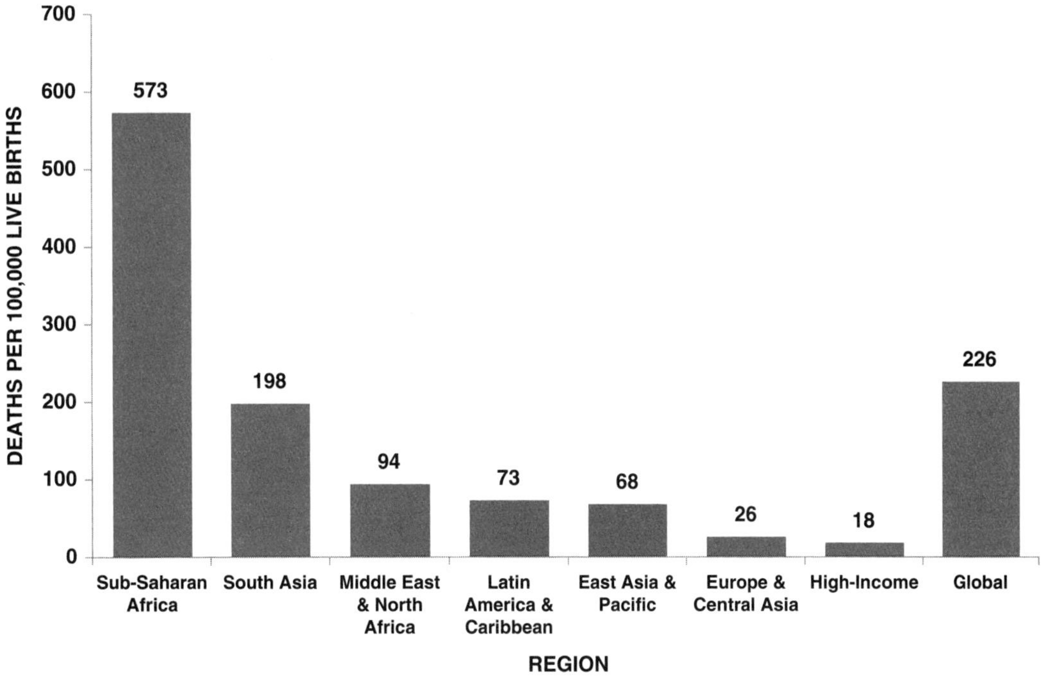

Figure 1.3 Maternal Mortality Ratios for World Bank Regions, High-Income Countries, and Globally 2013
Source: World Bank. World Development Indicators. http://wdi.worldbank.org/table/2.21

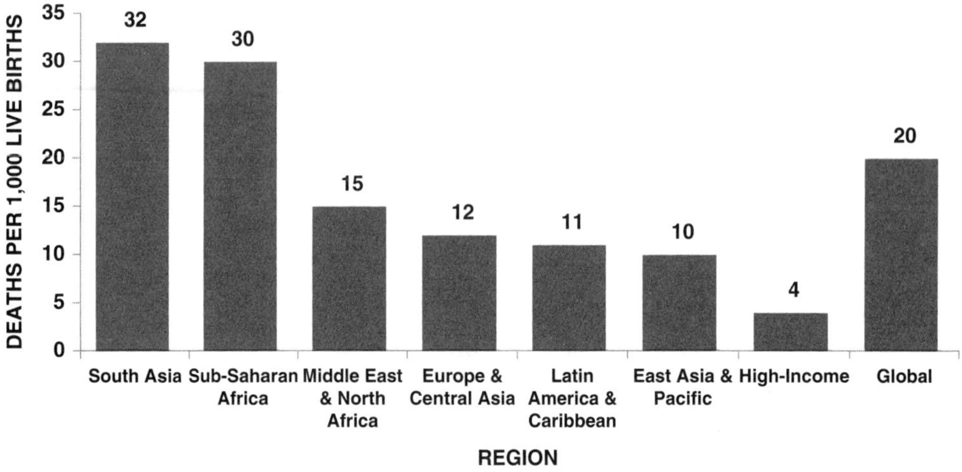

Figure 1.4 Neonatal Mortality Rates for World Bank Regions, High-Income Countries, and Globally, 2013
Source: World Bank. World Development Indicators. http://data.worldbank.org/indicator/SH.DYN.NMRT/countries/1W-8S-ZF-4E-XQ-XJ-XD?display=graph

ratio for the high-income countries, and the ratio in South Asia is 11 times the ratio for high-income countries.

It is essential to assess the age at which children die if one is to develop policies and programs to reduce child death. Figure 1.4 shows the rates of neonatal mortality by World Bank region and for the high-income countries. The neonatal mortality rate refers to the number of children under 28 days old who die for every 1,000 live births in a given year (World Bank, 2015c).

Once again we see that the rates of neonatal mortality are highest in sub-Saharan Africa and South Asia and that there is substantial variance across regions and country income groups. Children in sub-Saharan Africa and South Asia are about 8 times more likely to die during their first 28 days of life than are children in the high-income countries.

The infant mortality rate refers to children who die below one year of age, for every 1,000 live births in a given year (World Bank, 2015d). As expected, the rates of infant mortality follow a similar pattern to neonatal mortality rates, as shown in Figure 1.5.

Figure 1.5 clearly indicates that sub-Saharan Africa has a rate of infant mortality that is about three times, and South Asia about twice the rate of the next worst-off region, the Middle East and North Africa.

The under-five mortality rate is "the probability per 1,000 that a newborn baby will die before reaching age five, if subject to age-specific mortality rates of the specified year" (World Bank, 2015d). Figure 1.6 depicts under-five-child mortality by World Bank region.

Considered together, figures 1.4, 1.5, and 1.6 highlight the importance of neonatal deaths to all under-five child deaths. In the poorest regions of the world, children face almost equal risks of dying as neonates, between their first month and their first year, and between their first and fifth years of life. By contrast, in the middle- and higher-income countries, the risks of under-five

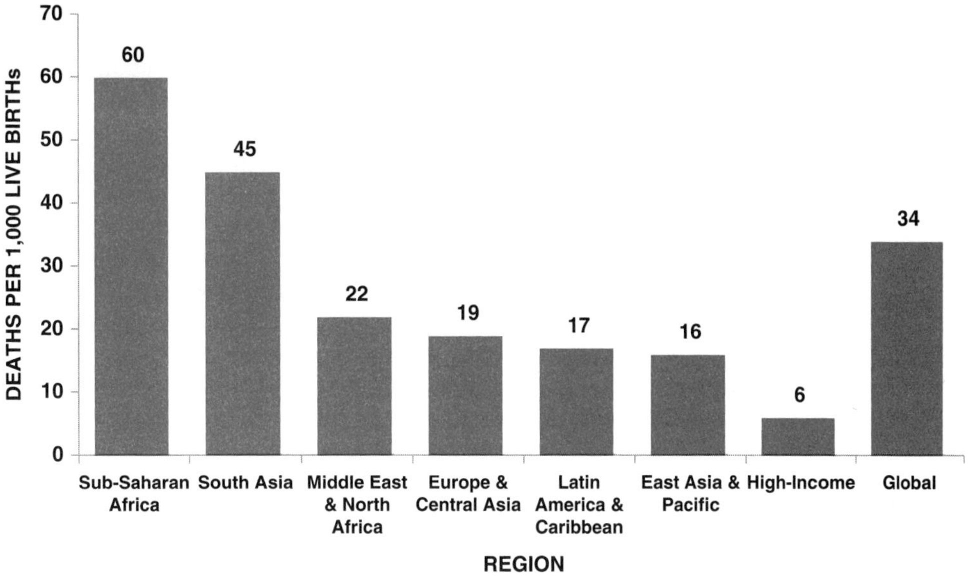

Figure 1.5 Infant Mortality Rates for World Bank Regions, High-Income Countries, and Globally, 2013
Source: World Bank. World Development Indicators. http://data.worldbank.org/indicator/SP.DYN.IMRT.IN/countries/1W-ZF-8S-4E-XJ-7E-XD?display=graph

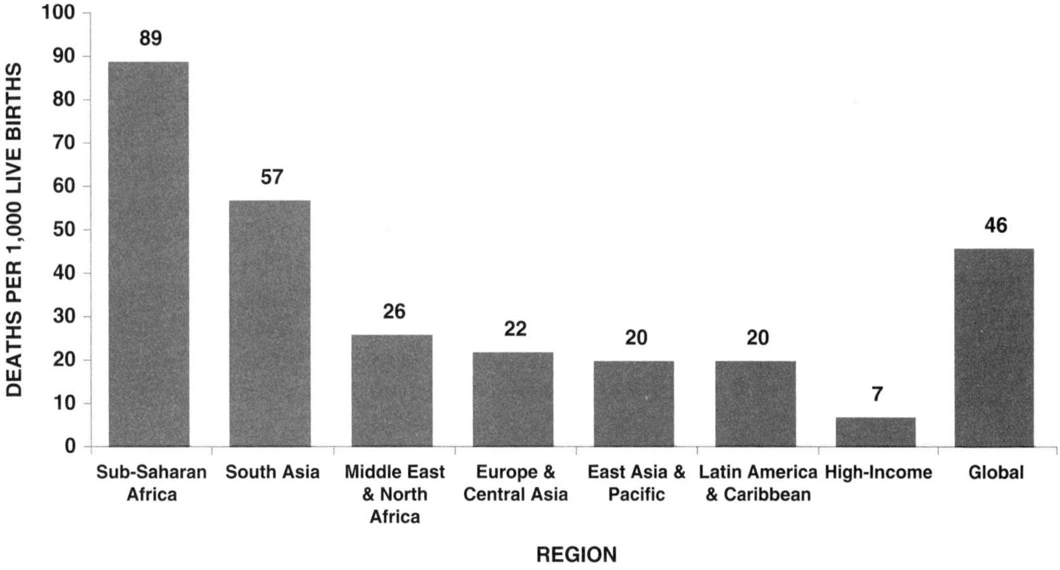

Figure 1.6 Under-Five Child Mortality Rates for World Bank Regions, High-Income Countries, and Globally, 2013
Source: World Bank. World Development Indicators. http://data.worldbank.org/indicator/SH.DYN.MORT/countries/1W-ZF-8S-XQ-XD-4E-XJ?display=graph

child death are greatest for neonates, and the rates of death of infants and children between the first and fifth years are very low.

When considering these data and the data on deaths and DALYs discussed in the next section, one must take into account not only the differences *between* countries, but also the differences in health status among different groups *within* countries. We should increasingly expect the health status of higher-income and better-educated people in low- and middle-income countries to be similar to that of high-income and well-educated people in high-income countries. By contrast, low-income and poorly educated people in low- and middle-income countries will generally have much worse health indicators than the better-off people in their own countries. We should also expect health status to vary not only by income and education status. In addition, it will vary with sex, ethnicity, location, and the extent to which people belong to marginalized groups, such as sexual minorities and prisoners. One of the main goals of health policy, of course, is to reduce these disparities.

Measuring Health Status

Life expectancy, and indicators of maternal, neonatal, infant, and child mortality are useful indicators of the health of a population. However, they fail to capture how healthy or unhealthy children and adults were when they lived. Say, for example, that there are two communities with 100 people each. In both communities, life expectancy at birth is 80 years. In one of the communities, the people stay completely healthy until they die. In the other, however, one-third of the adults get diabetes when they are 60. Nonetheless they still live 20 additional years—they just do so with a variety of complications of diabetes, including vision and wound problems and amputations of limbs. In this case, one society is clearly much "healthier" than the other, but the life expectancy indicator does not capture this difference.

Over the past several decades, therefore, those working in global health have primarily measured the health status of countries and regions in **disability-adjusted life years**, referred to as "DALYs." The DALY is a composite indicator that sums the years of healthy life lost to disability from illness or injury or the after effects of illness or injury (called years lived with disability or YLD) and the years of life lost due to premature death (YLL) (IMHE, 2013, pp. 6–14).

The years of life lost to death are calculated by assessing the gap between the age at which people die and their projected life expectancy at that age. Ideally, of course, all people everywhere would live just as long as any other group. Thus, the gap between the age at death and how long people "should have lived at that age" is calculated against a standard that is based on the group with the highest life expectancy in 2010 (IHME, 2013, pp. 10–14).

As a simplified example of how one calculates years of life lost to premature death, let's suppose a woman dies at 50 years of age. In principle, if she lived as long as the standard suggests she could have lived at age 50, then the woman should have lived until she was 83. Thus, the years of life lost to premature death would equal 33.

The years of life lived with disability (YLD) are calculated by multiplying the number of years that a person lives with a disability by a disability weight.

These weights have generally been derived from panels assembled by the World Health Organization, and they are periodically updated. GBD based them on 14,000 household surveys in a number of countries and 16,000 internet surveys. (Salomon, 2012).

As an example, let's suppose that someone aged 53 loses a leg to amputation because of complications of diabetes and then dies at 83 years of age. Let's further suppose that those who determine disability weights have assigned a disability weight of .5 to this disability. The person lived 30 years with disability. This would be equal to 15 DALYs, which is the number of years lived with disability, multiplied by the weight of that disability.

As noted previously, the DALY combines into a single metric the years of life lost to premature death and the years of healthy life lost due to disability. If everyone in a country lived until the normative standard life expectancy for the age at which they died and did so without any disability, the country would have no DALYs. By contrast, a low-income country like Liberia sees considerable premature death and a substantial number of disabilities from communicable and noncommunicable diseases and injuries. This would produce a substantial number of DALYs per person, indicating significant deviance from a population that "lives a healthy life until its time" and then dies.

The text that follows discusses both deaths and DALYs. This allows the reader to get a fuller appreciation for the state of the world's health than would be possible if only deaths were examined. In general, when the text refers to "burden of disease," it is speaking of DALY measures, as opposed to speaking only of deaths.

The IHME website on the burden of disease allows one to interactively manipulate the data by country, subregion, or a variety of different regions, such as those used by the World Bank and the World Health Organization. To simplify the presentation of burden of disease data below, most of the data has been organized into "representative" subregions from GBD, one for low-income, one for middle-income, and one for high-income countries. The text will also sometimes speak of these country income groups, rather than name the subregions that represent them. Those interested in more detail on burden of disease data should consult the IHME website (IHME, 2015).

Global Deaths and the Global Burden of Disease

The Leading Causes of Death Globally and Their Risk Factors

Causes of Death

The leading causes of death globally for all age groups and both sexes in 2010 were ischemic heart disease, stroke, chronic obstructive pulmonary disease (COPD), lower respiratory infections, and tracheal, bronchus, and lung cancers, as shown in Table 1.1. These were followed in the top 10 by HIV/AIDS, Alzheimer's disease and other dementias, road injuries, diarrheal disease, and tuberculosis (TB) (IHME, 2015).

Table 1.1 Ten Leading Causes of Death in Examples Low-Income, Middle-Income, and High-Income Sub-Regions and Globally, 2010

	Western Sub-Saharan Africa (Low-Income)		Southern Latin America (Middle-Income)		Western Europe (High-Income)		Global	
	Disease	**% of Total Deaths**	**Disease**	**% of Total Deaths**	**Disease**	**% of Total Deaths**	**Disease**	**% of Total Deaths**
1	Malaria	16.9	Ischemic heart disease	13.5	Ischemic heart disease	17.8	Ischemic heart disease	14.4
2	Lower respiratory infections	9.9	Stroke	9.4	Stroke	9.8	Stroke	11.5
3	HIV/AIDS	9.3	COPD	7.3	Alzheimer's disease and other dementias	8.4	COPD	5.2
4	Diarrheal diseases	5.9	Lower respiratory infections	7.0	Tracheal, bronchial, and lung cancers	5.8	Lower respiratory infections	4.9
5	Road injuries	4.0	Alzheimer's disease and other dementias	5.8	COPD	4.7	Tracheal, bronchial, and lung cancers	2.9
6	Stroke	3.9	Tracheal, bronchus, and lung cancers	3.3	Lower respiratory infections	3.9	HIV/AIDS	2.8
7	Preterm birth complications	3.5	Diabetes	2.8	Colon and rectum cancers	3.7	Alzheimer's disease and other dementias	2.8
8	Hemoglobinopathies and hemolytic anemias	3.4	Chronic kidney disease	2.7	Other cardio and circulatory diseases	2.3	Road injuries	2.6
9	Neonatal encephalopathy	3.2	Colon and rectum cancer	2.7	Diabetes	2.3	Diarrheal diseases	2.5
10	Protein energy malnutrition	3.1	Hypertensive heart disease	2.2	Breast cancer	2.1	Tuberculosis	2.4

Source: IHME. Global Burden of Disease Heatmap. Accessed December 18, 2015. Available at: http://vizhub.healthdata.org/gbd-compare/

As also shown in Table 1.1, and as discussed previously, the leading causes of death vary substantially by country income group and by the regions into which GBD data is organized. As generally expected, the higher the income per capita of the country or the region, the larger the share of deaths that is due to noncommunicable causes.

Risk Factors for Deaths

As part of GBD, calculations were also made of attributable risk factors for the causes of death and DALYs. As seen in Table 1.2, the five leading risk factors in 2010 for deaths globally were high blood pressure, smoking, high body-mass index, high fasting plasma glucose, and a diet high in sodium. These were followed by a diet low in fruit, household air pollution, ambient particulate matter pollution, alcohol use, and high total cholesterol (IHME, 2015).

As expected, the leading risk factors also vary by region and country income group. Generally, the lower the income of the country group, the more the leading risk factors will include risks related to undernutrition, such as childhood underweight and suboptimal breastfeeding. However, even in these low-income countries, some of the leading risk factors include those related to noncommunicable diseases such as high blood pressure, high body-mass index, and alcohol use (IHME, 2015).

DALYs and Their Attributable Risk Factors

Table 1.3 shows the top ten causes of the burden of disease in DALYs globally and in representative GBD subregions.

Table 1.2 Leading Risk Factors for Death in Low-Income, Middle-Income, and High-Income Sub-Regions and Globally, 2010

	Western Sub-Saharan Africa (Low-Income)	Southern Latin America (Middle-Income)	Western Europe (High-Income)	Global
1	Childhood undernutrition	High blood pressure	High blood pressure	High blood pressure
2	Unsafe sex	Smoking	Smoking	Smoking
3	High blood pressure	High body-mass index	High body-mass index	High body-mass index
4	Unsafe water source	High fasting plasma glucose	High total cholesterol	High fasting plasma glucose
5	Household air pollution	Alcohol use	Low physical activity	Diet high in sodium
6	Unsafe sanitation	Low glomerular filtration	Low glomerular filtration	Diet low in fruit
7	Suboptimal breastfeeding	High total cholesterol	Alcohol use	Household air pollution
8	Alcohol use	Diet low in fruits	Diet high in sodium	Ambient particulate matter pollution
9	High body-mass index	Diet low in vegetables	Ambient particulate matter pollution	Alcohol use
10	Ambient particulate matter pollution	Low physical activity	Low fruit in diet	High total cholesterol

Source: IHME. Global Burden of Disease Heatmap. Accessed December 18, 2015. Available at: http://vizhub.healthdata.org/gbd-compare/

Table 1.3 Ten Leading Causes of Burden of Disease in Low-Income, Middle-Income, and High-Income Sub-Regions and Globally, 2010

	Western Sub-Saharan Africa (Low-Income)		Southern Latin America (Middle-Income)		Western Europe (High-Income)		Global	
	Disease	**% of Total DALYs**	**Disease**	**% of Total DALYs**	**Disease**	**% of Total DALYs**	**Disease**	**% of Total DALYs**
1	Malaria	19.3	Ischemic heart disease	6.3	Low back and neck pain	9.5	Ischemic heart disease	5.9
2	Lower respiratory infections	9.2	Low back and neck pain	5.0	Ischemic heart disease	7.8	Lower respiratory infections	4.9
3	HIV/AIDS	7.0	COPD	4.8	Stroke	4.1	Stroke	4.5
4	Diarrheal diseases	6.0	Stroke	4.3	Tracheal, bronchus, and lung cancers	3.8	Low back and neck pain	4.1
5	Preterm birth complications	4.2	Depressive disorders	3.2	Sense organ diseases	3.5	Diarrheal diseases	3.2
6	Hemoglobinopathies and hemolytic anemia	3.9	Lower respiratory infections	3.2	Alzheimer's disease and other dementias	3.5	HIV/AIDS	3.2
7	Neonatal encephalopathy	3.8	Congenital anomalies	2.9	Falls	3.2	Malaria	3.2
8	Protein-energy malnutrition	3.4	Road injuries	2.9	Depressive disorders	3.2	Preterm birth complications	3.1
9	Meningitis	3.4	Skin diseases	2.5	COPD	3.0	Road injuries	3.0
10	Neonatal sepsis	2.9	Diabetes	2.4	Diabetes	2.9	COPD	2.8

Source: IHME. Global Burden of Disease Heatmap. Accessed December 18, 2015. Available at: http://vizhub.healthdata.org/gbd-compare/

Table 1.4 Leading Risk Factors for DALYs in Low-Income, Middle-Income, and High-Income Sub-Regions and Globally, 2010

	Western Sub-Saharan Africa (Low-Income)	Southern Latin America (Middle-Income)	Western Europe (High-Income)	Global
1	Childhood undernutrition	Smoking	Smoking	High blood pressure
2	Unsafe sex	High body-mass index	High blood pressure	Smoking
3	Unsafe water	High blood pressure	High body-mass index	Childhood undernutrition
4	Unsafe sanitation	Alcohol use	High fasting plasma glucose	High body-mass index
5	Suboptimal breastfeeding	High fasting plasma glucose	Alcohol use	High fasting plasma glucose
6	Household air pollution	Low glomerular filtration	High total cholesterol	Alcohol use
7	No handwashing with soap	High total cholesterol	Low glomerular filtration	Household air pollution
8	Alcohol use	Diet low in fruits	Low physical activity	Unsafe water
9	High blood pressure	Drug use	Diet high in sodium	Unsafe sex
10	Iron deficiency	Diet low in vegetables	Diet low in fruits	Diet low in fruits

Source: IHME. Global Burden of Disease Heatmap. Accessed December 18, 2015. Available at: http://vizhub.healthdata.org/gbd-compare/

Table 1.4 shows the top ten risk factors associated with those DALYs.

As seen in Tables 1.1 and 1.3, the main differences among the leading causes of deaths and DALYs globally in 2010 were the greater importance for DALYs than deaths of low back and neck pain, malaria, and preterm birth complications. At the same time, COPD, tracheal, bronchus and lung cancers, Alzheimer's and other dementias, and tuberculosis were more important for deaths than for DALYs (IHME, 2015).

Moreover, just as we would anticipate, major depressive disorders were ranked number 12 in DALYs globally, but were not in the top 25 causes of death globally. This reflects the fact that major depressive disorders create an enormous amount of ill health and disability but are not directly associated with much death. The neglected tropical diseases (NTD), discussed later, also rank higher in DALYs than deaths. They are not associated with much mortality, but in the poorest countries they are an important cause of disability, which is often severe and long lasting (IHME, 2015).

The most important risk factors for DALYs globally in 2010 were similar to those for death and included high blood pressure, smoking, high body-mass index, and high fasting plasma glucose. However, they also included childhood undernutrition, which is associated with a very large burden of excess morbidity and mortality (IHME, 2015).

Trends in Deaths, in the Burden of Disease, and in Risk Factors

As noted earlier in the chapter, there has been a substantial shift over the past two decades in the leading causes of death and in the leading causes of the burden of disease, measured in DALYs.

Table 1.5 Leading Causes of Deaths Globally, 1990 and 2010

1990		2010	
Rank	**Disease**	**Rank**	**Disease**
1	Ischemic heart disease	1	Ischemic heart disease
2	Stroke	2	Stroke
3	Lower respiratory infections	3	COPD
4	Diarrheal diseases	4	Lower respiratory infections
5	COPD	5	Tracheal, bronchial, and lung cancers
6	Tuberculosis	6	HIV/AIDS
7	Preterm birth complications	7	Alzheimer's disease and other dementias
8	Road injuries	8	Road injuries
9	Tracheal, bronchial, and lung cancers	9	Diarrheal diseases
10	Malaria	10	Tuberculosis

Source: IHME. Global Burden of Disease Heatmap. Accessed December 18, 2015. Available at: http://vizhub.healthdata.org/gbd-compare/

Table 1.5 shows the leading causes of deaths in 1990 and 2010, calculated as part of the 2010 GBD, using a consistent methodology.

Ischemic heart disease and stroke were the leading causes of death globally in 1990, and they remained so in 2010. However, beyond that, there were substantial changes in the leading causes of death, because almost all communicable causes and causes linked to the conditions of poverty fell and noncommunicable causes rose. The only exception to this was HIV/AIDS, a relatively "new" disease in 1990, which became, of course, a global pandemic (IHME, 2015).

Table 1.6 shows the leading causes of DALYS in 1990 and 2010.

Table 1.6 Leading Causes of DALYs Globally, 1990-2010

1990		2010	
Rank	**Disease**	**Rank**	**Disease**
1	Lower respiratory infections	1	Ischemic heart disease
2	Diarrheal diseases	2	Lower respiratory infections
3	Preterm birth complications	3	Stroke
4	Ischemic heart disease	4	Low back and neck pain
5	Stroke	5	Diarrheal diseases
6	Neonatal encephalopathy	6	HIV/AIDS
7	Tuberculosis	7	Malaria
8	Low back and neck pain	8	Preterm birth complications
9	Malaria	9	Road injuries
10	Congenital anomalies	10	COPD

Source: IHME. Global Burden of Disease Heatmap. Accessed December 18, 2015. Available at: http://vizhub.healthdata.org/gbd-compare/

The trends in DALYs over this period mirror those in deaths. The communicable causes of death and perinatal conditions, except for HIV/AIDS, became less important as causes of DALYs. Noncommunicable causes became more important, and those associated with substantial disability also became higher in the rankings. One of the most substantial changes over the two decades concerns measles. The progress in immunizing against measles moved measles from 15 to 62 in the leading causes of DALYs between 1990 and 2010 (IHME, 2015).

The composition of DALYs changed substantially between 1990 and 2010. Over this period the share of DALYs made up of years of life lost due to premature death declined and the share due to years lived with disability increased. These shifts reflect the facts that health status improved over this period, child death rates declined, and people lived longer than before. However, as people lived longer, they also suffered increasing amounts of disability (IHME, 2013a, pp. 25–30).

The Health of Women and Children

The health of women and children is a particular concern in the study of global health, especially those women and children in lower-income settings. The section that follows examines the most important causes of death and DALYs and their related risk factors for women and for children under five years of age.

The Health of Women

The five leading causes of death for women ages 15 to 49 globally in 2010 were HIV/AIDS, tuberculosis, ischemic heart disease, self-harm, and stroke. The sixth and seventh leading causes of death were road injuries and breast cancer (IHME, 2015).

Causes of death vary substantially by country income group and region. In the low-income countries of Western sub-Saharan Africa, for example, the five leading causes of death for women aged 15–49 in 2010 were HIV/AIDS, road injuries, tuberculosis, malaria, and "other maternal disorders." (This refers to causes other than hemorrhage, sepsis, hypertensive disorders, obstructed labor, and abortion; World Health Organization, n.d.). By contrast, in Western Europe, the five leading causes of death of women 15 to 49 were breast cancer, self-harm, lung cancer, road injuries, and ischemic heart disease (IHME, 2015).

The leading causes of DALYs in 2010 for this age group differed substantially from the leading causes of death, a difference that is critical for developing policies and programs. The five leading causes of DALYs globally for women ages 15–49 in 2010 were low back and neck pain, HIV/AIDS, depressive disorders, migraine, and skin diseases. The five leading causes of DALYs in Western Europe were low back and neck pain, depressive disorders, migraine, anxiety disorders, and skin diseases. In Western sub-Saharan Africa, the five leading causes of DALYs among women 15–49 globally in 2010 were HIV/AIDS, depressive disorders, road injuries, malaria, and low back and neck pain (IHME, 2015).

The most significant risk factors for deaths among women ages 15 to 49 globally in 2010 were unsafe sex, high blood pressure, high body-mass index, intimate partner violence, and alcohol use. However, the risk factors also vary, as we would expect, by country and regional income group and epidemiological status. In Western Europe, the five leading risk factors were alcohol use, smoking, high body-mass index, high blood pressure, and unsafe sex. In Western sub-Saharan Africa, the five most important risk factors for death were unsafe sex, intimate partner violence, alcohol use, unsafe water, and high blood pressure (IHME, 2015).

The most significant risk factors for DALYs globally among women in this age group do not differ substantially from the most significant risk factors for death, and include unsafe sex, high body-mass index, high blood pressure, intimate partner violence, and high fasting plasma glucose. As we move up the country income scale, such as in Western Europe, however, the five leading risk factors for DALYs change toward high body-mass index, alcohol use, smoking, high fasting plasma glucose, and low glomerular filtration. "In a low-income region such as Western sub-Saharan Africa, the five leading risk factors for DALYs for women in this age group were unsafe sex, iron deficiency, intimate partner violence, alcohol use, and unsafe water (IHME, 2015).

The pattern of deaths among women between 50 and 69 years of age is different from that for women 15 to 49. For women 50 to 69, the five leading causes of death globally in 2010 were are ischemic heart disease, stroke, COPD, diabetes, and breast cancer. In Western Europe, the five leading causes were breast cancer, lung cancer, ischemic heart disease, colorectal cancer, and stroke. For Western sub-Saharan Africa, the five leading causes of death of women in the 50 to 69 year old age group were stroke, HIV/AIDS, ischemic heart disease, lower respiratory infections, and tuberculosis (IHME, 2015).

For women 50 to 69 years of age, the five leading causes of DALYs were ischemic heart disease, stroke, low back and neck pain, diabetes, and COPD. In Western Europe, the five leading causes of DALYs among females in this age group were low back and neck pain, breast cancer, other musculoskeletal disorders, ischemic heart disease, tracheal, bronchial, and lung cancer. This pattern shifts dramatically, however, for low-income regions, such as Western sub-Saharan Africa. Here, the five leading causes of DALYs were HIV/AIDS, stroke, low back and neck pain, ischemic heart disease, and lower respiratory infections (IMHE, 2015).

The leading risk factors for death among women 50 to 69 years of age globally in 2010 all related to noncommunicable diseases: high blood pressure, high body-mass index, high fasting plasma glucose, a diet low in fruit and a diet high in sodium. In Western Europe, the leading risks were similar but smoking was the leading risk, followed by high body-mass index, high blood pressure, alcohol use, and high total cholesterol. For Western sub-Saharan Africa, the five leading risk factors for death were high blood pressure, unsafe sex, high body-mass index, household air pollution, and high fasting plasma glucose. These differences partly reflect the place of HIV/AIDS in parts of West Africa and the extent to which people cook there with biomass fuels on unventilated stoves (IMHE, 2015).

Implications for Health Promotion

A large share of the disability and premature deaths of women globally could be avoided by addressing the underlying risk factors and determinants of health. In the poorest countries of the world, women continue to die prematurely from communicable diseases such as HIV, TB, and malaria and from maternal disorders. The overwhelming majority of these deaths are preventable and treatable. Throughout the world, women are also increasingly dying prematurely of the most significant noncommunicable diseases, such as ischemic heart disease, stroke, COPD, and diabetes. By reducing tobacco smoking, alcohol use, and dietary risks, and increasing physical activity, women should be able to live longer with less disability while they are alive. Reducing exposure to indoor air pollution could also substantially reduce preventable female deaths in low-income settings. In each of these areas, there is an important role for health promotion and behavior change.

We also need to be attuned to the large number of DALYs among women that are attributable in most countries to musculoskeletal problems and to mental health conditions. To a large extent, these are not reflected in premature death, but they do cause very large amounts of disability and lost productivity. Given increasing life expectancy and the aging of populations, we need to promote measures to both prevent and treat these problems. If not, we will have more older women living longer, but doing so with disabilities that impose a substantial burden on them, their families, and society.

The Health of Children Ages 0 to 5

We saw earlier the rates at which neonates, infants, and under-five children die by region. However, improving the health of young children requires that we also understand what they get sick and die from, at what ages, and what are the key risk factors and determinants of those deaths. The section that follows examines children under five years of age. For young children, the DALY is a less useful concept than deaths, and this section looks only at child deaths and their related risk factors.

UNICEF estimated that about 6.3 million children under five years of age died in 2013. Given the dramatic differences in under-five child mortality between low- and high-income countries, it is clear that most of these deaths are preventable (UNICEF, 2014, p. 5).

UNICEF has also estimated that about 1 million, or about 16% of the under-five children who die each year, will die in their first day of life. UNICEF further estimates that about 2 million, or about 32% of the under-five children who die each year, will die in their first week of life and 2.8 million, or 44% of the annual under-five child deaths, occur in the first month of life (UNICEF, 2014, p. 6). Efforts to reduce young child deaths will clearly have to pay particular attention to neonatal deaths.

The GBD study estimates that the leading causes of under-five death globally are lower respiratory infections, preterm birth, neonatal encephalopathy, malaria, and diarrheal diseases. In Western sub-Saharan Africa, the five leading causes of under-five death are malaria, lower respiratory infections, diarrheal diseases, preterm birth, and neonatal encephalopathy. In Western Europe, four of the five leading causes of death of children this age mostly relate to neonatal conditions: congenital anomalies, preterm birth, neonatal encephalopathy, other neonatal conditions and sudden infant death syndrome (SIDS). Clearly, the global estimates are dominated by the fact that almost all of the young children who die are in low- and middle-income countries. We also see that as countries progress economically, child deaths from communicable causes and causes related to poverty decline and the causes related to neonatal conditions make up a larger share of total under-five child deaths (IMHE, 2015).

Given the importance of neonatal deaths to under-five child deaths, it is also valuable to note the leading causes of their death. The World Health Organization estimated in 2013 that the leading causes of neonatal mortality were preterm birth complications, birth asphyxia and birth trauma, and sepsis and other infections (World Health Organization, 2015a). As noted below, there are low-cost highly effective interventions that can be promoted and taken at the community level to address several of these issues, especially birth asphyxia and some infections.

Globally, the most important risk factors for young child death are dominated by deaths in low-income countries. Thus, they relate largely to the household environment, the nutritional status of the mother and the child, and the circumstances under which the birth occurs, such as whether or not it was assisted by a skilled attendant. In this light, the leading risk factors for young child death globally include childhood underweight, suboptimal breastfeeding, unsafe water, unsafe sanitation, and household air pollution. In high-income countries some of the most important risk factors for young child death may relate to tobacco, alcohol, and drug use among mothers, as well as poor maternal health and nutrition (IMHE, 2015).

Implications for Health Promotion

What share of the more than 6 million under-five child deaths each year are preventable? There will always be some children who die at young ages. However, the lowest rates of under-five child death occur in Iceland, which has an under-five child death rate of 2 for every 1,000 live births (World Bank, 2015b). This can be thought of as a lower boundary for child death rates. This compares with the worst under-five child death rate in the world—147 per 1,000 live births, in Chad (World Bank, 2015b). An important study done several years ago suggested that about two-thirds of the deaths of children under five globally could be prevented by scaling up a package of known and evidence-based interventions at a high level in low-income countries. Such interventions would include, for example, vaccines such as measles and *Haemophilus influenzae* type B (Hib), long-lasting insecticide-treated bednets, micronutrients, oral rehydration therapy, and breastfeeding (Jones et al., 2003, pp. 66–70). Another important study showed that 15% of the under-five child deaths globally could be averted through a package of 10 evidence-based nutrition interventions implemented at 90% (Bhutta et al., 2013). It is clear that fundamental to reducing child death rates is the need to promote a better understanding, especially in low-income and poorly educated communities, about the causes of child death, their risk factors, and how those risks can be prevented or mitigated. In principle, every country ought to aspire to bring its under-five child death rate down to the levels of today's highest-income countries, although it may take considerable time to achieve this.

Communicable Diseases

Although the share of the total burden of disease that is communicable is declining, communicable diseases remain an important part of the "unfinished agenda" among the poor everywhere, but especially in low- and middle-income countries. The section that follows offers some brief comments about the burden of HIV, TB, malaria, and the neglected tropical diseases. Because there are agencies responsible for addressing particular diseases, this section generally uses data from WHO or UNAIDS. However, it will complement that data with GBD data.

HIV

Incidence, Prevalence, and Deaths

About 35 million people in the world were living with HIV/AIDS in 2013. Of those who were infected with HIV, about 41% were men, 50% were women, and 9% were children under 15 years of age (UNAIDS, 2014, p. 1).

UNAIDS estimates that there were about 2.1 million people newly infected with HIV in 2013. About 1.86 million of these were adults, and the remaining 240,000 were children under 15. The number of new infections is a substantial decline from the 3.4 million new infections that were estimated to have occurred in 2001 (UNAIDS, 2014, p. 1).

In fact, the number of people newly infected globally with HIV each year has fallen, and following UNAIDS estimates, is now 38% lower than in 2001. Many countries in sub-Saharan Africa and the Caribbean have seen sharp declines in the number of new cases of HIV/AIDS between 2001 and 2013. However, the number of new infections continues to rise in some regions, particularly the Middle East and North Africa, Central Asia, and Eastern Europe (UNAIDS, 2014, p. 1).

The number of children newly infected with HIV has also fallen, with progress in the prevention of maternal to child transmission. Some highly affected countries, like Botswana, have made dramatic progress in stemming maternal to child transmission, even as some other countries have made only a start in reducing maternal to child transmission (UNAIDS, 2013, p. 30).

The overwhelming majority of new infections with HIV stem from sexual transmission, mostly heterosexual. In a number of places, however, the main route for the transmission of new infections is men who have sex with men or practice injecting drug use. Despite progress, maternal to child transmission remains an important share of the total number of new cases annually in a number of settings, overwhelmingly in sub-Saharan Africa (UNAIDS, 2013, pp. 38–45).

Over the past decade, the HIV/AIDS epidemic has also become "feminized," with an increasing share of the total cases among adults being among women. In sub-Saharan Africa, for example, almost 60% of the HIV-positive people are women (UNAIDS, 2014, p. 2).

UNAIDS estimates that about 1.5 million people died from HIV/AIDS in 2013 (UNAIDS, 2014, p. 1). There have been substantial declines in HIV-related deaths in sub-Saharan Africa, the Caribbean, and Oceania. However, the number of deaths annually from HIV has increased in Central Asia, Eastern Europe, and in the Middle East and North Africa (UNAIDS, 2014, pp. 2–4). As noted earlier, HIV remains among the top five causes of deaths for all ages combined in sub-Saharan Africa (IHME, 2015).

The prevalence of HIV/AIDS varies by region, by country, and by location within countries. Sub-Saharan Africa has the highest rate of adult prevalence, close to 5%. The Caribbean, Central Asia, and Eastern Europe have the next highest rates, at about 1%. However, there are a number of countries with very high rates of adult prevalence, including Botswana at 23%, South Africa at 18%, and Swaziland at 21% (UNAIDS, 2013, pp. A7, A8).

There has been dramatic progress in getting people on antiretroviral therapy, and the number of such people has increased to about 12.9 million in 2013. This is 37% of the people eligible under the WHO 2013 guidelines (UNAIDS, 2014, p. 10).

Implications for Health Promotion

Although there has been substantial discussion of "treatment as prevention" (Granich, Williams, & Montaner, 2013), in the short to medium term, behavior change is the key to reducing incidence and prevalence. This is made even more important by the fact that there is no HIV vaccine and little promise that a safe and effective HIV vaccine will be available in the near future. Some of the key interventions include promoting later sexual debut, fewer sexual partners, correct and consistent condom usage, the uptake of medical male circumcision, and being placed on and adhering to antiretroviral therapy. It will also be important to continue to address the stigma of HIV/AIDS. There is clearly a large role for health promotion in work on HIV/AIDS.

Tuberculosis

Prevalence and Deaths

There has been important progress in addressing the burden of TB. The rate of new infections has been falling for a decade. In addition, mortality from tuberculosis has been reduced by 47% since 1990 (WHO, 2015b). Nonetheless, TB remains a disease of exceptional significance, especially in low-income countries and countries with a high burden of HIV/AIDS. Indeed, as noted earlier, TB was the 10th leading cause of death globally in 2010, and in the GBD subregions of South Asia, Eastern sub-Saharan Africa and Southern sub-Saharan Africa, TB is among the top five causes of death (IMHE, 2015, p. 6).

WHO has estimated that there were about 9.6 million people infected with active TB disease in 2014 and that about 1.5 million people died from TB that year (WHO, 2015b). Although men are more likely to get TB than women, about one-third of the annual TB deaths are among women and TB remains a major killer of women of reproductive age (IMHE, 2015). It is difficult to diagnose TB in children, but WHO estimated that about 1 million children became ill with TB in 2014 and 140,000 children died that year of TB (IMHE, 2015).

TB is an opportunistic infection of HIV and TB/HIV co-infection is an important issue. It is estimated that about 13% of people with active TB disease in 2014 were co-infected with HIV, and about one-third of all deaths among people who are HIV-positive are from TB. About 75% of those who are co-infected are in Africa (WHO, 2015b).

Drug-resistant TB is a major issue in efforts to address TB. It is thought that about 480,000 of the 9.6 million cases of active TB disease were drug resistant 2014, but only about 20% of them have been identified and are being treated. The largest numbers of drug-resistant cases are in China, India, and Russia (WHO, 2015b).

Implications for Health Promotion

TB is treatable and curable, and proper treatment reduces the spread of TB and the development of drug-resistant TB. In principle, no one, certainly no one who is not immune compromised, should die of drug-susceptible TB. However, to avoid TB deaths, it is important to identify all people with TB and to seek to cure all of them. This is made more complicated by stigma against people with TB, the six-month course of therapy for drug-susceptible TB, and the even longer course of therapy for drug-resistant TB. Thus, progress against TB will require health promotion efforts aimed at helping people recognize the symptoms of TB, encouraging them to seek appropriate care as early as possible and to adhere faithfully to their drug regimen. In addition, it will be important to test all HIV positive people for TB and all people with TB for HIV.

Malaria

Incidence and Deaths

In 2010, malaria was the 12th leading cause of death globally. However, it was the first cause in the GBD subregions of Central and Western sub-Saharan Africa, the fourth cause in Eastern sub-Saharan Africa, and the ninth cause in Oceania (IMHE, 2015).WHO estimates that there were more than 200 million cases of malaria in 2012. The highest rates of malaria are found in Africa and six African countries: Nigeria, the Democratic Republic of the Congo (DRC), Tanzania, Uganda, Mozambique, and Cote'd'Ivoire, which account for nearly half of the malaria cases worldwide. Nigeria and the DRC alone account for about 40% of all malaria deaths (Roll Back Malaria, 2013).

WHO estimates that 627,000 people died of malaria in 2012 (Roll Back Malaria, 2013, p. 21). The overwhelming majority of the deaths, 77%, were in children under five years of age (Roll Back Malaria, 2013). However, malaria causes substantial risks for pregnant women in low-income countries and a significant share of the remaining deaths were among pregnant women (Roll Back Malaria, 2013). Adult male forest workers in some places in Southeast Asia and South Asia are also at risk for malaria.

Implications for Health Promotion

Many cases of malaria could be prevented through measures such as: the use of insecticide-treated bednets; indoor residual spraying; intermittent treatment of pregnant women; selected seasonal chemoprevention in young children; and, in some settings, larval and other environmental controls. Malaria can also be treated, which reduces transmission, provided that people recognize malaria symptoms, seek and receive appropriate care expeditiously, based on a confirmed diagnosis, and receive the correct drug. There are substantial gaps in each of these areas now and an important role for health promotion to help close them.

Neglected Tropical Diseases

The NTD Burden

The neglected tropical diseases (NTD) are a group of 17 diseases, some of which are highly prevalent but which did not garner much attention until the past decade. They include, for example, soil-transmitted helminths (worms), leprosy, schistosomiasis, lymphatic filariasis, onchocerciasis, and trachoma. They affect more than 1 billion people worldwide, about 90% in Africa, and many people suffer from more than one NTD at the same time (WHO, 2012, p. vii).

The NTDs are not associated with much mortality. However, many of the NTDs, such as lymphatic filariasis, can produce substantial morbidity, often for long periods of time or permanently. Estimates by those working on NTDs suggest that the burden of disease from the NTDs in DALYs may be greater than the burden from malaria and TB (Hotez, 2011, p. 104), although GBD suggests that NTDs cause about 30% of the burden of malaria and half the burden of TB (IMHE, 2015).

The largest number of NTD infections comes from soil-transmitted helminths. *Ascaris* (roundworm), for example, is estimated to infect about 1.2 billion people, *trichuris* (whipworm) about 800 million people, and hookworm about 740 million people. In addition, it is estimated that there are about 200 million cases of schistosomiasis, about 37 million cases of onchocerciasis, and about 84 million people actively infected with trachoma (Imperial College London—Schistosomiasis Control Initiative, 2015).

Implications for Health Promotion

Seven of the NTDs are now the focus of global attention: three soil-transmitted helminths, onchocerciasis, schistosomiasis, lymphatic filariasis, and trachoma. To combat these afflictions, a "Rapid Impact Package" of drug therapy is being promoted through mass drug administration at the community level.

This costs about US50 cents per person per year. This drug therapy can prevent the onset of these diseases in some cases and cure certain stages of the disease, as well. In addition, if mass drug administration is carried out effectively over an extended period, it should be possible to reduce transmission of some of these diseases in the affected locale. Reduction in transmission could also be aided if the people in endemic areas had greater knowledge of the diseases, their risk factors, and how to prevent those risk factors. This requires an effort to reduce the exceptional stigma attached to some of these diseases. There is a major role for health promotion in mobilizing communities around knowledge of the diseases and their risk factors, the need for participating in mass drug administration, and the need for early diagnosis and treatment if affected.

Noncommunicable Diseases

Two-thirds of the deaths that occurred in 2010 were due to noncommunicable causes. Ischemic heart disease and stroke caused almost 14 million deaths, or about 25% of total deaths. About 8 million people died from cancer and about 1.2 million from diabetes. Trachea, bronchus, and lung cancer accounted for about 1.5 million of those cancer deaths; however, if the deaths from all forms of cancer were combined, then cancer would have been the leading cause of death in 2010 (IHME 2015).

These figures represent a substantial change in the causes of death between 1990 and 2010, as noted earlier. In 1990, for example, the Group 1 diseases—communicable, maternal, neonatal, and nutritional causes—accounted for about 34% of all deaths. In 2010, however, they only accounted for 25% of all deaths. Today, these Group I causes are the predominant cause of death only in sub-Saharan Africa, in which they constitute about 75% of premature mortality (Lozano et al., 2012, p. 2096).

The total DALYs from all causes in 2010 is estimated to be about the same as in 1990. However, the composition of DALYs has changed significantly. First, the burden of disease has continued to shift from communicable to noncommunicable diseases. In 1990, communicable diseases were predominant, and noncommunicable diseases made up 43% of the total burden of disease. In 2010, however, noncommunicable diseases made up 54% of the burden of disease. Injuries as a share of the total burden of disease stayed about the same over the two periods, at around 11% (IHME, 2015).

The most important risk factors for deaths from noncommunicable diseases globally in 2010, for all age groups, are well known. These included high blood pressure, smoking, high body-mass index, high fasting plasma glucose, a diet high in sodium and low in fruit, household air pollution, ambient particulate matter, alcohol use, and high total cholesterol (IMHE, 2015).

Implications for Health Promotion

The links between behavior and noncommunicable diseases are clear, and there is an enormous role for health promotion in trying to reduce the burden of noncommunicable diseases. It may be most effective and efficient to tie health promotion efforts to the implementation of policies that also aim to encourage behavior change. This might include, for example, promoting healthier diets alongside better food labeling and taxes on unhealthy ingredients in processed foods. It could also include promoting a reduction in tobacco smoking, while raising tobacco taxes, or taking similar measures to reduce excessive alcohol use. Promoting better land use planning that encourages walking could also go hand in hand, for example, with efforts to promote more physical activity. In low- and middle-income settings, at least, it may also be necessary to mobilize communities to reduce the stigma of mental health and neuropsychiatric disorders and to engage them to provide psychosocial support to affected people.

Injuries

As noted earlier, about 9% of total deaths worldwide were associated with injuries in 2010. This was similar to the share of total deaths attributable to injuries in 1990. The share total DALYs attributable to injuries in 2010 was about 11%, also about the same as in 1990 (IHME, 2015).

The most important injuries in terms of their contributions to deaths and DALYs are road injuries, as also cited earlier, and almost 3% of all deaths in 2010 were related to such injuries. Road injuries that year were associated with about 50% more deaths than the next most important injury-related cause of death, which was self-harm, and about three times more deaths than the next largest injury-related cause of death, which was falls. Some of the other important causes of injury related deaths and DALYs are drowning, fire, and poisoning (IHME, 2015).

As expected, there is variance in injuries by location, age, and sex, among other factors. The rates of road traffic injuries vary considerably across regions, as is the likelihood that one will survive such an injury. Falls are of special importance for older people, drownings for younger people, and fires for women, especially in the South Asia region (IHME, 2015).

Implications for Health Promotion

Health promotion has an important role to play in efforts to reduce deaths and disability from injuries. At the simplest level, health promotion, often coupled with regulation, has played a very important role in reducing road injuries and deaths through encouragement of seat belt use and the use of motorcycle and bicycle helmets. Health promotion can also play a key role at the community level in promoting greater awareness of the risks of falls for older people and drowning for younger people and measures that can be taken to address them. This is also true of approaches to accidental poisoning, which is often the subject of health promotion efforts in high-income countries. Many countries face major gaps in their approach to mental health issues, including self-harm. Nonetheless, health promotion could also play an important role in reducing self-harm be helping to reduce the stigma of mental disorders and making individuals and communities more aware of such disorders and how they can get help for them.

Looking Forward

There are many factors that will influence the burden of disease in the future, in different communities, countries, and globally. Among the most important will be the pace of:

- their **epidemiological transition**
- their nutrition transition
- their **demographic transition**
- economic development
- urbanization
- increases in educational attainment, especially for girls
- technological change, especially in the health sector
- climate change

The possible outbreak of emerging and reemerging infectious diseases, of course, could also dramatically alter the future burden of disease, as epidemics have done historically and as HIV/AIDS has done more recently.

It is anticipated that most countries during the next few decades will continue to grow economically, become more urban, and that their children will achieve increasingly higher levels of educational attainment. It is also anticipated that fertility, even in today's high-fertility countries, will continue to fall, that people will live longer throughout the world, and that an increasing number of countries will have to deal with an aging population. Despite the stresses of urbanization, living in cities should increase longevity for most people. It can also be assumed that technological change in the health sector could lead to people living longer, as we are able to make use of better diagnostics, drugs, and vaccines. Increasing amounts are being written about the impact of climate change on health. Some of this change may hurt human health in some places, such as by enabling the spread of insect vectors that had been absent. However, it is certainly possible that in some places climate change might lead to a reduction in health risks.

In the absence of any major outbreak of infectious diseases, these factors are likely to lead, on balance, to continued reduction in fertility, the aging of populations, and an increase in the share of the population that is over 65 years of age. These changes *could* lead to healthier populations who live longer with less disability. However, this will also depend on the extent to which countries can avoid an increasing share of the globe becoming more exposed to "behavioral" risk factors, such as tobacco and obesity.

Projections of the future burden of disease have not yet been made in conjunction with the GBD. However, the World Health Organization in 2008 developed projections of the burden of disease to 2030. These projections suggest that there will be a continuing increase in the average age of death. In addition, the projections indicate that the burden of disease will continue to shift toward noncommunicable diseases. These projections further suggest that the three leading burdens of disease in 2030 would be unipolar depression, ischemic heart disease, and road traffic accidents. As expected, the projections also suggest that the burdens of disease we associate with poverty and underdevelopment will decrease, while those we associate with high-income settings and increasing age, such as vision and hearing loss, will increase. Of course, the pace of these changes will depend largely on the points noted earlier (WHO, 2008, p. 26).

Summary

The promotion of better health requires that we understand what people get sick, disabled, and die from. It is also important to understand how morbidity, disability, and mortality vary across groups, such as by sex, age, ethnicity, location, and socioeconomic status. In addition, we need to understand the risk factors and the social determinants that are associated with people falling ill from these causes.

There *has been* important progress in human health. People are living longer than ever before. The number of maternal deaths has decreased. The number of new TB and HIV infections have also decreased, and fewer people are dying of HIV/AIDS and TB than before. Many fewer young children are dying of diarrhea, pneumonia, malaria, or measles than ever before.

Despite this progress, there remains a substantial "unfinished agenda" of deaths from overwhelmingly preventable communicable, maternal, nutritional, and perinatal causes. These occur mostly in a range of low- and middle-income countries and especially among the poor. Moreover, they occur at highest rates in South Asia and sub-Saharan Africa, whose health indicators substantially lag those of the rest of the world.

At the same time, there is a growing burden of morbidity and mortality from noncommunicable causes. Today, the overwhelming majority of deaths and of the burden of disease measured in DALYs is linked with noncommunicable diseases. In fact, noncommunicable diseases are the predominant cause of both deaths and DALYs in all regions except sub-Saharan Africa. Moreover, over the past 20 years or so, DALYs related to noncommunicable causes as a share of total DALYs have increased from about 42% to 58%. The patterns of these noncommunicable causes vary among countries. However, as country incomes rise and lifestyles change, ischemic heart disease and stroke increasingly become the two leading causes of adult death. A large share of the deaths and DALYs associated with noncommunicable diseases are also preventable.

Injuries are also an important contributor to death and DALYs, and in 2010, about 9% of total deaths and 11% of total DALYs worldwide were attributed to injuries. These figures are about the same as they were in 1990. The importance of injuries to deaths and DALYs varies by location, sex, and age, among other things. It also varies with the ability in different places to both prevent and treat such injuries. Road injuries are the most important injury-related contributor to deaths and DALYs. However, self-harm, falls, drowning, fires, and poisoning are also important contributors to death and DALYs.

As populations have aged and people have lived longer, there has also been an increase in many settings in the number of years people are living with disability. In some settings, disability is also an increasing share of total healthy life years lost. The share of noncommunicable diseases in the overall burden of disease is expected to continue rising. Part of this rise is expected to follow substantial projected increases in the burden of ill health from conditions such as dementia, diabetes, and mental health disorders. These shifts will contribute to growing amounts of disability.

There is increasingly good evidence on the social determinants of and the risk factors for the unfinished agenda of communicable diseases, for noncommunicable diseases, and for injuries. To reduce child deaths, for example, there will have to be improvements in nutrition, access to safe water, improved sanitation, and handwashing with soap. In addition, child deaths could be reduced relatively rapidly if the affected countries could implement at scale a cost-effective package of evidence-based interventions, such as promotion of better birthing practices, improved caring behaviors for neonates, exclusive breastfeeding, and immunization.

Addressing the growing burden of noncommunicable diseases will require reductions in the use of tobacco and alcohol, dietary improvements, and more physical activity, among other things. These would also contribute to reductions in some of the conditions that are themselves risk factors for heart disease and stroke, such as diabetes and high blood pressure. Reducing deaths and DALYs from injuries will require efforts to reduce road injuries. These could include, for example, better enforcement of traffic, drunk driving, and seat belt and helmet laws. These could also include efforts to calm traffic, such as traffic circles and speed bumps.

There is a substantial role for health promotion in dealing with the agendas of all three "cause groups": communicable, maternal, perinatal, and nutritional (Group 1); noncommunicable (Group 2); and injuries (Group 3). On the Group 1 side, there is a need, among many other things, to mobilize families and communities to engage in a range of better health behaviors, such as more optimal breastfeeding, the feeding of a more diverse diet, safer use of water, the elimination of open defecation, and handwashing with soap. Families also need to be more knowledgeable, for example, about how to reduce exposure to malaria and diagnose and treat it effectively; how to recognize TB and seek appropriate care for it; and how to reduce exposure to HIV and to seek out testing for it. Promoting the immunization agenda will also continue to be important.

On the noncommunicable side (Group 2), many of the causes of morbidity and mortality are associated with behavioral factors. Among other things, it will be important to promote reduction in the use of tobacco and alcohol. It will also be important to encourage people to eat healthier and exercise more. People will also need to be encouraged to recognize early the risk factors for the most important noncommunicable diseases and to address them at an early stage.

We have known for many years that health promotion can play an extremely important role in preventing injuries.

For Group 3, in fact some of the most important measures will be to promote the use of seat belts in automobiles and helmets for motorcycles and bicycles. Health promotion at the community level, for example, can also be instrumental to reducing falls, drowning, and accidental poisonings. There is also a large and often forgotten agenda for health promotion to reduce self-harm and help to make people more aware of, more accepting of, and more willing to seek care for mental health disorders.

KEY TERMS

1. **Communicable diseases:** Illnesses that are caused by a particular infectious agent and that spread directly or indirectly from people to people, from animals to animals, from animals to people, or from people to animals
2. **Demographic transition:** The shift from high fertility and high mortality to low fertility and low mortality
3. **Disability-adjusted life years (DALYs):** A composite measure of premature deaths and losses due to illnesses and disabilities in a population
4. **Epidemiologic transition:** A shift in the pattern of disease from largely communicable diseases to noncommunicable diseases
5. **Morbidity:** Illness
6. **Mortality:** Death
7. **Noncommunicable diseases:** Illnesses that are not spread by any infectious agent
8. **Risk factor:** An aspect or personal behavior or lifestyle, an environmental exposure, or an inborn or inherited characteristic that, on the basis of epidemiologic evidence, is known to be associated with health-related conditions

REVIEW QUESTIONS

1. What is a DALY?
2. What is meant by the concept "the burden of disease"?
3. What are the three leading causes of death globally for all age groups and both sexes?
4. How would these causes vary by country income group?
5. How would the leading causes of death for women globally vary from that for men?
6. What are the three leading causes of death globally for under-five children?

7. How would the leading causes of death for under-five children vary across country income groups?
8. What types of health conditions might cause substantial numbers of years lived with disability but not be associated with many deaths?
9. What share of the burden of disease in a poor sub-Saharan African country today will be communicable diseases and how would you expect that to change during the next twenty years?

References

Bhutta, Z. A., Das, J. K., Rizvi, A., et al. for the Lancet Nutrition Interventions Review Group and the Maternal and Child Study Group. (2013). Evidence-based interventions for improvement of maternal and child nutrition: What can be done and at what cost? *Lancet, 382*(9890), 452–477.

Granich, R., Williams, B., & Montaner, J. (2013). Fifteen million people on antiretroviral treatment by 2015: Treatment as prevention. *Current Opinion in HIV and AIDS, 8*(1), 41–49.

Hotez, P. (2011). Enlarging the "audacious goal": Elimination of the world's high prevalence neglected tropical diseases. *Vaccine, 29* (Suppl. 4), 104–110.

Imperial College London-Schistosomiasis Control Initiative. (2015). *What are neglected tropical diseases.* Retrieved from http://www3.imperial.ac.uk/schisto/whatwedo/7ntds

Institute for Health Metrics and Evaluation. (2013). *The global burden of disease: Generating evidence, guiding policy.* Seattle, WA: Author.

Institute of Health Metrics and Evaluation. (2015). *GBD Compare|Viz Hub.* Retrieved from http://vizhub.healthdata.org/gbd-compare/

Jones, G., Steketee, R. W., Black, R. E., Bhutta, Z. A., Morris, S. S., and the Bellagio Child Survival Study Group. (2003). How many child deaths can we prevent this year? *Lancet, 362*(9377), 65–71.

Lim, S. S., Vos, T., Flaxman, A. D., et al. (2012). A comparative risk assessment of burden of disease and injury attributable to 67 risk factors and risk factor clusters in 21 regions, 1990–2010: A systematic analysis for the Global Burden of Disease Study 2010. *Lancet, 380*(9859), 2224–2260.

Lozano, R., Nagavi, M., Foreman, K., et al. (2012). Global and regional mortality from 235 causes of death for 20 age groups in 1990 and 2010: A systematic analysis for the Global Burden of Disease Study 2010. *Lancet, 380*(9859), 2095–2128.

Roll Back Malaria. (2013). *Key malaria facts.* Retrieved from http://www.rollbackmalaria.org/keyfacts.html

Salomon, J. A., Vos, T., Hogan, D. R., et al. (2012). Common values in assessing health outcomes from disease and injury: Disability weights measurement study for the Global Burden of Disease Study 2010. *Lancet, 380*(9859), 2129–2143.

UNAIDS. (2013). *Global report: UNAIDS report on the global AIDS epidemic 2013.* Geneva: Author.

UNAIDS. (2014). *2014 Fact Sheet.* Global Statistics. Geneva: Author.

UNICEF. (2014). *Committing to child survival: A promise renewed.* New York, NY: Author.

United Nations Statistics Division. (2015). *Millennium Development Goals Indicators.* Retrieved from http://mdgs.un.org/unsd/mdg/Metadata.aspx?IndicatorId=0&SeriesId=553

Wang, H., Dwyer-Lindgren, L., Lofgren, K. T., et al. (2012). Age-specific and sex-specific mortality in 187 countries, 1970–2010: A systematic study for the Global Burden of Disease Study 2010. *Lancet, 380*(9859), 2071–2094.

World Bank. (2015a). *Data; Life expectancy at birth, total (years).* Retrieved from http://data.worldbank.org/indicator/SP.DYN.LE00.IN

World Bank. (2015b). *Data; Mortality rate, infant (per 1,000 live births).* Retrieved from http://data.worldbank.org/indicator/SP.DYN.IMRT.IN http://data.worldbank.org/indicator/SP.DYN.IMRT.IN

World Bank. (2015c). *Data; Mortality rate, neonatal (per 1,000 live births).* Retrieved from http://data.worldbank.org/indicator/SH.DYN.NMRT

World Bank. (2015d). *Data; Mortality rate, under five (per 1,000 live births).* Retrieved from http://data.worldbank.org/indicator/SH.DYN.MORT

World Health Organization. (n.d.). *The Global Burden of Disease Study (2000–2002): Definition of cause categories in terms of international classification of disease (ICD) codes.* Retrieved from http://www.who.int/healthinfo/statistics/gbdestimatescauselist.pdf

World Health Organization. (2008). *The global burden of disease: 2004 update.* Geneva: Author.

World Health Organization. (2012). *Accelerating work to overcome the global impact of neglected tropical diseases.* Geneva: Author.

World Health Organization. (2013). *Global tuberculosis report 2013.* Geneva: Author.

World Health Organization. (2015a). *Global health observatory data repository.* Retrieved from http://apps.who.int/gho/data/view.main.CM300WORLD-CH17?lang=en.

World Health Organization. (2015b). *Tuberculosis. Fact sheet No. 104.* Updated October 2015. http://www.who.int/mediacentre/factsheets/fs104/en/

Ms. Lindsey Hiebert provided substantial assistance in the preparation of this chapter, including preparation of tables and figures and assistance in editing.

CHAPTER 2

GLOBAL HEALTH PROMOTION

The State of the Science

David V. McQueen

LEARNING OBJECTIVES

By the end of this chapter, the reader should be able to:

- **Acquire an overview of health promotion science from a global perspective**
- **Inform the reader that health promotion is not a static field, but a dynamic field that changes over time and the change varies in different parts of the globe**
- **Appreciate how health promotion science is conceptualized within the cultural context of different societies**
- **Understand the role and effect of sociocultural and political forces globally**
- **Consider how comparing and contrasting health promotion practice and research in diverse countries and regions as an approach to learning—it permits students and professionals to observe differences in the practice and research in the field**

The field of work that is health promotion is very diverse. This diversity is great in any single country, let alone globally. So at the beginning of this chapter there must be the caveat that not all of health promotion science can be surveyed and that not every country or region will get its due. Furthermore, in the spirit of self-reflexivity, a quality that all health promoters should possess, the view of health promotion science across the globe will highly reflect the author's experience in the field after more than four decades in academia, government, nongovernmental organizations (NGOs), and consultation.

The notion of a health promotion "science" should be broadly interpreted. There are those who would classify much of health promotion research and practice as nonscientific or at best as "soft" science. From the perspective of the philosophy of science this is highly questionable. Historically, science was always occupied with providing the best explanation for phenomena. Thus, the ancient Aristotelian writings on the physics of motion were the best science of the time, and remained so for many centuries to follow. Today Aristotelian mechanics are no longer adequate, yet modern physics and engineering still rely on 17th-century Newtonian mechanics at the non-quantum level. The everyday science and practice of health promotion relies on the same assumption, proceeding with confidence that it applies the best explanation of health-related phenomena at this point in time. Given that

For their advice on the case studies I heartily thank Mary Hall, Marie Claude-Lamarre, Vivian Lin, Hans Onya, Louise Potvin, and Alfred Rütten. Their advice was highly valuable; however, the content of the case studies is entirely my own responsibility. Many of the ideas in this chapter were taken from three chapters in McQueen, D. V. (Ed.). (2013). *Global handbook on noncommunicable diseases and health promotion*. New York, NY: Springer.

such widely accepted concepts such as *context* and *complexity* have entered into the explanations of causes in the understanding of health and illness, the science of health promotion is as modern and complicated as other scientific endeavors.

Why a Global Perspective Is Relevant Today

Another key characteristic is that science is not bounded by geography. It is a global phenomenon. Obviously some sciences are very similar globally in research and practice. One expects that molecular biological research in Atlanta is very similar to that in Tokyo, Buenos Aries, or Mumbai. But some sciences, and health promotion is in this category, have differences across the globe that reflect characteristics of localities, countries, regions, and continents. In addition, health promoters may be heard to refer to a Western approach or a Northern approach. Furthermore, the practitioners in the field may indeed perceive themselves as taking a Western approach or a Southern approach. In general the social science disciplines do relate to the cultures and contexts in which they work. Although this may even be subtly true in the so-called hard sciences, it is more apparent in the so-termed soft sciences. However, the contextual aspect of the work in a scientific field does not make it a lesser science.

The underlying institutional and organization structures that shape the practice of science globally are vital to the progress of health promotion science. As with the work in all sciences, although countries are important as foci of work in the field, there are other actors that shape the science that gets done in health promotion. International organizations, foundations, and national governmental institutions shape and influence what gets funded and what topics become relevant. These organizations and institutions themselves reflect the social and political forces found in the countries they are based in and the political constituencies they represent. Thus the Bill & Melinda Gates Foundation shapes research and practice in Africa. Similarly the **World Health Organization (WHO)**, embracing the FCTC (Framework Convention on Tobacco Control) or the **social determinants of health (SDOH)**, shapes health promotion thinking around the world. Powerful national agencies, for example, the US Centers for Disease Control (CDC), also help define what is done locally, nationally, and globally. This is not to be disparaged, but to be understood as one reality of modern-day science in any field.

Anthropology and sociology are social sciences that have long been concerned with the societal characteristics of countries and peoples. As a result there is now a better understanding of the nature of health promotion science as it occurs across the globe. Sociocultural characteristics shape the successes and failures of the health care systems in countries—an area of research that has been studied in detail (e.g., National Research Council and Institute of Medicine [NAS/IOM] Report, 2012). We need to assume that these same characteristics act on health promotion research and practice. Many of these characteristics may result in broad generalizations, but the cultural and societal emphasis on "individualism" that shapes the American spirit directly affects what is done and funded in health promotion. A similar case could be made for Canada, with its emphasis on population health over that of the individual. In Latin America, countries like Brazil have a health promotion science that is shaped by theoretical concepts coming from their theoretical champions such as Paulo Freire (1967). In the region and continent of Europe, one sees large difference in health promotion research and practice from the northern Scandinavian countries to the southern European countries. One can speculate that the variation may reflect differences arising from the classical separation of the Germanic and romance language bases, but such distinctions, though easy to assert, remain difficult to prove. Similarly, the continent of Africa has a mixture of diversity that rests on many forces, including colonialism and extensive poverty. Health promotion research and practice on that continent is also buffeted by the interest of powerful institutions from outside that area. Identifying a distinctive emerging "African-based" health promotion is challenging. Oceana, and notably the countries of New Zealand and Australia, has powerful and leading institutions of health promotion and in many ways leads the field of health promotion science beyond its population base. Global visibility of health promotion activities seems to remain a problem for Westerners; however, there is much health promotion activity in this diverse area. Finally, the large and highly populated Asian continent has enormous diversity of countries, resulting in varied research and practice. It is a region of economically advanced countries—for example, Singapore and Japan—to countries with outstanding poverty and inequities—for example, Bangladesh and Indonesia. The Middle Eastern region alone presents very different research and science challenges for modern-day health promotion.

The Impact of Language on the Conduct of Research

English is a language that ties most all of present-day science together globally. The science of health promotion is no exception. The major institutions, publications, and discussions on health promotion research occur largely in English. This is not to discount other languages, but at any point in time science communicates its findings in a common language. That helps make the pursuit of science universal. But there are strong educational aspects of this reliance on a common language, and it presents limitations to understanding the scope and output of health promotion science across the globe. The results of the practice of health promotion at the local level are often only accessible in the language of the locality. This language emphasis has perhaps greatly altered in recent years with the dependence on the Internet in scientific research. The Internet has helped to make accessible research and practice that in the past would have been unseen in the English-dominated world of science journals and publications. In addition, we now have powerful search engines that can find more obscure documents, even in languages other than English. We now possess fairly reliable online translation possibilities. The full impact of these fast-moving changes in technology remains to be seen.

Health promotion is a dynamic field that has changed markedly in the past 30 years. With regard to the scientific concepts of causality and evidence, health promotion has been very much affected in particular with the emergent idea of complexity. For health promotion research, the very simple idea that a single factor *x* causes a single outcome *y* is now regarded as far too simplistic. Multidimensional causality has become a commonplace notion in health promotion. Health promotion has also been infused with considerable ideology. This ideological orientation stems in part from such fundamental documents as the Ottawa Charter and others that have argued for a multicausal world (WHO, 1986, 2009; World Health Organization, Regional Office for Europe [WHO, EURO], 1984, 1998). At the same time that there was growing recognition of the complexity of causality there was a powerful movement toward what was termed "evidence-based medicine" (Sackett et al., 1996). As a result the field of public health, and in particular health promotion, was faced with showing evidence using increasingly complex models of causality.

Causality and causal thinking has a long and distinguished history in philosophy and science dating back to the ancient Greek world. In science and philosophy, discussions of causality have continued to modern times, with much of the underlying epistemological basis for modern-day evidence seeking resting on a number of assumptions about theory and observation. Complexity has many implications for health promotion as it relates to the notion of causality. In much of science, including public health science, causality has often been treated in a manner reflecting the tenets of causality set by logical positivism to fit an emergent view of science based on linear causality. Even as science, both social and physical, developed models of causation with many variables arranged in reciprocal and curvilinear structures, causality essentially was modeled on an underlying philosophical basis in logical positivism. The notion of complexity changed all this orientation. For health promotion science this has had many implications. It does not imply that causality cannot be understood, but that the understanding lies more with the interpreter of causality and with extrapolations of theory rather than with the events being described. For example, in trying to understand a phenomenon, scientists have often argued that complex systems might be broken down, or "reduced" to an understanding of the smaller causal units. That is, after one has understood all the single-factor causal units, the smaller units can be linked or "summed' in order to see the whole causal picture. On this basis it is seen as legitimate to understand pieces of the whole causal picture in order to understand the whole. However, the alternative notion that the "whole is the whole" and that the whole is complex, challenges this fundamental reductionist procedure in the practice of modern science. In health promotion science this is a critical issue, particularly when the underlying ideology of being holistic is being considered.

The Role of Context

Contemporary global health promotion has a major interest in understanding the context in which health promotion occurs. This concern with context in health promotion has led many in the field to rethink the methodological approaches of the field. This is particularly the case when applied to interventions. There is considerable debate over acceptable methods. For example, despite its general inappropriateness as a methodological approach for health promotion interventions, the **randomized controlled trial** (RCT) remains for many as an ideal to which intervention research should aspire. When control of a population receiving an intervention can be achieved for the period of the intervention, and where there is a focus on a simple intervention with an expected highly measurable outcome of success or failure, the RCT is a powerful design for intervention research in health promotion (Rosen et al., 2006). Thus the rejection of the RCT by many health promotion researchers has not convinced everyone. However, the strength of the RCT design is dependent upon meeting very restrictive assumptions of experimental design. When these severe design parameters are not met, the power of the RCT diminishes rapidly. Given the population-based interventions generally used in in health promotion, the misapplication of the RCT is highly probable (McQueen, 2007; McQueen & Jones, 2007). For example, in community-based health promotion interventions applied to **noncommunicable disease** (NCD), the separation of control and experimental populations is nearly impossible. It is part of the very nature of health promotion interventions that they operate in everyday life situations, involving changing aspects of the intervention as it is occurring; outcomes are often different from initial expectations and unanticipated consequences are common. However, there are lingering elements of the RCT design in many health promotion approaches, they just have a less strict model. The idea of experimental and control groups remain in studies and projects that use quasi-experimental designs, controls, and other subliminal trappings of the RCT. Unfortunately, for many at the so-called hard end of the hard-to-soft–science spectrum, a softer health promotion methodology may be viewed as a limitation of the field. The discussion and debate regarding conflicting ideas about how more ““rigid” methods, such as the RCT, should be applied to health promotion interventions in the population continues globally. Much of this debate is a product of the background orientation of the researchers and practitioners carrying out the health promotion research. The challenge for some is to provide a research infrastructure for health promotion that will not only satisfy those who revere the RCT, but also yield alternative intervention research designs that reflect the theoretical underpinnings of modern health promotion. This discussion on methods reveals a broader area of conflicting ideas and approaches in health promotion. In turn, this reflects a broader separation of ideas that characterizes public health in general.

How does health promotion fit into the broader world of public health? Over the years different orientations toward public health have developed in the health promotion research community. Roughly speaking, a separation exists between two views, which could be termed "biomedical public health" and "social public health." One may be seen as more disease oriented, concerned with prevention and control of disease. The other may be viewed as more health oriented, concerned with improving health, addressing the social contexts related to illness and the promotion of health. The underlying epistemologies are different but have considerable overlap. The orientation of the health promotion researcher toward these views may well determine the subjects of study and the methodologies applied. These two orientations are not necessarily conflicting, but they frequently give rise to differing interpretations of the underlying mission of public health and how those in health promotion perceive that mission. A public health steeped in the biomedical tradition tends to view epidemiology as the basic science of public health. It tends to view causation as linear and relies heavily on "evidence" gathered by methodological approaches that use mainly experimental designs and rely on a numerate tradition. Often the emphasis is on the individual as the focus of prevention programs, with the intent of influencing behavioral change. In contrast, a public health in the social tradition considers that there are many sciences that are "basic" to public health, and particularly relevant disciplines are the social sciences such as sociology, politics, and economics. In these disciplines direct causation is less relevant than patterns of change and complexity is expected; linearity in causality is not expected. Although this different orientation has been discussed in many sources (Kelly & Moore, 2012; Tones, 1997; Venkatapuram, 2011), there has yet to be a satisfactory resolution of the separation of views. Globally health promotion research and practice varies greatly depending on the orientation taken. One can particularly note these differing orientations in individual countries. As a generalization, those countries with a strong social orientation tend to favor a health promotion science that concentrates on issues such as **health in all policies** (HiAP), social justice, equity, and the social contexts of health.

The Emergent Role of Evidence in Global Health Promotion

Without doubt there is a major effort globally to provide evidence for the effectiveness of health promotion. In considering causality and evidence in health promotion there is one major challenge. Knowledge of the causes of poor health is not sufficient for health promotion action; one should also have a very good idea of how to alter the causes in order to improve health. However, when considering the role of social context in health promotion, it is a great challenge to show evidence that an intervention in the complicated causation process is effective. This is where complexity and dynamism of the real world makes the work of health promotion science very difficult. One problem is that the causation structure changes through time; and second, any intervention introduced into the whole context changes the causation structure through its action. This is neither an uncommon nor a trivial problem.

In the past two decades major institutions and organizations concerned with health promotion have sought to gain more understanding of interventions using an organizational response to assess evidence. Given the complexity of health-promotion-type interventions it was realized that assessing such complexity may well go beyond the abilities and resources of individual researchers in the field. Such a task requires an industrial effort to apply a systematic basis to showing evidence and effectiveness in health promotion. There is a huge literature accumulating from this collective work, and it continues to grow. Those who want greater insight into these efforts should consult the numerous websites, documents, and the considerable literature that has accumulated (e.g., http://www.cochrane.org/, http://www.thecommunityguide.org/, http://www.nice.org.uk/). In some cases organizational subsets of public health specialties have developed, as witnessed in the founding of the Canadian National Collaborating Centres for Public Health, which were established specifically to carry out knowledge synthesis and translate it into programmatic use for practitioners (http://www.nccph.ca/en/home.aspx). One center in particular, the National Centre for Methods and Tools (http://www.nccmt.ca/), conducts work that is highly relevant to the discussion found in health promotion research. In other cases, nongovernmental organizations such as the **International Union for Health Promotion and Education** (IUHPE) have developed **global programs on evidence and health promotion effectiveness** (GPHPE). These efforts and others have been accumulating knowledge on causality and evidence for years. Even with the greatly increased knowledge synthesis base provided by all these organizational efforts, there is still much to be done, and it would be wrong to assume that there is any completeness to this effort to assess evidence and effectiveness. The relevant topic areas for examination in health promotion are nearly boundless—everything from single diseases to issues of policy and climate change are potential subjects. It is important to note most of these efforts suffer significantly from lack of resources, and many have had to curtail activities.

In the United States, the Community Guide has produced a large body of works on the evidence and causality question. In the European region there have been a number of organizationally based efforts to assess the evidence of effectiveness of interventions. One effort was the IUHPE report to the European Commission that took an approach to evidence more rooted in health promotion ideology. The IUHPE-EC report concluded that (a) comprehensive approaches using all five Ottawa strategies are the most effective; (b) certain "settings" such as schools, workplaces, cities, and local communities offer practical opportunities for effective health promotion; (c) people, including those most affected by health issues, need to be at the heart of health promotion action programs and decision-making processes to ensure real effectiveness; (d) real access to information and education, in appropriate language and styles, is vital; and (e) health promotion is a key "investment"—an essential element of social and economic development (IUHPE, 1999). In the United Kingdom the continuing work of the **National Institute for Health and Care Excellence** (NICE) provides guidelines for public health interventions. Their systematic approach rests on a strong biomedical model of evidence and causality and has provided considerable insight into the basis for a health promotion science. This is explored in a seminal article by Kelly and Moore (2012) on the role of judgment in evidence-based medicine and technology assessment.

Sociocultural and Political Aspects of Global Health Promotion

For nearly five decades health promotion research and practice has been concerned with sociocultural and political forces as important considerations in determining the success and failure of practice and research. This observation is supported by the influence of the WHO report on the causes of the social determinants of health (WHOCSDOH, 2008), with its emphasis on inequity and its notion of searching for the "causes of the causes." However, there is another critical dimension related to this SDOH perspective in health promotion science, and that is the observation that health promotion research and practice itself is influenced by powerful social, cultural, and political forces. Every setting, whether a community or a nation, in which health promotion research is undertaken is influenced by these factors. Much of this diversity globally is summarized in a special issue of *Global Health Promotion* dedicated to global examples of seeking evidence (Potvin et al., 2011).

Four Case Studies

Given the great diversity of health promotion activity across the globe, it would be impossible to provide examples of all the diversity. However, it is possible to provide brief case studies of around 500 words each to illustrate some of this diversity. The four studies provided—Latin America, Thailand, Africa, Eastern Europe—are chosen to illustrate continental effects as well as institutional effects. It should be clear that the emphasis is on the science of health promotion and not just the total activity of health promotion work. For example, Case Study 2.2, on the Thaihealth experience, is not intended to be representative of the vast potential and work of health promotion foundations across the globe, but rather to illustrate a point about funding and institutional support for health promotion. Case Study 2.3, on Africa, does not take into account the enormous health promotion activity that is occurring with the heavily funded programs addressing AIDS on that continent; rather, it is focused on the underlying development of health promotion capacity to do science in the region. Thus, it is important for the reader to bear in mind that these are mere vignettes that demonstrate certain characteristics of modern-day health promotion and its efforts to become a more effective science.

Unfortunately, there does not exist a comprehensive database of all the work being carried out in the name of health promotion globally. Furthermore, given the wide range of subject matter that comes under the banner of health promotion, it is doubtful that such a database would ever be completed or successfully undertaken. Nevertheless, it would be highly useful if some international organization would provide a comprehensive database of the research that relates to health promotion. Although we do have quite comprehensive collections of efforts to assess effectiveness and also quite comprehensive summaries of work on specific risk factors related to disease, we lack a straightforward, nonjudgmental tabulation of the research being carried out in the name of health promotion.

CASE STUDY 2.1 LATIN AMERICAN EXAMPLE: THE SPECIAL CHARACTER OF LATIN AMERICAN HEALTH PROMOTION

Ligia de Salazar and Laurie Anderson (2008), in summarizing health promotion in Latin America, characterized it as highly related to the health promotion promulgated in Europe and North America during the 1970s and 1980s. But they also point out that even earlier the Latin American body of literature on social medicine had emphasized equity and social justice and in many ways had developed these notions critically before they became inculcated in North American and European health promotion. They argue that Latin American intellectual traditions influencing health promotion stemmed from both political and academic sectors. Already in the mid-20th century leaders such as the physician and politician Salvadore Allende in Chile asserted that poor health was a consequence of poverty and social injustice and put forward public measures to redistribute public resources. Political revolutions such as those in Cuba and Nicaragua had strong components of social justice related to health, housing, and the social environment. Most notably, in Brazil, Paulo Freire's writings were highly influential in shaping the educational movement toward empowerment, a concept that only later was emphasized in North American and European health promotion strategies. As Waitzkin et al. (2001) have pointed out, the Latin American region has had a strong emphasis on what would later be called the social determinants of health and in areas that would later characterize what came to be known as health promotion.

In producing the book *Health Promotion Evaluation Practices in the Americas: Values and Research* (Potvin & McQueen, 2008), the editors sought to explore the unique character of health promotion evaluation in the Americas. A basic assumption was there would be significant differences in the practice and evaluation of health promotion between the Anglophone North America and the non-Anglophone Americas. This assumption was based on the premise that health promotion is a context-based field. In reading through the documents and chapters written by health promoters from both Americas, it became clear that North American health promotion practice was dominated by a well-developed health education base, stemming largely from social psychology and the behavioral sciences. Furthermore, the scientific practice of the field emphasized experimental and quasi-experimental evaluation designs. Remarkably, the South American literature, particularly the strong methodological traditions in Brazil, for example, used methods that developed program systematization (Westphal & Fernandez, 2008) that were relatively unknown in what could be termed the Anglo-Saxon health promotion literature. This was not unique to the Brazilian literature, but was seemingly a characteristic of romance languages of the region. Although participatory action research (PAR) was attracting considerable interest in the field, its fundamental theoretical base in the work of such notables as Freire was seldom represented in the English literature base.

CASE STUDY 2.2 ASIAN EXAMPLE: HEALTH PROMOTION INSTITUTIONAL LEADERSHIP, THAIHEALTH

A major phenomenon in health promotion that aids the development of health promotion science is related to funding mechanisms and the subsequent support of health promotion institutions to manage this funding. One such institutional development is the funding of health promotion foundations. Notably, first among these globally was VicHealth in Australia, founded in 1987, and, more recently in the Asian region the Thaihealth Foundation, founded in 2001. Although VicHealth was created at the regional level within Australia and has served as a global inspiration for later health promotion foundations, Thaihealth Foundation has served an exemplary role for health promotion at both the country and the Asian regional levels, particularly in the Western Pacific Region of WHO (WPRO). Historically these foundations worldwide have generally arisen in response to the global concern with tobacco use and its negative health effects. As such, these efforts are illustrative of the power of a major public health focus on a major single causal agent, implicated in numerous noncommunicable diseases, to lead to funding a structured institutional response. Thaihealth is an excellent example of this. Its funding is based on a 2% excise tax on alcohol and tobacco which provides a very considerable sum of around US$50–$60 million per year. Using this base, the foundation funds many broad-based programs on health promotion with a strong focus on programs in settings such as community, school, and workplace. Obviously a significant percentage of funds are allocated to tobacco control and reduction. The underlying mission statements of Thaihealth reinforce the Ottawa Charter as a basis for action, and one significant advantage is the ability to both extend and reinforce health promotion programs carried out by government. One criticism of this type of funding approach for health promotion is that it tends to emphasize practice more than basic research in health promotion and, as is clearly related to the funding mechanism, an emphasis on individual behavioral change more than social change. Nonetheless, there has been considerable emphasis on broader policy issues in their work, particularly with relation to controlled substances. Obviously, with such strong financial support this foundation approach influences strategic thinking beyond the shores of Thailand, as witnessed by the foundation's heavy support of the IUHPE triennial world conference held in Pattaya in 2013.

It is perhaps too early to assess the impact of these funding mechanisms and foundations on the science of health promotion, and to date no critical examination of their impact on the field has been forthcoming. A cursory examination might examine to what extent the funding mechanisms themselves dictate the priorities given to different types of methodological approaches and underlying theoretical stances. Given the contrast between the health promotion orientation that emphasizes contextual factors and places heavy emphasis on social justice and equity issues and the orientation that emphasizes individual risk reduction, such an examination would be useful. Some might argue that this differing emphasis is a false dichotomy within the field and that most health promoters and arising institutions are concerned with both individual and social parameters in research and practice.

CASE STUDY 2.3 AFRICAN EXAMPLE: SYNTHESIZING AFRICAN REGIONAL RESEARCH

The science of health promotion has many challenges at this time. Perhaps the one continent where these are most harshly felt is Africa. Throughout the world, capacity building for health promotion has been an ongoing issue. In particular, funding for research and interventions has been very limited in many countries. In the so-called low- and middle-income countries (LMIC), funding for health promotion capacity building has been especially sparse. Whereas in most global continental areas there are bright spots in which government funding, university support, and strong NGOs allow for advancing the science of health promotion, Africa remains the exception. There are strengths, particularly in South Africa.

In 2003, David Nyamwaya, a key supporter of health promotion in the region, wrote hopefully about health promotion development in Africa:

> Over the last 20 years there has been a significant acceleration in the development of health promotion in Africa. This development has now acquired a steady pace and the use of health promotion as a means for increasing societal responsibility for health now exists in all African countries. The combined use of diverse approaches to health promotion programmes is becoming the norm rather than the exception, and use of the term "health promotion" per se is increasing. The development of health promotion can be seen, for example, in the comprehensive actions aimed at addressing the underlying causes of health problems, in the large number of professionals both inside and outside the health sector who describe themselves as practitioners, through professional associations which in one way or another include health promotion in describing their work.... (Nyamwaya, p. 85)

However, by the end of that decade the picture of the evidence for health promotion effectiveness in Africa was much more guarded (Amuyunzu-Nyamongo & Nyamwaya, 2009). The conclusion appeared to be that although a considerable amount of health promotion activity was taking place on the continent, the science of the field was lacking. Fortunately, there have been strong movements toward improving the situation in the region. There are health promotion strengths, particularly in South Africa, and the most important effort taking place throughout the region is addressing the fundamental issues of competency building for health promotion. This appears to be the ultimate hope for the full development of a science of health promotion in the region.

CASE STUDY 2.4 EASTERN EUROPEAN EXAMPLE: RESEARCH ON HEALTH PROMOTION POLICY IN PHYSICAL FITNESS

Health promotion science in the European region, particularly in the Northern European countries, has often emphasized physical activity as an area for emphasis. Whether emanating from a concern with obesity or simply befitting a strong historic orientation toward physical activity and sports science, physical activity promotion is a major focus of health promotion research and interventions throughout the region. One example is the European Union–funded project on building policy capacities for health promotion through physical activity among sedentary older people, titled PASEO. The project involved 15 European nations. As described by the project manager Alfred Rütten:

> The overall design of PASEO involved four main project phases based on the concept of co-operative planning (Rütten, 2001). In each country, the scientific partner started by teaming up with a large NGO or governmental organization, thus adding "political" credibility to the project work and tapping additional resources for the ensuing planning process (e.g., communication channels, meeting venues). In the second phase, both partners approached relevant organizations from the sport, healthcare, social care, and other sectors in order to engage them as partners for the planned alliance. In the third phase, the alliances conducted a planning process, moderated by the scientific partner, to build new policy capacities. In the final phase of the project, alliance partners moved on to implement the measures developed in the planning phase. This would contribute to capacity building either directly (for example if measures tackle networking, goal definitions, resource allocation and staff training) or indirectly (e.g., through pilot projects on specific topics, which in turn would improve capacities). (Rütten et al., 2013, p. 151)

In health promotion science this type of project illustrates several key characteristics of emergent health promotion today:

- the funding by a large multigovernment agency that seeks to develop a cooperative process that involves many countries in cooperation;
- an emphasis on an intervention specific to a certain segment of the population;
- an intervention that has multiple expected outcomes ranging from individual behavior change to policy shifts;
- an intervention that cuts across several sectors as well as levels of government;
- an intervention that adopts itself to each participating country context; and
- an intervention that develops from an academic conceptual and theoretical base that is highly regarded.

In all projects undertaken of this broad type, the overall state of research understanding of appropriate methodologies remains a critical area for study—study that most likely needs to be carried out in an academic institution.

Summary

Although it is changing, much of the research and practice in health promotion today is seen through a literature dominated by the English language. Even when not stemming from the British Isles, much of the European health promotion literature is in English, in particular the published literature; graduate studies and dissertations in Northern Europe are often written in English and defended in English. English writing in North America is dominant; in the Pacific the health promotion powerhouses of Australia, New Zealand, and Singapore carry out their work and publications primarily in English. This simple linguistic fact means that the bulk of the primary and secondary literature in the field is dominated by Western epistemologies and methodologies. Notable exceptions to this generalization are found in the Portuguese and Spanish literatures of Latin America and in the efforts of Francophone Canada. The IUHPE, in its constitutional mandate to be trilingual—English, French, and Spanish—regularly presents documents in all three languages in publications and conferences. Nonetheless, the quantity of presentations and publications in Spanish and French is quite small in comparison to those in English. Perhaps more critically, the crossover of readership appears problematic based on citations found in the scientific literature.

Without doubt there is considerable variation in what constitutes the science of health promotion globally today. There is little doubt that the field of health promotion was greatly enhanced and accelerated as a result of the widespread acceptance of the 1986 Ottawa Charter. The charter stated clearly that "the fundamental conditions and resources for health are: peace, shelter, education, food, income, a stable eco-system, sustainable resources, social justice, and equity."

Although such a statement may be readily understood presently as a baseline position for the field of health promotion, this was certainly not the case during the fourth quarter of the 20th century. There is a globally diverse history to be told of the development of the field since that time.

When Anderson et al. (1988) characterized the field in their book *Health Behaviour Research and Health Promotion*, the argument was largely one that started with concepts and research in health behavior and began to lead toward a broader concept that had a more social, cultural, political, and environmental perspective. More recently, John K. Davies (2013) nicely summarized the main threads of contemporary health promotion in a document prepared for the Health Promotion Forum of New Zealand. Among his conclusions is the view that the transition of health promotion from a concern with individual behavior to a social perspective is not only incomplete, but that the perspective found in the early 1980s remains current and the discussion of what is the science of health promotion continues. He writes:

> Health promotion is a discipline with its own ideology and ordered field of study. Its values relate to a holistic view of health that includes equity, autonomy/self-determination, social justice, participation and empowerment (Green & Tones, 2010). Health promotion is continually striving to maintain this value base and ethos, ensconced in the

> Ottawa Charter, and its socio-ecological focus on tackling the wider determinants of health (Wills and Douglas, 2008). Action needs to be grounded in the core values and principles of health promotion as it is "both a moral and political project, and is fundamentally values-based" (Smith, Kelleher and Fry, 2008). It needs to keep advancing its disciplinary and alliance base. The danger of a move away from Ottawa Charter based health promotion and a return to traditional public health approaches (based on pathogenic individual risk-factor disease prevention and lifestyles) will take the field backwards. Green and Tones (2010, p. 4) stress that health promotion "needs to re-engage with its radical agenda and core values and maintain its distinct identity and purpose." This allows freedom to experiment and try new approaches such as the healthy settings movement (cities, schools, workplaces, hospitals, prisons, for example), which demonstrates that health is produced and maintained in everyday life. Also these approaches have made substantive contribution to intersectoral action and healthy public policy approaches. Health promotion has in turn facilitated numerous policy statements and programmes in a variety of countries throughout the world. (p. 10)

This is a most interesting summary and nicely characterizes the discussions on what health promotion is that take place across the globe. Although Davies calls health promotion a discipline, this may be too narrow a classification for a field of effort that is characterized by being not only multidisciplinary, but also very much concerned with values. In present-day health promotion science, as practiced in research and practice, we witness an underlying concern with values. Particularly notable are values concerned with social justice and equity. But even in the methodologies that are generally proposed in health promotion research there is often an emphasis on participation and on an involvement between the researcher and the study population. There is a self-reflective recognition that the values of the researcher are intertwined with the subject of any study or intervention. These characteristics are what separate the science of health promotion from that of many other sciences. That these underlying values of the field vary across the globe is evident from the examples we have given, but the underlying principles remain quite similar.

Finally, upon reflection, the research, practice, and science that now take place under the rubric of health promotion are diverse in both content and methodology. However, this diversity cannot be seen as independent from the institutions in which it is conducted and the sources of funding that support the research. In essence there are four basic structural supports for the funding of health promotion research: government, global organizations, nongovernmental organizations, and academia. The nature of the health promotion science funded by these four pillars reflects the characteristics of each and yields a broad perspective that one could call health promotion science. Of course, these four pillars interact significantly with each other, particularly in financial support and capacity building for the field. For example, the academy might like to view itself as "independent" of other influences, but the reality of academic research funding is that it almost always follows the whims of government policies. The underlying value base of the field may not always provide a good fit to such whims, but the creative health promotion researcher will prevail.

KEY TERMS

1. **Global programme on health promotion effectiveness (GPHPE):** A program of the IUHPE in cooperation with WHO and many other agencies; http://www.iuhpe.org/index.php/en/global-working-groups-gwgs/gwg-on-hp-effectiveness-gphpe
2. **Health in all policies (HiAP):** A broad movement in which health promotion and health promotion values play a major role. The central idea is that all policies, across all government departments, have important health components. WHO has championed HiAP. It is very heavily tied conceptually to the SDOH area. http://www.who.int/social_determinants/hiap_statement_who_sa_final.pdf
3. **International Union for Health Promotion and Education (IUHPE):** A global health promotion and education NGO based in Paris, France; http://www.iuhpe.org/index.php/en/
4. **National Institute for Health and Care Excellence (NICE):** An organization that provides national guidance and advice to improve health and social care; http://www.nice.org.uk/
5. **Noncommunicable disease (NCD) (sometimes hyphenated):** General term for noninfectious diseases; examples are heart disease, cancer, diabetes, etc. It is complicated because many NCDs may have an infectious causation. An important concept in health promotion; refer to IUHPE and to CDC websites. http://www.cdc.gov/chronicdisease/
6. **Randomized controlled trial (RCT):** A type of scientific experiment used prominently in medicine for studying treatment efficacy. In the trial, participants are randomly allocated one or other of the different treatments under study. The RCT is considered by many to be a gold standard for evaluation. RCTs are seldom applicable in the evaluation of health promotion interventions.
7. **Social determinants of health (SDOH):** A concept championed in particular by WHO. Key concepts are found at http://www.who.int/social_determinants/thecommission/finalreport/key_concepts/en/
8. **World Health Organization (WHO):** Based in Geneva, the major global UN-based agency dealing with health. Regional offices also carry out the mission of WHO. http://www.who.int/en/

REVIEW QUESTIONS

1. What aspects need to be considered when looking at health promotion in different cultures and countries?
2. What are the key nonmedical sciences that need to be considered when approaching health promotion from a global perspective?
3. What is the idea of evidence in health promotion and why is it important?
4. What types of institutions are critical to the global health promotion perspective?
5. How has thinking about causality affected global discussions about health promotion?
6. Is there a "'science" of health promotion?

References

Amuyunzu-Nyamongo, M., & Nyamwaya, D. O. (Eds.) (2009). *Evidence of health promotion effectiveness in Africa*. Nairobi, Kenya: African Institute for Health and Development.

Anderson, R., Davies, J., Kickbusch, I., McQueen, D., & Turner, R. (Eds.). (1988). *Health behaviour research and health promotion*. Oxford: Oxford University Press.

Centers for Disease Control. (2015). http://www.thecommunityguide.org/

Davies, J. K. (2013). *Health promotion: A unique discipline?* Commissioned by HPF under its occasional paper series. Auckland: Health Promotion Forum of New Zealand.

de Salazar, L. & Anderson, L. (2008). Health promotion in the Americas: Divergent and common ground. In L. Potvin & D. McQueen (Eds.), *Health promotion evaluation practice in the Americas: Values and research* (pp. 13–24). New York, NY: Springer.

Freire, P. (1967). *Educação como prática de Liberdade*. Rio de Janeiro: Jorge Zahar.

International Union for Health Promotion and Education. (1999). *The evidence of health promotion effectiveness*. A report for the European Commission by the International Union for Health Promotion and Education, CSC-EC-EAEC. Brussels-Luxembourg: Author.

Kelly, M. P., & Moore, T. A. (2012). The judgement process in evidence-based medicine and health technology assessment. *Social Theory and Health, 10*, 1–19.

McQueen, D. V. (2007). The evaluation of health promotion practice: 21st century debates on evidence and effectiveness. In J. Douglas, S. Earle, S. Handsley, C. Lloyd, & S. M. Spurr (Eds.), *A reader in promoting public health: Challenge and controversy* (2nd ed., pp. 89–96). London: Open University/Sage.

McQueen, D. V., & Jones, C. M. (Eds.). (2007). *Global perspectives on health promotion effectiveness.* New York, NY: Springer Science & Business Media.

National Institute for Health and Care Excellence. (2008). *Social value judgements: Principles for the development of NICE guidance* (2nd ed.). London: Author. http://www.nice.org.uk/media/C18/30/SVJ2PUBLICATION2008.pdf

National Institute for Health and Care Excellence. (2009). *Methods for the development of NICE public health guidance* (2nd ed.). London: Author, http://www.nice.org.uk/aboutnice/howwework/developingnicepublichealthguidance/publichealthguidanceprocessandmethodguides/public_health_guidance_process_and_method_guides.jsp?domedia=1& mid=F6A97CF4-19B9-E0B5-D42B4018AE84DD51

National Research Council and Institute of Medicine. (2012). *U.S. health in international perspective: Shorter lives, poorer health.* Panel on Understanding Cross-National Health Differences Among High-Income Countries. S. H. Woolf & L. Aron (Eds.), Committee on Population, Division of Behavioral and Social Sciences and Education, and Board on Population Health and Public Health Practice, Institute of Medicine. Washington, DC: National Academies Press.

Nyamwaya, D. (2003). Health promotion in Africa: Strategies, players, challenges and prospects. *Health Promotion International, 18*(2), 85–87.

Potvin, L., Juneau, C. É., Jones, C. M., & McQueen, D. V. (2011). How is evidence used for planning, implementation and evaluation of health promotion? A global collection of case studies. *Global Health Promotion, 18*(1), 7–8.

Potvin, L., & McQueen, D. V. (Eds.). (2008). *Health promotion evaluation practice in the Americas: Values and research.* New York, NY: Springer.

Rosen, L., Manor, O., Engelhard, D., & Zucker, D. (2006). In defense of the randomized controlled trial for health promotion research. *American Journal of Public Health, 96*(7), 1181–1186.

Rütten, A. (2001). Evaluating healthy public policies in community and regional contexts. In I. Rootman et al. (Eds.), *Evaluation in health promotion: Principles and perspectives.* WHO Regional Publications, European Series No. 92. Geneva: World Health Organization. http://www.euro.who.int/__data/assets/pdf_file/0007/108934/E73455.pdf

Rütten, A. (2011). Evidence-based policy revisited: Orientation towards the policy process and a public health policy science. *International Journal of Public Health.* doi: 10.1007/s00038–011–0321–1

Rütten, A., Abu-Omar, K., Frahsa, A., & Gelius, P. (2013). Physical inactivity and health promotion: Evidence and challenges. In David V. McQueen (Ed.), *Global handbook on noncommunicable diseases and health promotion* (pp. 137–158). New York, NY: Springer.

Sackett, D. (1996, January 13). Editorial: Evidence based medicine: What it is and what it isn't. *British Medical Journal 312,* 71–72.

Tones, K. (1997). Beyond the randomized controlled trial: A case for judicial review. *Health Education Research, 12*(2), 1–4.

Venkatapuram, S. (2011). *Health justice: An argument from the capabilities approach.* Cambridge, UK: Polity.

Waitzkin, H., Iriart, C., Estrada, A., & Lamadrid, S. (2001). Social medicine then and now: Lessons from Latin America. *American Journal of Public Health, 91,* 1592–1601.

Westphal, M. F., & Fernandez, J. C. A. (2008). The contribution of a systematization evaluative approach to implement a health promotion project in Capelo Socorro, São Paulo, Brazil. In L. Potvin & D. V. McQueen (Eds.), *Health promotion evaluation practices in the Americas: Values and research* (pp. 269–285). New York, NY: Springer.

WHO, EURO. (1984). *Health promotion: A discussion document on the concepts and principles.* Copenhagen. http://apps.who.int/iris/handle/10665/107835?mode=full&submit_simple=Show+full+item+record

WHO, EURO. (1998). *Health promotion evaluation: Recommendations to policy-makers.* Copenhagen. Cf. http://whqlibdoc.who.int/euro/1998-99/EUR_ICP_IVST_05_01_03.pdf.

World Health Organization. (1986). *Ottawa Charter for health promotion.* Geneva: Author.

World Health Organization. (2009). *Milestones in health promotion: Statements from global conferences.* Geneva: Author. Cf. http://www.who.int/healthpromotion/Milestones_Health_Promotion_05022010.pdf

WHOCSDOH. (2008). *Closing the gap in a generation: Health equity through action on the social determinants of health.* Geneva: Author. http://whqlibdoc.who.int/publications/2008/9789241563703_eng.pdf

CHAPTER 3

GLOBAL HEALTH PROMOTION AND THE SOCIAL DETERMINANTS OF HEALTH

Kumanan Rasanathan and Alyssa Sharkey

LEARNING OBJECTIVES

By the end of this chapter, the reader should be able to:

- **Understand the concept of "social determinants of health" and the relationship between social determinants and health promotion**
- **Recognize major milestones in the field of social determinants**
- **Develop an appreciation for the contribution of global health promotion to action on the social determinants of health**
- **Have an in-depth examination of real-world experiences with strategies to act on social determinants through health promotion**

In this chapter, we discuss the contribution of global health promotion to action on the **social determinants of health** (SDH). Health promotion and the discourse on social determinants of health both have built on the common value base and legacy of the Declaration of Alma Ata (World Health Organization [WHO] & UNICEF, 1978). Eliminating health disparities and achieving high-profile health targets such as those within the Sustainable Development Goals are impossible without concerted action beyond the health sector on the social determinants of health. Here we consider the natural overlap between health promotion and action on social determinants, analyze how the potential of health promotion to address social determinants has not been fully realized, and discuss experiences in countries that illustrate how the field of health promotion can best contribute to effective policies and interventions to tackle social determinants to reduce health inequities.

The Relationship of Health Promotion to the Social Determinants of Health

The understanding that social conditions decisively influence health (Lee, 2005) and therefore that action across all sectors is required to promote health and well-being is not new. Such an understanding can be found in the discipline of social medicine developed in Latin America and Europe through the 20th century, focusing on the social construction of health. Similarly, the work of McKeown (1979) and Illich (1995) presented strong empirical evidence on the link between nonmedical interventions and health improvements in modern societies. The 1946 World Health Organization (WHO) Constitution recognized the need "to promote, in cooperation with other specialised agencies where necessary, the improvement of nutrition, housing, sanitation, recreation, economic or working conditions and other aspects of environmental hygiene" (WHO, 1948). Indeed, the awareness of the importance of social factors predates even the 20th century. Among a range of pioneers contributing to health progress in the 19th century by focusing on social, political, and environmental factors, the German pathologist Rudolf Virchow famously asserted that "medicine is a social science, and politics nothing more than medicine on a grand scale" (Mackenbach, 2009). Even earlier, the ancient Egyptians recognised the unequal impact of occupation and social status on health, as recorded in millennia old papyruses (Solar & Irwin, 2006) and indigenous peoples developed holistic views of health which implicitly understood the impact of social processes.

The Declaration of Alma Ata, adopted in 1978 by the International Conference on Primary Health Care (WHO & UNICEF, 1978), built on these understandings to codify the vision of primary health care. This vision had its origins in community-based health care efforts from around the developing world in the 1950s and 1960s. By the time of Alma Ata, experiences that extended beyond biomedical curative interventions to identify and address the basic causes of health and well-being were available from throughout the world and were being promoted both by WHO (Newell, 1975) and civil society actors such as the Christian Medical Commission of the World Council of Churches. The Alma Ata Declaration was explicit that health inequalities were a major driver for primary health care, and that primary health care involved "in addition to the health sector, all related sectors and aspects of national and community development, in particular agriculture, animal husbandry, food, industry, education, housing, public works, communications and other sectors; and demand[ed] the coordinated efforts of all those sectors".

There is strong correspondence between the principles of the 1986 Ottawa Charter for Health Promotion (WHO, 1986) (and the subsequent Health Promotion Statements) and the broad actions recommended by the WHO Commission on Social Determinants of Health (see Boxes 3.1 and 3.2) and the Rio Political Declaration on Social Determinants of Health ("Rio Political Declaration on Social Determinants of Health," 2011). Drawing from the Ottawa Charter, the principles of health promotion have always championed the importance of creating supportive environments for health, ensuring the participation of communities in decisions that affect their health, reorienting health services to emphasize promotion and prevention, building the individual capacity of people to live flourishing lives, and creating public policies that enhance rather than obstruct health. The settings approach of health promotion (for example, Healthy Cities and Health Promoting Schools) is highly compatible with action on social determinants. Moreover, health promotion has always had a fundamental commitment to **equity**, in particular to reducing inequities in health. Reflecting these commonalities, the Commission on Social Determinants of Health called for a strong health promotion approach to improve health equity (Commission on Social Determinants of Health, 2008).

Health promotion's apparent natural focus on social determinants, however, has not always translated into practice. Mainstream efforts at health promotion have often prioritized action on individual risk factors or individual actions (targeting "lifestyle") over addressing social factors and determinants, or diverged from engaging with health systems or public policy (Jackson, et al., 2013). The 2005 Bangkok Charter for Health Promotion in a Globalized World, 2006) can be seen as an attempt to correct this deviation from the core principles of health promotion and to engage social determinants in the global context (Ridde, Guichard, & Houéto, 2007). The charter thus "identifies actions, commitments and pledges required to address the determinants of health in a globalized world through health promotion," foreshadowing the work of the Commission on Social Determinants of Health.

Since the release of the Commission's final report in 2008, the WHO World Health Assembly (the annual gathering of ministers of health from around the world to decide upon the work of WHO) has twice—in 2009 and 2012—adopted resolutions urging global and national action on social determinants to reduce inequities ("Resolution WHA62.14. Reducing health inequities through action on the social determinants of health," n.d.). In 2011, WHO convened the World Conference on Social Determinants of Health, hosted by the government of Brazil, in Rio de Janeiro to catalyze commitment and understanding from countries on how to address social determinants and reduce health inequities. The conference resulted in the Rio Political Declaration on Social Determinants of Health (2011), which urged actions based around five key themes:

1. adopt better governance for health and development within countries, including transparency and inclusive decision-making processes, and effective, measurable, and fair policies;
2. promote participation in policy making and implementation particularly to engage communities and civil society;
3. further reorient the health sector toward reducing health inequities by strengthening accessibility, availability, acceptability, affordability, and quality of health care and public health services to promote equitable universal coverage;
4. strengthen global governance and collaboration with respect to international cooperation and solidarity in terms of developing norms and standards, identifying good practices, mobilizing financial and technical resources, and modifying negative policies and practices;
5. monitor progress and increase accountability through information systems that facilitate establishing relationships between health outcomes and social stratification variables, and through accountability mechanisms to guide policymaking across sectors.

In the rest of this chapter, we consider strategies required for action on social determinants linked to health promotion around each of these five themes and present experiences of implementation in low- and middle-income countries. We then reflect on how the global health promotion community can best contribute to supporting successful implementation of the required strategies to address social determinants at local, national, and global levels to reduce health inequities.

BOX 3.1 THE SOCIAL DETERMINANTS OF HEALTH

The social determinants of health are the social, political, economic, and environmental conditions and cultural forces in which people are born, grow, live, work, and age (Commission on Social Determinants of Health, 2008). These circumstances, which include the health system, are shaped by the distribution of money, power, and resources at global, national, and local levels, which are themselves influenced by policy choices. The social determinants of health are mostly responsible for health inequities—unfair and avoidable or remediable differences in health between populations within countries and between countries (Whitehead, 1992).

Over the past 25 years, there have been significant advances in understanding the social determinants of health (henceforth "social determinants") and their crucial role in generating health inequities. At the conceptual level, this work has been led by social epidemiologists such as Goran Dahlgren, Margaret Whitehead, and Michael Marmot (Dahlgren & Whitehead, 2006; M. Marmot et al., 2010; M. G. Marmot et al., 1991; Marmot & Wilkinson, 2005; Whitehead, 1990; Whitehead & Dahlgren, 2006), drawing attention to the wide inequities in health status within and between countries, and putting forward models of social processes to explain these inequities, rebutting the idea that they are reasonable or due to genetic, natural, or inevitable endowments.

There has been growing consideration of how global organizations and stakeholders can best contribute to action within countries on social determinants to reduce inequities. In 2005, the World Health Organization, responding to the trends of widening global health inequities and increased understanding of the importance of social determinants, convened the Commission on Social Determinants of Health, chaired by Michael Marmot. The Commission's main objectives were to gather and examine the evidence on social determinants and provide support to countries in tackling the social causes of poor health and health inequities. The Commission brought together a global network of policymakers, researchers, and civil society leaders with a three-year mandate (2005–2008) to identify what was needed to reduce health inequities within and between countries and to report its recommendations for action to the director-general of WHO. The Commission's final report, "Closing the Gap in a Generation," was released in 2008. This report presented 56 recommendations for policies across all sectors based around three overarching themes (Commission on Social Determinants of Health, 2008):

1. improve daily living conditions;
2. tackle the inequitable distribution of power, money, and resources;
3. measure and understand the problem and assess the impact of action (see Box 3.2).

Not all determinants are equally important. The most important are those that produce stratification within society—*structural* determinants—such as the distribution of income; discrimination on the basis of factors such as gender, ethnicity, or disability; and political and governance structures that reinforce rather than reduce inequalities in economic power

(WHO, 2011). These determinants establish hierarchies of power, prestige, and access to resources. Mechanisms that produce and maintain this stratification include formal and informal governance structures; education systems; market structures for labor and goods; financial systems; attention to distributional considerations in policymaking; and the extent and nature of redistributive policies, social provision, and social protection. These structural mechanisms that affect the differential social positions of individuals within hierarchies are the root cause of inequities in health. These differences shape individual health status and outcomes through their impact on *intermediary* determinants such as living conditions, psychosocial circumstances, behavioral and/or biological factors, and the health system itself. The Commission's final report used this framework (Solar & Irwin, 2010) (Figure 3.1) to inform its recommendations.

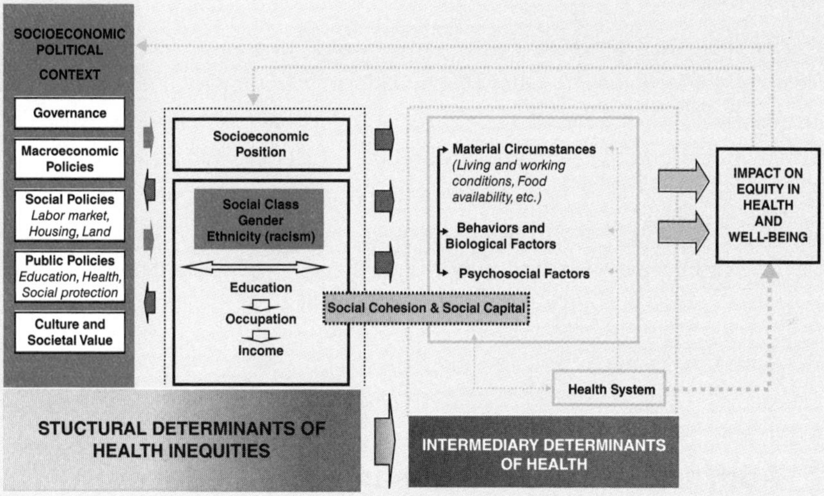

Figure 3.1 Commission on Social Determinants of Health Conceptual Framework

BOX 3.2 SUMMARY OF THE CSDH'S RECOMMENDATIONS

Overarching Recommendation No. 1: Improve Daily Living Conditions

Improve the well-being of girls and women and the circumstances in which their children are born, put major emphasis on early child development and education for girls and boys, improve living and working conditions and create social protection policy supportive of all, and create conditions for a flourishing older life. Policies to achieve these goals will involve civil society, governments, and global institutions.

Overarching Recommendation No. 2: Tackle the Inequitable Distribution of Power, Money, and Resources

In order to address health inequities, and inequitable conditions of daily living, it is necessary to address inequities—such as those between men and women—in the way society is organized. This requires a strong public sector that is committed, capable, and adequately financed. To achieve that requires more than strengthened government—it requires strengthened governance: legitimacy, space and support for civil society, for an accountable private sector, and for people across society to agree public interests and reinvest in the value of collective action. In a globalized world, the need for governance dedicated to equity applies equally from the community level to global institutions.

Overarching Recommendation No. 3: Measure and Understand the Problem and Assess the Impact of Action

Acknowledging that there is a problem, and ensuring that health inequity is measured—within countries and globally—is a vital platform for action. National governments and international organizations, supported by WHO, should set up national and global health equity surveillance systems for routine monitoring of health inequity and the social determinants of health and should evaluate the health equity impact of policy and action. Creating the organizational space and capacity to act effectively on health inequity requires investment in training of policymakers and health practitioners and public understanding of social determinants of health. It also requires a stronger focus on social determinants in public health research.

Address Social Determinants and Reduce Health Inequities

There are several actions that countries have taken to address the five key themes of the Rio Political Declaration.

Better Governance for Health and Development

As stated in the Rio Political Declaration, the achievement of health and development requires better governance strategies, including engaging various government actors in a coordinated and **intersectoral** way. In Asia, countries such as Cambodia, Fiji, Malaysia, Mongolia, and the Philippines have made strides in this regard by developing multisectoral coordination and partnerships around their programs for noncommunicable diseases (NCDs). One review of the NCD programs in these countries found that, between 2000 and 2011, each of the five countries moved from disease-based programs to integrated NCD programs with leadership provided through high-level multisectoral NCD coordination committees (Rani, Nusrat, & Hawken, 2012).

Brazil provides another example: in 2006, a high level National Commission on the Social Determinants of Health was created to produce and disseminate information on the relationships between the social determinants of health and health status (including within training programs for health professionals and for civil society organizations) and to improve policy and program design (WHO, 2011). This national Commission's leadership has no doubt played a key role in contributing to Brazil's recognition in recent years as an international leader in reducing inequities in health. Similarly, ministries of health in Argentina and Chile established national secretariats on social determinants of health, in 2007 and 2008, respectively, to provide national leadership on how to integrate strategies for responding to health problems (Rice, 2012).

Another key aspect of better governance for health and development outlined in the Rio Political Declaration is the need to "support all sectors in the development of tools and capacities to address SDH at national and international levels" (Section 11.2.vi). In Latin America, where numerous countries are working to address the SDH through health promotion and related initiatives, the Pan American Health Organization (PAHO) has developed tools, guides and resources to better demonstrate the effectiveness of these strategies. Examples of resources developed by PAHO for local policymakers and political leaders include (Rice, 2012):

- guidance on how to place health promotion on the local political agenda, build and strengthen intersectoral alliances in order to improve social and health conditions of the population, create healthy public policies, maintain healthy environments, and promote healthy lifestyles;
- recommendations on how to incorporate health promotion evaluation into policy and program development;
- suggestions on how to incorporate the Millennium Development Goals (MDGs) into local development plans with a focus on the social determinants of health;
- guides on how to implement participatory and economic evaluations (with suggested indicators for measurement).

Participation in Policymaking and Implementation

The second necessary action outlined in the Rio Political Declaration stresses the importance of participatory processes in both policymaking and implementation to address the social determinants of health. Among the countries that have prioritized the engagement of communities and civil society in their work to address the social determinants of health are Thailand and Brazil.

In Thailand, the National Health Assembly was established to involve all stakeholders in the country's efforts to support **health in all policies** (HiAP) (Rasanathan et al., 2012). The assembly has been held annually since 2008 and brings together representatives of government agencies, academia, civil society, health professions, and the private sector to discuss key health issues and produce resolutions to guide policymaking. Resolutions resulting from the assembly are credited with achievements such as "protection of budgets for universal health coverage, endorsement of strategies for universal access to medicines, and establishment of national commissions on health impact assessment and trade and health" (WHO, 2011).

In Brazil, strong social participation in health has been a priority since the 1988 constitution established the Unified Health System (SUS) and declared the right to participate in health governance as a human right for all (Fleury, 2011). Since then, Brazil has used legislation to establish national health councils and conferences (held every four years) at the national, state, and municipal levels. Both the councils and conferences engage users (50% of council members), health workers (25%), and health managers and service providers (25%), and work to assess the health situation, propose directives for health policies, and analyze health plans and management reports (Victora et al., 2011). In some jurisdictions the innovative practice of participatory budgeting has been institutionalized as well.

Reorientation of the Health Sector to Reduce Health Inequities

The third necessary action highlighted in the Rio Political Declaration, reorienting the health sector toward reducing health inequities, underscores that accessibility, acceptability, affordability, and quality of health care and public health services are essential to the enjoyment of the highest attainable standard of health.

In Chile, the government undertook several steps to achieve equity in health in response to the recommendations of the WHO Commission on Social Determinants of Health and in the context of the Chilean Social Protection System. A key objective was to reduce barriers to access to health care in the 96 most vulnerable counties and 68 most vulnerable urban neighborhoods in the country (Vega, 2011). Interventions were implemented that aimed to reduce the major barriers identified and prioritized by the local communities themselves. Many achievements resulted from this work, including reductions in health and social barriers among all participating districts (e.g., through expanding operating hours and the range of available services in remote settings); improved public awareness about, and participation in, available health and social protection programs; and infrastructural improvements (such as basic sanitation) to improve quality of life in these territories (Vega, 2011).

Programs designed to address structural barriers to reduce HIV and sexually transmitted infections (such as stigma, access to care, and violence perpetrated by intimate partners, clients, and police) underscore the importance of the physical, cultural, social, and policy contexts of the HIV risk environment and the need to take these factors into account in combination HIV-prevention strategies. In South Africa, for example, one randomized controlled trial sought to influence female sex workers' condom negotiation with their male clients and intimate male partners to empower them with new beliefs, skills, and confidence and change social norms within their networks (Strathdee et al., 2013). This study found that a combined approach incorporating individual-level sexual risk reduction, condom promotion, and improved access to sexually transmitted infection (STI) treatment with structural interventions, policy change, and empowerment can result in significant and sustained reductions in HIV/STI prevalence and incidence among vulnerable populations such as female sex workers (Strathdee et al., 2013) and has the potential to influence related problems such as addiction and gender-based violence.

Global Governance and Collaboration

The fourth necessary action outlined in the Rio Political Declaration stresses the importance of international corporation and solidarity to achieve improved health and development for all. In particular, signatories pledged to support the work of multilateral organizations to develop norms and standards, identify good practices, mobilize financial and technical resources, and review, and where appropriate, strategically modify negative policies and practices.

One activity related to this work is the establishment of "social protection floors" as defined by countries to address their specific needs and the ongoing work on social protection within the United Nations system, including the work of the International Labor Organization (ILO). Social protection floors are a fundamental strategy to extend social protection to all people and to support action on health inequities and other global priorities. The United Nations suggests social protection floors should consist of basic sets of social rights, services, and facilities (such as water and sanitation, health and education services, and essential cash or in-kind social transfers) (WHO, 2011).

The United Nations' Social Protection Floor Initiative (SPF-I) provides a framework for the systematic build-up of more comprehensive social protection systems and is gaining traction in a growing number of countries. To date, countries participating in the initiative have conducted social protection expenditure reviews, social budgeting, actuarial models, needs assessments, costing assessments, capacity building, and monitoring and evaluation activities as they work to build their own social protection floors. This SPF-I initiative provides a model for global intersectoral action, because it provides a common platform to further social determinants approaches and incorporates action on social determinants into key agreements and targets.

Progress and Accountability

The fifth and final action outlined in the Rio Political Declaration is to monitor progress in health equity and to increase accountability to guide policymaking in all sectors. Among the pledges signatories agreed to was to "establish, strengthen and maintain monitoring systems that provide disaggregated data to assess inequities in health outcomes as well as in allocations and use of resources" (Rio Political Declaration, 2011, Section15.2.i) and to "improve universal access to and use of inclusive information technologies and innovation in key social determinants of health" (Rio Political Declaration, 2011, Section 15.2.xii).

In Uganda, a communications technology developed by UNICEF Uganda in 2011, called Ureport, is an innovative approach that aims to improve inclusiveness in health and social program monitoring and in social mobilization efforts (World Health Organization & Government of South Australia, 2010). The initiative enables any mobile phone user to be a volunteer "Ureporter" who can share her or his observations and ideas in response to a question prompted on their phones via SMS text. Questions have covered a wide range of development issues, including female genital mutilation, outbreaks of disease, access to medications, safe water, early marriage, education, health, and inflation. The technology is straightforward: UNICEF sends a question on a specific topic via SMS text to Ureporters, who can respond toll-free either with a simple menu-based reply or with personal messages. UNICEF Uganda and a team of partners then analyze and interpret Ureporter responses, sharing the results and often following up with additional questions or suggestions. The findings can be stratified by area, or by characteristics of the Ureporters such as gender or age. Ureporter responses are then used both in weekly radio talk shows to create discussion on community issues and shared among UNICEF and other aid organizations to provide a better picture of how services work across Uganda.

The program was designed to establish and enforce new standards of transparency and accountability in development programming and services. Within one year, the population of Ureporters in Uganda grew to more than 89,000, with an estimated 400 to 500 new Ureporters joining the network daily. Since its inception, UNICEF has been working to increase access to the Ureport technology by creating versions of the app in different languages spoken in Uganda, as well as by working with telecommunication companies to equip telephone booths with Ureport service for those without access to a mobile phone.

The Way Forward

The global health promotion community can contribute to addressing SDH and reducing health inequities, while fostering better adherence to the principles of the Ottawa and Bangkok Charters, and Statements of the other Global Health Promotion Conferences.

It has been argued that the HiAP approach, as articulated in the Adelaide Statement on Health in All Policies (World Health Organization & Government of South Australia, 2010) is the next wave of health promotion (Kickbusch, 2010). Advancing this approach is both the first theme of the Rio Political Declaration (on improving governance for action on SDH) and the focus of the WHO Global Health Promotion Conference held in Helsinki, Finland in mid-2013. Intersectoral action is vital to primary health care, health promotion and addressing SDH, but has proved extremely difficult to implement in practice, despite isolated excellent examples. Assisting countries and communities to implement a HiAP approach thus represents the key strategic focus that global health promotion can contribute to reducing inequities through action on SDH and to moving forward on health promotion itself.

WHO and the International Union on Health Promotion and Education (IUHPE) have the major global stewardship role in ensuring that global health promotion moves forward in this way. Both organizations are already progressing in this direction. Work on health promotion and SDH within WHO is increasingly (but still incompletely) aligned, with the Helsinki conference, supported by the Government of Finland, a clear signal of this. IUHPE similarly prioritizes SDH as one of its key strategic directions. Both organizations are attempting to build guidance and tools for countries to implement HiAP, and to facilitate networks for capacity building.

Other actors can contribute to this effort as well. The Pan-American Health Organization (PAHO) has a strong focus and networks in this area. Many academic institutions, along with non-governmental organizations and civil society groups, also play a significant role in advancing health promotion at both the national and global levels.

Yet there remains a critical shortage of expertise and capacity to implement HiAP, even independent of the political challenges in doing so, particularly in low- and middle-income countries, that reflects overall insufficient capacity for health promotion. Accelerating the building of networks and the development of tools is thus an urgent priority. "South-south cooperation" is increasing (for example, the sharing of experiences in Latin America, especially catalyzed by countries such as Brazil, Chile and Mexico), but global health promotion could do more to support this.

Moreover, there is a need to move beyond the "usual suspects" to ensure that capacities are strengthened in the countries with the greatest need. This will require redistribution of global health promotion resources. Health promotion remains strongest in high-income countries in the "West" and in a small vanguard of middle-income countries such as Brazil and Thailand. These, unsurprisingly, are also the countries making the most progress with HiAP. Global health promotion can lead a reflection as to why, after over thirty years of the health promotion movement, this remains the case. HiAP is not a luxury approach for wealthy countries. The health problems for which it is essential are most acutely found in countries that face the greatest health challenges, such as so-called "fragile" states enmeshed or emerging from conflict. Global health promotion needs to help ensure that the resources of the health promotion community are instead concentrated in these countries. In this regard, the convening of the WHO Global Health Promotion Conferences in Nairobi, Kenya and in Helsinki, Finland (in 2009 and 2013, respectively) has been a welcome development. The Nairobi Call for Action, which emerged from this meeting, made a number of recommendations on strengthening health promotion in Africa, and on advancing HiAP approaches, and this was more explicitly built upon in Helsinki, where the conference was dedicated to discussions on HiAP, culminating in the Helsinki Statement on Health in All Policies. However, it remains unclear to what degree the intentions of these statements have been implemented. Documentation and dissemination of these experiences would help clarify progress made since these conferences, as well as challenges and lessons learned.

At the same time, the development of health promotion efforts in low- and middle-income countries can learn from the experiences of health promotion in high-income countries – not only to adapt positive strategies but also to learn from the challenges that health promotion has faced, and in particular avoid the tendency to focus on individual based approaches. That is, by focusing on building capacity to address SDH and implement a HiAP approach at global, national and community levels, global health promotion can assist low- and middle-income countries to transcend current experiences in implementing health promotion.

To achieve this aim, global health promotion can contribute to continuing the reorientation of the health promotion workforce, including training, towards a greater focus on SDH and HiAP, away from overemphasis on individual strategies. National institutes of public health and consortiums of schools of public health are important allies in this endeavor.

Finally, global health promotion can contribute to action and advocacy on global processes which are beyond national jurisdictions. These processes include addressing global SDH such as trade. For example, fulfilling the pledges of the Political Declaration on Noncommunicable Diseases will require addressing the global food supply and the forces that encourage the consumption of energy-dense, low nutrition food.

Similarly, the launch of the Sustainable Development Goals requires a change of paradigm in health to incorporate the concept of sustainable development. For health this can be conceived as "Healthy Planet, Healthy People"(Horton et al., 2014). Global health promotion is best suited to considering how health promotion, which is also supportive of a sustainable approach, can in practice realign itself in implementation to not only new goals, but also to show how health promotion is an essential contribution to health and other priorities in the post-2015 era by addressing SDH and facilitating intersectoral action on linked priorities on sustaining the environment and improving health.

Summary

Health promotion is essential to effective action on the social determinants of health, and strategies to address social determinants are a fundamental part of the practice of health promotion. Health promotion and the social determinants of health are thus inextricably linked. However, intersectoral action on primary health care, health promotion, and social determinants has proved difficult to implement in practice. Assisting countries and communities to implement a health in all policies approach thus represents the key strategic focus that global health promotion can contribute to reducing inequities through action on social determinants and to moving forward on health promotion itself.

KEY TERMS

1. **Equity:** The absence of avoidable or remediable differences among groups of people, whether those groups are defined socially, economically, demographically, or geographically.
2. **Health in all policies (HiAP):** An approach to public policies across sectors that systematically takes into account the health implications of decisions, seeks synergies, and avoids harmful health impacts, in order to improve population health and health equity.
3. **Intersectoral:** The promotion and coordination of the activities of different sectors such as agriculture, education, housing, public works, communication, and so on.
4. **Social determinants of health (SDH):** The social, political, economic, and environmental conditions and cultural forces in which people are born, grow, live, work, and age.

REVIEW QUESTIONS

1. Explain why structural determinants are particularly influential factors with respect to health.
2. What do you think are some of the key challenges that countries face in developing strategies to address social determinants of health?

References

The Bangkok charter for health promotion in a globalized world. (2006). *Health Promotion International, 21*(Suppl 1), 10–14. Retrieved from doi.org/10.1093/heapro/dal046

Commission on Social Determinants of Health. (2008). *Closing the gap in a generation: Health equity through action on the social determinants of health.* Commission on Social Determinants of Health final report. Geneva: World Health Organization.

Dahlgren, G., & Whitehead, M. (2006). *Levelling up (part II): European strategies for tackling social inequities in health.* Liverpool: WHO Collaborating Centre for Policy Research on Social Determinants of Health, University of Liverpool, 2006 (No. 3). (p. 138). Copenhagen: WHO Regional Office for Europe. Retrieved from http://www.euro.who.int/__data/assets/pdf_file/0018/103824/E89384.pdf

Fleury, S. (2011). Brazil's health-care reform: Social movements and civil society. *Lancet, 377*(9779), 1724–1725. doi.org/10.1016/S0140-6736(11)60318-8

Horton, R., Beaglehole, R., Bonita, R., Raeburn, J., McKee, M., & Wall, S. (2014). From public to planetary health: A manifesto. *Lancet (London, England), 383*(9920), 847. doi.org/10.1016/S0140-6736(14)60409-8

Illich, I. (1995). *Limits to medicine: Medical nemesis: The expropriation of health.* London: M. Boyars.

Jackson, S. F., Birn, A.-E., Fawcett, S. B., Poland, B., & Schultz, J. A. (2013). Synergy for health equity: Integrating health promotion and social determinants of health approaches in and beyond the Americas. *Revista Panamericana De Salud Pública = Pan American Journal of Public Health, 34*(6), 473–480.

Kickbusch, I. (2010). Health in all policies: The evolution of the concept of horizontal health governance. In I. Kickbusch & K. Buckett (Eds.), *Implementing health in all policies: 2010* (pp. 11–23). Adelaide: Department of Health, Government of South Australia. Retrieved from http://www.who.int.ezproxy.auckland.ac.nz/entity/sdhconference/resources/implementinghiapadel-sahealth-100622.pdf

Lee, J.-W. (2005). Public health is a social issue. *Lancet, 365*(9464), 1005–1006. doi.org/10.1016/S0140-6736(05)71115-6

Mackenbach, J. P. (2009). Politics is nothing but medicine at a larger scale: Reflections on public health's biggest idea. *Journal of Epidemiology and Community Health, 63*(3), 181–184. doi.org/10.1136/jech.2008.077032

Marmot, M., Allen, J., Goldblatt, P., Boyce, T., McNeish, D., Grady, M., & Geddes, I. (2010). *Fair society, healthy lives: Strategic review of health inequalities in England, post-2010, the Marmot Review.* London: UCL.

Marmot, M., & Wilkinson, R. (Eds.). (2005). *Social determinants of health* (2nd ed.). Oxford: Oxford University Press.

Marmot, M. G., Smith, G. D., Stansfeld, S., Patel, C., North, F., Head, J., … Feeney, A. (1991). Health inequalities among British civil servants: The Whitehall II study. *Lancet, 337*(8754), 1387–1393.

McKeown, T. (1979). *The role of medicine: Dream, mirage, or nemesis?* Princeton, NJ: Princeton University Press.

Newell, K. (Ed.). (1975). *Health by the people.* Geneva: World Health Organization.

Rani, M., Nusrat, S., & Hawken, L. H. (2012). A qualitative study of governance of evolving response to non-communicable diseases in low- and middle-income countries: Current status, risks and options. *BioMed Central Public Health, 12,* 877. doi.org/10.1186/1471-2458-12-877

Rasanathan, K., Posayanonda, T., Birmingham, M., & Tangcharoensathien, V. (2012). Innovation and participation for healthy public policy: The first National Health Assembly in Thailand. *Health Expectations, 15*(1), 87–96. doi.org/10.1111/j.1369-7625.2010.00656.x

Resolution WHA62.14. Reducing health inequities through action on the social determinants of health. (n.d.). World Health Organization. Retrieved from http://apps.who.int/gb/ebwha/pdf_files/WHA62-REC1/WHA62_REC1-en-P2.pdf

Rice, M. E. (2012). Effective global health promotion achievements, tools, and strategies used in the Americas over the past decade. *Health Promotion Practice, 13*(3), 313–319. doi.org/10.1177/1524839912443243

Ridde, V., Guichard, A., & Houéto, D. (2007). Social inequalities in health from Ottawa to Vancouver: Action for fair equality of opportunity. *Promotion & Education, Suppl 2,* 12–16, 44–47.

Rio Political Declaration on Social Determinants of Health. (2011). Presented at the World Conference on Social Determinants of Health, Rio de Janeiro: World Health Organization. October 19–21, 2011. Retrieved from http://www.who.int/entity/sdhconference/declaration/Rio_political_declaration.pdf

Solar, O., & Irwin, A. (2006). Social determinants, political contexts and civil society action: A historical perspective on the Commission on Social Determinants of Health. *Health Promotion Journal of Australia, 17*(3), 180–185.

Solar, O., & Irwin, A. (2010). *A conceptual framework for action on the social determinants of health.* Social determinants of health discussion paper 2 (policy and practice). Geneva: World Health Organization. Retrieved from http://whqlibdoc.who.int/publications/2010/9789241500852_eng.pdf

Strathdee, S. A., Wechsberg, W. M., Kerrigan, D. L., & Patterson, T. L. (2013). HIV prevention among women in low- and middle-income countries: Intervening upon contexts of heightened HIV risk. *Annual Review of Public Health, 34,* 301–316. doi.org/10.1146/annurev-publhealth-031912-114411

Vega, J. (2011). *"Steps toward the health equity agenda": 2008-2010: Ministry of Health and Regional Health Authorities in Chile.* Background paper prepared prepared for the World Conference on Social Determinants of Health. http://www.who.int/sdhconference/resources/draft_background_paper25_chile.pdf

Victora, C. G., Barreto, M. L., do Carmo Leal, M., Monteiro, C. A., Schmidt, M. I., Paim, J., ... Barros, F. C. (2011). Health conditions and health-policy innovations in Brazil: The way forward. *Lancet, 377*(9782), 2042–2053. doi.org/10.1016/S0140-6736(11)60055-X

Whitehead, M. (1990). *The concepts and principles of equity and health.* Copenhagen: World Health Organization Regional Office for Europe.

Whitehead, M. (1992). The concepts and principles of equity and health. *International Journal of Health Services: Planning, Administration, Evaluation, 22*(3), 429–445.

Whitehead, M., & Dahlgren, G. (2006). *Levelling up (part 1): A discussion paper on concepts and principles for tackling social inequities in health.* Copenhagen:

WHO Regional Office for Europe. Retrieved from http://www.euro.who.int/__data/assets/pdf_file/0010/74737/E89383.pdf

World Health Organization. (1948). *Constitution of the World Health Organization.* Geneva: Author.

World Health Organization. (1986). Ottawa Charter for Health Promotion. Presented at the First International Conference on Health Promotion, Ottawa. 21 November 1986.

World Health Organization. (2011). *Closing the gap: Policy into practice on social determinants of health.* Discussion paper for the World Conference on Social Determinants of Health. 19-21 October 2011 Geneva: Author. Retrieved from http://www.who.int/entity/sdhconference/Discussion-Paper-EN.pdf

World Health Organization & Government of South Australia. (2010). *Adelaide statement on health in all policies.* Adelaide: Author.

World Health Organization & UNICEF. (1978). Declaration of Alma-Ata. Presented at the International Conference on Primary Health Care, Alma-Ata, USSR. 6-12 September 1978.

CHAPTER 4

MODELS OF HEALTH BEHAVIOR CHANGE

International Applications

Rick S. Zimmerman, Zhiwen Xiao, Purnima Mehrotra, and Charles Roy

Much has been written about models of health behavior change that have been primarily developed and tested in the United States and Western Europe. But we have seen very little discussion about the testing of these models in low- and middle-income countries. Our own experience in South Africa was hearing from local researchers that they expected that these largely individual-focused models would not work very well in the more collectivist-oriented developing world cultural contexts. In this chapter, we review five groups of models: "classic" health behavior models, other (more recently developed and less well-known) health behavior models, expanded health behavior models, interpersonal or community-level models, and socioecological and structural-level models. For each type of model, after presenting descriptions of key constructs, we present examples of the use of these models in low- and middle-income country contexts.

LEARNING OBJECTIVES

By the end of this chapter, the reader should be able to:

- Describe classical social psychological theories of behavior change, more recent social psychological theories, expanded social psychological theories, and structural and ecological theories
- Define and explain the usefulness of health behavior change theories and models and how they can help us understand the determinants of health behavior change
- Identify the best theory for a health behavior for a target population in a particular context
- Describe some examples of international applications of health behavior change theories
- Summarize the usefulness of health behavior change theories in the international context

"Classic" Social Psychological Models

Five "classic" theories or models emerged as the most frequently used. They are the Health Belief Model, the Theory of Reasoned Action, the Theory of Planned Behavior, Social Cognitive Theory, and the Transtheoretical Model.

The Health Belief Model

The **Health Belief Model** (HBM) was developed in the 1950s by a group of social psychologists who worked for the US Public Health Service to explain the widespread failure of a screening program for tuberculosis (Janz, Champion, & Strecher, 2002). The underlying assumption of the original

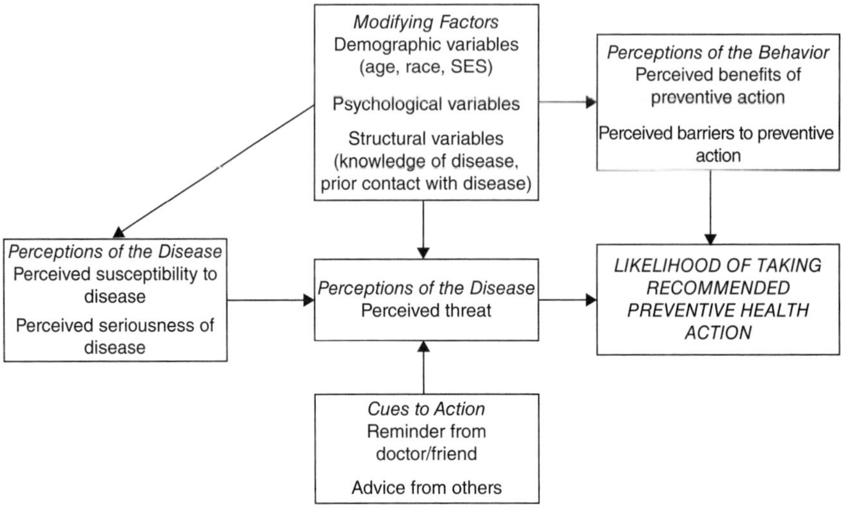

Figure 4.1 Health Belief Model
Source: Adapted from Becker, 1974.

HBM is that health behavior is determined by an individual's perceptions or beliefs about a disease or health condition and strategies to reduce the threat (Hochbaum, 1958). The main constructs include *perceived susceptibility,* an individual's belief regarding the likelihood of contracting a disease or getting a condition; *perceived severity,* a person's belief of how serious a condition or disease and its consequences are; *perceived benefits,* a person's belief in the efficacy of a certain advised action to avert the risk of a threat; *perceived barriers,* one's belief in the costs of performing the advised behavior to reduce the perceived threat; and *cues to action,* any stimuli that can trigger one to enact an appropriate health behavior. The model was expanded (Figure 4.1) to explain not only simple behaviors of a one-shot nature (such as taking immunization or screening tests) but also preventive behaviors, sick-role behaviors, and clinic visits (Janz & Becker, 1984). Self-efficacy was added to the original HBM to respond to evolving research evidence that self-efficacy successfully predicts one's execution of the advised behavior (Rosenstock, Strecher, & Becker, 1988).

A number of systematic reviews of research with the HBM demonstrate that the four primary dimensions (perceived susceptibility, perceived severity, perceived benefits, and perceived costs) can provide consistent predictions of a variety of health behaviors, including influenza inoculations, high blood pressure screening, smoking cessation, seatbelt use, breast self-examination, PAP screening behavior, and HIV/AIDS prevention, among diverse populations (see Harrison, Mullen & Green, 1992; Janz & Becker, 1984; Zimmerman & Vernberg, 1994).

Application of HBM in International Settings

Located in sub-Saharan Africa, Benin, West Africa, is representative of a region where systemic condom use remains low. With limited access to antiretroviral medications, prevention holds the primary position in limiting HIV/AIDS transmission. Using a cross-sectional survey and a total of 251 participants, Hounton, Carabin, and Henderson (2005) utilized a structured questionnaire to identify factors associated with condom use. The results were unforeseen in that despite satisfactory knowledge on HIV/AIDS transmission, participants were still at elevated risk of contracting the disease. Using HBM, high-perceived vulnerability and perceived severity of HIV was present in the population, yet it did not encourage condom use. Condom use in this experiment was dependent on perceived quality and perceived efficacy. Perceived severity of HIV and fear did not serve as a deterrent in this population.

Volk and Koopman (2011) applied the HBM in Kisumu, Kenya, to examine specific cultural beliefs and knowledge and its relation to condom use. Out of 223 participants, 75% engaged in intercourse with less than 20% utilizing a condom. The results of the study indicated that a high percentage of the subjects had false beliefs regarding condoms. A segment of the population (47%) endorsed the belief that HIV can pass through the pores in the condom, and 44% reported that condom lubricants might contain HIV. The only component of the HBM that was found to be significant in condom use was perceived barriers where respondents stated that condoms are difficult to use (40%) and that their partners do not like to use it (70%). In this study, greater perceived barriers were related to less frequent condom use, suggesting that future interventions should aim at educating patients to overcome barriers to condom use.

In a telephone interview survey of 1,004 participants, Sung et al. (2007) applied the HBM model to further investigate barriers and perceived notions concerning colorectal cancer. The purpose was to increase public participation in CRC prevention by exploring the attitudes, and beliefs of the at-risk population. In variables pertaining to HBM, 20.4% did not know whether they were at risk, and the majority (68%) considered themselves not at risk for CRC at all. Nearly one-third (29.2%) perceived a high level of negative consequences of CRC on personal and family life, with nearly one-third of the respondents (27.5%) skeptical about the accuracy of the available tests for screening CRC. Overall, knowledge of CRC symptoms, knowledge of CRC risk factors, a physician's recommendation, and having health insurance are positively associated with the uptake of screening tests. As discovered by the HBM, the significant association between knowledge of the disease and compliance to CRC testing requires interventions in the form of educational initiatives. More specifically, the availability and effectiveness of different types of tests to help screen for CRC should be promulgated. This model highlighted the significant role a family physician plays; his or her recommendation increases the likelihood of clients complying with CRC screening by 23-fold. The HBM was able to successfully predict barriers and behaviors in this population and remains a key tool in developing interventions for CRC prevention.

Lymphatic Filariasis (LF) is the second most common cause of physical disability worldwide, with the WHO targeting it for elimination globally by 2020. India alone holds 40% off the world's LF burden, with mass drug administration (MDA) as one of the main solutions. For India to meet this timeline, a high coverage of 85% is required to achieve the interruption of transmission in four to six years. One of the major barriers to this goal is medication compliance. Nujum et al. (2012) utilized the HBM in this case to further understand medication compliance and how India can better implement MDAs in the future. The goal of the study was to identify factors related to awareness, acceptability, and attitude in determining compliant behavior to MDA. Employing self-administered questionnaires, Nujum et al. (2012) discovered that there was no significant association of compliance with awareness of LF, experience of LF, or MDA awareness. Health workers were the most common source of knowledge regarding MDA (48.5%), followed by television (20.7%) and newspapers (10.1%). Perceived benefits and self-efficacy were significantly associated with compliance, whereas side effects as perceived barriers were not a significant factor in determining compliance. Significant association was found between noncompliant status and low drug administrator acceptability. Only 42% of the drug administrators believed that the drugs must be taken. Using the HBM, it was found that the effect of low drug administrator acceptability had been confounded by the effect of perceived benefits. In conclusion, the HBM provided a successful framework in this study, elucidating the fact that the individual giving the drug to the beneficiary is the most important person, whose attitude and acceptability determines compliance.

A study conducted by Kashfi and colleagues in Shiraz, Iran, in 2012 highlighted another successful intervention based upon the HBM for control of blood sugar in Type 2 diabetic patients. It is believed that most diabetic patients in the region are not aware of the role of exercise, especially jogging, in the control of their illness. In a quasi-experimental intervention, 100 patients were randomly divided into two groups: experimental and control. The experimental group received three sessions (60 minutes each) of training on jogging and control of sugar. Using a questionnaire three months prior and three months after, data were collected according to the HBM categories, including the patient's hemoglobin (HbA_1C) and fasting blood sugar (FBS) levels.

Findings emphasized the significant difference between the mean score of HBM variables (susceptibility, severity, benefit, and perceived obstacles) in the experimental group compared to the controlled group (all $ps < .001$). In addition, levels of HbA_1C and FBS improved significantly among the experimental group versus the control (down 0.32% for the experimental group, up 0.46% for the control group, $p < .001$).

Theory of Reasoned Action and Planned Behavior

The **Theory of Reasoned Action** (TRA), first introduced from the social psychology setting by Fishbein in 1967, concerns the relationship between attitudes and behavior. The TRA posits that the most important determinant of behavior is an individual's *behavioral intention,* which is a person's intention to enact the behavior. Behavioral intention is a function of a person's *attitude* toward the behavior and the person's *subjective norms* regarding the behavior. Attitude toward a behavior is determined by *behavioral beliefs,* the individual's beliefs about the likelihood of a certain outcome of performing a behavior, weighted by the person's evaluation (i.e., good or bad) of the outcome. One's subjective norm is determined by his or her *normative beliefs,* a person's perception about whether significant others approve or disapprove of enacting the behavior. Normative beliefs are weighted by the individual's *motivation to comply* with their significant referents.

The ability of the theory to explain behavior is determined by the degree to which the individual can exercise volitional control over the behavior (Montano & Kasprzyk, 2002). However, when individuals are not under full volitional control, the TRA constructs might not be sufficient to predict behaviors (Kippax & Crawford, 1993). Therefore, Ajzen and associates (Ajzen, 1988; Ajzen & Driver, 1991) extended the TRA to the **Theory of Planned Behavior** (TPB) by adding *perceived behavioral control* to account for environmental factors that are not under a person's volitional control but may influence his or her performance of behavior (Figure 4.2). Perceived behavioral control is determined by *control beliefs* that are weighted by the *perceived power*. Control beliefs are an individual's beliefs about the presence of factors that facilitate or hinder performance of the behavior. Perceived power is the impact of each factor on facilitating or inhibiting the behavior. Perceived behavioral control is considered synonymous with self-efficacy by many researchers (Sheeran & Taylor, 1999).

There has been a large body of research supporting the utility of TRA and TPB in understanding health behaviors such as HIV/AIDS prevention, smoking, drinking, signing up for treatment programs, using contraceptives, dieting, wearing seatbelts or safety helmets, exercising regularly, and breastfeeding. A relatively recent meta-analysis concluded generally moderate relationships between model variables and prospective prediction of behavior. Over 237 prospective predictions in 206 articles, average correlation between intention and behavior was .43, between attitude and behavior was .31, between subjective norm and behavior was .21, and between perceived behavioral control and behavior, .31. (McEachan, Conner, Taylor, & Lawton, 2011). Results were found to be stronger when physical activity or dietary behaviors were the outcomes, and weaker when risk, disease screening, safer sex, and abstinence from drugs were the outcomes.

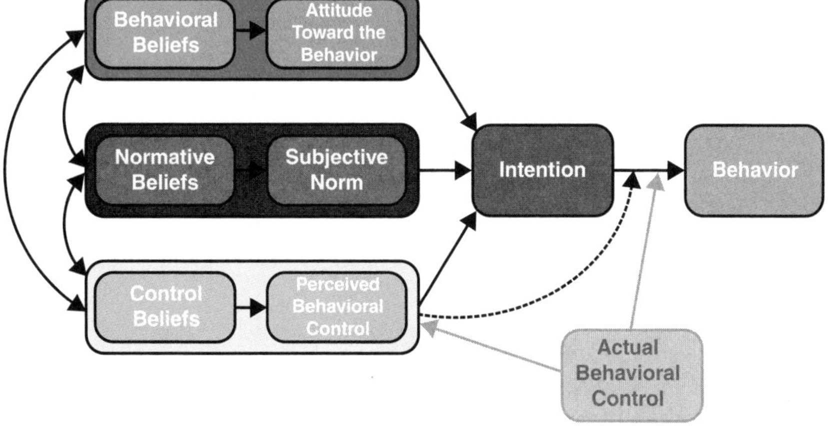

Figure 4.2 Theory of Planned Behavior
Source: Copyright © 2006 Icek Ajzen.

Application of Theory of Planned Behavior in International Settings

A study of 721 health workers in South Africa discovered an HIV/AIDS prevalence of 15.7% (Shisana et al., 2004). Questionnaires administered contained cognitive variables, demographic information, and information regarding HIV counseling and testing. Specifically, opinions, individual pros and cons, and beliefs regarding voluntary counseling and testing (VCT) services were obtained. Results indicated that most health professionals tested their own blood for fear of disclosure of HIV-positive status (Shisana et al., 2001). The findings failed to establish a link between sociodemographic status and intention to use VCT. The intentions to use VCT service were primarily due to subjective norms, attitudes, and perceived social pressure; perceived behavioral control was statistically irrelevant. Subjective norm was the most important predictor of all other components of TPB. The components of TPB independently explained the variance in intention to VCT by 30.3%. Strategies that empower health professionals on social pressure resistance and changing negative attitude on VCT will be beneficial as interventions in this population.

Protogerou and colleagues (2013) also affirmed TPB in its applicability and sustainability in Cape Town, South Africa. This group utilized the model to determine intentions of condom use among undergraduate students in a university in the Western Cape province of South Africa. Both direct and indirect variables of TPB were tested and demonstrated impressive correlations. The study clearly supported the use of TPB in the study of condom use in South Africa by noting 43.2% of the variance of intentions to use condom among the sexually active sample, and 31.1% of the variance among the sexually inactive. In terms of actual condom use, the model accounted for 56.7% of the variance in intentions.

Social Cognitive Theory

Bandura's **Social Cognitive Theory** (SCT; Bandura, 1986, 1997, 2001) dates back to the 1970s and has its roots in behaviorism but has evolved into cognivitism in its present form (Luszczynska & Schwarzer, 2005). SCT has been characterized as an "agentic framework" (Bandura, 2001) for studying human behavior as a "triadic, dynamic, and reciprocal" (Baranowski, Perry, & Parcel, 2002, p. 165) interaction of personal factors, behavior, and the environment. The primary components of the theory are reciprocal determinism (individual's behavior, his or her characteristics, and the environment interact and influence each other simultaneously), environment, situation, behavioral capability, expectations, expectancies, self-control, observational learning (also called "vicarious learning"), reinforcements, self-efficacy, and emotional coping responses. However most studies have employed only the three constructs of outcome expectancies, observational learning, and self-efficacy (Luszczynska & Schwarzer, 2005; McAlister, Perry, & Parcel, 2008).

Self-efficacy is perhaps the most important contribution of the SCT to health behavior; it has now been integrated in almost all important theories of health behavior (Luszczynska & Schwarzer, 2005; McAlister et al., 2008). Health-protective behavior results from a process of cognitive appraisal by which people integrate knowledge about a disease, outcome expectancies associated with adopting preventive behaviors, and social influences. The result of this integrative process is a judgment of "self-efficacy" or an estimate of how well one will be able to cope with a difficult situation, which moderates behavior (Baranowski et al., 2002).

Outcome expectations or the consequences of a behavior can be portrayed as physical (pleasant or unpleasant sensory experiences); social (pleasant or unpleasant social consequences such as approval or censure of a behavior by important others); and self-evaluative (behaviors that give a sense of self-worth or satisfaction versus those that do not).

Observational learning is a concept that is central to the SCT and depends on four processes: attention, retention, production (or adaptation of behavior), and motivation (Bandura, 2002). According to Bandura (2001), "To a large extent people act on their images of reality," provided by the symbolic environment created by the media as well as the behavior of important others in one's life. Observational learning has been extensively employed in influencing health behaviors (O'Leary et al., 2012; Li et al., 2008), including in entertainment education in the United States and elsewhere (Hinyard & Kreuter, 2007; Singhal & Rogers, 1999; Wilkin et al., 2007).

Application of Social Cognitive Theory in International Settings

Li et al. (2008) applied SCT in Nanjing, China, in 2008 with a pilot study evaluating the efficacy of the cultural adaptation of an SCT-based HIV risk reduction program delivered among college students. Given the technological shift and the recent exposure of the Chinese population to the Westernized way of life, college students are at the center of a major cultural paradigm transition (Zhang et al., 2004). The study consisted of an SCT-based HIV prevention curriculum ("Focus on Kids") and a control group consisting of 380 students total (186 in SCT intervention and 194 control). Participants were provided an initial and six-month follow-up questionnaire designed to assess various elements such as intention of engaging in risk behavior and knowledge of HIV/STD and condom use. The results failed to establish a connection between the SCT-based intervention and behavioral effects, but it may effectively reduce future sexual risk among adolescents and young adults because of the significant increase in knowledge of HIV/AIDS and condom use among students. The lack of influence on sexual behaviors can be attributed to relatively low rates of sexual activities in the population, even before the intervention was initiated. Overall, it is concluded that an SCT-based intervention for HIV risk reduction for young adults is effective in altering HIV perceptions and intentions in China (Li et al., 2008).

O'Leary et al. (2012) utilized an SCT-based intervention titled "Let Us Protect Our Future" as a sexual risk reduction intervention for sixth-grade adolescents in Mdantsane and Berlin, South Africa. Similar to former studies, two interventions were planned with focus groups that included 89 sixth-grade students, 34 parents, and 12 teachers. The sexual risk reduction intervention was directed to (a) increase knowledge of HIV and other STDs, (b) enhance expected outcomes that support abstinence and condom use, and (c) increase skills to use condoms and self-efficacy to negotiate abstinence and condom use. The health promotion intervention controlled nonspecific features such as group interaction and special attention with an emphasis on heart disease, hypertension, stroke, diabetes, and certain cancers. Assessments were in the form of questionnaires given immediately post, 3, 6, and 12 months subsequently after interventions. Evaluations demonstrated that living at home with fathers, high parental strictness, and religiosity all moderated the efficacy of the intervention in reducing unprotected intercourse. Derived from SCT, self-efficacy to avoid risky situations and expected parental disapproval of sexual experiences greatly mediated abstinence. This is the first study to demonstrate SCT variables serving a crucial role in sexual risk reduction intervention among South African adolescents.

The Transtheoretical Model

The **Transtheoretical Model** (TTM) was developed in the late 1970s; authors credited with the development of the model are Prochaska, DiClemente, Norcross, and Velicer, who initially examined why some smokers were capable of quitting smoking on their own (Prochaska, & DiClemente, 1983). They concluded that people quit smoking when they were ready to do so. Based on their findings, these authors stated that traditional action-oriented prevention interventions would not work for the majority of at-risk populations because the individuals are not ready for action. The researchers posit that behavioral change progresses through a sequence of stages, and no single theory can explain the complexities of different stages of behavior change. Therefore, there should be an integrative or *transtheoretical* model of behavior change that integrates processes and principles of behavior change from across other theories.

The TTM assumes that people must go through five stages of change: precontemplation, contemplation, preparation, action, and maintenance. Hence, the TTM is also called the Stages of Change Model (Prochaska, Redding, & Evers, 2002). Transitions between different stages are affected by a set of independent variables known as the processes of change. That is, people employ 10 cognitive, affective, and evaluative processes to progress through the stages of change, including consciousness raising, dramatic relief, self-reevaluation, environmental reevaluation, self-liberation, helping relationships, counterconditioning, reinforcement management, stimulus control, and social liberation (Prochaska, & Velicer, 1997). In addition, the model incorporates a number of intervening or outcome variables, which include decisional balance (the pros and cons of change), self-efficacy (self-confidence in the ability to change across a variety of situations), situational/contextual temptations to engage in the problem behavior, and problem behaviors (Prochaska et al., 2002). Other physiological, psychological, environmental, cultural, socioeconomic, and biochemical variables are also included in the model (Prochaska et al., 2002).

The TTM has evolved through initial studies on smoking behavior to a wide range of health and mental health behaviors, including HIV/AIDS prevention, alcohol and substance abuse, anxiety and panic disorders, mammography screening, eating disorders, obesity, sedentary lifestyle, and unwanted pregnancy prevention, to mention a few (Prochaska et al., 2002).

Application of Transtheoretical Model in International Settings

TTM provided the basis for Naar-King et al. (2008) in their approach when evaluating and predicting risky behavior in HIV-positive youth in Thailand. Seventy HIV-infected youth (ages 16–25) were interviewed regarding their sexual practices and readiness to "practice safer sex" with answers recorded on a Likert scale. The results demonstrated that 65% of the participants engaged in intercourse in the previous 30 days, with 44% having at least one intercourse act without a condom (Naar-King et al., 2008). Surprisingly, rates of substance abuse in the previous 30 days were low (7%). Overall, self-efficacy was not correlated with unprotected intercourse acts. Readiness to change was correlated and mediated unprotected intercourse acts and self-efficacy. Readiness to change directly predicted risk behavior, while self-efficacy for practicing safer sex indirectly influenced unprotected sexual intercourse. The results supported the effectiveness of the TTM for HIV-positive youth in Thailand with some variations relative to applications in US samples. This data suggest utilization of interventions that improve readiness to change may be successful for Thai youth who are HIV-positive.

Another application of the TTM was studied by Ha, Rohan, and Owen (2003) in the Hai Phong province of Vietnam. The TTM was used by the group to examine men's involvement in general contraception and intrauterine device (IUD) use by their wives, with a sample of 201 married men ages 19–45 years who lived with their wives in the same house during the previous three months. The measures were five in-depth elicitation interviews and two focus group discussions dedicated to contraceptive use and IUD use. A questionnaire was provided that assessed the three main constructs from the TTM (stage of change for IUD use, pros and cons, and self-efficacy). For this purpose, the contemplation and preparation stages of the models were combined to precontemplation as well as action and maintenance into action/maintenance. A total of 25.8% of men were in the precontemplation stage, 10.5% in the contemplation/preparation stage, and 63.7% in the action/maintenance stage. These results reflected the dominant pattern of IUD use in Vietnam at 56.0% (National Committee for Population and Family Planning, 2000). Disadvantage of IUD use for men in precontemplation were markedly increased than those in the action/maintenance stages. The reverse was true for self-efficacy for convincing the wives to utilize an IUD. Interventions that target stage of change, seek to reduce cons, and increase self-efficacy may have significant potential to increase male involvement in IUD adoption by their wives.

Other Social Psychological Models

In addition to classic models, some other social psychological models, such as the Information-Motivation-Behavioral Skills Model and Extended Parallel Process Model, are emerging as important theoretical frameworks to compete for attention and application.

Information-Motivation-Behavioral Skills Model

The **Information-Motivation-Behavioral Skills Model** (IMB) (Fisher & Fisher, 1992) was developed specifically for studying HIV prevention behaviors and is based primarily on the TRA. The notion of health risks is extremely important here; it is derived largely from the construct of perceived susceptibility of HBM. This model posits that (HIV) prevention behavior is determined by (HIV) prevention behavioral intentions, which in turn are determined by prevention information and prevention motivation. The construct of information includes knowledge; motivation includes attitudes about behavior, social norms, and perceived risk; and behavioral skills include actual and perceived skills.

HIV preventive information should be precise, relevant, and easy to translate into behavior for the given population in the particular context in which those individuals live. Information or knowledge about the negative health consequences of behavior is considered a prerequisite for forming opinions on the behavior rather than a motivator of actual behavior change (Bandura, 2001). The variable of perceived susceptibility brings in the notion of fear appeals into the IMB. The other variables in this model—that is, attitudes and behavioral skills—are similar to attitudes in the TPB and self-efficacy in the SCT.

Fisher and Fisher (1992) first introduced this model for changing HIV-related risk behaviors. This model has been used fairly extensively for studying at-risk populations and designing HIV prevention, care, and treatment interventions. The IMB is a parsimonious model, with well-defined relationships and clear instructions on operationalization of its three main constructs. However some of its limitations include the weak and inconsistent predictive ability of the construct of information and lack of environmental and cultural constructs for predicting behavior (much like the other social psychological models).

Application of Information-Motivation-Behavioral Skills Model in International Settings

The utilization of this model has yielded disparate results in two parts of the world vastly affected by HIV. Cornman et al. (2007) worked with truck drivers in India to analyze the usefulness of the IMB model in contrast with an information-only control condition in a randomized trial. The IMB intervention consisted of a single-session group workshop with five interactive activities designed to address HIV prevention and motivate condom use (Cornman et al., 2007). One IMB strategy entitled "Picture Your Health" utilized flashcards with images of objects, scenes, and people to influence constructive and meaningful discussions on HIV transmission and prevalence. Other pertinent topics addressed included negative attitudes about condoms, high prevalence of HIV among truck drivers, and the fact that HIV serostatus cannot be determined based on appearance. The information-only control workshop provided a prewritten HIV prevention curriculum that addressed general points on HIV/AIDS, such as the functions of the immune system and the stages of HIV progression. The focus of this workshop was exclusively on knowledge advancement and not increasing motivation or behavioral skills training. Starting with a baseline of 250 truck drivers with 125 in each of the two workshops, survey findings of 194 participants 10 months later affirmed the increased effectiveness of IMB-based interventions versus knowledge-based interventions. Significantly fewer participants from the IMB intervention (83%) than the control (94%) reported having sex with a commercial sex worker in the previous 4 months ($p < .05$). Individuals who were in the IMB-based intervention group also reported a striking increase in condom use with marital partners ($p < .001$), although it is imperative to note that condom use overall was still low.

Employing the IMB, Eggers et al. (2014) attempted to predict the use of condoms in 13 Cape Town, South Africa, high schools (involving 1,099 students) through survey responses at baseline, at 6 months, and then 14 months later (685 students). Five domains were assessed though the questionnaires (attitude, subjective norm, self-efficacy, intention, and condom use) with the six-month results indicating intentions on using a condom at the next intercourse high, at 81.3%, between sexually active teens. At 14 months, the results elucidated that having knowledge about STI transmission and condom use practice was directly related to future behavior and that no other cognitive factor was significantly involved (Eggers et al., 2014). However, evidence establishing a direct link to self-efficacy and condom use was absent, indicating a contradiction of the IMB model that posits motivational and information factors have indirect effects on behavior via self-efficacy beliefs (Fisher, Fisher, & Harman, 2003).

Extended Parallel Processing Model

The **Extended Parallel Process Model** (EPPM) (Witte, 1992) is a fear appeal theory in which fear arousal (perceived susceptibility) is the primary motivator of precautionary behavior. The EPPM evolved from three major groups of fear appeal theories: (1) drive models (Hovland, Janis, & Kelly, 1953; McGuire, 1968); (2) parallel process models (Leventhal, 1970); and (3) subjective expected utility models (e.g., Rogers's Protection Motivation Theory, 1975). Witte (1992) in the Extended Parallel Process Model, brought together concepts from all of these traditions in the fear appeals literature to explain how efficacious (danger control) or avoidance (fear control) pathways are activated as a result of a fear appeal. In the EPPM fear arousal (perceived susceptibility) leads to one of three behavioral pathways:

1. danger control, that is, when a perceived health threat appraised as serious and relevant, combined with high self-efficacy to deal with it leads to active precautionary behavioral measures;
2. fear control, that is, when a perceived health threat is appraised as serious and relevant but due to low self-efficacy of dealing with it, leads to denial or "defensive avoidance" (Witte, 1992) of the seriousness of the threat and continuation of risky behaviors;
3. and last if a threat is perceived as low severity and irrelevant, it is simply ignored.

The EPPM has been predominantly employed as a message design theory for promoting health-related information and has been most extensively used in HIV prevention. A meta-analysis by Witte and Allen (2000) recommends that that using strong fear appeals that produce high levels of perceived severity and susceptibility in combination with high-efficacy messages result in the greatest behavior. However according to other researchers, including Albaraccin, Kumkale, and Johnson (2005) and Bandura (2001), scaring people into practicing health behaviors has not been a very effective strategy. Another recent review of the EPPM literature shows that operational definitions of some constructs are inconsistent, some propositions have not been explicitly tested, and none has "unequivocal empirical support" (Popova, 2012, p. 455).

Application of Extended Parallel Process Model in International Settings

A number of studies have tested the EPPM in middle- or low-income country contexts. We present two here: one reviewed components of the EPPM in messages about over-the-counter (OTC) medicine advertisements in China; the other tested hypotheses derived from the EPPM related to HIV beliefs and behaviors in Namibia.

Sheer and Chen (2008) conducted a textual (content) analysis of print advertisements for OTC medicines in China to assess the correspondence between the messages and components of the EPPM, as well as some potential additional cultural values in China. In particular, the authors were concerned that there had been little research on the kinds of themes expressed in fear messages outside of experimental settings, and whether the individualistic perspective inherent in fear theories including the EPPM would be reflected in a collectivistic culture, that is, China. The authors investigated the types of fear messages, types of threats, susceptibility, response efficacy, and personal efficacy messages expressed in Chinese fear-based print OTC ads and what collectivist cultural values are expressed in those ads. The authors found that "the four components [severity, susceptibility, response efficacy, and personal efficacy] for fear message construction likely boasts a high degree of cross-cultural validity" (p. 950). They also found some infusion of Chinese cultural values influencing the components of the model, with messages targeted at concerns about others (e.g., shame on family) added to those about self, and the addition of the efficacy of others' behavior as well as one's own.

Muthusamy, Levine, and Weber (2009) tested their hypothesis that, consistent with the EPPM, use of fear appeals in Namibia (where high fear already existed about HIV/AIDS) would be ineffective because the perceived threat would exceed efficacy. The authors conducted a 2 (high threat, low threat) × 2 (high efficacy, no efficacy) experiment with an independent groups factorial design, with a no-message control group and a high self-efficacy-only condition. A total of 374 undergraduate students at the University of Namibia were randomly assigned to these six experimental conditions. Participants read the message associated with the cell to which they were assigned in the design, underlining important passages, to increase attention. They then completed an immediate post-questionnaire on their reactions to the message, as well as demographic information. Two weeks later, the students completed a post-study questionnaire, eliciting responses about behavior related to condom use since they read the message in the first part of the study. Results indicated that, in fact, fear of HIV was very high (4.31 on a five-point scale). Consistent with this result, high-threat messages had no impact on perceived fear of HIV. A low-threat message did reduce fear. Level of threat in the message also had little impact on attitudes and behavioral intentions related to condoms. Given that the level of threat was higher than that of efficacy, these findings were consistent with the EPPM. However, threat and efficacy did not interact to affect outcomes as predicted by the model.

Expanded Social Psychological Models

The past three decades have witnessed vast advances in the development of social psychological theories in health promotion. However, most of these theories have narrow scopes, and simply "focus on smaller, manageable, and measurable components that contribute to a specific health behavior, leaving planners of health promotion (HP) programs with a puzzle that had scores of pieces (variables), different ways of putting the pieces together (theories) and different sections of the puzzle complete or incomplete. Unfortunately, this predicament leads to considerable confusion and little agreement about how to design HP programs" (Flay, Snyder, & Petraitis, 2009, p. 453). Therefore, researchers indicate that more expanded and comprehensive theories of health behaviors are needed to reduce such confusion and help look at "the big picture" of any behavior (DeKay & Buss, 1992). "That picture must be based on a comprehensive and integrative analysis of (a) the broad social environment or cultural milieu surrounding the behavior, (b) the more immediate social situation or context in which the behavior occurs, (c) the characteristics or dispositions of the person performing the behavior, (d) the behavior itself and closely related behaviors, and (e) the interaction among all of these" (Flay et al., 1995, p. 3). Though we would consider including both Flay's Theory of Triadic Influence (Flay et al., 1995; Flay & Petratis, 1994) and the Multiple Domain Model (Zimmerman et al., 2007), we have included only the latter here because we have found no examples of international applications of the former.

Multiple Domain Model

The **Multiple Domain Model** (Zimmerman et al., 2007) was based on the integrated model that was proposed by Fishbein (2000). The MDM integrates social psychological constructs derived from the TRA/TPB (i.e., attitudes, social norms, intentions, self-efficacy), and additional factors that predict sexual behaviors, including social structural factors (e.g., gender, age), social environmental factors (e.g., factors at the family, school, and individual levels), personality/individual difference factors (e.g., sensation-seeking and impulsivity), situational/contextual factors (e.g., alcohol use, relationship status), and preparatory behaviors (e.g., being in sexual situations). Zimmerman et al. (2007) proposed that situational/contextual variables and preparatory behaviors are

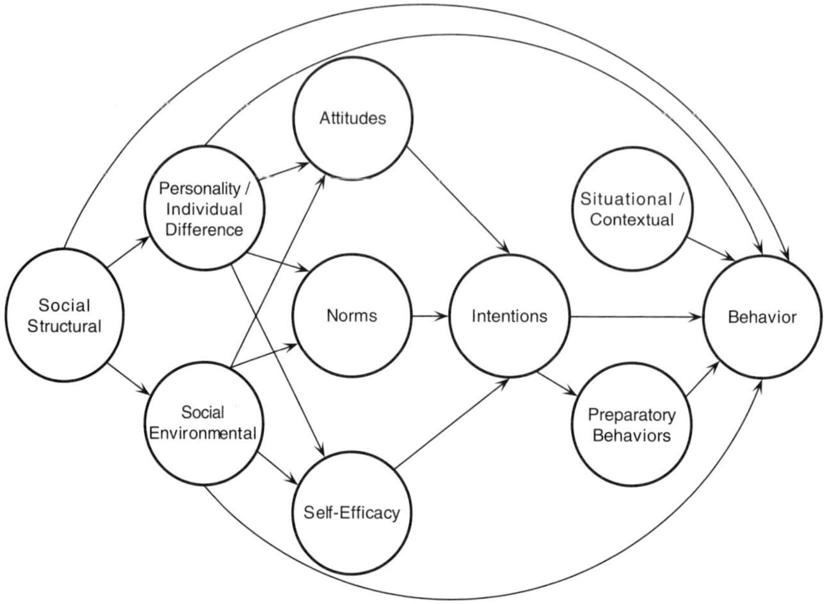

Figure 4.3 Multiple Domain Model
Source: Zimmerman et al., 2007.

the most proximal factors that influence sexual behaviors. The next most proximal factors are the psychosocial variables, followed by personality, social environmental, and structural variables (Figure 4.3).

In a longitudinal study to understand predictors of condom use among 511 urban high school students in the United States, a structural equation model using the MDM fit the data well (Zimmerman et al., 2007). Specifically, condom use was significantly and directly predicted by a situational variable (hormonal contraceptive not used), preparatory behavior (a scale summing having items about having condoms and talking about condoms with partners), and intentions to use a condom, with a total R^2 of .28. Preparatory behaviors were predicted by gender (males were more likely to engage in these), use of birth control, and intentions to use condoms. Use of hormonal contraceptives was in turn more likely to be reported by females. Positive condom attitudes, peer condom norms, and condom self-efficacy all predicted condom intentions.

Application of MDM in International Settings

Two studies have now been conducted in non-Western settings, testing adapted versions of the Multiple Domain Model. In a cross-sectional test of the model with Chinese college students, Xiao et al. (2010) found that two situational variables (relationship length and alcohol use) and impulsivity were all negatively associated with condom use, and that preparatory behaviors, peer norms, condom self-efficacy, and positive condom attitudes were all positively associated with condom use. In addition, condom self-efficacy had an indirect positive effect on condom use through its effect on preparatory behaviors and

HIV information exposure (added to the MDM in this study) had a positive indirect effect on condom use through self-efficacy.

Mehrotra et al. (2013) tested the MDM cross-sectionally with unmarried young adults in India. Key predictors of ever having had sex included preparatory behaviors (being alone without adults in potentially sexual situations more frequently), peer norms supportive of sexual activity, negative attitudes about waiting to have sex, and having a more masculine gender role identity. In turn, the model variable most associated with peer norms was the personality variable sensation-seeking; the model variables most associated with frequency of being in sexual situations were attitudes about waiting to have sex, peer norms supportive of having sex, and higher socioeconomic status. Personality variables (impulsivity and sensation-seeking) were the strongest (negative) correlates of positive attitudes about waiting to have sex; other variables related to attitudes about waiting included gender (females had more positive attitudes about waiting) and a social psychological environment variable, parental monitoring/control related in a negative way to positive attitudes about waiting.

Interpersonal- or Community-Level Models

A number of theories have developed at the mid-range or meso- or community level, but we were unable to find non-Western applications of a number of these theories, including community coalition theory (Butterfoss, Goodman, & Wandersman, 1993; Butterfoss, 2007) and the theory of gender and power (Connell, 1987; Wingood & DiClemente, 2002). Thus we describe and present international applications of the two theories for which we have found such applications: Social Capital Theory and Diffusion of Innovations Theory.

Social Capital Theory

Social Capital Theory has been employed to help public health researchers and professionals to better understand how to enhance the effectiveness of community-based health promotion (Kreuter & Lezin, 2002). Social capital, concerning the value of social networks, bonding similar people, and bridging between diverse people (Dekker & Uslaner 2001; Uslaner 2001), is generally seen as "the ability of actors to secure benefits by virtue of membership in social networks and other social structures" (Portes, 1998, p. 6). A number of theorists have offered a variety of definitions of social capital (e.g., Portes, 1995; Putnam, 1995). All of these conceptualizations or categorizations focus on some central themes such as the relations an actor has with other actors and the structure of relations among actors within a collectivity (Adler & Kwon, 2002). Some of the key ingredients of social capital include social support, social influence, social control, social participation, material resources, and trust (Eriksson, 2011).

The concept of social capital has also been categorized into different forms (Krishna & Shrader, 2000). For example, cognitive social capital refers to the more intangible concept such as norms of trust, solidarity, and reciprocity. Structural social capital refers to the composition and activities of networks. Another important distinction is the differences between bonding, bridging, and linking social capital. Bonding social capital is to combine and strengthen commonalities and functions within a network to serve as a source of support and help for members. Bridging social capital is linking people from different networks together to become important resources. Linking social capital refers to vertical ties between people in different power hierarchies. Social capital can be conceptualized at both individual and collective levels (Eriksson, 2011). Individual social capital is defined in terms of resources and support that are embedded within individual's social network. Contextual social capital emphasizes the resources that can be drawn upon by individuals to pursue collective aims by being interconnected. Strengthening individual social capital can be an important health promotion strategy. Mobilizing collective social capital is also linked to health promotion.

Diffusion of Innovation Theory

Diffusion of Innovation Theory was originally developed by Rogers (2003) to explain how innovations were diffused through networks of farmers in Iowa and widely or less widely adopted as new planting methods and seeds were developed. More generally, the theory explains how an innovation ("idea, practice, or object that is perceived as new by an individual or other unit of adoption") is diffused ("communicated through certain channels over time among the members of a social system") within social networks to be potentially adopted, implemented, and ultimately institutionalized to become the typical practice. Rogers' theory also proposed characteristics of both innovations and social systems that make it more or less likely that the innovation will ultimately be adopted, implemented, and/or institutionalized.

This theory has most often been applied with regard to innovative devices or practices in health care (e.g., Berwick, 2003) and with regard to key individuals within social networks diffusing messages about HIV prevention (e.g., Sikkema et al., 2000; Kelly et al., 1997). Since this chapter is about health behavior rather than about health care or health systems, we will focus on the latter use of the theory. Here we present the use of the theory in implementing an HIV preventive intervention in the United States. In the next section, we discuss two examples of its use for HIV prevention in non-Western settings.

In a relatively large community-level randomized trial of the "Popular Opinion Leader" (POL) intervention, based on ethnographic reports, popular gay men were recruited to be POLs consisting of approximately 15% of the estimated number of patrons in gay bars in each of the 4 small US intervention communities (populations less than 180,000 residents overall; Kelly, et al., 1997). Recruitment and data analysis focused on men without exclusive partners. The POL intervention included a multi-session training for the POLs in sharing HIV prevention-supportive messages with their friends. POLs reported the number of conversations they had with friends or acquaintances for the three weeks after the training sessions. Data were collected over a 3-day period in each bar in all 8 communities (4 intervention and 4 control) at baseline (before the intervention) and 1 year after the intervention was implemented. Results showed that, at the city level, there was a significant reduction in average frequency of unprotected anal sex in the past two months from baseline to follow-up (from 1.68 to 0.59) and a significant increase in the proportion of anal sex episodes during which condoms were used (from 0.45 to 0.67). The odds ratio of a control-city population member engaging in unprotected anal sex at follow-up compared with baseline was 2.08 times the odds ratio among men in the intervention city.

Applications in International Settings

Social Capital Theory has been pertinent in sub-Saharan Africa with antiretroviral therapy and HIV transmission in Zimbabwe.

Social Capital Theory According to Binagwaho and Ratnayake (2009), the role of social capital in adherence to antiretroviral therapy (ART) is absolutely crucial. In fact, it is higher in sub-Saharan Africa that it is in the United States (Mills et al., 2006). Africans overcome economic obstacles in obtaining ART by begging and borrowing funds from their community and even health care providers. Funds allocated for food or care of their sick child may be utilized for transportation such that adherence remains high. One reason as to why social capital remains high in Africa may be because the social atmosphere is not as individualist as the United States. Taking ART in Africa is a community effort and survival is contingent upon dependence on others.

A study of HIV vulnerability in woman of Zimbabwe also demonstrated the high effectiveness of social capital in the population. Women who had increased participation in community groups had lower incidence of new HIV infections and adopted safer sexual behaviors, even after accounting for difference in sociodemographic composition (Gregson et al., 2011). However, this was not true for men due to the possibility of interactions focused on developing and demonstrating masculinity instead of engaging in educational conversations about HIV.

Diffusion of Innovation Theory Kelly et al. (2006) conducted a POL intervention with young Roma men in Bulgaria. They conducted the study in a settlement of about 35,000 primarily poor Romas. Local staff conducted ethnographic research to determine the number of and membership in "social circles," and identified 55 social networks, of which 52 (comprising 286 men) participated. Sociometric data about fellow members of their social network were used to choose the social network leaders to participate in the intervention. A multisession training was conducted for the popular opinion leaders of all of the groups about how to have HIV prevention–supportive conversations with friends and acquaintances, and then multiple booster sessions. Assessments were conducted at baseline, and 3 and 12 months after the intervention. Results indicated significant differences in reductions in the percentage of men engaging in unprotected intercourse with casual partners, as well as fewer incident cases of gonorrhea in the intervention than control group.

A massive, five-country trial by NIMH Collaborative in 2010 involving a total of 18,147 individuals in China, India, Peru, Russia, and Zimbabwe, with a total of 138 venues matched and randomized within each country

(20 to 40 venues each) implemented this model with significant results. In each country, target populations and venues for recruiting them were chosen based on HIV epidemiology and ethnographic research. In China, food market stall owners and workers were selected for the study; in India, male patrons of wine shops and at-risk women congregating near those shops were included. Young men and women from lower socioeconomic barrios (neighborhoods) included the following groups: *esquineros,* unemployed young men who drink alcohol heavily and have sex with men and women; *movidas,* "loose girls" open to having sex with men in their neighborhood for money; and self-identified homosexuals. The subjects in St. Petersburg, Russia were young adult students in trade and vocational school; and individuals ages 18–30 who patronized venues such as bottle stores or markets in "growth points," areas targeted for economic development in rural areas.

The diffusion of innovation-based (Community-Popular Opinion Leader, C-POL) model was implemented, selecting popular social network or venue members to be trained to share personal-based messages about HIV prevention messages with friends and acquaintances (NIMH Collaborative HIV/STD Prevention Trial Group, 2007). In each country, networks or venues were randomly assigned within matched pairs to the C-POL intervention or AIDS education comparison condition. Surprisingly disappointing results were found from the point of view of POL interventions for HIV prevention: both the control and intervention groups showed declines of around 30% in self-reported unprotected intercourse and around 20% reduction in STD incidence. These are excellent results for a behavior change intervention, but the AIDS education control condition, which included individual-level risk reduction counseling, multiple interview assessments about risk behavior, treatment for current STDs, and condoms, showed results as strong as the C-POL intervention. The results were interpreted as indicating that a relatively intensive HIV education intervention, with risk-reduction counseling, STD treatment, detailed behavioral interviews, and condoms may also be effective at reducing risk behavior and STD outcomes.

Ecological and Structural Models

Ecological models are posited on the fact that behaviors are derived from outside influences and factors.

Ecological Models

There has been a marked increase in theorization and application of **ecological models** for guiding large-scale behavior change programs to maximize the effect of public health interventions on large populations. This comprehensive approach to behavior change, combining interventions targeted at individual, social, environmental, and policy levels, is credited with bringing about the steady decline in tobacco use in the United Stated and is increasingly being applied to many public health problems such as obesity.

The primary thesis of ecological models is that individuals' behavior is determined by multiple levels of influence including "intrapersonal (biological, psychological), interpersonal (social, cultural), organizational, community, physical environmental, and policy" (Sallis, Owen, & Fisher, 2008, p. 466). Ecological models provide an understanding and framework of how these multiple levels of determinants interact and influence individuals' behavior. Sallis et al. (2008) specify four principles of ecological models: (1) multiple influences on health behaviors include those at the intrapersonal, interpersonal, organizational, community, and public policy levels; (2) these multiple influences interact at different levels; (3) ecological models should be specific to a behavior; (4) multilevel interventions should be most effective in changing behavior.

The term *ecology* refers to the study of the relationship between organisms and their environment (Lewin and Cartwright, 1951). The origins of ecology lie in the study of the relationship between the "biologic processes and the geographic environment" (Stokols, 1996) referred to as human ecology. Social ecology on the other hand, which emerged in the 1960s and 1970s, focuses on the social, economic, and cultural contexts of the environment and its relationship with humans. There are a number of models which might be classified as ecological and some of those most used in the health behavior arena and described by Sallis et al. (2008) include

- Moos's Social Ecology (1980), which identifies four categories of influences on human behavior: physical environment, organizational settings, sociocultural characteristics of people in one's environment, and supportive social setting for a behavior;
- Bronfenbrenner's Systems Theory (1979), which specifies three levels of environmental influences: *microsystem,* entailing interactions with family and colleagues at work; *mesosystem,* including family, school, and work; and *exosystem,* which includes the larger system of economics, culture, and politics;
- Glass and McAtee's Ecosocial Model (2006), which theorizes that the social and physical environment provide opportunities and constraints while biological processes regulate expression of behavior;
- Hovell and colleagues' Behavioral Ecological Model (Hovell, Wahlgren, & Adams, 2002); and
- McLeroy et al.'s Ecological Model of Health Behavior (1988), which proposes five sources of influence on behavior: intrapersonal, interpersonal, institutional, community, and public policy.

One of the greatest advantages of ecological models is to effect sustained population-wide behavior change as through policy-level change, in the case of tobacco use, unlike those interventions in which participation is voluntary or are time bound (Glanz & Mullins, 1988). However, there are several weaknesses associated with ecological models as well, such as lack of specific testable hypotheses, poorly or undefined interrelationships between the various levels of influence, lack of specificity about how the broader levels of influence operate, difficulties in manipulating the various levels of influence in an experimental design, and logistical and financial difficulties in collecting data based on multiple levels of determinant.

Application of Ecological Models in International Settings

A telephone survey was conducted with 2,576 South Koreans chosen via a stratified random sampling procedure to assess factors associated with receiving gastric cancer screening, including variables at intrapersonal, interpersonal, community, and public policy levels using the socioecological model (Bae et al., 2008). Among the 985 who responded, 402 (41%) had received gastric cancer screening. Intrapersonal variables included demographic variables (gender, age, education, marital status, area of residence), anxiety about cancer, fear about results of screening, perceived effectiveness of screening, cost burden for screening, and access to health care. Interpersonal factors included recommendation by family for screening, family practices related to screening, and doctor recommendations. Community factors included having experienced health education or a campaign and social norms. Public policy included knowledge of guidelines and awareness of government policy. Age was the only related demographic variable related to having been screened, with individuals in their 50s and 60s more likely than others to have done so. At the intrapersonal level, access to health care was related to screening. At the interpersonal level, family members recommending they get screened and family habit of routine cancer screening were significantly related. At the community or policy level, those with regular education about cancer screening or with stronger feelings that cancer screening is necessary were also more likely to have been screened.

A multilevel intervention to promote physical activity, based on ecological models, called *Agita* (a word that encompasses "the desire for physical activity, but also includes considerations of the mind, social health and citizenship") *São Paulo* was implemented in São Paulo State, Brazil, and its first five years of implementation (1996–2001) were evaluated in 2002 (Matsudo et al., 2002). Activities to increase activity to 30 minutes on most days of the week were encouraged at home, in transportation, and in leisure time. In addition to mass media, social marketing, and linkage of messages to the local culture, health educational programs and activities were implemented throughout the region; also, "mega-events," including special days of the year in which public school students discuss active living and 6,000 students walk annually through the streets of their communities; more than 5 million employees have participated in Active Worker Day; and an annual short walk in local parks for the elderly population. A dosage-response analysis suggested that levels of physical activity were more likely adequate among those who were familiar with the purpose and objectives of the *Agita* message than those who were not familiar with the program. The proportion of sedentary adults and adolescents have both declined significantly, with some evidence to support the link between involvement in *Agita*-related programs and these broad behavior changes.

The social-ecological model was the theoretical framework within which 20 couples living with HIV in Malawi were interviewed to understand barriers to their access to sexual and reproductive health services (SRHS,

Gombachika et al., 2012). Barriers at the individual level included limited skills in reading and writing, stigma and discrimination related to persons living with HIV, gender and cultural beliefs about reproductive health, and past negative experiences related to attempts to access these services. At the intrapersonal level, attitudes, beliefs, and knowledge about SRHS, misinformation and disapproval from friends, family structure and disapproval from family were all mentioned as barriers. Organizational-level barriers were inconvenient service hours, disapproval from health workers, geographical inaccessibility, inadequate counseling from health workers, and lack of privacy. Barriers at the community level included rigid gender roles, loss of support from traditional cultural allies, and economic hardships. Finally, at the societal level, respondents indicated that national policies on SRHS and HIV, lack of free services for a portion of SRHS, and conflicting information from health institutions and the media were all reported as barriers. The authors concluded that the three key focuses for intervention should be (1) bringing services closer to couples living with HIV, (2) empowering formal and informal information gatekeepers with knowledge about SRHS, and (3) coordinating information between Malawi government health providers and formal and informal organizations about SRHS and HIV.

Cassel (2010) conducted a review of 25 studies that assessed factors related to obesity in Samoan populations using the socioecological model as a framework. The authors concluded that "recent political and socioeconomic changes, combined with specific Samoan cultural and biological dynamics" (p. 397) have contributed to recent trends toward poorer health generally and toward higher rates of obesity in Samoans. After colonization, subsistence fishing and agriculture intended for local use was replaced by industrial agriculture and fishing exported to foreigners. Instead, foreign foods, including many calorie-dense foods, came to be seen as "classy," and their consumption has greatly increased, while the consumption of much healthier local fish and agricultural products has diminished. Further, because Western Samoa is less economically developed and less far along the "epidemiologic transition" from infectious to chronic disease than American Samoa, higher income is associated with higher cardiovascular disease (CVD) risks in American Samoa, and lower income is associated with higher CVD risks in Western Samoa (similar to other developing countries like Brazil, South African, and Mexico). Several studies have identified two potential cultural factors related to obesity in Samoans: some (but not all) studies suggest a larger body size is associated with higher social status; a careful analysis of traditional Samoan cultural ideology suggests that disease prevention concepts are not present within that ideology.

The social-ecological model was used as an organizing framework to review the literature of factors related to physical activity for indigenous Australian populations (Nelson, Abbott, & Macdonald, 2010). Structural factors included "those influences that occur at a political, historical, cultural and institutional level" (p. 501), with colonization as primary among these factors. Structural environmental factors primarily involve the physical environment. Individual characteristics include psychosocial factors that "encompass the stress caused by the long-term impact of colonization" (p. 503). Socioeconomic and behavioral factors are considered other individual-level factors in this model. From the literature review, specific variables within the social-ecological model considered to influence indigenous people's engagement in physical activity included colonization history, discrimination, difference and diverse cultural meanings of physical activity (all structural factors); availability of resources, very hot climate, dependence on cars, and feeling unsafe (structural environmental factors); external (nonindigenous) control of programs, family members as key influencers of physical activity, and physical activity and sport as providing opportunities for social connection (social connections); physical activity as managing stress, critical perspectives of sport as panacea for socioeconomic issues, physical activity as a way to escape or prevent at-risk behavior, competition as encouraging or inhibiting participation (individual characteristics); and critical perspectives of race as a biological construct (genetic characteristics). According to the authors, all of these levels of variables must be taken into account when developing programs to increase physical activity in indigenous Australians.

Structural Models

All of the funding for interventions related to HIV, stable incidence in HIV in the United States for more than 10 years despite massive infusion of HIV-prevention programs, and minorities and those in poverty increasing in the percentage of those contracting HIV have led to calls for more **structural models** to help understand HIV transmission and prevention. Unfortunately, most of the researchers funded to construct "structural" interventions around structural models have been psychologists, with little participation by sociologists, economists, and political scientists who have constructed significantly more "macro" models but few interventions. Even some of the best-known interventions that have focused on systems broader than interpersonal (e.g., keeping girls in school, Hallfors et al., 2011; housing people living with HIV with co-morbidities such as mental health or substance abuse issues, Buchanan et al., 2009; and microfinance for women in low-income countries to provide them some autonomy from men with respect to sexual behavior; Pronyk et al., 2006) do not refer to theories or models related to the mechanisms that would lead these interventions to reduce HIV incidence within their respective populations. Kaufman et al. (2014) identified several structural models that have been proposed: the Network-Individual-Resource Model (Johnson et al., 2010); the Dynamic Social Systems Model (Latkin et al., 2010); and Friedman's work on "big events" and horizontal communication alliances (Friedman, Rossi, & Braine, 2009 and Friedman et al., 2014). So far, however, as best we can tell, none of these have been tested in middle- or lower-income countries. Thus we do not present any international examples of structural models in this chapter.

Future Directions

With few exceptions, tests of the various kinds of health behavior models, from the classic psychological ones, to more recent or expanded social psychological models, to interpersonal, to community and ecological models, supported the models. This may reflect the fact that models are rarely compared to one another to assess which one(s) explain behavioral outcomes better (Noar & Zimmerman, 2005); instead, various portions of models may be tested, or models may "adequately" fit the data, whether or not they explain much of the variance in outcomes. In particular, because they are not in testable form, ecological models were only partly tested, in fact, primarily involved literature reviews to assess whether any variables at levels higher than the individual level were found in any studies to be correlated with behavior. Those were generally fairly easy tests to pass. Perhaps importantly, unlike the predictions of some of our colleagues, the relatively individual-focused Western-developed models were not found to be inapplicable in low- and middle-income countries due to the more "collectivist" nature of these countries.

We hope that many other authors begin to seriously look at the potential usefulness of health behavior models in low- and middle-income countries. In particular, how these models might be improved by adding variables that may reflect important cultural differences with higher income countries, such as attitudes about gender roles and equality for men and women, the importance of family and community perceptions, and more difficult economic contexts. We do also hope, as we have begun to argue elsewhere (Kaufman et al., 2014), both in high-income and lower-income countries, that ecological models are improved so that they are testable, and structural and multi-level models are developed and tested using multi-level analysis techniques, to help us understand the joint and interactive effects of variables at multiple levels from that of the individual to communities and entire cultural groups or societies.

Summary

This chapter reviewed a variety of models/theories of health behavior change, including classic social psychological models (Health Belief Model, Theory of Planned Behavior, Social Cognitive Theory, and the Transtheoretical Model), newer social psychological models (Information–Motivation–Behavioral skills and Extended Parallel Processing models), expanded social psychological models (Multiple Domain Model and Theory of Triadic Influence), and several structural and ecological models. We then reviewed some examples of research studies that have used the models in international (i.e., low- or middle-income country) settings. The Theory of Triadic Influence and structural and ecological models (i.e., used in testable rather than merely taxonomic ways) have been tested little outside of Western country contexts, and structural and ecological models need much further development to be tested rigorously in either Western or low- or middle-income countries. We found that a variety of models seemed to be as useful and predictive of health behavior and health behavior change in low- and middle-income countries as in higher-income countries. We also conclude that models should be compared more and that structural and ecological models need significantly more development and testing using complex statistical methods, especially in their use in international contexts.

KEY TERMS

1. **Diffusion of Innovation Theory:** An interpersonal-level health behavior change model that focuses on the diffusion of new behavior change ideas from opinion leaders to members of their social network
2. **Ecological models:** Health behavior change models that point to a variety of levels that need to be attended to: individual, family, neighborhood, community, social structure, and nation
3. **Extended Parallel Processing Model (EPPM):** Health behavior change model that proposes that susceptibility and severity (combined as threat) *and* efficacy (response efficacy and self-efficacy) are both required to produce behavior change, and that threat only will instead produce resistance to the message
4. **Health Belief Model (HBM):** Health behavior change model that includes perceived severity and susceptibility to an illness or disease, perceived benefits and barriers to engaging in the preventive behavior, cues to action, (and in later versions of the model) self-efficacy
5. **Information–Motivation–Behavioral Skills Model (IMB):** Health behavior change model that suggests that information, motivation (including behavioral attitudes and perceived norms), and behavioral skills (including both self-efficacy and actual experienced behavioral success) all combine to predict behavior and behavior change
6. **Multiple Domain Model (MDM):** Health behavior change model that adds social structure, social environment, personality, situation, self-efficacy, and preparatory behaviors to the theory of reasoned action
7. **Social Capital Theory:** A community-level health behavior change model that focuses on the relationship between social cohesion and collaboration within communities and the health outcomes in those communities
8. **Social Cognitive Theory (SCT):** Theory that includes variables related to both the individual (like self-efficacy) and a variety of measures related to others' behavior
9. **Structural models:** Health behavior change models that focus on variables at levels higher than the individual (such as social structure and economic state, community, national culture), largely untested and generally not yet well developed in the health behavior change arena
10. **Theory of Planned Behavior (TPB):** Theory initially developed as an extension of the Theory of Reasoned Action, includes attitudes about behavior, social norms, and perceived behavioral control

11. **Theory of Reasoned Action (TRA):** Theory posits that the most important determinant of behavior is an individual's *behavioral intention*, which is a function of a person's *attitude* toward the behavior and the person's *subjective norms* regarding the behavior.
12. **Transtheoretical Model (TTM):** Health behavior change model focused on the importance of classifying individuals into different stages of change (precontemplation, contemplation, preparation, action, maintenance) to determine what kinds of interventions will be most likely to succeed

REVIEW QUESTIONS

1. What are the key variables that make up the Theory of Planned Behavior?
2. Describe some models of behavior change that go beyond the individual level.
3. Why might structural or ecological models be more useful in changing behavior than the other models described in this chapter?
4. How useful have health behavior change models been in explaining or predicting health behavior in low- or middle-income countries?
5. Which models have not been tested much to date in low- or middle-income country contexts?

References

Adler, P. S., & Kwon, S. W. (2002). Social capital: Prospects for a new concept. *Academy of Management Review*, *7*(1), 17–40.

Albarracin, D., Kumkale, G.T., & Johnson, B.T. (2004). Influences of social power and normative support and condom use decisions: A research synthesis. *AIDS Care*, *16*(6), 700–723.

Ajzen, I. (1988). *Attitudes, personality, and behavior*. Chicago, IL: Open University Press.

Ajzen, I. (1991). The theory of planned behavior. *Organizational Behavioral and Human Decision Processes*, *50*, 179–211.

Ajzen, I., & Driver, B. L. (1991). Prediction of leisure participation from behavioral, normative, and control beliefs: An application of the theory of planned behavior. *Leisure Sciences*, *13*, 185–204.

Bae, S. S., Jo, H. S., Kim, D. H., Choi, Y. J., Lee, H. J., Lee, T. J., & Lee, H. J. (2008). Factors associated with gastric cancer screening of Koreans based on a socio-ecological model. *Journal of Preventive Medicine and Public Health, 41(2),* 100–106.

Bandura, A. (1986). *Social foundations of thought and action: A cognitive social theory.* Englewood Cliffs, NJ: Prentice-Hall.

Bandura, A. (1997). *Self-efficacy: The exercise of control.* New York, NY: W. H. Freeman.

Bandura, A. (2001). Social cognitive theory: An agentic perspective. *Annual Review of Psychology, 52,* 1–26

Bandura, A. (2002). Social cognitive theory of mass communications. In J. Bryant & D. Zillman (Eds.), *Media effects: Advances in theory and research* (2nd ed., pp. 121–153). Hillsdale, NJ: Erlbaum.

Baranowski, T., Perry, C. L., & Parcel, G. S. (2002). How individuals, environments, and health behavior interact. In K. Glanz, B. R. Rimer, and Lewis, F. R. (Eds.), *Health behavior and health education* (pp. 165–184). San Francisco, CA: Jossey Bass.

Berwick, D. M. (2003). Disseminating innovations in health care. *Journal of the American Medical Association, 289*(15), 1969–1975.

Binagwaho A., & Ratnayake N. (2009). The role of social capital in successful adherence to antiretroviral therapy in Africa. *Public Library of Science (PLOS) Medicine, 6*(1): e18, doi:10.1371/journal.pmed.1000018.

Bronfenbrenner, U. (1979). *The ecology of human development.* Cambridge, MA: Harvard University Press.

Buchanan, D., Kee, R., Sadowski, L. S., & Garcia, D. (2009). The health impact of supportive housing for HIV-positive homeless patients: A randomized controlled trial. *American Journal of Public Health, 99*(S3), S675–S680.

Butterfoss, F. D. (2007). *Coalitions and partnerships in community health.* San Francisco, CA: Jossey-Bass.

Butterfoss, F. D., Goodman, R., & Wandersman, A. (1993). Community coalitions for prevention and health promotion. *Health Education Research, 8,* 315–330.

Cassel, K. D. (2010). Using the social-ecological model as a research and intervention framework to understand and mitigate obesogenic factors in Samoan populations. *Ethnicity and Health, 15*(4), 397–416.

Connell, R. W. (1987). *Gender and power.* Stanford, CA: Stanford University Press.

Cornman, D. H., Schmiege, S. J., Bryan, A., Benziger, T. J., & Fisher, J. D. (2007). An information-motivation-behavioral skills (IMB) model-based HIV prevention intervention for truck drivers in India. *Social Science and Medicine, 64*(8), 1572–1584.

DeKay, W. T., & Buss, D. M. (1992). Human nature, individual differences, and the importance of context: Perspectives from evolutionary psychology. *Current Directions in Psychological Science, 1*(6), 184–189.

Dekker, P., & Uslaner, E.M. (2001). Introduction. In E. M. Uslaner (Ed.), *Social capital and participation in everyday life* (pp. 1–8). London: Routledge.

Eggers, S. M., Aaro, L. E., Bos, A. E., Mathews, C., & de Vries, H. (2014). Predicting condom use in South Africa: A test of two integrative models. *AIDS & Behavior, 18*(1), 135–45.

Eriksson, M. (2011). Social capital and health: Implications for health promotion. *Global Health Action, 4,* 5611.

Fishbein, M. (Ed.). (1967). *Readings in attitude theory and measurement.* New York: Wiley, 1967.

Fishbein, M. (2000). The role of theory in HIV prevention. *AIDS Care, 12,* 273–278.

Fishbein, M., Middlestadt, S., & Hitchcock, P. (1994). Using information to change sexually transmitted disease-related behaviors: An analysis based on the theory of reasoned action. In R. DiClemente & J. Peterson (Eds.), *Preventing AIDS: Theories of methods of behavioral interventions* (pp. 61–78). New York, NY: Plenum Press.

Fisher, J. D., & Fisher, W. A. (1992). Changing AIDS risk behavior. *Psychological Bulletin, 111,* 454–474.

Fisher, W. A., Fisher, J. D., & Harman, J. (2003). The Information-Motivation-Behavioral skills model: A general social psychological approach to understanding and promoting health behavior. In J. Suls & K. A. Wallston (Eds.), *Social psychological foundations of health and illness* (pp. 82–106). Malden, MA: Blackwell.

Flay, B. R., & Petraitis, J. (1994). The theory of triadic influence: A new theory of health behavior with implications for preventive interventions. In G. S. Albrecht (Ed.), *Advances in medical sociology, Vol. IV: A reconsideration of models of health behavior change.* Greenwich, CT: JAI Press.

Flay, B. R., Phil, D., Petraitis, J., & Hu, F. B. (1995). The theory of triadic influence: Preliminary evidence related to alcohol and tobacco use. In J. B. Fertig & J. P. Allen (Eds.), *Alcohol and tobacco: From basic science to clinical practice* (pp. 37–57). Darby, PA: Dianne Publishing.

Flay, B. R., Snyder, F., & Petraitis, J. (2009). The theory of triadic influence. In R. J. DiClemente, M. C. Kegler, & R. A. Crosby (Eds.), *Emerging theories in health promotion practice and research* (2nd ed., pp. 451–510). San Francisco, CA: Jossey-Bass.

Friedman, S. R., Downing, M. J., Smyrnov, P., Nikolopoulous, G., Schneider, J. A., et al. (2014). Socially-integrated transdisciplinary HIV prevention. *AIDS and Behavior, 18,* 1821–1834.

Friedman, S. R., Rossi, D., & Braine, N. (2009). Theorizing "Big Events" as a potential risk environment for drug use, drug-related harm and HIV epidemic outbreaks. *International Journal of Drug Policy, 20*(3), 283–291.

Glanz, K., & Mullins, R. M. (1988). Environmental interventions to promote healthy eating: A review of models, programs, and evidence. *Health Education Quarterly, 15,* 395–415.

Glass, T. A., & McAtee, M. J. (2006). Behavioral science at the crossroads in public health: Extending horizons, envisioning the future. *Social Science and Medicine, 62*, 1650–1671.

Gombachika, B. C., Fjeld, H., Chirwa, E., Sundby, J., Malata, A., & Maluwa, A. (2012). A socioecological approach to exploring barriers to accessing sexual and reproductive health services among couples living with HIV in southern Malawi. *International Scholarly Research Network.* Article ID 825459, doi:10.5402/2012/825459

Gregson, S., Mushati, P., Grusin, H., Nhamo, M., Schumacher et al. (2011). Social capital and women's reduced vulnerability to HIV infection in rural Zimbabwe. *Population and Development Review, 37*(2), 333–359.

Ha, B. T., Rohan, J., & Owen, N. (2003). Male involvement in family planning in rural Vietnam: An application of the Transtheoretical Model. *Health Education Research, 18*(2), 171–180.

Hallfors, D., Cho, H., Rusakaniko, S., Iritani, B., Mapfumo, J., & Halpern, C. (2011). Supporting adolescent orphan girls to stay in school as HIV risk prevention: Evidence from a randomized controlled trial in Zimbabwe. *American Journal of Public Health, 101*(6), 1082–1088.

Harrison, J. A., Mullen, P. D., & Green, L. W. (1992). A meta-analysis of studies of the health belief model with adults. *Health Education Research, 7*, 107–116.

Hinyard, L. J., and Kreuter, M. W. (2007). Using narrative communication as a tool for health behavior change: A conceptual, theoretical, and empirical overview. *Health Education and Behavior, 34*(5), 777–792.

Hochbaum, G. M. (1958). *Public participation in medical screening programs: A sociopsychological study.* PHS publication no. 572. Washington, DC: Government Printing Office.

Hounton, S., Carabin, H., & Henderson, N. (2005). Towards an understanding of barriers to condom use in rural Benin using the Health Belief Model: A cross-sectional survey. *Biomed Central Public Health, 5*, 8.

Hovell, M. F., Wahlgren, D. R., & Adams, M. (2009). The logical and empirical basis for the Behavioral Ecological Model. In R. J. DiClemente, R. A. Crosby, & M. Kegler (Eds.), *Emerging theories in health promotion practice and research: Strategies for improving public health* (2nd ed., pp. 415–449). San Francisco, CA: Jossey-Bass.

Hovland, C., Janis, I., & Kelly, H. (1953). *Communication and persuasion.* New Haven, CT: Yale University Press.

Janz, N. K., & Becker, M. H. (1984). The Health Belief Model: A decade later. *Health Education Quarterly, 11*, 1.

Janz, N. K., Champion, V. L., & Strecher, V. J. (2002). The Health Belief Model. In K. Glanz, B. K. Rimer, & F. M. Lewis (Eds.), *Health behavior and health education: Theory, research, and practice* (pp. 45–66). San Francisco, CA: Wiley.

Johnson, B.T., Redding, C.A., DiClemente, R.J., Mustanski, B.S., Dodge, B.M., Sheeran, P., ... Fishbein, M. (2010). A network-individual-resource model for HIV prevention. *AIDS & Behavior.14(Supp2)*, 204–221.

Kashfi, S. M., Jeihooni, A. K., Rezaianzadeh, A., & Amini, S. H. (2012). The effect of health belief model educational program and jogging on control of sugar in Type 2 diabetic patients. *Iranian Red Crescent Medical Journal, 14*(7), 442–446.

Kaufman, M. R., Cornish, F., Zimmerman, R. S., & Johnson B. T. (2014). Health behavior change models for HIV prevention and AIDS care: Practical recommendations for a multi-level approach. *Journal of Acquired Immune Deficiency Syndrome, 66*(Suppl 3), S250–S278.

Kelly, J. A., Amirkhanian, Y. A., Kabakchieva, E., Vassileva, S., Vassilev, B., McAuliffe, T. L., … Dimitrov, B. (2006). Prevention of HIV and sexually transmitted diseases in high risk social networks of young Roma (Gypsy) men in Bulgaria: randomised controlled trial. *British Medical Journal, 333*, 1098–1101.

Kelly, J. A., Murphy, D. A., Sikkema, K. J., McAuliffe, T. L., Roffman, R. A., Solomon, L. J., … Kalichman, S. C. (1997). Randomised, controlled, community-level HIV-prevention intervention for sexual-risk behavior among homosexual men in US cities. *Lancet, 350*(9080), 1500–1505.

Kippax, S., & Crawford, J. (1993). Flaws in the theory of reasoned action. In D. Terry, C. Galloios, & M. McCamish (Eds.), *The theory of reasoned action: Its application to AIDS-preventive behavior* (pp. 253–269). Exeter, UK: Pergamon.

Kreuter, M. W., & Lezin, N. (2002). Social Capital Theory: Implications for community-based health promotion. In R. J. DiClemente, R. A. Crosby, & M. C. Kegler (Eds.), *Emerging theories in health promotion practice and research: Strategies for improving public health* (pp. 228–254). San Francisco, CA: Jossey-Bass.

Krishna, A., & Shrader, E. (2000). *Cross-cultural measures of social capital: A tool and results from India and Panama*. Social Capital Initiative, Working Paper no. 21. Washington, DC: World Bank.

Latkin, C., Weeks, M. R., Glasman, L., Galletly, C., & Albarracin, D. (2010). A dynamic social systems model for considering structural factors in HIV prevention and detection. *AIDS and Behavior, 14*(Suppl 2), 222–238.

Leventhal, H. (1970). Findings and theory in the study of fear communications. In L. Berkowitz (Ed.), *Advances in experimental social psychology* (Vol. 5, pp. 119–186). New York, NY: Academic Press.

Lewin, K., & Cartwright, D. (1951). *Field theory in social science*. New York, NY: Harper.

Li, X., Stanton, B., Wang, B., Mao, R., Zhang, H., Qu, M., … Wang, J. (2008). Cultural adaptation of the focus on kids program for college students in China. *AIDS Education and Prevention, 20*(1), 1–14.

Luszczynska, A., & Schwarzer, R. (2005). Social Cognitive Theory. In M. Conner & P. Norman (Eds.), *Predicting health behaviour* (2nd ed. rev., pp. 127–169). Buckingham, England: Open University Press.

Matsudo, V., Matsudo, S., Andrade, D., Araujo, T., Andrade, T., de Oliveira, L. C., & Braggion, G. (2002). Promotion of physical activity in a developing country: The Agita Sao Paulo experience. *Public Health Nutrition, 5*(1A), 253–261.

McAlister, A. L., Perry, C. L., & Parcel, G. S. (2008). How individuals, environments, and health behaviors interact: Social cognitive theory. In K. Glanz, B. K. Rimer, K. Viswanath (Eds.), *Health behavior and health education: Theory, research, and practice* (4th ed., pp. 169–188). San Francisco, CA: Jossey-Bass.

McEachen, R. R. C., Conner, M., Taylor, N. J., & Lawton, R. J. (2011). Prospective prediction of health-related behaviors with the Theory of Planned Behaviour: A meta-analysis. *Health Psychology Review, 5(2),* 97–144.

McGuire, W. J. (1968). Personality and susceptibility to social influence. In E. Borgatta & W. Lambert (Eds.), *Handbook of personality theory and research* (pp. 1130–1187). Chicago, IL: Rand McNally.

McLeroy, K. R., Bibeau, D., Steckler, A., & Glanz, K. (1988). An ecological perspective on health promotion programs. *Health Education Quarterly, 15,* 351–377.

Mehrotra, P., Zimmerman, R. S., Noar, S. M., & Dumenei, L. (2013). A test of an adapted multiple domain model in predicting sexual behaviors in unmarried young adults in India. *Journal of Sex Research, 50*(2), 116–127.

Mills, E. J., Nachega, J. B., Buchan, I., Orbinski, J., Attaran, A., Singh, S., ... Rachilis, Bangsberg, D. R. (2006). Adherence to antiretroviral therapy in sub-Saharan Africa and North America: A meta-analysis. *Journal of the American Medical Association, 296*(6), 679–690.

Montano, D. E., & Kasprzyk, D. (2002). The theory of reasoned action and the theory of planned behavior. In K. Glanz, B. Rimer, & F. M. Lewis (Eds.), *Health behavior and health education* (pp. 67–98). San Francisco, CA: Jossey-Bass.

Moos, R. H. (1980). Social-ecological perspectives on health. In G. C. Stone, F. Cohen, & N. E. Adler (Eds.), *Health psychology: A handbook* (pp. 523–547). San Francisco, CA: Jossey-Bass.

Muthusamy, N., Levine, T., & Weber, R. (2009). Scaring the already scared: Some problems with HIV/AIDS fear appeals in Namibia. *Journal of Communication, 59*(2), 317–344.

Naar-King, S., Rongkavilit, C., Wang, B., Wright, K., Chuenyam, T., Lam, P., & Phanuphak, P. (2008). Transtheoretical model and risky sexual behaviour in HIV + Youth in Thailand. *AIDS Care, 20*(2), 198–204.

National Committee for Population and Family Planning. (2000). *Demographic and Health Survey 1997.* Retrieved from: http://dhsprogram.com/pubs/pdf/FR104/FR104.pdf.

Nelson, A., Abbott, R., & Macdonald, D. (2010). Indigenous Australians and physical activity: Using a social-ecological model to review the literature. *Health Education Research, 25*(3), 498–509.

NIMH Collaborative HIV/STD Prevention Trial Group. (2007). Selection of populations represented in the NIMH Collaborative HIV/STD prevention trial. *Journal of Acquired Immune Deficiency Syndrome, 21*(Suppl 2), S19–S28.

NIMH Collaborative HIV/STD Prevention Trial Group. (2010). Results of the NIMH Collaborative HIV/STD Prevention Trial of a Community Popular Opinion Leader Intervention. *Journal of Acquired Immune Deficiency Syndrome, 54*(2), 204–214.

Noar, S. M., & Zimmerman, R. S. (2005). Health behavior theory and cumulative knowledge regarding health behaviors: Are we moving in the right direction? *Health Education Research: Theory and Practice, 20*(3), 275–290.

Nujum, Z. T., Remadevi, S., Nirmala, C., Rajmohanan, K., Indu, P. S., & Nair, S. M. (2012). Factors determining noncompliance to mass drug administration for lymphatic filariasis elimination. *Tropical Parasitology, 2*(2), 109–115.

O'Leary, A., Jemmott, J. B. III, Jemmott, L. S., Bellamy, S., Ngwane, Z., Icard, L., & Gueits, L. (2012). Moderation and mediation of an effective HIV Risk-reduction intervention for South African adolescents. *Annals of Behavioral Medicine, 44*(2), 181–191.

Popova, L. (2012). The extended parallel process model: Illuminating the gaps in research. *Health Education and Behavior, 39*(4): 455–473. doi: 10.1177/1090198111418108.

Portes, A. (1995). Economic sociology and the sociology of immigration: A conceptual overview. In A. Portes (Ed.), *Economic sociology of immigration: Essays on networks, ethnicity, and entrepreneurship* (pp. 1–41). New York: Russell Sage Foundation.

Portes, A. (1998). Social capital: Its origins and applications in modern sociology. *Annual Review of Sociology, 24*, 1–25.

Prochaska, J. O., & DiClemente, C. C. (1983). Stages and processes of self-change of smoking: Toward an integrative model of change. *Journal of Consulting and Clinical Psychology, 51*, 390–395.

Prochaska, J. O., DiClemente, C. C., & Norcross, J. C. (1992). In search of how people change: Applications to addictive behavior. *American Psychologist, 47*, 1102–1114.

Prochaska, J. O., Redding, C. A., & Evers, K. E. (2002). The Transtheoretical Model and stages of change. In K. Glanz, B. K. Rimer, & F. M. Lewis (Eds.), *Health behavior and health education: Theory, research, and practice* (pp. 99–120). San Francisco, CA: Wiley.

Prochaska, J. O., & Velicer, W. F. (1997). The Transtheoretical Model of health behavior change. *American Journal of Health Promotion, 12*, 38–48.

Pronyk, P. M., Jargreaves, J. R., Kim, J. C., Morison, L. A., Phetla, G., Watts, C., … Porter, J. D. H. (2006). Effect of a structural intervention for the prevention of intimate-partner violence and HIV in rural South Africa: A cluster randomized trial. *Lancet, 368*, 1973–1983.

Protogerou, C., Flisher, A. J., Wild, L. G., & Aarø, L. E. (2013). Predictors of condom use in South African university students: A prospective application of the theory of planned behavior. *Journal of Applied Social Psychology, 43*, E23–E36.

Putnam, R. D. (1995). Bowling alone: America's declining social capital. *Journal of Democracy, 6*, 65–78.

Rogers, R. W. (1975). A protection motivation theory of fear appeals and attitude change. *Journal of Psychology, 91*, 93–114.

Rogers, E. (2003). *Diffusion of innovation* (5th ed.). New York, NY: Free Press.

Rosenstock, I. M., Strecher, V. J., & Becker, H. M. (1988). Social learning theory and the health belief model. *Health Education Quarterly, 15,* 175–183.

Sallis, J., Owen, N., & Fisher, E. (2008). Ecological models of health behavior. In K. Glanz, B. Rimer, & K. Viswanath (Eds.), *Health behavior and health education: Theory, research, and practice.* (4th ed., pp. 465–482). San Francisco, CA: Jossey-Bass.

Sheer, V. C., & Chen, L. (2008). Intrinsic characteristics of health-related fear appeals from Chinese print OTC ads: Implications for fear message construction. *International Journal of Communication, 2,* 936–958.

Sheeran, P., & Taylor, S. (1999). Predicting intentions to use condoms: A meta-analysis and comparison of the theories of reasoned action and planned behavior. *Journal of Applied Social Psychology, 29,* 1624–1675.

Shisana, O., Hall, E., Maluleke, R., Chauveau, J., & Schwabe, C. (2004). HIV/AIDS prevalence among South African health workers. *South African Medical Journal, 94*(10), 846–850.

Sikkema, K. J., Kelly, J. A., Winett, R. A., Solomon, L. J., Cargill, V. A., Roffman, R. A., ... Mercer, M. B. (2000). Outcomes of a randomized community-level HIV prevention intervention for women living in 18 low-income housing developments. *American Journal of Public Health, 90*(1), 57–63.

Singhal, A., & Rogers, E. A. (1999). *Entertainment-education: A communication strategy for social change.* Hillsdale, NJ: Erlbaum.

Stokols, D. (1996). Translating social ecological theory into guidelines for community health promotion. *American Journal of Health Promotion, 10*(4), 282–295.

Sung, J. J., Choi, S. Y., Chan, F. K., Ching, J. Y., Lau, J. T., & Griffiths, S. (2007). Obstacles to colorectal cancer screening in Chinese: A study based on the health belief model. *American Journal of Gastroenterology, PMID*: 18047545 [Epub ahead of print].

Uslaner, E. M. (2001). Volunteering and social capital: How trust and religion shape civic participation in the United States. In E. M. Uslaner (Ed.), *Social capital and participation in everyday life* (pp. 104–117). London: Routledge.

Volk, J. E., & Koopman, C. (2001). Factors associated with condom use in Kenya: A test of the health belief model. *AIDS Education and Prevention, 13*(6), 495–508.

Wilkin, H. A., Valente, T. W., Murphy, S., Cody, M. J., Huang, G., & Beck, V. (2007). Does entertainment-education work with Latinos in the United States? Identification and the effects of a telenovela breast cancer storyline. *Journal of Health Communication, 12*(5), 455–469.

Wingood, G. M., & DiClemente, R. J. (2009). The theory of gender and power: Constructs, variables, and implications for developing HIV interventions for women. In R. J. DiClemente, R. A. Crosby, & M. C. Kegler (Eds.), *Emerging theories in health promotion practice and research: Strategies for improving public health* (2nd ed., pp. 393–413). San Francisco, CA: Jossey-Bass.

Witte, K. (1992). Putting the fear back into fear appeals: The extended parallel process model. *Communication Monographs, 59*, 329–349.

Witte, K., & Allen, M. (2000). A meta-analysis of fear appeals: Implications for effective public health campaigns. *Health Education and Behavior, 27*(5), 591–615.

Xiao, Z. W., Palmgreen, P., Zimmerman, R. S., & Noar, S. (2010). Adapting and applying a Multiple Domain Model of condom use to Chinese college students. *AIDS Care, 22*(3), 332–338.

Zhang, H., Stanton, B., Li, X., Mao, R., Sun, Z., Kaljee, L., ... Qu, M. (2004). Perceptions and attitudes regarding sex and condom use among Chinese college students: A qualitative study. *AIDS and Behavior, 8*(2), 105–117.

Zimmerman, R. S., Noar, S. M., Price, S. F., Dekthar, O., Cupp, P. K., Anderman, E., & Lock, S. (2007). Longitudinal test of a multiple domain model of adolescent condom use. *Journal of Sex Research, 44*(4), 380–394.

Zimmerman, R. S., & Vernberg, D. (1994). Models of preventative health behavior: Comparison, critique, and meta-analysis. *Advances in Medical Sociology, 4*, 45–67.

CHAPTER 5

TWO HEALTH COMMUNICATION APPROACHES

Communication for Behavioral Impact (COMBI) and Entertainment Education

Everold N. Hosein, May G. Kennedy, and Sandra de Castro Buffington

As shown by the inclusion of a chapter on health communication in the United States' Healthy People objectives in both the 2010 and 2020 editions (Parrott, 2004) and a variety of other evidence, communication-based approaches are being used more often in health promotion globally, due at least in part to their "emphasis on combining theory and practice in ... changing human behaviour" (Rimal & Lapinski, 2009). Consistent with the greater emphasis on communication approaches in public health, this chapter focuses on two health communication approaches that have been implemented in many international settings: **Communication for Behavioral Impact** and **entertainment education**.

LEARNING OBJECTIVES

By the end of this chapter, the reader should be able to:

- Explain the need to go beyond traditional health communication approaches
- Describe the Communication for Behavioral Impact (COMBI) approach to behavior change
- Compare and contrast COMBI and social marketing
- List some health areas and countries in which COMBI has been applied
- Know how entertainment education (EE) has been defined and the major formats it has used
- Explain the way EE is thought to work
- Summarize the knowledge base regarding EE effectiveness
- Describe some of the crossnational influences of and on EE
- List top applied research priorities for EE

Communication for Behavioral Impact

Communication for Behavioral Impact is a 10-step strategic communication planning method that focuses sharply on achieving clearly defined behavioral results.

COMBI Rationale

One dilemma in public health globally is the fact that people know what to do to improve their health status, but do not take the necessary action. The fundamental challenge confronting the prevention and control of diseases is having individuals (within the context of families and communities) adopt and maintain healthy behaviors. It is often presumed that this challenge will be met once "everything else is in place," once the drugs and other health interventions are available. For example, when antiretroviral therapy is readily and freely available for the HIV-infected, what could be easier than having someone come in for the HIV test and the free drugs? The low response to available testing and treatment services in several African countries attests to the challenge (cf. Doherty, McCoy, & Donohue, 2005; Matovu & Makumbi, 2007). Indeed, quality health systems, trained staff, and health services and products need to be in place. Yet superb medical–technical solutions to health problems do not sell themselves, even when readily available. Sixty years of public health experience offer one example after the other of this quandary. Examples abound of the wide gap between knowledge of and access to health products and services and use of these products and services. Whatever the healthy behaviors, they remain elusive (Gulliford et al., 2002; Haines, Kuruvilla, & Borchert, 2004; Badcock-Walters, Kelly, & Gorgens, 2004).

The public health communication and education response has been to keep improving people's knowledge of diseases and preventive behaviors. But increased awareness and education about healthy behaviors have been notoriously insufficient bases for individual or family action, although they are essential steps in the process toward healthy behavior practice. The cliché is appropriate: It is one thing to *know,* another to *do.* There is the classic story of a pregnant woman in Caprivi, Namibia, receiving a free insecticide-treated bednet during an antenatal visit but instead of sleeping under it at night, she gives it to her husband to go and fish with it. And the gap is not going to be bridged by the production of more posters, radio jingles, pamphlets, and T-shirts dedicated to increasing public awareness of a disease. With the ultimate goal of achieving behavioral impact in health, ministries of health and their health education, communication, and promotion departments now desperately search for new ways of achieving desired behavioral results in health, with a keen awareness that they need to go beyond the ineffectual tools of producing more posters and pamphlets. A different approach to health communication and social mobilization is necessary and one which focuses rigidly on achieving behavioral impact and outcomes and not just increased awareness or knowledge impact.

What Is COMBI?

COMBI (Communication for Behavioral Impact) is a 10-step strategic communication planning method for designing communication programs to engage individuals, families, communities, and nations to consider and take action on specific recommended behaviors which could make a difference in the quality of their lives (Hosein, Parks, & Schiavo, 2009; World Health Organization [WHO], 2012). COMBI begins with a precise focus on the behavioral result(s) expected in relation to people's needs, wants, or desires. A COMBI planning mantra (Mantra #1) is "Do nothing—produce no T-shirts, no posters, no pamphlets, no videos … until one has set out precise, specific behavioral objectives" (SBOs). Another COMBI planning mantra (Mantra #2) has a similar ring but focuses on market research: "Do nothing—produce no T-shirts, no posters, no pamphlets, no videos … until one has carried out a **situational market analysis** in relation to the desired behavioral results, until one has listened to the 'consumer' with regard to the offered recommended behavior." This situational market analysis (SMA) involves listening to people and learning about their perceptions and grasp of the offered behavior; the factors that would constrain or facilitate adoption of the behavior; and their sense of the costs (time, effort, money) in relation to their perception of value of the behavior to their lives. The SMA also facilitates the search for **communication keys** (CK) for opening of the door of engagement with the consumer for better consideration of behavioral options offered. This combination of SMA and CK has led to the acronym SMACK as a way of referring to the process of conducting market research and listening to the consumer.

COMBI effectively integrates five communication action areas: (1) administrative mobilization/public relations/advocacy; (2) community mobilization; (3) advertising, promotion, and incentives; (4) personal selling/interpersonal communication/counseling; and (5) point-of-service promotion.

- *Administrative mobilization/public relations/advocacy,* when the recommended health behavior and its associated COMBI program are put on the agendas of various groups of people from whom we seek enthusiastic implementation support. First, the focus is on administrative and management staff in the public sector and public–private sector partnerships who will facilitate implementation of the COMBI plan. This is done by sharing an administrative memorandum with all staff and partners, coupled with meetings and discussions with various categories of government and community leadership, service providers, and administrators. Next we put the recommended behavior on the agenda of the wider public via non-advertising use of mass media and social media. Finally, we put the recommended behavior and associated program on the agenda of policymakers, legislators, and private sector–public sector partnerships, via various consultations and meetings.
- *Community mobilization,* including use of participatory research, community group meetings, partnership meetings, traditional media, music, song and dance, road shows, community drama, leaflets, posters, pamphlets, videos.
- *Advertising, promotion, and incentives,* via radio, television, newspapers, social media, and other available media, engaging people in reviewing the merits of the recommended behavior vis-à-vis the "cost" of carrying it out. Incentives, such as free samples and small gifts, are used to motivate people to consider the suggested behavior; so too is branding the behavior or associated product or service and promoting the brand.
- *Personal selling/interpersonal communication/counseling* at the community and household level via community-selected volunteers, in schools and involving schoolchildren as "personal sellers" to their parents, and particularly at service points via health staff, with appropriate informational literature and additional incentives, and allowing for careful listening to people's concerns and addressing them.
- *Point-of-service promotion,* emphasizing easily accessible and readily available solutions to health problems at places where health services are available and where people go for other services (supermarkets, small shops, hair dressing salons, banks, post offices).

COMBI strives for an integrated, synchronized strategy that judiciously blends various communication actions appropriate to the behavioral outcome desired. It recognizes that no single type of communication intervention is all-powerful but acknowledges the critical importance of personal selling and interpersonal communication for behavioral impact.

The Key Steps in Designing a COMBI Plan

COMBI planning applies a 10-step process in designing a strategic health communication plan. These 10 steps are presented in the following annotated summary form.

Special note is taken of the two principal mantras that were mentioned earlier and that guide the process of COMBI design.

Step 1: Set Out the Overall Goal

This is a statement of the overall, long-term program goal that the COMBI plan will help achieve. For example: To contribute to the elimination of lymphatic filariasis in Zanzibar by the year 2020. Such long-term goals are usually already enunciated in government health planning documents. They are presented as Step 1 so as to remind the COMBI planner or COMBI planning group of the ultimate program result desired.

Step 2: Set Out Preliminary, Tentative, Specific Behavioral Objectives

This is a statement of Specific, Measurable, Appropriate, Realistic, and Time bound **(SMART) behavioral objectives**. The statement is best expressed in the 4W format: exactly *Who* will do precisely *What, Where,* and *When.* COMBI strategic thinking argues that ultimately what matters in health communication is whether the intended behavioral result was attained. As a consequence, effective communication planning cannot proceed without a clear definition of intended behavioral results. Hence, in COMBI design, the sharp behavioral focus emerges as the first original step in strategic communication planning, presuming that Step 1 has already been done by health planners. It is in this step that Mantra 1 is put into play: "Do nothing—produce no T-shirts, no posters, no leaflets, no videos, etc … until one has set out clear, precise, specific behavioral objectives (SBOs)."

Step 3: Carry Out a Situational Market Analysis

This is a "consumer-focused" exploration of the factors influencing the attainment of the behavioral objectives that will inform the communication strategy and plan of action. It is in this step that Mantra 2 is applied. In its simplest formulation, it can succinctly be presented as: "Listen to the consumer."

A wide range of SMACKing tools are used in this step, which is perhaps the most time consuming of the 10 steps. Two noteworthy ones are a HIC-DARM (Hear, Informed, Convinced-Decision, Action, Reconfirmation, Maintain; see Figure 5.1), and 4 Cs analysis (defined in the section on COMBI and social marketing following; also see a more detailed explanation in Hosein,

©HIC-DARM: BEHAVIOR ADOPTION

First, we	**H**ear about the new behavior
then, we become	**I**nformed about it
and later	**C**onvinced that it is worthwhile.
In time, we make the	**D**ecision to do something about our conviction.
and later we take	**A**ction on the new behaviour.
We await next	**R**e-confirmation that our action was a good one
and if all is well, we	**M**aintain the behavior.

Figure 5.1 HIC DARM
Source: © Everold Hosein.

Parks, & Schiavo, 2009). Step 3, as can be seen from the myriad of tools to be used, is the most vital and most time consuming of all the steps in COMBI planning.

Step 4: Present the Communication Strategy

Based on the SMACKing exercise, one now presents the overall communication strategy for achieving the stated behavioral result(s):

a. Restate specific behavioral objective(s);
b. Set out "communication objectives" that will need to be achieved in order to secure the desired behavioral result(s);
c. Outline communication strategy. Here one provides an outline of the proposed communication actions for results in terms of the five communication actions areas alluded to by the 4 Cs (see the COMBI and social marketing section following).

Step 5: Present the COMBI Plan of Action

This is a detailed listing of the integrated communication actions to be undertaken. The activities described in general terms in Step 4(c) are now laid out in specific operational detail. For example: Prepare draft of administrative memo for review by minister of health; arrange meeting with minister of health for review of draft memo; finalize administrative memo; print 60,000 copies of the administrative memo; and so on.

Step 6: Manage and Implement the COMBI Plan

This a description of how COMBI will be managed, specifying the multidisciplinary planning and implementation team, including specific staff or collaborating agencies (e.g., local advertising firms and research institutions), designated to coordinate communication actions and other activities such as monitoring. Also included are any technical advisory groups or government body from which the management team receives technical support or to whom it should report.

Step 7: Monitor Implementation

This is a description of the process **indicators** to be used in tracking the reach and effect of the communication actions, including a description of how monitoring data will be gathered, shared, and used.

Step 8: Assess Behavioral Impact

This provides details of the behavioral indicators to be used, methods for data collection, analysis, and reporting.

Step 9: Develop Calendar/Timeline/Implementation Plan

This provides a detailed work plan with time schedule for the preparation and implementation activities required to execute each communication action as described in Step 5. This could be presented in a PERT or GANTT chart, or simply a repeat of Step 5 in a smaller font with two additional columns, specifying who is responsible for execution and by when.

Step 10: Prepare the Budget

A detailed listing of costs for the various activities described in Steps 5, 6, 7, and 8.

COMBI in Practice: 2000–2013

During the past 13 years, WHO has applied the COMBI approach successfully to mass drug administration for lymphatic filariasis elimination in Zanzibar, Sri Lanka, Kenya, the Philippines, and the State of Tamil Nadu in India; to dengue in Malaysia, Laos, Cambodia, Indonesia, and several Latin American and Caribbean countries; to leprosy in India and Mozambique; to tuberculosis in Kerala/India, Kenya, Bangladesh, and Namibia; to malaria in Ghana, Sudan, Mozambique, and Afghanistan; to HIV/AIDS in Sudan, Myanmar, Moldova (with UNICEF), Kazakhstan (with UNICEF), Albania, Namibia (with UNFPA), Swaziland, the Caribbean, and the Ukraine; to exclusive breastfeeding in the Philippines, Laos (with UNICEF), Papua New Guinea, Vietnam, and China; to Guinea worm eradication in South Sudan; to avian influenza in Indonesia; and to chronic noncommunicable diseases in the South Pacific, the Caribbean, and Vietnam.

COMBI in Malaysia

Dengue fever is the most prevalent arbovirus infection in the world, as well as the most prevalent infectious disease in the tropics after malaria (Gubler, 1998). In January 2001, the Ministry of Health in Johor Bahru (MOHJB) decided to apply COMBI's integrated model to its strategic communication efforts with assistance from WHO. The trial followed COMBI's 10-step planning model and consisted of a 12-week pilot project in Malaysia. Launched in August 2001 after a comprehensive situational market analysis, the project intended to affect behavioral change among residents of Johor Bahru City, the state's capital (approximately 1.2 million people).

Research data helped identify the following behavioral objectives: (a) to prompt family members in every home to conduct a weekly 30-minute home inspection (both inside and outside) on Sundays to look for potential mosquito larval habitats and, if needed, take specific action to rid infested areas of these habitats; (b) to prompt the creation of a Dengue Volunteer Inspection Team (DeVIT) that would conduct a weekly larval site inspection of community surroundings (not within the definition of homes) and take specific action to rid the area of these habitats; (c) to prompt every individual with fever symptoms to suspect DF and go immediately (at least within one day) to the nearest health clinic for diagnosis and treatment.

The COMBI plan relied on the integration of its five communication action areas and included:

- advocacy and public relations activities to engage key local stakeholders, including politicians;
- the creation of social mobilization units such as (a) 48 DeVITs, which included 615 volunteers and were instrumental in providing advice to 100,956 people, distributing 101,534 flyers and inspecting 1,440 vacant lots; and (b) bicycle riding teams (D'RIDERS), including local youth who were responsible for promoting the project and were accompanied by a van equipped with a public announcement system. At each location, local community leaders and residents greeted the team;
- a comprehensive advertising and public service announcement (PSA) strategy, including 2,000 vertical buntings posted along selected streets of Johor Bahru, a radio PSA in Malay and Chinese, a series of print ads that were carried by local newspapers and featured recommended behaviors;
- a school-based program that provided children and their parents with a single, two-sided self-instructional worksheet/checklist on how to deal with Aedes breeding sites at home was prepared in four languages (Malay, Chinese, English, and Tamil);
- radio talk shows hosted by local doctors to promote COMBI and provide listeners with information on dengue. Listeners were also encouraged to call in with questions; and
- point-of-service promotion sites that were staffed by physicians and other health care providers to explain the behavioral goals of the project to every patient who attended the clinic for any given reason.

At the end of the 12-week campaign, a post-intervention questionnaire survey was used to compare results against baseline data collected before the implementation of COMBI. Respondents were either household heads or anyone above the age of 18 years. Out of 1,712 post-intervention respondents, 926 were considered "paired" respondents. That is, they were the same respondents who had been interviewed during the baseline survey. (Almost all [99%] of the respondents interviewed in the post-survey claimed that they had performed household inspections on Sundays, compared to 71% in the pre-survey.) Short questionnaires were also developed to gather data on treatment-seeking behaviors among patients admitted and diagnosed with dengue in all government hospitals throughout Johore state. Patients admitted into Sultanah Aminah Hospital and Kulai Hospital (government hospitals serving Johor Bahru district) were considered as "cases," while those admitted in hospitals in other districts served as "controls." It was assumed that people who resided in other districts had not been exposed or involved in all the COMBI mobilization and communication activities.

During the 12-week study period, a total of 134 patients admitted into the two government hospitals in Johor Bahru district as well as 146 patients admitted into government hospitals in other districts participated in the study's interviews. Patients admitted into private hospitals were not interviewed. Results show that 59% of those admitted into Johor Bahru government hospitals sought treatment within 24 hours of the onset of the fever compared to 42% among those from control areas ($p > 0.01$). Apart from "exposure to COMBI," there were no associations between other variables and the time between the onset of fever and hospital admission. It was also noted that there was a slight decline in the number of cases in areas where DeVITs were established. No decline was measured in the non-DeVIT areas (Suhaili et al., 2004). A key lesson learned from COMBI's application in dengue prevention and control is that intersectional coordination and active community involvement can be effectively stimulated but must also be accompanied by improvements in the public health infrastructure, epidemiological and entomological surveillance, effective clinical management, emergency preparedness, and reinforcement of health policy and legislation (Parks et al., 2004).

COMBI at UNICEF

Although the WHO experiences are all in the field of health, they provide useful lessons in achieving any kind of behavioral objective in the social development arena. Recently, various UNICEF country offices (UNICEF/Moldova, UNICEF/Kazakhstan, UNICEF/Georgia, UNICEF/Jordan, UNICEF/Cambodia, UNICEF/Albania, UNICEF/Mozambique, and UNICEF/China) have applied the COMBI approach in a variety of programs. They include promotion of iodized salt, perinatal care, antenatal care and tetanus toxoid elimination, youth HIV/AIDS prevention, early childhood development, children and violence, immunization, safe motherhood, infant and young child feeding, environmental education, and juvenile justice. COMBI training has also been carried out for various other UNICEF country and regional offices.

COMBI has also been incorporated in the work of other UN agencies (UNFPA, UNAIDS, UNDP). COMBI programs have also been developed for seasonal flu in France (with the Ministry of Health) and anti-littering in Singapore (with the ministry of the environment and the National Environmental Agency). One of the more compelling stories of COMBI's results is presented in a final evaluation report on an antenatal behavior change intervention using the COMBI approach in Cambodia (Peou & Ram, 2011). It documented a 600% increase (from 6% to nearly 36%) in the percentage of pregnant women who came in for their first antenatal visit within the first 8 weeks of their pregnancy during a year-long COMBI program.

COMBI and Social Marketing

COMBI and social marketing (SM) are both derivatives of the private sector's approach to marketing and marketing communications. Though they share similarities, there are some key differences, which can make for wider acceptability of COMBI in the public sector world of social development. Traditional marketing revolves around the concept of the **4 Ps**: Product, Price, Placement, and Promotion. SM has stuck to this language and the approach implied. One version of SM that has been widely applied in the developing world has been use of the techniques of marketing to sell price-subsidized products treated as "social products," such as condoms, mosquito nets, and oral rehydration salts. This type of SM practice led to an emphasis on branding the subsidized product and then massive promotion of the brand to drive sales, with due attention to Placement. Prices were set at levels that would make the products accessible to major segments of the target audiences and the products' distribution sustainable over time (Agha, Do, & Armand, 2006). Success was measured by amount of sales and awareness of the brand but not necessarily accompanied by use. For example, in Cambodia, everyone will know the name of the top condom brand (the subsidized No.1 condom) and there might even be significant sales, but the consistent use of condoms remains dismally low (Sopheab et al., 2008).

Charging impoverished people any price for the health products they need has been controversial (Sachs, 2006). The SM approach has another limitation when it is applied to behaviors not linked to a tangible product. For example, if we wanted to tackle the mother's behavior of exclusive breastfeeding of babies under six months of age, or "handwashing before feeding your infant," and if we began using the language of "what is the product" we are "selling," the language alone can put off health colleagues. Finally, branding and massive promotion of product benefits would lead to increasing awareness of the brand but not likely lead to massive adoption of the recommended behavior if it faces substantial interpersonal, environmental, or policy barriers. And yet the behavioral communication inherent in marketing can be very useful to achieving behavioral results if marketing can be made more relevant to health communication colleagues in language that goes beyond the 4 Ps, and in a communication strategy that focuses on behavioral results (use, for example) and not just brand recognition or sale of product.

COMBI draws on a different view of marketing: integrated marketing communication (IMC), as described by Robert Lauterborn (in Schultz, Tannenbaum, & Lauterborn, 1993) and refined by Everold Hosein, in relation to health and social development themes. Instead of the language of the 4 Ps and inherent conceptual limitations when applied to health and social development behaviors, IMC offers the language of the **4 Cs**. The 4 Cs are conversationally much more engaging with health and social development professionals than the 4Ps.

Instead of talking about product, one talks about how the recommended behavior, exclusive breastfeeding, serves the first C: the Consumer's (read "mother's") need, want, or desire. We are not selling anything; we are offering a behavior in response to the consumer's sense of her need, want, or desire. This drives us to explore with the mother what are her needs, wants, and desires vis-à-vis her baby, which in turn shapes how we engage and communicate with her. Of course, this approach is fully consistent with best practice social marketing, as exemplified by successful breastfeeding promotion in the context of US Women, Infants and Children's (WIC) clinics (Lindenberger & Bryant, 2000).

Instead of talking about Price, which triggers thoughts of money, we talk about the second C: Cost. Cost is a more embracing term and incorporates money but with some behaviors the far more important concerns of time and effort involved in carrying out the behavior and what some refer to as "opportunity costs." This is much better language with health and social development colleagues as we explore what it "costs" the mother to wash her hands with soap and water before feeding her baby.

Instead of Placement we talk about the third C: Convenience. How convenient is it for the mother to continue exclusive breastfeeding when she needs to go help her husband in the rice field within weeks of coming home with her new baby?

Instead of Promotion, which suggests a one-way beating over the head with the brand name and the virtues of the brand, we talk about integrated, engaged two-way Communication as the fourth C. It indicates a willingness to listen to the consumer and engage. And with the fourth C, COMBI stresses that there is no magical communication intervention and that a primary reliance on mass media promotion is a mistake. Although many SM programs have marvelous media promotion campaigns, COMBI puts the stress on personal selling and interpersonal, door-to-door communication, along the lines of Mary Kay Cosmetics, Avon, and the Church of Latter-day Saints. It also integrates communication actions from health education and social mobilization efforts such as structured community mobilization and involvement and fully engaging all staff of government in executing a COMBI plan.

Above all, just as social marketing practitioners are encouraged to do by experts in the field (Andreasen, 1994), COMBI focuses forcefully on behavioral results and not just sales and brand recognition. When we are exploring in the field why people know what to do but do not act, we find the barriers imbedded in the 4 Cs: we fail to connect what we are offering behaviorally to what the consumer needs, wants, or desires; we fail to explore how the consumers see the costs we ask them to bear in relation to the value of the behavior we promise; we fail to consider how convenient or inconvenient it is for the consumer to carry out a recommended behavior; we fail to engage with consumers at a personal, face-to-face level and listen to their concerns and queries. The foundation of SM and COMBI is in marketing; but COMBI takes a different tack.

Future COMBI Trends

COMBI initially focused on behavioral outcomes in health as part of the social mobilization work of the World Health Organization back in 2000. But over the years, the methodology has been effectively used with regard to an extensive array of non–health-related behavioral expectations. Much of this non-health work has been with UNICEF and UNDP, and one anticipates further expansion of COMBI utilization in other dimensions of social development. One expects to see the COMBI approach used wherever specific behavioral results are desired, whether in society at large with reference to a broad range of social programs, or in large institutions (such as a government ministry itself), or just among networks of policymakers.

With UNICEF, COMBI has been used for achieving behavioral results in a broad range of non-health programs: Juvenile Justice in Moldova and Albania (getting judges and prosecutors not to send juveniles to adult jail but use alternative sentencing); Violence Against Children/Child Protection in Moldova and Albania; Jordan (getting teachers not to hit children or verbally abuse them in the classroom but to adopt alternative nonviolent means to maintain classroom discipline); Environmental Education in Albania (encouraging schoolchildren and their parents to collect plastic bags for recycling); Early Childhood Development in Albania and Moldova (getting parents to read to their infants and young children), and in Albania attempting to get more Roma children enrolled in kindergarten. With UNDP, COMBI has been used in efforts to reduce domestic violence. A major behavior challenge upon us is climate change that raises a host of behavioral expectations on the part of the community and families. One expects that in the future COMBI will be increasingly used in encouraging families and communities to adopt responsible environmental behaviors.

Another future area of COMBI application is in dealing with behavioral issues that confront an increasingly urbanized world. Health and social development programs take on a different shape when implemented in urban settings. The COMBI blend of integrated, synchronized communication actions will need to be reexamined and modified when applied to the urban environment of emerging societies. COMBI in the future will also need to examine carefully and cautiously the use of social media in emerging societies with respect to achieving desired behavioral outcomes. While we have seen the behavioral impact of social media in political mobilization, we have only just begun exploring social media's efficacy with regard to behavioral results in health and social development. Another area of COMBI implementation that will need to be addressed in the future is management of implementation. COMBI plans require exquisite management. In emerging societies, these management skills are often available in the private sector but at a high cost. They are available in some parts of the public sector and are often available in political campaigning. We will need in the future to determine how to insert sharp implementation and managerial capacities in COMBI plans.

And finally, much more detailed attention will need to be paid to measuring the behavioral impact of COMBI. Although there have been a few carefully documented impact studies, too often impact is perceived anecdotally, and there is little financial interest in pursuing deliberate studies of behavioral impact. The ultimate end goal of almost all of our social development initiatives are behavioral: we want somebody to do something. In health communication and promotion, the behavioral imperative is paramount. We hope the application of

COMBI will expand in response to these health-related behavioral challenges, going beyond knowledge and information to action.

Entertainment Education

The second major communication approach described in this chapter is entertainment education (EE). EE (in its original and best-studied form) uses engaging fictional stories to teach audience members about (a) a health or social problem, (b) actions they could take to avoid or solve the problem, and (c) possible barriers to and consequences of those actions.

What Is EE?

Man has been described as *homo narrans*, the story-telling animal (Fisher, 1984). Narratives have the power to make experiences coherent and memorable, to shape attitudes and perceptions, and to influence transactions between people (Bruner, 1990; Schank & Berman, 2002). In turn, a narrative can be reinforced or edited in the course of social interaction (Bruner, 1990).

Individuals and societies are headed for trouble if they cannot adapt their narratives to respond to new threats and opportunities (Galavotti et al., 2005). One way to encourage large audiences to adapt their narratives in positive ways is to employ the EE approach. It has been defined as "purposely designing and implementing a media message to both entertain and educate, in order to increase audience members' knowledge about an educational issue, create favorable attitudes, shift social norms, and change overt behavior" (Singhal & Rogers, 2004, p. 5).

EE interventions can take multiple forms (see Table 5.1). To date, however, some of the most broadly reaching and best known EE applications have been serialized, fictional, dramatic narratives that were broadcast on radio or television. Internationally, health and its social determinants (e.g., women's equality) have been key EE topics.

How Does EE Fit With COMBI?

After planners have taken the initial steps of the COMBI process (i.e., after they have specified a behavioral objective, and conducted **formative research** to understand target audience motivations and constraints), EE can be considered as a communication vehicle. EE broadcasts can either stand alone or be part of a multipronged communication intervention that includes face-to-face interaction. Analogous to the COMBI tenet that mounting communication interventions at several system levels has a synergistic effect, EE is thought to work best when it is supplemented two ways. First, exposure to the health or development message should be amplified by encouraging or actually structuring face-to-face discussions of the health issue depicted in the broadcast storyline. Second, services relevant to the EE topic should be made more accessible and user friendly. Mobilizing interpersonal discussion opportunities and health services has been described as the "ground cover" that complements the broadcast "air cover" in an EE intervention (Singhal et al., 2004).

Table 5.1 Technology Theme: Examples of Media Used for EE Other Than Radio and Television

Medium	Country	Story/Show	Health Topic[1]
Folk performance[2]	India	*Taru*[4]	Reproductive health care Educating lower-caste children
Animated cartoon	Bangladesh, and on to much of South Asia	*Meena*[5]	Nutritional needs of girls
Comic book[3]	Aboriginal Canada	*It Takes a Village*[6]	Healthy pregnancies
Puppetry	South Africa	*Puppets Against AIDS*[7]	How HIV infection occurs, other facts about HIV/AIDS
Computer game	United States	*Heart Sense Game*[8]	Cardiovascular disease symptom recognition
Tweet	United States	*Army Wives*[9]	Traumatic brain injury[12]
Popular song	United States	*Dog Doggety*[10]	Picking up dog litter
Internet	United States	*Retratos de la Vida Real (Photographs of real life)*[11]	Breast cancer screening among Hispanic women

[1] Several stories or shows dealt with multiple topics.
[2] One of a number of subcategories within EE theater, which comprises such formats as street theater, clown theater, teen theater, and interactive/participatory theater.
[3] Similar to the longer, nonserialized graphic novel format.
[4] Singhal et al. (2004).
[5] McKee, Aghi, and Shahzadi (2004).
[6] Hunt (2012).
[7] Skinner et al. (1991).
[8] Silverman et al. (2003);
[9] *Hollywood, Health & Society (HH&S)(a,b)*,(n.d.).
[10] Luther (n.d.).
[11] Jibaja et al. (2000).
[12] One of several transmedia elements (i.e., Facebook page, website content, links to vetted information sources) included with a six-episode story arc on the *Army Wives* TV series as a result of an HH&S collaboration.

One key difference between EE and most other candidate COMBI communication strategies is that EE *emphasizes* entertainment *over* education, at least in terms of explicit content. The EE approach is thought to work best when a health message is introduced only after an audience has become involved with characters and engaged by a plot (Barker & Sabido, 2005).

How Did EE Start?

The idea that broadcasts should educate as well as entertain goes back at least as far as 1922 when the British Broadcasting Corporation (BBC) received its royal charter, but it was not until the early 1970s that a systematic set of steps for narrative EE was laid out. Miguel Sabido, a Mexican television executive, observed a phenomenal audience response to a telenovella (a six-to-nine-month soap opera series) called *Simplemente Maria* that was broadcast on a commercial station in Peru. The melodrama depicted an illiterate girl who comes down from her mountain village to work as a maid in Lima. Maria becomes pregnant when she is seduced by a young medical student, who then abandons her. She learns to read in night classes and begins a sewing business. Overcoming a variety of challenges, Maria raises her child successfully, prospers financially, and eventually marries her reading teacher who has been a quietly loyal friend and advocate for decades (Singhal, Obregon, & Rogers, 1994). What caught Sabido's attention was that people who saw *Simplemente Maria* enrolled in literacy classes in record numbers, and sales of sewing machines skyrocketed (Singhal & Rogers, 1989a).

Realizing that this type of story could be employed with the purpose of encouraging positive audience behaviors, Sabido mapped out a formula for a behavior-change melodrama (Barker & Sabido, 2005). Along with guidance for formative research (which he considered essential) and prescriptions for artistic elements such as dramatic tone and story arc, the Sabido method includes (a) a positive role model character who practices a recommended behavior, (b) a negative role model character who resists the recommendation and suffers a harsh fate, and (c) a transitional character who is initially resistant but eventually decides to adopt the behavior, overcoming a series of barriers to perform it successfully. The transitional character's action is rewarded by positive, culturally valued consequences.

Sabido executed this formula for the first time in 1977 in a nine-month series called *Acompáñame* (*Accompany Me*); during the year of the broadcasts, there was a 33% increase over the previous year in enrollment in Mexican family planning clinics (Poindexter, 2004). After producing several other Mexican television and radio dramas that dealt with family planning, Sabido and some of his international colleagues met with Prime Minister Indira Gandhi and convinced her of the potential value of such a series in India. Beginning in July 1984, *Hum Log* (*We People*) ran for 18 months, with as many as 90% of potential viewers tuning in for key episodes. Approximately 70% of viewers who were later surveyed said that they had learned lessons about the status of women and limiting family size from the show (Singhal & Rogers, 1989b). Since then, with support from technical assistance organizations and international donors, hundreds of EE series have been developed and broadcast in many places in the developing world, including Africa, South America, the Caribbean, the Philippines, Southeast and Southern Asia, and China.

Theorists Explain EE Effects Mechanisms

Social cognitive theory (SCT, originally social learning theory) influenced EE from the outset (Bandura, 1977). The theory is complex and continues to evolve, as detailed in chapter 4. In simple terms, early versions of SCT predicted that if an individual believes that (a) most other people behave a certain way, (b) a behavior would be possible with effort, and (c) the benefits of the behavior outweigh its costs, then the intention to perform the behavior would form, and the behavior itself would be likely to follow. The three beliefs are fostered by observation of a role model who attempts the behavior, eventually succeeds after overcoming barriers, and enjoys positive consequences. It is readily apparent that the arc of the health subplot in a Sabido-style drama mirrors this early version of SCT, providing viewers with an opportunity for observational or **vicarious learning**.

Later versions of SCT (Bandura, 1997) address vicarious learning also on a community scale, arguing that (a) simultaneous exposure to the role model can provoke discussions (and perhaps reinterpretations) of the observed events, (b) such discussions can lead to changes in collective norms and efficacy and positive outcome expectancies (i.e., the perceptions that collective action is appropriate, possible, and likely to succeed), and (c) these changes can lead to collective behavior. Collective action (which can extend into the public policy arena) can loop back to shape individual behavior, an iterative process that Bandura called "reciprocal determinism." Evidence from several recent studies supports the predictions about collective behavior, attitudes about policy, and concrete policy activity that one would make on the basis of SCT (see discussion on Soul City below) (Kennedy et al., 2011; Marcus et al., 2010; Murphy et al., 2012; Nahm et al., 2010; Slater, Rouner & Long, 2006).

EE researchers have also applied (or invoked post hoc) general theories of behavior change other than SCT. For example, Kennedy and colleagues (2004) maintained that the original version of the Health Belief Model (HBM) (Rosenstock, Stretcher, & Becker, 1988), a simpler theory than SCT, was sufficient to explain dramatic spikes in calls to the HIV/STD hotline that followed two episodes of *Bold & Beautiful* (B&B), an afternoon soap opera in the United States. In HBM, when people perceive themselves to be at risk of a health problem and consider it serious, they are likely to take action to reduce their risk, especially when prompted or cued to do so. The first B&B episode featured Tony, a non–drug-using heterosexual man who was diagnosed with HIV. The second episode included Tony's disclosure of his HIV status to his fiancée Kristen. Most American audience members already believed that HIV infection was a serious health problem and had the ability to make a phone call, but may not have had a personalized sense of HIV risk. The HIV plot points may have increased perceptions of risk among heterosexual audience members, the majority of whom were women, and hotline public service announcements on the show may have served as cues to action. If increases in health information-seeking behavior can be explained by a relatively simple theory, more shows might be able to accommodate EE elements.

Recently, in the hope of strengthening EE effectiveness in the future, scholars have turned to communication theory for insights into the mechanisms of narrative effects. One theory, the Transportation Imagery Model (TIM) (Green & Brock, 2000), holds that transporting narratives, those that are so engaging that they impart a sense of being carried away into a fictional world, are the ones that have the power to change knowledge, attitudes, and behavior. TIM originally dealt with written narratives, but the findings of several recent studies of televised EE have been consistent with TIM predictions (Kennedy et al., 2011; Murphy et al., 2011; Murphy et al., 2012). A similar theory, the Extended Elaboration Likelihood Model (Slater & Rouner, 2002), adds emphasis on becoming involved with the character, which has been referred to as developing a "parasocial" relationship. Indeed, identifying with or liking/respecting a character has been linked empirically to an openness to persuasive health messages embedded in a story (e.g., Moyer-Gusé, Chung & Jain, 2011; Sharf et al., 1996; Wilkin et al., 2007).

In the past few years, some attention has been paid to the effects of genre (e.g., comedy vs. drama) within the broader narrative category. Genre effects appear to be complicated. For example, although humor may have some advantages, particularly for a frightening subject like cancer, there is some evidence that humor can trivialize the importance of a health issue, at least among certain audience segments (Moyer-Gusé, Mahood, & Brookes, 2011). Nonetheless, in the United States, televised situation comedy series such as *Desperate Housewives* and *Girlfriends* have been receptive to consultation with health experts and have broadcast storylines about serious illnesses such as HIV and lymphoma. The genre of so-called "reality television" presents another quandary in that it is obviously based on formulas (if not completely scripted) and is very popular worldwide, but does not always count positive role models among its array of characters (Singhal & Rogers, 2004).

Additional theories that have been used in EE scholarship were listed by Sood, Menard, and Witte in a 2004 review; they also noted a need for new theoretical and empirical studies of EE effects on the emotions of an audience member and on community empowerment.

Furthermore, there is debate about the relative merits of using one intact theory versus variables from various theories to guide formative research, script development, and EE outcome evaluation. In at least one instance, a composite theoretical model proved useful for evaluation purposes. Several authors integrated the transtheoretical or "stages of change" model (DiClemente & Prochaska, 1985) with SCT and other theories in their evaluation of *Twende na Wakati*. They generated a six-stage model of communication effects that reflects the fact that many social and behavioral changes are processes that take place gradually over time. A staged outcome measure allowed them to detect change in the treatment district (i.e., significant movement through stages of adoption of family planning) that was not observed in the comparison district.

EE and Entertainment Industry Outreach in the United States

In many developing countries, broadcast content is under the control of a governmental ministry of culture charged with enhancing public well-being. In the United States, by contrast, the content of broadcast shows is controlled by the entertainment industry and is largely driven by profit motives. Air time on major television network and cable channels in the United States can be bought in some cases, but it is extremely expensive. Thus, instead of creating an entire EE series to convey health information and securing air time to broadcast the series, American health experts have engaged in **entertainment industry outreach**. Its goal is to collaborate with the writers and producers of ongoing commercial television series to include health storylines in one or more episodes.

This kind of EE reaches millions of viewers in the United States, including regular viewers who are most prone to learn about health topics from television (Beck & Pollard, 2000). However, the collaborations are often on an uncomfortably tight timeline, at least from the perspective of a methodical scientist. In addition, entertainment industry partners retain complete creative control over show content, and this can be anxiety provoking to health experts accustomed to extensive peer review and/or audience testing prior to any public release of information.

Nonetheless, experts on both sides of the art–health science exchange have described their interactions as productive and satisfying (Hollywood, Health & Society [HH&C(b)], n.d.). Injury, disease, and death are compelling topics with inherent drama. Many Hollywood writers and producers write about these topics routinely, and appreciate getting relevant, timely, credible, and understandable health information from health experts. The "creatives" also benefit from new health story ideas. For their parts, health experts need introductions to entertainment professionals who are considering or working on stories with health themes. Health experts may also need assistance in translating scientific or medical knowledge into less technical terms.

In the United States, a number of entities have facilitated exchanges between health experts and the entertainment industry. Some of these organizations and agencies focus on one or two health issues. For example, the Entertainment Industries Council was founded in 1983 to promote inclusion of information about substance abuse and mental health issues in entertainment offerings. The Kaiser Family Foundation and the White House Office of National Drug Control Policy offer information on the topics of sexual health and drug abuse, respectively. By contrast, Hollywood, Health & Society (HH&S), a program of the Norman Lear Center of the University of Southern California's Annenberg School for Communication and Journalism, has supported public health–entertainment industry exchanges on a wide range of health topics since 2001. More recently, the Fielding School of Public Health at the University of California at Los Angeles (UCLA) established the Media Center for Impact on Global Health specifically to promote and support the development of entertainment and news stories with the potential to make a difference in international health outcomes.

Data on HH&S activities are available for online examination; examining just these records, it becomes apparent that many creative professionals have been open to public health outreach. In the past several years, HH&S staff have made or organized hundreds of presentations and briefings, led several story tours for entertainment media professionals (including tours to South Africa and India), written scores of tip sheets, and worked with more than 91 series, resulting in 877 confirmed air dates [HH&S, c, d] n.d.). Moreover, HH&S outreach to Telemundo, a major Spanish language station, has expanded EE programming to resident and migrating Hispanics in the United States and audiences in other Latin American countries (e.g., Wilkin et al., 2007). Finally, in several cases, HH&S has been successful in arranging for the on-show promotion of public service announcements, toll-free information numbers, websites, and/or social media offerings (e.g., Nahm et al., 2010), thereby linking viewers to more in-depth, personalized, interactive health information.

There are EE promotion organizations in Europe and elsewhere in the developed world as well. However, compared with their US counterparts, they typically function on a smaller scale and are organized around the academic interests and professional consultations of individual EE researchers. Nonetheless, they have made very important contributions to EE research, theory, and practice in both their home countries and internationally. One prize-winning example is the Center for Media and Health in the Netherlands, headed by Dr. Martine Bouman.

Long-Running Shows

Several shows have made long-term commitments to educating the public on health issues. An early example is the BBC's *The Archers,* which has been broadcast in Great Britain since 1951 (Singhal & Rogers, 2004). A prime example in the United States is *Sesame Street;* via its Muppets (puppets created by Jim Henson), generations of American children have learned for example, that eating fruits and vegetables is important and can be fun (Kotler, Shiffman, & Hanson, 2012).

Similarly, the developing world has long-running programs in the EE genre, which they refer to as "edutainment." Beginning in 1994 in South Africa, 12 *Soul City* television series have been broadcast by the Soul City Institute for Health Development Communication. Each series has a health focus such as HIV transmission from mother to child, violence against women, or alcohol abuse. Extensive formative research is conducted on the topic prior to crafting the episodes to maximize their potential for increasing public awareness of the issue and changing relevant attitudes and behavior. The institute also sponsors community activities connected to the year's topic. In 1999, the fourth *Soul City* series modeled a neighborhood response to domestic violence: encircling the perpetrator's home during an incident of abuse and banging loudly on pots and pans to shame him. Evaluations of the show detected effects on several levels; it built self-efficacy with regard to escaping abuse among abused women, prompted a tremendous increase in the numbers of calls to a domestic abuse help line, raised self-awareness of the inappropriateness of abuse among perpetrators, and spurred **collective efficacy** in communities that had previously had a norm of silence around physical abuse. After the series aired, other patrons of a township pub banged bottles when a man beat his girlfriend in the bar. The storyline also prompted police training in taking domestic violence seriously (Soul City, 2000; Usdin et al., 2004).

The Soul City Institute has branched out to offer another ongoing multimedia program, *Soul Buddyz,* to promote the well-being and aspirations of preteen youth. In addition, the institute provides technical assistance in EE to other countries in the region. Native-language *Soul City* broadcasts and related activities are now underway in several countries in southern Africa.

For younger children, the *Sesame Street* model has been recreated and adapted for local audiences in more than 150 countries around the world with technical assistance from the Writer's Workshop. Data indicate that children in Tanzania who were exposed to *Kilimani Sesame* (the local version of *Sesame Street*) knew significantly more about malaria than other children in that country (Borzekowski & Macha, 2010). The South African version of the show, *Takalani Sesame,* features Kami, a little girl Muppet described as "fun-loving" and "HIV+" (Sesame Workshop, n.d.). Researchers found that, compared to children who did not see the show (which is thought to reach 70% of urban children and 50% of rural children), young viewers were four times more likely to have accurate information about HIV and five times more likely to think

HIV should be destigmatized (e.g., that one should play with a child who is HIV-positive; Khulisa Management Services, 2005).

Syndication, Cross-Fertilization, and Diffusion Initiatives

To date, most of the international dissemination of the Sabido-style EE approach has resulted from the remarkable work of a handful of researchers (e.g., Everett Rogers and Arvin Singhal), nongovernmental organizations (e.g., Population Communications International), and major university-based centers (e.g., the Johns Hopkins University Center for Communication Programs, https://www.jhuccp.org/). But increasingly, entertainment professionals and television shows cross national boundaries and influence the diffusion of information and perspectives. For example, after a 2012 tour of South Africa sponsored by HH&S for American writers and producers, an episode of the broadcast television series *Touch* on the US Fox channel portrayed a community response to domestic abuse in South Africa (de Castro Buffington, 2012), clearly reflecting the *Soul City* storyline described previously. There is also potential for "grassroots" influence in the other direction, that is, from the US entertainment industry to foreign audiences. The top US prime time shows are eventually syndicated in reruns in approximately 100 countries (de Castro Buffington, 2012).

An assessment of the effects of this diffused exposure is in its infancy. It has been observed that residents of Botswana who were exposed to an HIV/AIDS storyline on the syndicated soap opera *Bold & Beautiful* scored significantly lower on a scale of AIDS stigma than others in that country who had not seen the show (O'Leary et al., 2007). In addition, viewing an episode of *Law & Order: Special Victims Unit* that dealt with rape in the Republic of Congo was found to be associated with knowledge gains and discussions about global health among audience members in the United States who identified with one of the characters, and support for international aid among viewers who were transported by the narrative (Murphy et al., 2012). Based on the scant available data, the effects of such "EE without borders" appear to have been positive, but more technical support for and study of these imported and exported offerings is needed.

Several universities have established or assisted new centers to address this need. HH&S recently helped create centers for EE in India and Nigeria (de Castro Buffington, 2012). These centers link local formative research and in-country creative expertise in the major media markets that serve their respective developing countries. UCLA's new Center for Impact on Global Health will reach out to these markets and others (e.g., in Latin America). The objective of increasing EE capacity in "Bollywood" and "Nollywood" and other entertainment industry capitals is to produce entertainment storylines that are rich in socially provocative content and appropriate for local cultural contexts.

EE Research and Evaluation

Several evaluations of EE broadcasts are summarized next. The EE effects uncovered by this research, the soundness of the research designs employed, and some of the important questions that remain unanswered are outlined.

Effects of Sabido-Style EE in Low- and Middle-Income Countries

Special surveys, routine indicator surveillance, and sales data have typically shown temporal associations between EE broadcasts in the developing world, and gains in outcomes such as valuing smaller family sizes and sales of contraceptives (Poindexter, 2004). Admittedly, the EE narratives were probably not solely responsible for the large-scale changes in attitudes and behaviors that have been observed. Simultaneous efforts to promote family planning were being undertaken by governments and nongovernmental organizations. However, the rare evaluation rigorous enough to disentangle the effects of EE broadcasts from the effects of concurrent social and behavior change strategies has tended to support the view that Sabido-style EE has made a unique contribution to change in developing countries.

One early example of a well-controlled study of Sabido-style EE outcomes was the evaluation of *Twende na Wakati* (*Let's Go With the Times*), an HIV/AIDS prevention radio series broadcast in Tanzania between 1993 and 1997. For the first two years, the show was aired in all districts of the country but one, which constituted a comparison field site in a natural quasi-experiment. Random sample surveys with adults were conducted by personal interview; sample sizes each year exceeded 2,500. Compared with the comparison area, significant increases in HIV/AIDS knowledge, discussion of the issue with others, the perception of being at risk personally, self-efficacy with regard to taking a prevention measure, and actual adoption of a preventive behavior (especially limiting the number of sex partners) were observed in the "treatment" area (Vaughan et al., 2000).

Effects of EE in the United States

Research has shown that, in the United States, viewers of health storylines integrated into ongoing afternoon soap operas and evening dramas learn about health from the shows, change their attitudes accordingly, seek more health information, and change (or intend to change) their behavior to promote health and well-being. In addition to examples of findings cited elsewhere in this chapter, there have been documented increases in knowledge about emergency contraception (Brodie et al., 2001), intentions to be tested for syphilis (Whittier et al., 2005), intentions to be tested for the BRCA gene for breast cancer (Hether et al., 2008), and intentions to donate organs (Morgan, Movius, & Cody, 2009). Many of the study designs have been subject to threats to validity, especially self-selection of exposure to the shows. Still, the conclusion that EE effects are reliably detectable, at least in the short-term aftermath of the shows, is warranted by the accumulated body of evidence.

Consensus-Based Applied EE Research Agendas

More research is needed to deepen our understanding of psychosocial mechanisms of EE effects in order to make the technique more powerful in the future. Some practical questions of interest to developers of EE products and sponsors of EE outreach to the entertainment industry have also been raised. Two expert panels were convened by (CDC) the Centers for Disease Control

Table 5.2 Behavior Change Theme: Expert Recommendations for Priority Topics for Applied Research in EE

Source	Priority Research Question
General audience agenda	In what ways are health issues and concerns portrayed in entertainment programming?
	What is the potential for "mixed messages" when health topics are portrayed in entertainment programs?
	What are the separate and combined effects of EE, structured interpersonal communication accompanying EE messages, and integration of EE messages with other communication vehicles such as the Internet?
	What EE "dosage" is necessary for adoption of pro-health practices?
	How can we promote community discussion of EE offerings?
	How can we increase the duration of EE effects?
	How can we reduce oppositional or "boomerang" effects of EE exposure?
Multicultural agenda	What is the "right" kind of humor, i.e., culturally sensitive humor that can take the edge off taboo topics, increase attention, comprehension, and recall?
	How many distinct audiences exist and how many is it feasible to target?
	What impact will acculturation have on EE efforts?

and its partners to come to consensus on EE research priorities from a pragmatic public health perspective (Greenberg et al., 2004; Murphy & Cody, 2003; Salmon, 2000). See Table 5.2 for examples of the questions highlighted by the expert panelists.

Since 2003, the first question in the general audience section of Table 5.2 has been addressed by the HH&S monitoring project, which has tracked treatment of 70 health topics in the shows that are most popular among general, African American, and Hispanic audiences in the United States according to Nielsen ratings. The researchers overseeing the project have published revealing reports on depictions of specific issues such as sex roles, as well as general surveys of health content (Hether & Murphy, 2010; Murphy, Hether, & Rideout, 2008; Pariera et al., 2014).

Future EE Research Directions

As communication satellites proliferate, and high-speed Internet becomes more accessible and reliable, the reach of broadcast EE will continue to expand. In addition, interactive EE formats are likely to grow in number and popularity. These emerging media trends raise both narrowly focused and very general questions. It would be helpful to know, for example, whether allowing audience members to make choices about characters and plots—thereby blurring the line between audience and story-teller—affects engagement with the narrative and, in turn, the influence the narrative will have on health knowledge, attitudes, and behaviors. Thinking broadly, health policymakers will want to understand how to avoid diluting the effectiveness of EE through overuse, and whether strategic national EE priorities would hamper creativity and thus diminish possible benefits.

EE Evaluation Challenges

There are three basic challenges to broadcast EE evaluation. The first is that exposure to the broadcasts is elected by viewers, not randomly assigned.

This means that there is no adequate comparison group for research purposes. Viewers may well be different from nonviewers in ways that matter with regard to a desired health outcome, both before and after the show. The second challenge is that viewers talk to nonviewers about the show's content, and other shows or community services provide information on the focal same health topic, thus "contaminating" a "no-treatment" comparison group. A third challenge is that it is usually too expensive or too difficult logistically to identify and follow over time enough individual viewers to examine long-term effects of EE exposure on health behaviors. This is especially true if the behaviors must be repeated over time (e.g., wearing condoms or eating fruits and vegetables). Of course, cost and practical challenges are compounded when measuring EE effects on actual health conditions, particularly those like cancer, that can take decades to develop.

In general, research design strategies that address any one of these challenges are still subject to the other threats to the validity of their findings. For example, one could add a question about exposure to an EE broadcast to an already funded national health survey conducted at regular intervals. That would generate a large, longitudinal sample inexpensively, but the survey findings based on a large sample size obtained by adding a question about having seen an EE storyline would still be marred by viewer self-selection bias. Conversely, addressing self-selection bias by doing a small controlled experiment (e.g., by randomizing with college students to either a show-exposed or a show-unexposed condition) would invite charges that the findings were irrelevant to large groups at risk in the real world.

Because EE is such an efficient way to reach so many high-risk audience members, evaluators are looking to fields like econometrics for innovative evaluation solutions. One possible solution for the self-selection problem in data from large surveys involves devising a statistical model of the likelihood (or "propensity") for an audience member to be exposed to a show and then controlling for this propensity in subsequent models of the effects of exposure on health outcomes (Yanovitzky, Zanutto, & Hornik, 2005). Even the propensity scoring approach has its critics. They argue that (a) the variables required for a robust propensity model are hard to predict in advance and absent from or poorly measured in most large data sets, (b) the final models are still essentially correlational and do not justify causal claims, and (c) findings based on models with propensity scores rarely turn out to be very different from models without those scores (Weitzen et al., 2005).

In the end, practitioners and funders will probably have to judge EE effectiveness by means of evidence triangulation. That is, they must assemble findings from various study designs with complementary strengths and weaknesses to form a mosaic picture of the impact of this health promotion approach. Commendably, some researchers have already begun to use multiple and complementary research methods within single evaluation studies, at the same that they bring to bear new approaches (e.g., using local ratings of other TV shows to control for geographic propensity to be exposed to an EE offering) (Kearney & Levine, 2015).

Finally, as we seek to understand how EE works in traditional and new media formats, we should bear in mind that a series of sound scientific findings does not add up to a good story. Cultural competence and artistic talent provided by members of EE teams from the creative arts will remain indispensable. Collaborations between health experts and the entertainment industry should continue to be supported around the world.

Summary

This chapter has described two approaches to health communication, COMBI and EE, that draw insights for motivating health behavior change from the broadly successful commercial marketing and entertainment spheres. The approaches overlap to some degree, in that EE can be the format that COMBI planners select for conveying a health message. Furthermore, both approaches emphasize collaboration with stakeholders and audience research. Moreover, both COMBI and EE are based on the understanding that, in many if not most cases, simply imparting factual information about health risks is insufficient to change relevant human behavior, at least over the long term. By treating human emotions, desires, and circumstances as centrally important, both COMBI and EE have accumulated impressive track records of behavior change. If health communication resources are to be managed wisely, COMBI and EE have key roles to play.

KEY TERMS

1. **Collective efficacy:** The jointly held view that a group of people would be capable of successfully performing a certain action, if attempted
2. **Communication for Behavioral Impact (COMBI):** A complex, multilevel approach to behavior change that incorporates an integrated marketing perspective
3. **Communication keys (CK):** Communication content and other strategies for opening the door to audience engagement in consideration of behavior change
4. **Entertainment education:** The practice of transmitting a media message designed to both entertain and educate, in order to increase audience members' knowledge about an educational issue, create favorable attitudes, shift social norms, and change overt behavior
5. **Entertainment industry outreach:** Activities undertaken by public health entities to encourage commercial entertainment providers to disseminate health messages in the course of their regular programming
6. **Formative research:** Also called formative evaluation, exploratory research conducted prior to an intervention in order to inform its content and structure
7. **4 Cs:** Factors to take into account in planning a COMBI offering, including the consumer's needs/wants/desires; the tangible and intangible cost of behavior change; convenience; and communication

8. **4 Ps:** Factors involved in traditional marketing: product, price, placement, and promotion
9. **Indicators:** Measures of a program's activities or outcomes, often drawn from routinely collected information
10. **Situational market analysis:** A consumer-focused approach that involves learning from audience members about their perceptions and understanding of a behavior and its costs, benefits, barriers, and facilitators
11. **SMART behavioral objective:** A statement of the desired outcome of an intervention that is specific, measurable, achievable, realistic, and time bound
12. **Vicarious learning:** Learning that takes place when one person has the opportunity to observe another person behaving in a certain way and reaping certain rewards or punishments

REVIEW QUESTIONS

1. Using the example of using antimalarial bednets, what are some of the situational barriers to health behavior change that a consumer in the developing world might face?
2. Beyond the individuals who stand to avoid health problems by practicing a new behavior, who should be included in research and planning for a COMBI intervention?
3. What were the various elements of the dengue prevention COMBI project in Malaysia?
4. What are some foreseeable future trends in the practice of COMBI?
5. How are COMBI and EE alike and how do they differ?
6. What forms does EE take internationally and in the United States?
7. Which theories have been used to explain the mechanisms of EE effects?
8. How is EE in the developing world relevant to public health in the United States and vice versa?
9. What questions do trends toward media interactivity raise for EE practitioners and theorists?
10. From which field may EE evaluators draw analysis techniques to reduce bias in studies of the effectiveness of EE offerings, and what is an example of such a technique?

References

Agha, S., Do, M., & Armand, F. (2006). When donor support ends: The fate of social marketing products and the markets they help create. *Social Marketing Quarterly, 12*(2), 28–42.

Andreasen, A. R. (1994). Social marketing: Its definition and domain. *Journal of Public Policy and Marketing, 13*(1), 108–114.

Badcock-Walters, P., Kelly, M., & Gorgens, M. (2004). *Does knowledge equal change?* Paper commissioned for the Education for All Global Monitoring Report 2005, The Quality Imperative. New York, NY: UNESCO.

Bandura, A. (1977). *Social learning theory.* Englewood Cliffs, NJ: Prentice Hall.

Bandura, A. (1997). *Self-efficacy: The exercise of control.* New York, NY: Freeman.

Barker, K., & Sabido, M. (Eds.). (2005). *Soap operas for social change to prevent HIV/AIDS: A training guide for journalists and media personnel.* Shelborne, VT: Population Media Center. Retrieved from http://www.populationmedia.org/wp-content/uploads/2008/01/unfpa_training_guide.pdf

Beck, V., & Pollard, W. (2000). *Soap opera viewers and health information: 1999 Healthstyles survey executive summary.* Presented at the 128th APHA meeting. Boston, MA. November 12–16.

Borzekowski, D.L.G., & Macha, J. E. (2010). The role of *Kilimani Sesame* in the healthy development of Tanzanian preschool children. *Journal of Applied Developmental Psychology, 31*, 298–305.

Brodie, M., Foehr, U., Rideout, V., Baer, N., Miller, C., Flournoy, R., & Altman, D. (2001). Communicating health information through the entertainment media. *Health Affairs, 20*(1), 192–199. PubMed PMID: 11194841

Bruner, J. S. (1990). *Acts of meaning.* Boston, MA: Harvard University Press.

de Castro Buffington, S. (2012, November). Storytelling is strong medicine: Entertainment becomes a force for global social change. *Monthly Development*, 1–4. Retrieved from https://hollywoodhealthandsociety.org/sites/default/files/whats-new/strong_medicine.pdf

DiClemente, C. C., & Prochaska, J. O. (1985). Processes and stages of change: Coping and competence in smoking behavior change. In S. Shiffman & T.A. Willis (Eds.), *Coping and substance abuse* (pp. 319–334). San Diego, CA: Academic Press.

Doherty, T. M., McCoy, D., & Donohue, S. (2005). Health system constraints to optimal coverage of the prevention of mother-to-child HIV transmission programme in South Africa: lessons from the implementation of the national pilot programme. *African Health Sciences, 5*, 213–218.

Fisher, W. R. (1984). Narration as a human communication paradigm: The case of public moral argument. *Communication Monographs, 51*(March), 1–22.

Galavotti, C., Petraglia, J., Harford, N., Kraft, J. M., Pappas-DeLuca, K. A., & Kuhlman, A. S. (2005). New narratives for Africa: Using stories to fight HIV-AIDS. *Story-telling, Self and Society, 1*(2), 26–37.

Green, M. C., & Brock, T. C. (2000). The role of transportation in the persuasiveness of public narratives. *Journal of Personality and Social Psychology, 79*(5), 701–721.

Greenberg, B. S., Salmon, C. T., Patel, D., Beck, V. & Cole, G. (2004). Evolution of an EE research agenda. In A. Singhal, M.J. Cody, E. M., Rogers, & M. Sabido (Eds.), *Entertainment-education and social change* (pp. 191–206). Mahwah, NJ: Erlbaum.

Gubler, D. J. (1998). Dengue and dengue hemorrhagic fever. *Clinical Microbiology Reviews, 11*(3), 480–496.

Gulliford, M., Figueroa-Munoz, J., Morgan, M., Hughes, D., Gibson, B., Beech, R., & Hudson, M. (2002). What does "access to health care" mean? *Journal of Health Services Research and Policy, 7*(3), 186–188.

Haines, A., Kuruvilla, S., & Borchert, M. (2004). Bridging the implementation gap between knowledge and action for health. *Bulletin of the World Health Organization, 82*(10), 724–732.

Hether, H. J., Huang, G., Beck, V., Murphy, S. T., & Valente, T. W. (2008). Entertainment-education in a media-saturated environment: Examining the impact of single and multiple exposures to breast cancer storylines on two popular medical dramas. *Journal of Health Communication, 13*(7), 808–823.

Hether, H. J., & Murphy, S. T. (2010). Sex roles in health storylines in prime time television: A content analysis. *Sex Roles, 62*, 810–821.

Hollywood, Health & Society. (a). (n.d.). *Transmedia outreach.* Retrieved from http://hollywoodhealthandsociety.org/transmedia-outreach

Hollywood, Health & Society. (b). (n.d.). *Testimonials.* Retrieved from http://hollywoodhealthandsociety.org/about-us/industry-talk

Hollywood, Health & Society. (c). (n.d.). *History and stats.* Retrieved from http://hollywoodhealthandsociety.org/about-us/history-stats

Hollywood, Health & Society. (d). (n.d.) *Calendar.* Retrieved from http://hollywoodhealthandsociety.org/events/?event_type=2

Hosein, E., Parks, W., & Schiavo, R. (2009). Communication-for-Behavioral-Impact: An integrated model for health and social change. In R. J. DiClemente, R. A. Crosby, & M. Kegler (Eds.), *Emerging theories in health promotion practice and research* (2nd ed., pp. 536–550). San Francisco, CA: Jossey-Bass.

Hunt, C. A. (2012, September 6). Comic book teaches healthy pregnancy to Canadian Aboriginals. *Examiner.* Retrieved from http://www.examiner.com/article/comic-book-teaches-healthy-pregnancy-to-canadian-aboriginals

Jibaja, M. L., Kingery, P., Neff, N. E., Smith, Q., Bowman, J., & Holcomb, J. D. (2000). Tailored, interactive soap operas for breast cancer education of high-risk Hispanic women. *Journal of Cancer Education, 15*(4), 237–242. PubMed PMID: 11199243

Kearney, M. S., & Levine, P. B. (2015). Investigating recent trends in the teen birthrate. *Journal of Health Econimics, 41*, 15–29.

Kennedy, M. G., O'Leary, A., Beck, V., Pollard, K., & Simpson, P. (2004). Increases in calls to the CDC National STD and AIDS Hotline following AIDS-related episodes in a soap opera. *Journal of Communication, 54*, 287–301.

Kennedy, M. G., Turf, E. E., Wilson-Genderson, M., Wells, K., Huang, G. C., & Beck, V. (2011). Effects of a television drama about environmental exposure to toxic substances. *Public Health Reports, 126*(Suppl. 1), 150–159. PMID: 21563723

Khulisa Management Services. (2005). Impact assessment of *Takalani Sesame* season II programme. Johannesburg, South Africa: Author.

Kotler, J. A., Schiffman, J. M., & Hanson, K. G. (2012). The influence of media characters on children's food choices. *Journal of Health Communication, 17*(8), 886–898.

Lindenberger, J. H., & Bryant, C. A. (2000). Promoting breastfeeding in the WIC program: A social marketing case study. *American Journal of Health Behavior, 24*(1), 53–68.

Luther, M. *Dog doggety*. Retrieved from http://www.pugetsoundstartshere.org/scoop-poop/

Marcus, P. M., Huang, G. C., Beck, V., & Miller, M. J. (2010). The impact of a primetime cancer storyline: From individual knowledge and behavioral intentions to policy-level changes. *Journal of Cancer Education, 25*(4), 484–489. PMID: 20300910

Matovu, J. K. B., & Makumbi, F. E. (2007). Expanding access to voluntary HIV counseling and testing in sub-Saharan Africa: Alternative approaches for improving uptake, 2001–2007. *Tropical Medicine and International Health, 12*(11), 1315–1322.

McKee, N., Aghi, M., & Shahzadi, N. Cartoons and comic books for changing social norms: Meena, the South Asian girl. In A. Singhal, M. J. Cody, E. M. Rogers, & M. Sabido (Eds.), *Entertainment-education and social change* (pp. 331–349). Mahwah, NJ: Erlbaum.

Morgan, S. E., Movius, L., & Cody, M. J. (2009). The power of narratives: The effect of entertainment television organ donation storylines on the attitudes, knowledge, and behaviors of donors and nondonors. *Journal of Communication, 59*, 135–151.

Moyer-Gusé, E., Chung, A.H. & Jain, P. (2011). Identification of characters and discussion of taboo topics after exposure to an entertainment narrative about sexual health. *Journal of Communication, 61*(3), 387–406.

Moyer-Gusé, E., Mahood, C., & Brookes, S. (2011). Entertainment-education in the context of humor: Effects on safer sex intentions and risk perceptions. *Health Communication, 26*(8), 765–774.

Murphy, S., Frank, L., Moran, M., & Woodley, P. (2011). Transported or emotional? Exploring the determinants of change in knowledge, attitudes and behavior in entertainment education. *Journal of Communication, 61*(3), 407–431.

Murphy, S. T., & Cody, M. (2003). *Summary report: Developing a research agenda for entertainment education and multicultural audiences*. Retrieved from https://hollywoodhealthandsociety.org/developing-research-agenda-entertainment-education-and-multicultural-audiences

Murphy, S. T., Hether, H. J., Felt, L. J., & de Castro Buffington, S. (2012). Public diplomacy in prime time: Exploring the potential of entertainment education in international public diplomacy. *American Journal of Media Psychology, 5*, 5–32.

Murphy, S. T., Hether, H. J., & Rideout, V. (2008). How healthy is prime time? An analysis of health content in popular prime time television shows. Kaiser Family Foundation report. September. Retrieved from http://kff.org/other/report/how-healthy-is-prime-time-an-analysis-of-health-content-in-popular-prime-time-television-programs/

Nahm, S., Le, K., de Castro Buffington, S., Schiman, N., Raider, S., & Resko, S. (2010). Engaging youth through partnerships in entertainment education. *Cases in Public Health Communication and Marketing, 4*, 57–78.

O'Leary, A., Kennedy, M. G., Pappas-DeLuca, K. A., Nkete, M., Beck, V., & Galavotti, C. (2007). Association between exposure to an HIV storyline in *The Bold and the Beautiful* and HIV-related stigma in Botswana. *AIDS Education and Prevention, 19*(3), 209–217. PMID: 17563275

Pariera, K. L., Hether, H. J., Murphy, S. M., Buffington, S. C., & Baezconde-Garbanati, L. (2014). Portrayals of reproductive and sexual health issues on primetime television. *Health Communication, 29*, 698–706.

Parks, W. J., Lloyd, L. S., Nathan, M. B., Hosein, E., Odugleh, A., Clark, G. G., …, & Renganathan, E. (2004). International experiences in social mobilization and communication for dengue prevention and control. *Dengue Bulletin, 28* (Suppl.), 1–7.

Parrott, R. (2004). Emphasizing "communication" in health communication. *Journal of Communication, 54*, 751–787.

Peou, E., & Ram, P. (2011). *End-of-project evaluation of Health Behaviour Change Communication Project in Cambodia*. Cambodia: UNICEF.

Poindexter, D. O. (2004). A history of entertainment-education, 1958–2000. In A. Singhal, M. J. Cody, E. M. Rogers, & M. Sabido (Eds.), *Entertainment-education and social change* (pp. 21–36). Mahwah, NJ: Erlbaum.

Rimal, R. N., & Lapinski, M. K. (2009). Why health communication is important in public health. *Bulletin of the World Health Organization, 87*, 247.

Rosenstock, I. M., Strecher, V. J., & Becker, M. H. (1988). Social learning theory and the health belief model. *Health Education Quarterly 15*(2), 175–183.

Sachs, J. D. (2006). How to help the poor: Piecemeal progress or strategic plans? *Lancet, 367*(9519), 1309–1310.

Salmon, C. (2000). *Setting a research agenda: Entertainment-Education Conference*. Centers for Disease Control and Prevention, Office of Communication. Retrieved from http://www.cdc.gov/healthcommunication/toolstemplates/entertainmented/researchagenda.html

Schank, R. C., & Berman, T. (2002). The pervasive role of stories in knowledge and action. In M. C. Green, J. J. Strange, & T. C. Brock (Eds.), *Narrative impact: Social and cognitive foundations* (pp. 287–313). Mahwah, NJ: Erlbaum.

Schultz, D. E., Tannenbaum, S. I., & Lauterborn, R. (1993). *Integrated marketing communications: Putting it together and making it work*. New York, NY: McGraw-Hill.

Sesame Workshop. Retrieved from http://www.sesameworkshop.org/what-we-do/our-results/health-and-wellness.htm

Sharf, B. F., Freimuth, V. S., Greenspon, P., & Plotnick, C. (1996). Confronting cancer on thirtysomething: Audience response to health content on entertainment television. *Journal of Health Communication, 1*, 157–172.

Silverman, B. G., Mosley, J., Johns, M., Weaver, R., Green, M., Holmes, J., …, & Holmes, W. (2003). Computer games may be good for your health: Shifting healthcare behavior via interactive drama videogames. *American Medical Informatics Association Annual Symposium Proceedings*, 1075. PubMed PMID: 14728578

Singhal, A., Obregon, R., & Rogers, E. M. (1994). Reconstructing the story of *Simplemente Maria,* the most popular telenovella in Latin America of all time. *Gazette, 54,* 1–15.

Singhal, A., & Rogers, E. M. (1989a). Educating through television. *Populi, 16*(2), 38–47.

Singhal, A., & Rogers, E. M. (1989b). *India's information revolution.* Thousand Oaks, CA: Sage.

Singhal, A., & Rogers, E. M. (2004). The status of entertainment-education worldwide. In A. Singhal, M. J. Cody, E. M. Rogers, & M. Sabido (Eds.), *Entertainment-education and social change* (pp. 21–36). Mahwah, NJ: Erlbaum.

Singhal, A., Sharma, D., Papa, M., & Witte, K. (2004). Air cover and ground cover mobilization: Integrating entertainment-education broadcasts with community listening and service delivery in India. In A. Singhal, M. J. Cody, E. M. Rogers, & M. Sabido (Eds.), *Entertainment-education and social change* (pp. 351–375). Mahwah, NJ: Erlbaum.

Skinner, D., Metcalf, C. A., Seager, J. R., de Swardt, J. S., & Laubscher, J.A. (1991). An evaluation of an education programme on HIV infection using puppetry and street theatre. *AIDS Care, 3*(3), 317–329. PubMed PMID: 1932196

Slater, M. D., & Rouner, D. (2002). Entertainment education and elaboration likelihood: Understanding the processing of narrative persuasion. *Communication Theory, 12,* 173–191.

Slater, M. D., Rouner, D., & Long, M. (2006). Television dramas and support for controversial public policies: Effects and mechanisms. *Journal of Communication, 56,* 235–252.

Sood, M., Menard, T. & Witte, K. (2004). Theory behind entertainment-education. In A. Singhal, M. J. Cody, E. M. Rogers, & M. Sabido (Eds.), *Entertainment-education and social change* (pp. 117–149). Mahwah, NJ: Erlbaum.

Sopheab, H., Morineau, G., Neal, J. J., Saphonn, V., & Fylkesnes, K. (2008). Sustained high prevalence of sexually transmitted infections among sex workers in Cambodia. *BiomedCentral (BMC) Infectious Diseases, 8,* 167.

Soul City. (2000). *The evaluation of Soul City 4: Methodology and top-line results.* Paper presented at the Third International Entertainment-Education Conference for Social Change. Arnheim, The Netherlands. September 17–22.

Suhaili, M. R., Hoscin, E., Mokhtar, Z., Ali, N., Palmer, K., & Isa, M. M. (2004). Applying Communication for Behavioural Impact (COMBI) in the prevention and control of dengue in Johor Bahru, Johore, Malaysia. *Dengue Bulletin, 28*(Suppl.), 39–42.

Usdin, S., Singhal, A., Shongwe, T., Goldstein, S., & Shabalala, A. (2004). No short cuts in entertainment-education: Designing *Soul City* step-by-step. In A. Singhal, M. J. Cody, E. M. Rogers, & M. Sabido (Eds.), *Entertainment-education and social change* (pp. 153–175). Mahwah, NJ: Erlbaum.

Vaughan, P. W., Rogers, E. M., Singhal, A., & Swalehe, R. M. (2000). Entertainment-education and HIV/AIDS prevention: A field experiment in Tanzania. *Journal of Health Communication, 5(*3*),* 81–100.

Weitzen, S., Lapane, K. L., Toledano, A. Y., Hume, A. L., & Mor, V. (2005). Weaknesses of goodness-of-fit tests for evaluating propensity score models: The case of the omitted confounder. *Pharmacoepidemiology and Drug Safety, 14*(4), 227–238.

Whittier, D. K., Kennedy, M. G., St Lawrence, J. S., Seeley, S., & Beck, V. (2005). Embedding health messages into entertainment television: Effect on gay men's response to a syphilis outbreak. *Journal of Health Communication, 10*(3), 251–259. PubMed PMID:16036732

Wilkin, H. A., Valente, T. W., Murphy, S. T., Cody, M. J., Huang, G. C., ..., & Slan, L. (2007). Does entertainment-education work with Latinos in the United States? Identification and the effects of a telenovela breast cancer storyline. *Journal of Health Communication. 12*(5), 455–469.

World Health Organization. (2012). *Communication for Behavioural Impact (COMBI): A toolkit for behavioural and social communication in outbreak response.* Luxembourg: Author.

Yanovitzky, I., Zanutto, E., & Hornik, R. (2005). Estimating causal effects of public health education campaigns using propensity score methodology. *Evaluation and Program Planning, 28*(2), 209–220.

CHAPTER 6

GLOBAL HEALTH PROMOTION IN THE CONTEXT OF HUMAN RIGHTS

Elvira Beracochea and Lubna Ahmed

Global health promotion (GHP) is an essential component of global health projects and programs because effective global health promotion program is the only way to prevent disease and improve health status in developing nations. Timely treatment and quality health care delivery save individual lives but do not have the impact that GHP has at the population level, keeping the majority of the population healthy in the communities where they live and work. The **effectiveness** of GHP programs is enhanced if we use a human rights–based approach (RBA) to identify the health needs of the population in every community in every nation, particularly the needs of the marginalized or unserved. Every human being is entitled to have his or her **human rights,** as defined in the Universal Declaration of Human Rights (1948) respected, protected and, fulfilled. An RBA allows public health professionals to plan and implement prioritized and needed health promotion interventions and services to meet the unique needs of every group whose rights are not being fulfilled. The **right to health** is essential for human beings to reach their potential and live fulfilling lives. GHP programs must address the priority needs of every population and be incrementally implemented, reaching at least 10% of the unserved population every year. This chapter describes global health promotion, the human rights legislation that is the basis for developing global health programs that have GHP components as well as GHP programs that are adapted and implemented at country level and that are monitored and evaluated to meet effectiveness and quality standards. Accounting for the health needs of those whose rights are not fulfilled and ensuring that global health programs reach all are not a matter of philanthropy or charity, they are a human rights issue and the challenge of the next generation of global health professionals. This chapter can help you get started.

LEARNING OBJECTIVES

By the end of this chapter, the reader should be able to:

- **Describe the international legal framework for the right to health and what a rights-based approach is**
- **Understand the unique role of GHP to help protect and fulfill the right to health**
- **Discuss various rights-based approaches to GHP and applications**
- **Propose ways the reader may engage in and apply rights-based approaches to GHP**

The Case for GHP in the Context of Human Rights

In a village in rural India, or northern Nigeria, or in the slums of Nairobi, a human being is coughing in the middle of the night. He has been coughing for more than three weeks and every night the same thing happens. His cough does not let him sleep or rest and awakens the infant who shares the same room; the infant starts crying and awakes the other older children who sleep in the same room too. His wife starts breastfeeding the infant, who stops crying and the man steps outside to let his wife and the children go back to sleep. He lights up a cigarette. Smoking seems to stop the cough for a while. He is tired; he has not been able to sleep well for many nights because of the cough. As he goes back to sleep, he looks at the clock on the table. In a couple of hours, he will start his 12-hour shift unloading trucks in the local market. The nearest clinic closes at 4:00 p.m. He would have to ask his boss for unpaid time off to go see the nurse at the clinic to get something for his cough. He does not have money to pay the clinic fees and buy medicine, so he rejects that idea. Better yet, he decides to stop at one of the drug outlets in the market and ask the clerk what to get for his cough, and he will buy whatever medicine the clerk recommends.

As a global health professional, you read this story and are happy the infant is breastfed, but you are also thinking the infant's father may have tuberculosis (TB), or even lung cancer because he is a smoker, in which case the most likely only breadwinner in this household is at risk. You are also thinking he will probably waste his money buying a cough medicine in the market because he will likely get a counterfeit product from an unlicensed street seller. If he has TB, you are wondering how he will find the time to go to the clinic for testing and get the long course of medicines. You are also thinking of the children exposed to his cough, and of how he will afford the treatment for them too. How will he get help to quit smoking? All this thinking makes you feel overwhelmed and wonder whether anything can help this family. What can you and global health promotion do for him and his family and others like them? This is the question we answer in this chapter.

Global health is increasingly thought of through the lens of human rights, and not as part of a global charity effort. We can now say that global health is the public health field that looks at ways to realize the right to health of all human beings on this planet by promoting healthy practices, preventing disease, and delivering quality and timely treatment to international standards. Global health includes the practice of medicine and nursing and all the sciences of public health and health system reform, in addition to international human rights legislation and the effective work of international development assistance industry that addresses the most prevalent diseases as well as the social determinants of health. International development assistance is the more or less organized and effective response to fulfill the responsibility of developed countries to assist developing nations to respect, protect and fulfill two human rights: the right to health and the **right to development**, as defined in the Declaration on the Right to Development (1986). The international development assistance is a multinational industry that consists of multilateral donors such as the World Bank and the Global Fund Against Malaria, TB and HIV/AIDS; bilateral donors such as USAID, academic institutions, and foundations that support a number of implementing organizations such as nonprofit organizations and other grantees, as well as consulting companies and contractors. All these strengthen, support, and complement the work country governments do with varied degrees of success to improve health care in developing countries. All this is loosely, with more or less success, coordinated by the World Health Organization (WHO) in accordance with its constitution, which states that "the enjoyment of the highest attainable standard of health is one of the fundamental rights of every human being without distinction of race, religion, political belief, economic or social condition" (http://www.who.int/governance/eb/who_constitution_en.pdf). The objective of WHO is "the attainment by all peoples of the highest possible level of health" (article 1 of the WHO constitution). The constitution was adopted by the International Health Conference held in New York from June 19 to July 22, 1946, signed on July 22, 1946, by the representatives of 61 states (*Off. Rec. Wld Hlth Org.*, 2,100), and entered into force on April 7, 1948. Amendments adopted by the 26th, 29th, 39th, and 51st World Health Assemblies (resolutions WHA26.37, WHA29.38, WHA39.6, and WHA51.23) came into force on February 3, 1977, January 20, 1984, July 11, 1994, and September 15, 2005, respectively, and are incorporated in the present text.

GHP programs are, therefore, essential to enjoy the "highest attainable standard of health" and to the effective work of the international development assistance industry.

If you remember those two rights—the right to health and the right to development—and that your role as a global health professional is to help realize those two rights, your job will be clear and simple—not easy, but simple and focused on what matters and makes a difference. Your job will include studying, planning, implementing, and evaluating promotion and health care delivery programs that prevent disease and deliver solutions to the challenges of realizing these two rights at a global scale. Excited? Hope so.

Global Health Promotion From a Human Rights Perspective

Like all public health sciences, global health promotion must be available to all people at all times in accordance with every community's epidemiological patterns of risk factors and prevalent conditions, as opposed to medical care that must be available and accessible when you need it. Healthy behaviors and preventive services must be promoted all the time, taught in schools, in the workplace, at community events, and in household visits by community public health nurses and workers, as well as through mass and social media. The family in our story needs to have the right information to stay healthy, raise healthy children, and prevent common conditions in their geographic area. They and the other families in their community all must have enough healthy food, sleep under mosquito nets to be protected from malaria, and have safe drinking water and sanitation. GHP programs ensure that all infants are breastfed, well nourished when weaned, vaccinated, and protected from accidents in the household. Women need to know where to get care during pregnancy and delivery and education to care for newborns and infants. Men and women need GHP programs that empower them to access family planning services to space and time births and to be protected from prevalent communicable conditions in their communities, such as trachoma, AIDS, TB, and malaria; and noncommunicable conditions such as tobacco addiction, obesity, diabetes, cancer, and cardiovascular conditions. All this must happen by design and needs planners, managers, evaluators, epidemiologists, health surveillance professionals and health care providers to work in a coordinated manner to make sure no one's right to health is denied. The right to health ensures they *all* have access to the highest standard of health care, including effective and well-managed health promotion programs. That is where GHP programs come in as part of an effective health care delivery program that meets the needs of the population. They are the basis on which every country can create its own public health promotion programs and include health promotion activities as part of all of its disease prevention and control programs. Furthermore, the Millennium Development Goals (MDGs) and Sustainable Development Goals (SDGs) agendas indicate the need to progressively expand health promotion and health care services to all and thus progressively achieve the right to health of all in every country.

At the time of this writing, West African nations are emerging out of the largest Ebola Viral Disease (EVD) outbreak in history, which proved the importance of GHP programs to help countries develop effective disease prevention and control programs as well as effective health systems that deliver promotive, preventive, and curative care. The EVD outbreak was important not only because of its magnitude or its approximate 50% mortality rate, because other diseases such as TB and malaria affected and killed many more people in West Africa during that time, but because it reminded WHO and the international development assistance industry of the need to develop effective GHP programs and public health prevention and disease control programs for all prevalent conditions as well as the need to progressively improve the health system that implements and manages these programs in every country. The outbreak also showed the importance of health promotion programs and preventing contact with infected animals as well as of changing traditional burial practices to stop transmission. This was not new. Any textbook of infectious disease will teach you how to prevent and control EVD. What was missing was the GHP program to prevent it, detect it quickly, and use the disease surveillance system that could have detected it quickly and stopped it. What was also missing was a long-term relationship between health workers and the communities they serve that is built on mutual trust and effective health promotion programs. In short, EVD reminded us all that our job is to respect, protect, and fulfill the right to health of everyone everywhere; of the need for effective health promotion, surveillance, and epidemic control programs; and that we need to have globally and regionally coordinated programs because viruses and bacteria do not need passports to cross borders.

Like Ebola, the drama of the family in our short story can be prevented and controlled with effective GHP programs and country-specific health promotion programs. For example, a community health worker (CHW) should have visited this household and helped them make the necessary changes to promote the health of everyone in the family (Beracochea, Evans, & Weinstein, 2011). The CHW would have linked the father to a smoking cessation program that would have saved him money and protected him against preventable diseases. The CHW would have helped the couple choose a family planning method to space the births of their children and allow them the time and resources to take care of them; even, as in some countries, CHWs also deliver birth control pills and condoms as necessary. And, a CHW would have suspected TB and helped arrange for an evening appointment at the local clinic to have the father and even the whole family tested. Deliberately designed and implemented GHP programs do that. This is not by chance or good will. It is people's right and it must be by design.

To further support the need for effective GHPs that build trust and positive relationships between health workers and the communities they serve, I use the case of the nine health workers who were shot in northern Nigeria (BBC, 2013) while they were providing vaccines to children. Lack of appropriate information and support for effective health interventions such as immunization programs causes these effective health promotion and life-saving programs to fail. In addition to the senseless loss of life, this act proves the need to develop health systems that are tailored and meet the needs of the populations they are to serve. In addition, the rights of the children who would not be immunized as a result of these senseless acts of violence were not to be fulfilled. They faced increased chance of sickness and death. Promotion for the highest attainable standard of care must be ensured in every community and accurate information through trusted sources must be provided all of the time to every person and by every public health professional. GHP ensures the programs that fulfill the right to health work.

What Are Human Rights?

There is international legislation endorsed by most countries that defines a number of rights that all human beings are entitled to by the mere fact of being human. The Universal Declaration of Human Rights (UDHR, 1948) was adopted by the General Assembly (GA) of the United Nations (UN) on December 10, 1948, just a few years after the end of World War II; it is a visionary document that states that the rights are universal; everyone has them; and that all rights are equally important, inalienable, and interdependent. Being free is not more important than being healthy or having access to health services, or clothing, or housing. In fact, how can a human being be free if he or she is uneducated and sick? Particularly Article 25 (see Box 6.1) talks about the right to health and health care, protection even if unemployed or sick, and that women and children are entitled to special care, assistance, and protection. In 1988, General Comment 14 about the right to the highest attainable standard of health (General Comment 14, 1988) was adopted to further define what was meant by Article 25 of the UDHR. General Comment 14, a 10-page document that every GHP and international development professional must read and reread often, defines the right to health, the importance of availability, accessibility, acceptability, and quality of the care to be provided. In short, General Comment 14 is the main to-do list of every global health professional.

BOX 6.1 UNIVERSAL DECLARATION OF HUMAN RIGHTS

Article 25.

1. Everyone has the right to a standard of living adequate for the health and well-being of himself and of his family, including food, clothing, housing and medical care and necessary social services, and the right to security in the event of unemployment, sickness, disability, widowhood, old age or other lack of livelihood in circumstances beyond his control.
2. Motherhood and childhood are entitled to special care and assistance. All children, whether born in or out of wedlock, shall enjoy the same social protection.

Access to quality health care is not something only those who can afford it can have; it is everyone's right, and this is why health promotion makes its most significant contribution. By promoting access to services and their acceptability, self-care and family care improves as well as the timely utilization of health services increases.

Human rights are also important in global health promotion because they not only define the rights of all human beings, also known as "right holders," but also the responsibilities of the "duty bearers," that is, the corresponding governments of the countries where the right holders live. Governments are not required to *deliver* health services to all, but some countries, such as the Netherlands, United Kingdom, and Cuba, have chosen to do so. Governments are required to *ensure* that access to quality services is possible to all. Many countries have a mix of government-run and private for-profit and nonprofit health care and treatment services. Governments are required to *ensure* that whoever provides health services is accredited and delivers safe health care; and that if a citizen is prevented for whatever social, economic, or geographic reason from accessing those services, the government is responsible for providing the service and implementing programs that systematically provide the services needed. For example, Australia has flying doctors go to remote areas, and many countries have mobile clinics and providers such as Peru's health brigades, who visit isolated rural communities to give vaccines and promote healthy practices such as handwashing and good nutrition and family planning. They do it in an integrated way, providing services such as immunizations for children and pregnant women, and provision of basic care and treatment for common diseases. Neither of these services is perfect and reaches everyone all the time, but it is the government's responsibility to find better ways to do so and incrementally and continuously improve services according to changing epidemiological needs. This is what universal health coverage, the main target of Sustainable Development Goal 3, is all about: the progressive realization of the right to health of every citizen.

Further international legislation also supports the important role of health promotion in global health: the International Covenant on Economic, Social and Cultural Rights (ICESCR, 1966); the Convention on the Elimination of all forms of Discrimination Against Women (CEDAW, 1979); the Convention of the Rights of the Child (CRC, 1989); the Declaration on the Right to Development (1986); and the Millennium Declaration (2000) also support global health promotion as one of the main and effective strategies to achieve development goals.

The legislation described is the basis for fairness and social justice as well as professional effectiveness in our work as global health promotion and public health professionals. This is the reason we strive to reach the vulnerable and underserved, the uninsured, the marginalized, and improve our country's health system and global health systems. The human beings in our story are right holders of all the above rights. Their government is the duty bearer that must respect their rights, pass and enforce legislation to protect them, and implement programs to fulfill them. Friendly developed countries that have the knowledge, technology, and resources to solve the problems in realizing the right to health of families in developing countries, like the one in our story, also become duty bearers when they sign international cooperation agreements. To "respect, protect and fulfill" the right to health is what a health professional must do about the family in the story and all the families in each one of our areas of work. In the next sections, we discuss various rights-based approaches and applications to respect, protect, and fulfill the right to health of various groups through effective health promotion programs and effective health systems.

Health Systems, Global Health Promotion Programs, and Human Rights

A health system is the way each country organizes itself to take care of the health of its citizens and fulfill their right to health. Most countries have more or less organized ways to ensure access to quality health care, preventive and promotion services, and protect the public's health. Few have well-designed systems that respect, protect, and fulfill the right to health of all their citizens. And even fewer countries ensure the continuum of care that includes promotion, prevention, early diagnosis, care, and treatment and rehabilitation and palliative care services for all their citizens. However, this is a great time to work in public health and particularly health promotion. Now is the time to ensure health promotion programs are based on the right to health of all citizens and part of the health system that promotes healthy practices and ensures the access to quality health care delivery and treatment services to all.

There are many global health promotion initiatives, and most global disease control strategies include some health promotion component. There is GAVI (http:/www.gavialliance.org/) to improve access to vaccines; Stop TB (http:/www.stoptb.org) to improve diagnosis and treatment of TB; the Global Fund (http:/www.theglobalfund.org), which funds grants for countries to fight HIV/AIDS, malaria, and TB; foundations such as the Bill & Melinda Gates Foundation and the Bill, Hillary, and Chelsea Clinton Foundation have programs; the United States and other donors also have global health programs (http://www.usaid.gov/globalhealth) that include promotion of various healthy behaviors such as family planning, breastfeeding, use of mosquito nets, and so on. Many European countries have global health programs, and countries such as Korea, Russia, Brazil, China, and India are entering the global health assistance field. The main challenges are the lack of coordination when planning and implementing health promotion programs, lack of common goals that result in competing agendas, the need for attribution to each funding organization that creates parallel information and monitoring systems, and the overall lack of **accountability** for results in terms of the contribution made to improve the country's health system and leave sustainable improvements when the aid ends. For example, the community-based acute malnutrition program in Malawi has more than 30 different stakeholders. A recent evaluation of the efforts to promote healthy infant and child nutrition, including promotion of breastfeeding, showed the need for all these organizations to improve how they coordinate their work to ensure all the districts were covered and that all donors and organizations use the same communication messages and materials as well as that all strengthen the existing health facilities and support to community-based nutrition prevention activities (Beracochea et al., 2012).

We know what works in health promotion and that health surveillance systems tell us what needs to be promoted based on the epidemiological disease patterns in each community. We know that our "zip code" is an indicator of our life expectancy in the United States and that in each country the people have different life expectancies based on current mortality rates. With this information, we can start creating global and country-specific health promotion programs that progressively and transparently respect, protect, and fulfill the right to health of every person wherever he or she lives. We can do it through GHP programs that promote lifestyle changes that help people stay healthy and seek care when necessary.

Another challenge global health professionals face now is to scale up and expand programs to ensure they reach everyone and meet their right to health. Let's take a look at this challenge in the context of global health promotion programs for children, women, and men from a rights-based approach.

Rights-Based Approach to Global Health Promotion

Global health requires realizing the right to health of all, improving how health care is delivered and better health **outcomes** for all, no matter what country they live in or their condition, particularly when a way to prevent or cure exists. For that reason, global health must include programs that help every country achieve the right to health in annual increments over the next 10, 15, or 20 years. Global health promotion is essential to achieve the right to health through the SDG3 agenda by promoting healthy practices to all, everywhere, consistently through programs that ensure the fulfillment of the right to health of all, including minorities, marginalized populations, the poor, the abused, the disabled, and anyone who cannot speak for themselves. To develop appropriate and effective programs we must work with other public health professionals to conduct community health diagnoses, analyze health surveillance data and other databases and information sources to identify priorities, and then, design or improve how health promotion programs and health facilities work worldwide, that is, at a global scale.

With the advent of the new "Sustainable Development Goals" (SDGs) and targets for 2030, it is essential that every country, developed and developing, plan to progressively expand their health promotion programs as part of the overall GHP programs that must effectively be coordinated by the WHO. The WHO must develop a culture of results in GHP that goes beyond legislation or creating technical guidelines that are not implemented worldwide and only trying to help countries when they are in trouble. Effective GHP coordination strategies and structures help countries work together and demonstrate improvements of their GHP indicators. For the past 30 years or more, the WHO has been part of charters (WHO, 2009) that have not been fully implemented, including the targets of the Millennium Development Goals. It is essential that WHO play an effective coordinating role of the many actors in GHP and in the international development assistance industry. Otherwise the Helsinki Statement Framework for Action of the Eighth Global Conference on Health Promotion (WHO, 2013a) will be just another unkept promise. Now is the time to take global health and GHP to higher level of effectiveness and accountability for realizing the right to health of all on this planet.

Rights-Based Global Health Promotion Approaches for Children

The Convention on the Rights of Child (CRC, 1989) was approved by the UN Assembly in November 1989. At the time of this writing, the CRC was entering its 25th anniversary. Many countries have signed it but not ratified it, including the United States. Why? It is a commitment and it means accepting the responsibility of the duty bearer to respect, protect, and fulfill the rights of every child. The US government would have to respect, protect, and fulfill the right to health of every child in America. The Affordable Care Act has moved the needle in this regard, but the debate on health reform is ongoing in the United States and will probably go on for many more years, because health is considered a commodity that only those who can afford it can buy, and not a right of every American. Health promotion, on the other hand, is a public health function that benefits all, so the government can have a much bigger impact in keeping young Americans healthy. Other governments have ratified the CRC but have not enforced it or reformed their programs to ensure they really respect, protect, and fulfill the rights of every child. Particularly, countries in sub-Saharan Africa with high HIV/AIDS prevalence and AIDS orphans, children's right to health must be respected, protected, and fulfilled by all stakeholders through effective health promotion and health care delivery programs. Following are some examples of how health organizations and health promotion programs can be improved by using the CRC and other rights-based approaches.

UNICEF (http://www.unicef.org) is an example of a rights-based organization. All UNICEF's programs are designed, managed, and monitored to ensure they help countries advance the progressive realization of children's rights; the rights to health, food, clothing, and safety are part of its programs. Save the Children (http://www.savethechildren.org) is another rights-based organization that advocates for children's rights. One may argue about the actual impact of these organizations, numbers of lives actually saved, and the many orphans who do not yet live in safe and healthy conditions. In any case, their efforts offer many examples of what works and what needs to scaled up and changed.

Some countries have laws and programs that protect children's lives, such as the prohibition against telling parents the sex of the baby in India to prevent female feticide, and food supplementation programs to pregnant women that benefit the mother and the child, particularly for teen mothers. Other countries have free antenatal care to all women and free care to all children until five years of age. Honduras, for example, has community health workers that visit newborns at home within 24 hours of the birth even in rural areas and that educate the mother about breastfeeding and monitor the baby's growth monthly. The United States has the Women and Children Program (http://www.wicprogram.org/). All these programs must be monitored to ensure they reach all they need to serve and that they are effective and provide quality health services and information. In the UK, there are health promotion programs that have public health nurses visit the elderly and assess their needs and mothers to help them breastfeed and take care of the baby; in France, as well.

Particularly, **school-based programs** deliver relevant and practical health promotion messages. From teaching children how to use a mosquito net, how to say no to smoking or inappropriate touching, how to mix oral rehydration salts (ORS), how to eat healthy and exercise, and to how to use medicines safely and correctly, school-based programs offer the opportunity to have a continuous health promotion curriculum that can be reinforced and deepened as the children grow older and develop stronger self-care skills. In addition, children bring these practices home and teach parents and siblings and prepares them for when they are parents themselves.

In global health, on a worldwide scale, it is our job to empower children to address health problems they may find in the school and home, from playing safely and handling bullying to taking care of themselves and younger siblings while parents are at work, and when to tell a grown-up when a fellow teen is depressed and at risk of suicide or may be a victim of abuse. Standards need to be set by government agencies and their partners for programs to be adapted, implemented, monitored, and evaluated to ensure they are effective and achieve the intended results. Every school in the world must have a health promotion program that protects and improves the health of children of all ages. We will progressively and incrementally achieve this goal by working in partnership with various stakeholders, local leaders, parents, and organizations to achieve the goal of having effective promotion programs and safe playgrounds by at least 10% of the country's schools per year.

Rights-Based Global Health Promotion Approaches for Women

Women, because of their reproductive role, have specific health needs, and therefore need specific health promotion programs and services during their childbearing years. Health promotion programs need to be developed to reach every woman and address the prevalent problems women have in that population or geographic area, before, during, and after their childbearing years. We must remember women are not just baby-carrying beings, they are human beings and have health, physical, mental, and social needs beyond their reproductive role and require services such as cancer prevention, obesity reduction, and prevention of cardiovascular conditions. In most countries, you will see that health centers have a coverage area, conduct a community diagnosis, and develop integrated healthcare delivery and community-based programs that educate professional community health workers, volunteers, or village health workers to promote messages about various health services and healthy practices and behaviors such as family planning, antenatal care, supervised deliveries, and breastfeeding; and how to prevent health problems such as date rape, physical, psychological, and verbal abuse; and cancer prevention through regular health promotion, check-ups and screening programs. We must ensure that these programs reach and affect the health of every woman worldwide; that these programs meet quality standards and are effective and progressively expanded to reach at least 10% of the women not covered every year. Progressive expansion of global health promotion programs is essential to empower women to realize their right to health as defined in CEDAW and then reaffirmed in the Millennium Declaration and in the UN Sustainable Development Goals agenda. The "Every Woman, Every Child" program (http://everywomaneverychild.org/) is an example of a start in the right direction, that if coupled with firm commitments and accountability, may achieve the unfinished agenda of the MDGs and contribute to universal health coverage of the highest attainable standard of care, including promotion, prevention, timely diagnoses and treatment, rehabilitation and palliative care, for every woman and child on our planet. We must ensure that all initiatives are coordinated so they do not overlap and account for increasing health promotion and healthcare delivery coverage by 10% every year for the next 10 years.

Approaches for People With Infectious Diseases and Noncommunicable Diseases

Specific health promotion programs must be developed to reach patients with infectious diseases (IDs) and noncommunicable diseases (NCDs) worldwide. It is the job of the state in every country, that is, government and non-governmental organizations as well as private health providers, donor agencies, and foundations, and of the global health professionals who work in them to ensure that human beings like the one in our story at the start of this chapter know how to protect their health, get help to overcome nicotine addiction and quit smoking, know that buying medicines from a drug outlet is not going to help because the clerks usually are untrained and medicines are cheaper because they are expired or fake. Having access to the right diagnosis and treatment is part of the right to health, and those who cannot afford it must have access to services as well. Health is not a commodity; it is a human right, and, therefore, if health information had been readily available, the man in the story would have known about the risk of smoking, suspecting TB when cough lasts more than two weeks, and about how to access care after hours and fee exemptions for those who cannot pay. If a community health worker had visited their household and conducted a health diagnosis, these services could be provided. Community diagnosis and/or health surveillance information programs are essential to plan and implement health promotion and health care programs that meet the needs of the communities and the health facilities that serve them.

Let's take a look at some of these NCD country profiles (http://www.who.int/nmh/countries/en/) to see the need for effective GHP programs at a global scale. An analysis of these needs is beyond the scope of this chapter but should encourage you to look for innovative ways to reach at least 10% of the unserved every year for the next 10 years with effective GHP messages and services.

Global health professionals are at a fork in the road. Turning points like this in the development of health sciences seem to happen in every generation because needs, health knowledge, and resources improve and/or change. Global health professionals, therefore, must change programs and break with business as usual and use rights-based legislation to ensure they get the job done through effective GHP and health care delivery programs. Now it is the turn of this generation of global health professionals and the organizations they work for to take GHP programs to a higher level of impact in the next 15 years. If we do our work right, by 2030, every family will have had their right to health fulfilled. Hope you will have played your role in getting us there!

CASE STUDY 6.1 MAHBOUBA'S RIGHT TO HEALTH

Case Study Instructions

Form groups of no more than four students and read the following case. Then answer the questions below and identify what global health promotion program(s) needs to be developed or improved to meet Mahbouba's right to health.

Mahbouba is a tall and beautiful young lady who grew up in western Ethiopia. As a child of divorce, she was raised by her aunt who treated her as a servant and did not educate her. Mahbouba one day decided to run with her sister and worked as a maid in exchange for room and board. She was then lied to and sold to a man who beat and raped her at age 13. The man was 60 years old and married. The couple beat her and would never let her get out of the house. She found out she was pregnant and in her 7th month of pregnancy she was finally able to run away. She wanted to go drown herself in the river but a man rescued her and provided shelter in a hut near their house. Mahbouba could not afford a midwife so she tried to give birth on her own. Unfortunately, her pelvis did not accommodate the baby's head and he got stuck for 7 days and died. Mahbouba lost consciousness and was finally brought to a hospital after 7 days and found out that the baby had rotted away and she found out she had developed fistula and could not walk as a result. (Kristof & Wudunn, 2010)

Case Study Questions

1. What human rights are not being fulfilled in Mahbouba's situation?
2. What objective should a global health promotion program include to prevent this from happening again?
3. Whose responsibility is it to address the health needs of young girls like Mahbouba?
4. What other ideas for practice will you apply in the future?
5. Why should women's right to health not be left only to charity organizations or missionaries in the post-2015 era? What else can be done?

Conclusion

This chapter provides a preliminary introduction to the concept, principles, and practices related to human rights–based approaches—or RBA, for short—and to global health promotion as an essential and integral part of global health practice and health care service delivery. No attempt is made to provide a comprehensive review of such programs worldwide. However, several illustrative case studies are provided to highlight the complexities and challenges as well as the opportunities of RBA-based health promotion programs within global contexts. References to relevant UN treaties and other international declarations and statements on human rights and global health that provide the legal and foundational basis for RBA-based government policies, strategies, and programs for global health promotion and global health services are included to guide the students toward further reading and research.

In summary, global health can be defined as the field in public health that globally deals with the right to health for every human being by encouraging healthy practices and the highest attainable quality standard of health care delivery through effective and efficient health systems. The two essential human rights that global health professionals need to concentrate on are the right to health and the right to development. To fulfill these rights, global health promotion must be available at all times as an integral part of every disease prevention and control program and health care delivery services, and not in an ad-hoc basis. The lack of awareness and knowledge of healthy behaviors causes effective programs like immunizations and TB and HIV/AIDs control to fail due to stigma, lack of access and use. Effective health promotion ensures their global health impact.

Human rights are rights that all humans are entitled to as defined by the Universal Declaration of Human Rights and other treaties and conventions as approved by the UN General Assembly and ratified by most countries. The UDHR states the right to health for the first time in history, and General Comment 14 goes further into defining it as access to the highest attainable standard of health. Governments, particularly those of fragile and poor countries, are not obligated to provide health care services to everyone, but they are required to use all resources available, their own and those of international development assistance, to progressively protect, respect, and ensure access to healthcare is available for all. For that reason, in this chapter we advocate for progressive expansion of GHP program to at least 10% of those who need them and are not covered yet, over the next 10 years, until 2025.

The next generation of GHP programs must include the promotion of evidence-based healthy practices to everyone, everywhere consistently to thus ensure the fulfillment of the right to health of all including minorities, marginalized populations, the poor, the abused, the disabled, and anyone who cannot speak for themselves. Governments and donors must give priority to children's right to health, particularly newborns, so their rights are respected, protected, and fulfilled by all stakeholders. Women's right to health must address their physical, mental, and social needs, not only reproductive health needs, and for that reason, GHP programs need to be expanded to reach as much of the population as possible. Women's rights are defined in CEDAW and the MDG and SDG declarations. More targeted health promotion programs need to be developed to reach and fulfill the right to health of patients with preventable and treatable IDs and NCDs worldwide.

RBA is a new concept for global health promotion and global health care service delivery. Based on the authors' personal experience with RBA programs, the challenges and rewards are hugely satisfying and enduring, both personally and professionally. It is the fervent hope of the authors that this admittedly brief and preliminary introduction to the concept, principles, and practice of rights-based approaches will raise the curiosity and interest of current and future students of global health for the benefit of the poor majority, both in the developed and developing nations to advance the achievement of the post-2015 SDG agenda by 2030 and that they do not repeat the mistakes of the past.

KEY TERMS

1. **Accountability:** The professional responsibility to demonstrate results, good and bad, and transparency in the means to achieve them; essential to improving poor health outcomes
2. **Effectiveness:** A quality of public health programs and health care delivery that ensures that they achieve the planned result or outcome
3. **Human rights:** International legislation that protects, respects, and fulfills the rights of every human being as established in the Universal Declaration of Human Rights of 1948 and subsequent treaties, conventions, and declarations

4. **Outcomes:** Measures of health and disease that are quantifiable and demonstrate improvement in the status of the health of an individual or population leading to positive impact on the status
5. **Right to development:** The collective right of every country to participate in the development of the well-being of the people of that country as defined in the Declaration of the Right to Development
6. **Right to health:** The right of every individual to the highest attainable standard of health care as established in the General Comment 14
7. **School-based programs:** Programs that are designed and implemented by school staff, parent volunteers, and the students themselves to improve the knowledge and health practices of children, teachers, and parents in order to improve the children's physical, mental, and social well-being

REVIEW QUESTIONS

1. What are the implications of applying a rights-based approach to the promotion of health in a state in the United States?
2. What are the implications of applying the same approach in a developing country in sub-Saharan Africa?
3. How would you advocate for a rights-based approach in your organization or GHP program?
4. What actions must governments take to plan and implement effective health promotion programs?
5. What must be the role of the World Health Organization in global health promotion?
6. Why does global health promotion matter in the SDG 2030 agenda?

References

Beracochea, E., Evans, D., & Weinstein, C. (2011). *Rights-based approaches to public health.* New York, NY: Springer.

Beracochea, E., Tisch, S., Webber, S., Bickel, D., Zanera, D., & Mandalira, A. (2012). Final evaluation of the institutionalization of community-based therapeutic care of malnutrition in Malawi. *Social Impact.* Retrieved from http://pdf.usaid.gov/pdf_docs/pdacy084.pdf

British Broadcasting Company. (2013). Retrieved from http://www.bbc.co.uk/news/world-africa-21381773

Convention on the Elimination of all forms of Discrimination Against Women. (1979). Retrieved from http://www.un.org/womenwatch/daw/cedaw/

Convention of the Rights of the Child. (1989). Retrieved from http://www.ohchr .org/EN/ProfessionalInterest/Pages/CRC.aspx

General Comment 14. (1988). Retrieved from http://www.unhchr.ch/tbs/doc.nsf/ %28Symbol%29/40d009901358b0e2c1256915005090be?Opendocument

International Covenant on Economic, Social and Cultural Rights. (1966) Retrieved from http://www2.ohchr.org/english/law/cescr.htm

International Initiative on Maternal Mortality and Human Rights. (2010). *Human rights-based approaches to maternal mortality, India*. Retrieved from http:// righttomaternalhealth.org/sites/iimmhr.civicactions.net/files/IIMMHR% 20Field%20project%20booklet.pdf

Kristof, N., & Wudunn, S. (2009). *Half the SKY: Turning oppression into opportunity for women worldwide*. New York, NY: Vintage.

Millennium Declaration. (2000). Retrieved from http://www.un.org/millennium/ declaration/ares552e.htm

Right to Development. (1986). Retrieved from http://www2.ohchr.org/english/law/ rtd.htm

Universal Declaration of Human Rights. (1948). Retrieved from http://www.un .org/en/documents/udhr/index.shtml

World Health Organization. (2009). Retrieved from http://www.who.int/health promotion/milestones/en/ accessed

World Health Organization. (2013). Retrieved from http://www.healthpromotion 2013.org/conference-programme/framework-and-statement

CHAPTER 7

eHEALTH AND GLOBAL HEALTH PROMOTION

Sheana S. Bull, Gretchen Domek, and Deborah Thomas

Technology is pervasive throughout society, becoming so commonplace that it is almost hard to imagine a time without access to a computer or the Internet. Even though digital technologies are not equally accessible or available to all, the cell phone is bridging the digital divide in ways not imaginable even 5 or 10 years ago. People can access cell phones even in seemingly remote areas. To be sure, we live in a technological era, and the possibilities for health promotion are immense. In particular, computers and the Internet have evolved to facilitate social interaction through social media and to incorporate location for place-based applications (applications that integrate **geographic information systems** [GIS], for example, mapping applications to help identify resources nearby). Notably, they have become portable, making access to computers and the Internet nearly ubiquitous.

Ultimately, the increasing access to the Internet and mobile phones has revolutionized global health promotion. We now have several decades of examples that illustrate the promise for computers and the Internet to be marshaled to reduce risk factors for disease and facilitate healthy behavior. Throughout this chapter, we use the term "global **eHealth** promotion" to encompass all of these technologies.

Although burgeoning technology applications throughout global health are encouraging, they are not uniformly effective and should be viewed with a critical eye. Technology for technology's sake only squanders scare resources. As such, this chapter explores the use of technology in global eHealth promotion, critically highlighting key approaches that can foster successes in enhancing health behaviors and, as a consequence, health. After providing a brief history of the rapid evolution of computers and the Internet, this chapter presents a review of scientific evidence of how computers, the Internet, mobile phones and **short message service (SMS)**, and initial studies on social media have been rigorously investigated and demonstrate efficacy in health

LEARNING OBJECTIVES

By the end of this chapter, the reader should be able to:

- Have an appreciation for the rapid evolution of technology in the context of global eHealth promotion
- Describe how computers, the Internet, and mobile devices are beginning to come together as part of a single field
- Have an understanding of the scientific evidence for using technology in global eHealth promotion
- Have an understanding of what specific technologies have proven efficacious for global eHealth promotion
- Name at least two new technological advances related to global eHealth promotion
- Name at least two promising adaptations of global eHealth promotion to technology

promotion globally. The next section then highlights some of the emerging technologies, including geographic information systems, **smartphones,** and **social media,** that have great potential but that have not been evaluated in carefully designed studies. The chapter concludes with an overview of some overarching considerations for the implementation of technology for global eHealth promotion.

The Rapid Evolution of Computers, the Internet, and Mobile Phones

Although modern computing and electronic communication has grown exponentially in the past two decades, the technology has been evolving for over 75 years. Konrad Zuse, a construction engineer, is credited with developing the original prototypes for our modern personal computers with the electronic calculators he invented in the late 1930s, which led ultimately to the personal computer in the early 1970s. What we now know as the World Wide Web or Internet, linking personal computers globally, began in 1969 with the Advanced Research Projects Agency (ARPA) net, which was the first attempt to link computers together to share information. ARPANet evolved into local area networks (LAN) and then the US-based National Science Foundation network (NSFnet), linking supercomputers together (Bellis, 2010).

Linking supercomputers together allowed individuals to post information online where others could read and review it—this process of interaction between an individual and the computer has come to be known as **Web 1.0** and represents a static process of human–machine interaction. **Web 2.0** is a term credited to Dale Dougherty of O'Reilly Media, who used the term in 2003 to represent the process whereby people interact with each other using the Internet as a medium of communication (Nations, 2012). Although functions such as chat rooms and threaded discussions that we consider central to Web 2.0 communication predate the label "Web 2.0," these functions coincide with social media such as MySpace and Facebook, which were established in 2003 and 2004. On these sites users develop personal profiles, link to other users they consider "friends," and subsequently engage with each other through activities such as threaded discussion, chatting, sharing links to websites, and posting photos (called "user-generated" content) (Lenhart et al., 2007).

Since the 1980s, there has been a rapid increase globally in mobile telephone use in both developed and developing countries. In fact, developing countries now have the majority of world mobile phone subscribers, and it has been argued that the so-called **digital divide** among socioeconomic classes may be more relevant for communication mediums such as computers and the Internet compared to mobile telephones, which seem to be viewed as a more affordable and necessary means of communication even in resource-poor areas (Forestier, Grace, & Kenny, 2002).

In the late 1990s, we began to see handheld computers and devices such as the PalmPilot™ and others that allowed for users to access word processing, accounting, databases, scheduling, address books, and other software features on a small handheld computer. As early as the 1970s, we saw prototypes of mobile phones and two-way pager systems. These early mobile phones were very simple, with only voice capabilities for making and receiving telephone calls. However, mobile phones have evolved over four decades to be highly sophisticated, allowing for calls, short message service (SMS, also known as text messaging), access to the Internet, and storage of files, photos, and music. Mobile phones have essentially contributed to the obsolescence of the handheld computer device and now incorporate computing applications and telephone communications in a single device called a smartphone.

The increasing portability of computers has meant that users can more often access the Internet through mobile devices. The number of US adults who use their mobile devices to connect to the Internet has doubled in three years (Brenner, 2013); in the Middle East and Africa, over 70% of mobile phone users go online with their phone at least weekly (Wiltfong, 2013).

Geospatial technologies include a wide range of activities from remote sensing to geographic information systems to global positioning systems (GPS). A GIS is essentially a computer mapping systems with analytical capabilities and incorporates information from GPS and remote sensing. In the health context, GIS is used for improving health care delivery, disease surveillance, and evaluating links between environment and health. The extensive ability to integrate numerous types of data into a single software platform conveys data in an extremely accessible manner, with maps being a common language. In fact, these technologies have been around for decades with early applications predominately in natural resources, military, urban planning, and agriculture, and then expanding rapidly more broadly starting in the 1990s, including public health applications, with the wide availability of the personal computer. The Internet and smartphones have continued the growth and adoption of **place-based health**.

The Internet has not always been accessible equally for users globally. In fact, early challenges with Internet technology illustrated evidence of a "digital divide," making access to the Internet unequal with greater access afforded to those countries with infrastructure to support the computer equipment and bandwidth initially needed for Internet access. With the advent of mobile and cellular technologies, land lines for telephone and desktop computers are no longer critical for Internet access; this means the digital divide is shrinking as globally more and more people are connected to the Internet through a mobile device. However, we need to remain cognizant of who we reach with our programs and carefully consider whether we are reaching those most in need of health promotion. Globally, this suggests that ongoing assessment of who has access to computers, the Internet, and mobile and social media is critical to planning and delivery of global eHealth promotion.

Technology for Global eHealth Promotion—What Works?

In this section, we review scientific evidence that supports the utilization of computers, the Internet, mobile phones/SMS, and some initial encouraging findings on **social media** for global eHealth promotion, particularly focusing on randomized control trials that provide the strongest evidence of effective uses. Using technology to facilitate live communication and care delivery is important and critical (often referred to as "telemedicine"). Because it is considered a field in and of itself, we touch on it in a limited fashion here, primarily to illustrate key successes. Although the field remains relatively young, there have been a growing number of studies that distinctly support the promise of these tools for health promotion through their use of rigorous methodology in randomized controlled trials. Table 7.1 offers an overview for the technologies reviewed in this section, highlighting some available features, along with consideration of some pros and cons associated with each and example applications to health promotion from the literature.

Table 7.1 Evidence-Based Technology Tools for Global eHealth Promotion

Tools	Description	Pros/Cons	Examples
Computers and Internet			
Computer- based Programs	User inputs information and algorithm generates tailored feedback (e.g., height + weight calculates BMI)	Pros: Can reach potentially larger numbers of people than otherwise possible; can be accessed when convenient Cons: Digital divide suggests those with greater need may not have access	De & Brug, 1999; Kreuter et al., 2000; Kukafka, et al., 2002
Internet	Websites with information, tailored feedback, testimonial stories, chat rooms, threaded discussions	Pros: Reach; convenient access; additional social support Cons: Digital divide	Gustafson et al., 2002; Gustafson et al., 2005
E-mail	Two-way communication with provider or educator re: health behavior	Pros: Greater access to care provider Cons: Provider burden may increase	Tate, Wing, & Winett, 2001
Mobile Phone/SMS			
Mobile Phone SMS	Short message service texts that allow for interactive two-way communication between users	Pros: Greater access to resource-limited settings; relatively inexpensive; easy to use; highly portable; relatively good evidence for global eHealth promotion Cons: Unable to use with illiterate populations; confidentiality and data security concerns	Lester et al., 2010; Rodgers et al., 2005; Zurovac et al., 2011
Social Media			
Social Media (SM) Pages	Users can create profiles and invite friends and others to view what they post; then they post information that others can see	Pros: Evidence shows that exposure to SM sites can help people maintain healthy behavior Cons: Rigorous evidence of efficacy for health promotion is limited; evidence that networks of friends can reinforce unhealthy behaviors	Bull, Levine et al., 2012; Christakis & Fowler, 2007

Computers: E-mail and the Internet

Initially, with Web 1.0 and computers prior to social networking, the advantages offered to primary prevention of disease (i.e., health promotion) via computers were through the use of tailored messaging that could create individualized information for a consumer. There is a substantial body of research that shows computer-based programs for health promotion can be effective, and one meta-analysis of computer-based efforts for HIV prevention that demonstrate computerized sexual health promotion is as effective as face-to-face education efforts (Noar, Black, & Pierce, 2009).

A study conducted in Belgium across multiple worksites utilized tailored messages related to reduction in fat consumption; researchers offered users access to a computer kiosk in the workplace where they could input personal information on dietary practices and receive feedback that was personally tailored to help them reduce fat consumption. Those receiving tailored information were better able to reduce total fat consumption compared to those receiving generic nontailored information (De Bourdeaudhuij, et al., 2007). The Activ-O-Meter program is one that offers users tailored feedback on their individual level of physical activity—persons regularly log their physical activity either manually or through tools such as pedometers and cyclometers; when tested with adolescent school children across six countries in Europe, it was shown to increase moderate and physical activity as well as cycling for transportation (De Bourdeaudhuij et al., 2010).

Prior to the advent of social networking, the use of e-mail for communication became commonplace and has been effectively integrated into health promotion efforts. Consider, for example, the simple approach to enhance care delivery offered when persons can communicate via e-mail with a nutritionist. This approach was one of the early efforts shown to have efficacy for weight loss. Persons enrolled in a nutrition education program could send messages and communicate via e-mail with a counselor at regular intervals (Tate, Wing, & Winett, 2001).

Other examples of using the Internet for health promotion globally have recently emerged. Ybarra et al. demonstrated that a six-session, Internet-based comprehensive sexuality education program with interactive games designed for secondary school students in Uganda was effective in reducing sexual activity among intervention participants (Ybarra et al., 2013). The program is tailored to deliver different programs to boys and girls and to those who are and are not yet sexually active.

With regard to self-management of disease, computer and Internet-based initiatives have also been widely studied. A US-based meta-analysis of more than 11,000 individuals enrolled in 22 studies that examined the effects of Internet-based chronic disease self-management interventions compared to those that were non-Internet based. The data reveal that Internet-based self-management programs are at least as effective as those delivered in person, and in some cases more so. Specific benefits from participation in these studies among persons with chronic illness included increased exercise time, increased access to medical care, increased awareness of nutrition status, reduced decline in health status, and improved weight loss (Wantland et al., 2004).

Mobile Phones: Short Message Service

Given the ubiquitous nature and relative affordability of mobile phones, these devices have enormous potential to improve health outcomes in developing countries. Mobile phone-based health interventions, also called **mobile health** or **mHealth**, are now being rapidly integrated into health care delivery and global eHealth promotion.

As mobile phone technology has advanced, even basic devices are now equipped with short message service (SMS) capabilities, which consist of the ability to send short text messages of generally 160 characters in length asynchronously to other mobile users at any time or place—meaning that such messages can be accessed immediately or at a later time that is personally convenient for the receiver. SMS is now the most widely used data application in the world, with great potential for global health promotion given its lower bandwidth and lower cost compared to other mobile phone functions. SMS text messages have the added advantages of being able to be customized to individuals as well as allowing for interactive two-way communication between users (which may consist of researchers, health care professionals, patients, and the general population), both of which can be important features in increasing the efficacy of health-related interventions. Indeed, several studies have explored the use of short message service to improve disease prevention (Cole-Lewis & Kershaw, 2010; Fjeldsoe, Marshall, & Mille, 2009; Krishna, Boren, & Balas, 2009; Wei, Hollin, & Kachnowski, 2011), including specifically in developing countries (Déglise, Suggs, & Odermatt, 2012; Gurman, Rubin, & Roess, 2012). There is a growing body of evidence to support SMS applications for both managing chronic diseases—such as HIV/AIDS (Lester et al., 2010), diabetes (Franklin et al., 2006), and asthma (Ostojic et al., 2005)—and promoting behavior modification—such as clinic attendance reminders (Car et al., 2012; Chen et al., 2008), vaccine compliance (Ahlers-Schmidt et al., 2012; Stockwell et al., 2012a; Stockwell et al., 2012b; Vilella et al., 2004), smoking cessation (Whittaker et al., 2012), breast self-examination reminders (Khokhar, 2009), promoting skilled birth attendance (Lund et al., 2012), sunscreen use (Armstrong et al., 2009), weight management (Patrick et al., 2009), and physical activity (Hurling et al., 2007).

The first large randomized control trial to evaluate behavior change using mobile phone text messaging was done in New Zealand with a smoking cessation program (Rodgers et al., 2005). This study included 1,705 young adult smokers who owned mobile phones. The participants were randomized to an intervention group that received regular, personalized text messages promoting smoking cessation (quitting advice, educational support, distraction messages) and to a control group that did not receive any smoking cessation text messages. Participants allocated to the intervention group received five messages per day starting one week prior to a personally established quit date and for the following four weeks. The text messages were then reduced to three per week until the end of a six-month follow-up period. At six weeks follow-up, more than double the number of participants in the intervention group had successfully quit smoking compared to the control group (28% vs. 13%, $p < 0.0001$; number needed to treat [NNT] = 13—meaning one additional quitter for every 13 in the intervention), with a random sample of self-reports confirmed by salivary cotinine verification tests. This treatment effect was similarly observed after 12 weeks (29% vs. 19%, $p < 0.0001$), but between-group differences were less clear after 26 weeks secondary to incomplete follow-up (25% vs. 24%, $p = 0.4$).

As mobile phone SMS interventions became more widely appreciated for their health promotion potential, the first large randomized clinical trial to evaluate SMS in a resource-limited setting was conducted at multiple sites in Kenya (Lester et al., 2010). This study randomized 538 HIV-positive adults initiating antiretroviral therapy (ART) to either an intervention group receiving weekly SMS messages or a control group receiving standard care alone. The intervention group received a text message each week from a clinic nurse inquiring how they were doing (to serve as both a medication reminder and support message). Participants were required to reply to these messages, and the clinic nurse would further call the patient if problems were identified. Self-reported ART adherence (measured as taking > 95% of prescribed doses in the past 30 days) was assessed at 6 and 12 month follow-up visits, and plasma HIV-1 viral RNA load suppression (measured as < 400 copies per mL) was measured at 12 months. Intention-to-treat analysis indicated that ART adherence (62% vs. 50%, $p = 0.006$, NNT = 9) and viral suppression (57% vs. 48%, p = 0.04, NNT = 11) were both significantly better in the intervention group than in the group of patients who received the standard care alone; no further analyses such as dose response were conducted to assess the effects of the number and frequency of message views. Study participants in the intervention group overwhelmingly reported the SMS program to be valuable and said they would recommend it to a friend (98%).

SMS interventions can also be used with target audiences other than patients. A large cluster-randomized control trial in Kenya was the first such study to use text messages to improve health workers' adherence to national guidelines for the management of outpatient pediatric malaria (Zurovac et al., 2011). This study was conducted at 107 rural health facilities and included 119 health workers who were randomized to either an intervention group that received text message reminders regarding malaria case management or a control group that did not receive any text messages. The intervention group received two text messages daily for five days a week during a six-month period; 2,269 children were treated over the course of the study. Intention-to-treat analysis showed that the correct artemether-lumefantrine treatment for malaria, according to the Kenyan national guidelines, improved by 25% ($p = 0.003$) six months after the trial period ended. The authors concluded that text messages could be used in resource-limited settings to improve health worker performance and case-management practices. Additionally, a follow-up study showed that the text messages were well received by the health workers involved in the intervention (Jones et al., 2012).

There are many advantages to using mobile phones for global eHealth promotion. These devices are more affordable than other mediums of telecommunication and often have pay-as-you-go plans offered in many resource-limited settings. Mobile phones are also increasingly more portable with their small size, low weight, and rechargeable and long-life battery. People are therefore able to carry mobile devices wherever they go, providing nearly constant access. Mobile phones are now able to reach remote and otherwise inaccessible areas that do not have access to the Internet, consistent electricity, or cumbersome fixed land lines—reaching populations previously limited by the digital divide.

Mobile telecommunication with text messaging provides new and exciting opportunities for health promotion. However, such technology is not without its disadvantages—namely, that interventions cannot go into depth with small mobile screens and short messaging allowances, a potential lack of confidentiality with potential device sharing, difficulties ensuring anonymity and data security, the for prohibitive SMS and mobile device costs, high mobile phone turnover rates, mobile network fluctuations, and an inability to reach illiterate populations. Additionally, the evaluation of SMS interventions has generally not been done consistently or rigorously (Gurman et al., 2012). There currently is only limited empirical evidence of efficacy surrounding these interventions because sample sizes have often been small and study designs have not been consistently rigorous. There is a need for a greater number of studies evaluating SMS with sound methodology and sufficient statistical power (Fjeldsoe et al., 2009). Most research evaluating mHealth interventions has historically been done in developed countries (Cole-Lewis & Kershaw, 2010). There remains a need for more studies based in resource-limited settings, especially with regard to large-scale implementation and the evaluation of cost-effectiveness. Finally, there is a lack of evidence for the long-term maintenance of SMS interventions. An immediate need exists for ongoing and long-term evaluations of such mHealth programs. Although the use of cellular telephones and text messaging still remains in its infancy in many parts of the world, the potential for this medium of communication to promote health outcomes is gaining important momentum with a growing body of evidence toward its positive impact on global health.

Social Media

Although there has been substantial interest in and use of social media, through which people use the computer and Internet as a way to interact with friends and acquaintances, we know of only one intervention to date that has established efficacy for improvements in health behavior using this tool. In a study exploring the use of the popular social networking site Facebook, investigators randomized participants to "like" a page focused on increasing condom use for prevention of sexually transmitted infections, including HIV (intervention—called the "Just/Us" study, an attempt to convey that sexual health content for youth was "just" for them) or a control page with content related to celebrity and music news. Those exposed to the intervention page were significantly more likely to have a higher proportion of sex acts protected by condom use and a higher proportion of persons who used condoms at last sex than to the controls. The majority of this intervention was delivered through RSS feed, sending regular, short messages to participants' Facebook pages about the importance of condom use (see examples in Figure 7.1) (Bull, Levine, Black, Schmiege, & Santelli, 2012).

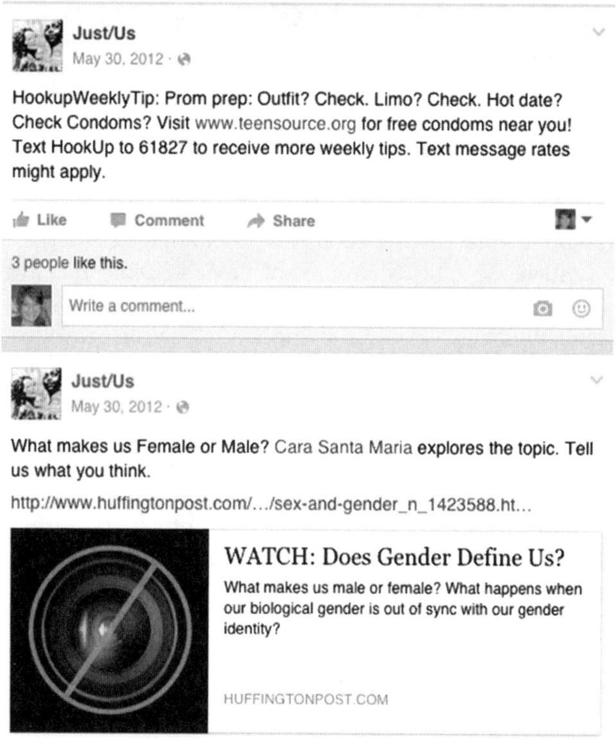

Figure 7.1 Examples of RSS Feed on Facebook re: Sexual Health

As with the Internet and mobile devices, the use of social media for global eHealth promotion promises substantial reach to populations at risk for negative health outcomes beyond what is typically available in traditional health promotion programs. Additionally, social media provides access to not only individuals, but those within their social networks. Given strong evidence that social support (Christakis & Fowler, 2007; Sanders, Lim, & Sohn, 2008; Väänänen et al., 2008) can facilitate or hinder adoption of healthy behavior as well as the presence of "important others," "role models," and "popular opinion leaders" (Friedman et al., 2007; Kelly, 2004; Moreira, Smith, & Foxcroft, 2010) online social networks accessible through social media offer an unprecedented opportunity to explore whether we can indirectly influence members of online social networks through education of influential persons online.

Although social media use is substantially widespread across the globe, it is not universal, and considerations for whether particular audiences for a given health promotion program utilize social media are important. For example, China has banned Facebook, but local social media companies are developing there. Beyond China, however, the access to and use of social media sites such as Facebook globally are staggering. The company has more than a billion users, and a 2011 report indicated there were only seven countries in the world where Facebook was not the most popular social media site (Radwanick, 2013).

Emerging Technologies in Global eHealth and mHealth

Over time, technologies become increasingly adopted or fall by the wayside. As they evolve, new uses and applications may become established. Many of the technologies described in the previous section were reviewed distinctly, but the reality is they are becoming increasingly integrated, and particularly so when examining emerging technologies. Technologies emerge, evolve, and sometimes dissolve, so quickly in current environments that the following section can only provide a snapshot of the possibilities. Also, the ways in which these technologies inform and support global eHealth promotion are only beginning to be understood. Though the possibilities are immense and the imagination can only begin to realize promising opportunities, they should be critically approached. Ethical considerations abound, and technology is not effective for health promotion just because it is new and exciting. The following section presents a series of emerging technologies with great promise for health promotion, but their effectiveness is not yet established. Table 7.2 provides a brief summary of the technologies reviewed in this section, including smartphones, social media, and place-based systems.

Smartphone Applications

During the past decade, mobile phones and tablets have become much more sophisticated in their capacity—both in terms of their operational speed and increased versatility. Mobile technologies have moved beyond basic voice and text messaging communication to become compact, handheld computers with telephone capabilities. Such devices now typically include additional services, such as wireless Internet capability, high-resolution touchscreens, increased memory, multimedia players, digital cameras, video recorders, geopositioning, and other various downloadable applications or "apps." Apps are diverse programs designed to run on a smartphone operating system that can be downloaded from several mobile app markets and vary both in function and price (some are free downloads, a one-time purchase price, or periodic subscriptions). Although primitive versions of smartphones were developed in the early 1990s (the IBM Simon Personal Communicator marketed by BellSouth), more advanced devices were not created for nearly another decade. Starting in 1996, Nokia developed the Nokia Communicator line, which began to incorporate personal digital assistants (PDAs) with mobile phones. In 2000, Ericsson coined the term *smartphone* when it unveiled the R380 Smartphone, the first phone to use an open operating system (Symbian). Other companies soon followed with the Palm OS Treo and RIM's BlackBerry released in 2002, Apple's iPhone in 2007, Google's Android in 2008, and Samsung's Bada-based phone and Microsoft's Windows Phone in 2010. Further advancements in the functioning of smartphones have completely revolutionized the way we communicate and access information and have made this technology an emerging method of global eHealth promotion.

Though smartphones certainly hold promise, this technology is very much in its infancy, with little evidence to support its widespread use as a means

Table 7.2 Emerging Tools With Potential for Global eHealth Promotion

Tools	Description	Pros/Cons	Examples
Smartphones			
Smartphone Applications ("apps")	Diverse programs designed to run on a smartphone operating system that can be downloaded from several mobile app markets and vary both in function and price	Pros: Highly sophisticated and portable; able to reach remote areas Cons: Expensive devices that will likely be limited by the digital divide; lack of regulatory oversight for content	Boulos et al., 2011; Hicks, 2012; Kreatsoulas, 2010; Kroemer et al., 2011; Rajput et al., 2012
Social Media			
Weblogs/Blogs	Online journals that anyone can create and post on any topic; have been used to describe personal experiences with illness; share information about accessing care; outbreaks	Pros: May allow for (a) qualitative assessment of online content; (b) understanding of what engages users Cons: No quality guidelines or uniformity in posting; difficult to ascertain whether post is valid	Health Weblogs http://www.mdanderson.org/cancerwise http://www.hioti.org
RSS Feed	Information that is "pushed" to social media users by their friends and organizations directly to their social media page	Pros: Users do not have to leave their own page and navigate elsewhere online to obtain content on topics they are interested in Cons: Users must "opt in" to get information through RSS	Just/Us Facebook http://www.facebook.com/justusisis?ref=ts&fref=ts
Message Boards	Online bulletin boards where people can post comments to ongoing discussions; also known as threaded discussions	Pros: Users can participate on their own homepages in discussions or can do this on a project specific space; they can interact in dialogue and obtain helpful guidance from other users on a topic Cons: Users may have to navigate away from their own pages to participate; no way to identify credibility of post or person posting	Everyday Health Message Boards http://www.Everydayhealth.com http://www.Healthboards.com
Video	Users and professionals can develop videos on health related topics and post them to a video sharing site (e.g., YouTube, Vimeo)	Pros: Digital storytelling is developing as a recognized method for conveyance of health information; tools are widely available for public use Cons: Nonetheless, not all users comply with standards in development; no way to identify credibility of post/person posting	Digital Storytelling for Health http://tinyurl.com/HepC-Colorado; http://www.youtube.com/watch?v=-iUJxlzxUTw&list=PL580CF813CAF66FE2; http://www.youtube.com/watch?v=0gJ183CbGNI

(*continued*)

Table 7.2 *(Continued)*

Tools	Description	Pros/Cons	Examples
Place-Based Systems			
Mapping & Data Exchange	Static (paper and digital) and interactive mapping based on a dataset in place	Pros: Can be used for surveillance, evaluation, hypothesis generation, risk communication Cons: Data is collected for a specific purpose and may not be useful in other contexts; issues of updating, maintenance, completeness, consistency and time period	Global Health Atlas http://www.who.int/globalatlas/ US CDC's Atlas of Mortality: http://www.cdc.gov/nchs/products/other/atlas/atlas.htm Dartmouth Atlas of Health Care: Regional Disparity in Medicare Spending http://dartmouthatlas.org/interactive_map.shtm
Community-Based, Participatory Mapping	Mapping done in close collaboration with the community, whereby the community sets priorities and collects data; paper and/or digital	Pros: Garners detailed information; community buy-in; data that is not collected otherwise; local concerns emerge; can be used for advocacy and empowerment Cons: Participatory processes can take on many forms that in turn can produce divergent information; ethical issues around ownership, who is represented, who is empowered	Transparent Chennai http://www.transparentchennai.com/ Map Kibera http://mapkibera.org/
Interactive Mapping (Data Generation)	Crowdsourcing integrating information using SMS, e-mail, Twitter, and the Web integrated with mapping	Pros: Innovative data not obtainable through traditional sources; creative approaches to deriving mapped data Cons: Ethical considerations around privacy and confidentiality; data verification and validity; credibility of people contributing; credibility of information	Ushahidi: http://www.ushahidi.com/ Who is Sick?: http://www.whoissick.org/sickness/
Mapping & Data Exchange	Static (paper and digital) and interactive mapping based on a dataset in place	Pros: Can be used for surveillance, evaluation, hypothesis generation, risk communication Cons: Data is collected for a specific purpose and may not be useful in other contexts; issues of updating, maintenance, completeness, consistency and time period	Global Health Atlas: http://www.who.int/globalatlas/ U.S. CDC's Atlas of Mortality: http://www.cdc.gov/nchs/products/other/atlas/atlas.htm Dartmouth Atlas of Health Care: Regional Disparity in Medicare Spending http://dartmouthatlas.org/interactive_map.shtm

Source: Table material on social media adapted from Korda, H., and Itani, Z. (2011). Harnessing Social Media for Health Promotion and Behavior Change. *Health Promotion Practice*. [Epub ahead of print] http://hpp.sagepub.com/content/14/1/15.long

of promoting health. As shown earlier in this chapter, there is relatively good evidence to support using mobile phones for text messaging interventions to promote behavior changes such as smoking cessation (Rodgers et al., 2005; Whittaker et al., 2012). Similar large, randomized controlled studies with smartphone apps do not currently exist. In a 2011 review Abroms et al. explored smartphone applications for smoking cessation; They concluded that not only is there a lack of evidence surrounding the efficacy of such applications, but these apps also rarely adhere to proven strategies and established guidelines for smoking cessation. The article further concluded that future smartphone applications for behavior change should be developed around evidence-based practices and should undergo much more rigorous evaluation by public health professionals before being used as a method of health promotion.

The traditional health care delivery model, where patients present to health care providers, has often been inadequate in developing countries where clinics may be sparse, trained specialty physicians are rare, and travel is more difficult. Smartphones have the potential to improve this paradigm in multiple ways. A home-based counseling and testing program was developed in a resource-limited setting in western Kenya to collect health information, offer rapid HIV testing as well as sputum collection for tuberculosis testing, and provide focused clinical care when needed (Rajput et al., 2012). This Android-based mHealth program, called "Open Data Kit Collect," was shown to have high user satisfaction by the community health workers and was determined to be a cost-effective method of large-scale data collection and population surveillance (as compared to pen-and-paper collection and comparable to PDA methods). Smartphones are also revolutionizing **telehealthcare**, which is the delivery of health-related services via telecommunication technologies (Bashshur et al., 2014). The eCAALYX (Enhanced Complete Ambient Assisted Living Experiement) Android smartphone app is a European Union-funded project to monitor elderly patients with multiple chronic medical conditions (Boulos et al., 2011). The patient wears a small garment with wireless health sensors (such as accelerometers measuring motion and gait and infrared detectors measuring body temperature and heart rate) that send information through the smartphone's Internet connection to health care providers so that they can remotely monitor each patient's well-being (such as fall risk) and help manage the patient's multiple medical problems (such as heart disease). Similarly, a mini-feasibility trial conducted in Belfast showed positive results for the INNSULIN (Intelligent Neural Network for Suggesting Unambiguous Levels of Insulin via Needle) application that uses a glucometer linked to a smartphone to help diabetic patients manage their glucose levels and insulin dosing with the help of a remote endocrinologist (Curran et al., 2010). Though no clinical trials have yet to be conducted on these applications, they show promise as emerging methods of telehealthcare.

Additionally, the camera phone function of smartphones has important implications for telemedicine. Pilot studies have shown positive results for the remote diagnosis and management of extremity wounds via consultation with a plastic surgeon (based on a pilot study with 60 patients conducted by Tsai et al., 2004), the remote diagnosis and triaging of digital soft-tissue injuries via consultation with a plastic surgeon (based on a pilot study with 45 patients conducted by Hsieh et al., 2004), and the remote diagnosis of malignant skin tumors via consultation with a dermatologist (based on a pilot study with 88 patients conducted by Kroemer et al., 2011). A portable RetCam Shuttle, which is a wide-field digital retinal fundus camera, is being used to take retinal images in premature infants. These images are then transmitted via cellular phones to a consulting ophthalmologist who is able to diagnose retinopathy of prematurity in a resource-limited setting in India through a tele-ophthalmology program called KIDROP (Karnataka Internet-Assisted Diagnosis of Retinopathy of Prematurity) (Kreatsoulas, 2010). New smartphone technology is now exploring the possibility of the remote diagnosis of malaria via the Lifelens smartphone app, which uses a magnified image from a patient's blood smear (prepared from a finger prick with a specific marker dye) to identify the malaria parasite (Hicks, 2012), as well as the remote diagnosis of acute otitis media via a clip-on smartphone attachment called the Remotoscope, which allows parents to take images of their child's tympanic membrane to send to a physician to diagnose ear infections (Atlanta Pediatric Device Consortium, 2013).

Smartphone technology is also being increasingly used by both laypersons and health care providers in daily clinical care. Smartphone apps exist for providing patient education and self-assessment tools (including patient handouts, physician directories, and other reference tools), continuing professional development for health care professionals and students (including virtual procedures, training games, board review material, logbooks, and instructional videos), aiding clinical decision making with quick reference tools for health care providers (including textbooks and journals, established guidelines and algorithms, drug guides such as *Epocrates*, outbreak surveillance such as H1N1 influenza apps during the 2009–2010 pandemic, and various medical calculators), and accessing patient records and administrative tools (including electronic medical records and billing apps). Thousands of medical apps already exist, including applications for eye surgeons (Bastawrous, Cheeseman, & Kumar, 2012), general surgeons (Dala-Ali, Lloyd, & Al-Abed, 2011), plastic surgeons (Mohan & Branford, 2012), orthopedic surgeons (Franko, 2011), neurosurgeons (Kubben, 2010), anesthesiologists (Kraidin, Ginsberg, & Solina, 2012), otolaryngologists (Pope, Silva, & Almeyda, 2010), urologists (Abboudi & Amin, 2011), radiologists (Choudhri & Radvany, 2011), medical residents (Franko & Tirrell, 2012), dermatologic diseases (Hamilton & Brady, 2012), colorectal diseases (O'Neill & Brady, 2012), pain management (Rosser & Eccleston, 2011), and infectious diseases (Oehler, Smith, & Toney, 2010). The number of medically related smartphone applications will only continue to increase as this technology becomes more prevalent and accessible.

Many challenges exist surrounding the use of smartphones for global eHealth promotion, including those previously expressed for SMS interventions. When compared to basic mobile phones, however, smartphone devices and data packages for more advanced features may be cost-prohibitive for many low-income populations, and interventions utilizing these devices will likely not circumvent the digital divide in the same way in which we saw SMS technology. The battery life in areas of weak cellular signal is also likely to be a problem. Additionally, when smartphones are used as medical devices, there are concerns related to interference with other clinical equipment, surface contamination of the phone, and regulatory oversight. The US Food and Drug Administration (FDA) has regulated medical devices for many years, and there is a growing acknowledgement that such regulations will also need to be applied to mobile applications similarly functioning as medical devices (Barton, 2012; Merrell & Doarn, 2011). In fact, the FDA issued draft guidance regarding the regulation of mobile medical applications in July, 2011 (US FDA, 2011) and final guidance for developers of mobile medical apps in September 2013 (US FDA, 2015). Similarly, there is a very concerning lack of regulation or guidelines related to the content of smartphone applications, especially in their use among lay consumers, resulting in unknown validity and reliability of smartphone programs (Rosser & Eccleston, 2011). Many applications either do not include or do not specify any medical professional involvement in their design, and there is currently no capacity for critical peer review, leading to obvious patient safety concerns (Visser & Buijink, 2012). No randomized controlled trials exist in the literature for using smartphone apps in global eHealth promotion, and there is an obvious need to explore the evidence and evaluate the effectiveness of specific apps already in use. As smartphone applications continue to advance, it will be important to balance the need for regulatory oversight with the promotion of further innovation so that neither technological advancement nor patient safety are compromised.

Social Media and Social Networking

Some researchers posit that "social media is a communications tool and not a causal factor in behavior change or health status" (Neiger et al., 2013 p. 159) and is instead an opportunity to raise awareness, promote a brand (e.g., for a health promotion campaign), expand campaign reach, and foster engagement between professionals and the public on key health topics. We would disagree with the assessment that social media cannot be a causal factor in behavior change given evidence to the contrary discussed from the Just/Us study demonstrating the efficacy of using social media to affect sexual health behaviors. It is certainly the case, however, that there are as of yet few other examples that demonstrate efficacy of the medium for behavior change.

Although publications attending to the use of social media for health promotion have come from the United States, there is indication that social media is increasingly popular globally, particularly media that allows for access on mobile devices (Bull et al., 2012; Houghland 2013; Moreno et al., 2011). Given this popularity, we consider that social media has potential for benefit with regard to health promotion and that future work should focus on establishing its effects. Evidence shows that interaction with social media is primarily focused on posting comments on friends' social media pages, sharing photos and sending group messages (Lenhart et al., 2007). Consideration of these activities and the potential they hold for health promotion have been outlined in greater detail in Table 7.2. With each element we offer consideration of the potential pros and cons and examples of its use to promote health.

In the face of limited evidence of social media efficacy for health promotion, researchers have focused on the need to identify appropriate indicators that can demonstrate efficacy. Neiger et al. call for the development of key performance indicators (KPI) for social media that would be similar to the Web-based analytics used in industry settings that document traffic to webpages and engagement with content (Neiger et al., 2013). Their argument is that these KPI would help establish important process data to demonstrate that site users are engaging with content. Our own perspective is that the assumption that engagement in the form of posting, or commenting on posts or sharing material, is a necessary factor in promoting behavior change is as of yet an empirical question. It may be that simple exposure to content without active engagement is sufficient to affect behavior; in the case of the Just/Us study, even though there was significantly higher condom use among those in the intervention group compared to controls, only 10% of those in the intervention group actually posted on the Facebook page; all others were exposed to content only through the RSS feed (Bull, Walker, & Levine, 2012). This suggests we have more to understand about what type of engagement with social media is needed to affect behavioral outcomes; indeed, multiple researchers argue for the importance of understanding what elements of social media are critical to include in effective health promotion campaigns (Gold et al., 2013).

One element of social media that has substantial potential yet has not been explored for health promotion is the capacity to engage and influence networks of users. In particular, social media sites allow friends to stay connected, and as such, these networks represent groups of people who have a priori influence on others in their network. This influence likely goes beyond what may be possible for any teacher or health professional interacting with individuals online. Christakis et al. showed retrospectively how network members influenced each other's weight gain over time (Christakis & Fowler, 2007). We posit that an as-yet unexplored but critical area for exploration is how we can prospectively spread information on health through networks using social media. The tool would allow for rapid and almost instant access to large numbers of people who may be more influential among their friends than any professional could hope to be.

Ultimately the role of social media in global eHealth promotion hinges on access and utilization of these tools. As mentioned, access to mobile phones is much higher than access to the Internet; as long as there remains a digital divide for access to the Internet we face limitations in the extent to which we can realize the potential for these tools to fundamentally influence health.

Place-Based Technologies

People are increasingly familiar with place-based (spatial) technologies through popular interfaces such as GoogleMap, MapQuest, or even mapping technologies embedded within cell phone applications. Mapping technologies have almost become a part of everyday life for many using Internet and smartphones, and in fact are becoming increasingly common on mobile platforms. The development of the technologies is incredibly rapid, far outpacing our ability to assess and evaluate effectiveness. The ways in which basic mapping supports health promotion is not well documented in research studies so understanding the interface with other technologies becomes an even greater challenge. However, we do have numerous examples of emerging innovations with place-based technology that show promise for facilitation of global eHealth promotion.

GIS is increasingly utilized throughout many public health activities, including disease surveillance, identifying contributing factors to illness, examining health disparity, and even to evaluate healthcare access (Comber, Brunsdon, & Radburn, 2011; Cromley, 2003; McLafferty, 2003). The use of GIS for detecting, monitoring, and designing interventions for infectious diseases is also widely applied (Sueur & Tanser, 2002), including cholera (Ali, et al., 2002; Emch et al., 2009), malaria (Caldas de Castro, Sawyer, & Singer, 2007; Kelly et al., 2012), HIV (Torugsa et al., 2003; Wand, Whitaker, & Ramje, 2011), among numerous others. Community health mapping (Ansumana et al., 2010) and participatory health mapping (Rambaldi et al., 2006) are also becoming more common approaches. GIS and spatial analysis provide tools for examining how various aspects of location (for example, altitude, pollution, or even social context) are associated with a variety of diseases and health outcomes. The WHO's Global Health Atlas (WHO, n.d.) is but one example of the numerous online platforms that integrates standardized data from numerous sources to support work in a variety of health areas.

Many of the social networking and information sharing technologies presented in the other portions of the chapter now automatically collect some type of geographic location, though not all in a complete manner. In other words, information can be tied directly to maps, which is termed georeferenced information. When information is crowdsourced or volunteered from the public or a defined group of experts with this geographic element, the ability to incorporate onto maps becomes possible. An example includes photographs taken from a smartphone uploaded to Facebook, which are posted to all sorts of sites that now have a geotag (now referenced to a map). Ushahidi has emerged as a leading open-source GIS package that supports the input of crowdsource information, and has frequently been used in health and disaster applications (Ushahidi, n.d.), with examples from monitoring the swine flu to the generation of crisis maps during the Russian fires or the Pakistan floods. In these cases, people volunteer SMS information into a central location, which then produces a picture of events that is useful for organizing response efforts and identifying places for intervention.

Another platform, Google.org's Flu Trends captures Google searches in different parts of the world to estimate influenza activity (Google.org, n.d.) and illustrates another type of technology integration only recently possible. Web mashups are automated functions for combining data or functionality from a variety of sources to create new information. While revealing vast potential for public health applications, this application also highlights challenges with the emerging place-based technologies. Privacy, monitoring, confidentiality, data quality, and confirmation all emerge as significant ethical considerations.

Selecting Appropriate Technologies

In global eHealth promotion, the continual emergence of new technologies can be seductive. A new technology can certainly be admired for its innovation, but we caution that choices to develop and implement a global eHealth promotion endeavor should be driven primarily by whether it will reach the intended audience, whether they will use it, and whether it can be sustained in that environment. If, for example, there is an effective, highly interactive, bandwidth-intensive program designed for delivery on the Internet, it may not be appropriate for a setting where Internet service is limited; where electricity is sporadic; and where few people own the computer hardware to access the program. Similarly, a peripheral device to electronically monitor medication adherence may be costly, easily lost or broken. If we know that self-report of medication compliance via text message can work equally well to facilitate compliance with medication among patients, this relatively lower technology solution can reach more people and be more easily sustained over time.

The key considerations for selecting appropriate technologies in global eHealth promotion include:

- Will the technology help us reach a larger number of people than we are currently reaching?
- Are these people in greater need or currently not accessing services or programs we provide?
- Can people access the program elements using the technologies they currently have? (e.g., their current phone?)

Consideration of Privacy, Confidentiality, and Data Ownership

The advent of computers, the Internet, mobile phones, place-based technology, and social media is accompanied by heightened awareness of consumer privacy and confidentiality. Any effort to promote health that includes collection of personal data and information opens up the possibility that individual privacy or confidentiality may be compromised. To that end, it is critical to consider whether it is even necessary to collect or maintain any personally identifying information in the implementation of a program. If documentation of personally identifying information is necessary for a program, then careful attention to computer security and systems that limit access to such information are needed. Additionally, a full disclosure to any program participant about how personal information will be managed and shared represents standard practice for any program.

There have been important questions raised about data ownership when technologies such as mobile phones, GIS, and social media are being used. For example, if a person receives a text message encouraging them to test for HIV, and then GIS from their phone shows they are in the vicinity of a clinic, should that information be accessible to the program sending the original text? Questions about ownership of photos posted on social media have emerged in the media, and continue to spark debate about this issue. Health promoters need to consider how to negotiate data ownership in a way that is fair and ethical to their constituents (Levine et al., 2011).

The key considerations for privacy, confidentiality, and data ownership include:

- Dialogue before a program starts on what types of data are critical and necessary

- Dialogue before a program starts on who "owns" data and has rights for using it
- Transparency; being open and clear about what data are being collected for a program and why, who has access to it and how it will be protected

Program Evaluation

A continual concern expressed about global eHealth promotion is that evaluation of program efficacy lags behind new technological innovations. We are challenged to ensure that our systems for evaluation can be efficient and timely. We can do more to shorten the timeline for research on program efficacy, and to improve systems to disseminate information beyond academia so that more practitioners have access to timely information about what works for global eHealth promotion. Additionally, we can reconsider approaches for evaluation that are more agile than a randomized controlled trial (RCT), such as quasi-experimental evaluation, modeling, and simulations (Bennett & Glasgow, 2009). This could make research more responsive in a fast-paced technologic environment, particularly to help developers in rapidly prototyping their applications. However, the RCT does represent the gold standard in methodological rigor, and ultimately the best practices to demonstrate evidence of efficacy and effectiveness. There are methodological trade-offs that may be needed for agility and rapid responsiveness.

The key considerations for evaluation of global eHealth promotion include:

- Shortening the timeline for evaluation to ensure that programs aren't obsolete by the time we determine they work
- Disseminate evaluation information on "what works" quickly, capitalizing on the technologies described here to do so
- Consider options beyond the RCT to facilitate more accessible evaluation

Summary

In this chapter, we have oriented the reader to the use of computers, the Internet, mobile phones, place-based systems, and social media in global eHealth promotion. These rapidly evolving technologies offer fundamental advantages in reaching unprecedented numbers of people, allowing for access to desired health information at the most relevant times, and facilitate both social support for and delivery of health promotion programming in new and exciting ways. We have shared the most current information available related to "what works," using these technologies as well as what is emerging in this field. We reviewed critical considerations for anyone wishing to integrate technology into their health promotion endeavor: the need to select appropriate technologies and to consider resources, cost, and the ability to maintain technology based efforts to promote health among those who are in the greatest need. They include the need for careful consideration of privacy and confidentiality of individual information and for consideration of ownership of data and information shared via technology.

Technology has revolutionized global health promotion. We have seen a growing number of innovations that can exponentially expand the reach of our programs and have the potential to substantially impact the health of communities worldwide. With every new month there are exciting new technological advances that can be applied to health. Our work in the coming years will be to recognize their value for health promotion, and be prepared to quickly evaluate their effectiveness for impacting health outcomes.

KEY TERMS

1. **Digital divide:** The divide between those who have access to computer hardware and software and those who do not, who are generally poor and with fewer resources
2. **eHealth:** The use of technology of any kind, including computers, the Internet, mobile, and social media to promote health and healthy behavior
3. **Geographic information systems (GIS):** Computer software that captures, manages, analyzes, and displays spatial (geographic) data
4. **Mobile health (mHealth):** The use of using mobile telecommunication technology (such as text messaging, video messaging, voice calling, and Internet connectivity) for health-related purposes
5. **Place-based health:** The set of geographic technologies (global positioning systems: GPS, GIS, remote sensing) that assist in understanding how social, environmental, economic, and other conditions in a given place contribute to various health outcomes
6. **Short message service (SMS):** A simple transfer of data between mobile phones that is usually limited to 160 characters in length (also known as *text messaging*)
7. **Smartphone:** A cellular phone built on a mobile operating system that integrates computer capabilities such as wireless Internet, multimedia player, digital camera, video recorder, geopositioning, and other various downloadable applications or "apps"
8. **Social media:** Use of a mobile or desktop computer to interact with others through chat, posting pictures, participating in discussion, or games
9. **Telehealthcare:** The delivery of health-related services via telecommunication technologies
10. **Web 1.0** and **Web 2.0:** The evolution of the Internet; Web 1.0 refers to earlier days of the Internet when users would obtain information and resources online; Web 2.0 refers to the added capacity to interact not only with the Internet but with others (e.g., friends, family) via the Internet.

REVIEW QUESTIONS

1. What evidence is there to suggest that computers, the Internet, and mobile devices can be used to support global health?
2. What is an example of a specific program that has utilized an eHealth element with proven success in global health?
3. What is at least one example of an emerging strategy using eHealth for global health promotion?
4. What are at least two key considerations for privacy and confidentiality in the delivery of eHealth promotion in global health?

References

Abboudi, H., & Amin, K. (2011). Smartphone applications for the urology trainee. *British Journal of Urology International, 108*, 1371–1373.

Abroms, L. C., Padmanabhan, N., Thaweethai, L., & Phillips, T. (2011). iPhone apps for smoking cessation: A content analysis. *American Journal of Preventive Medicine, 40*(3), 279–285.

Ahlers-Schmidt, C. R., Chesser, A. K., Nguyen, T., Brannon, J., Hart, T. A., Williams, K. S., & Wittler, R. R. (2012). Feasibility of a randomized controlled trial to evaluate Text Reminders for Immunization Compliance in Kids (TRICKs). *Vaccine, 30*, 5305–5309.

Ali, M., Emch, M., Donnay, J. P., Yunus, M., & Sack, R. B. (2002). Identifying environmental risk factors for endemic cholera: A raster GIS approach. *Health & Place, 8*(3), 201–210.

Ansumana, R., Malanoski, A. P., Bockarie, A. S., Sundufu, A. J., Jimmy, D. H., ... Stenger, D. A. (2010). Enabling methods for community health mapping in developing countries. *International Journal of Health Geography, 9*, 56.

Armstrong, A., Watson, A., Makredes, M., Frangos, J., Kimball, A., & Kvedar, J. (2009). Text-message reminders to improve sunscreen use: A randomized, controlled trial using electronic monitoring. *Archives of Dermatology, 145*(11), 1230–1236.

Atlanta Pediatric Device Consortium. (2013). *Remotoscope*. Retrieved from http://pediatricdevicesatlanta.org/remotoscope

Barton, A. J. (2012). The regulation of mobile health applications. *BMC Medicine, 10*, 46.

Bashshur, R., Shannon, G., Smith, B., Alberson, D., Antoniotti, N., Barsan, W., ... Yellowlees, P. (2014). The empirical foundations of telemedicine for chronic disease management. *Telemedicine Journal of e-Health. 20*(9): 769–800.

Bastawrous, A., Cheeseman, R. C., & Kumar, A. (2012). iPhones for eye surgeons. *Eye, 26*, 343–354.

Bellis, M. (2010). Inventors of the modern computer. *About.com.* Retrieved from http://inventors.about.com/library/weekly/aa050298.htm

Bennett, G., & Glasgow, R. (2009). The delivery of public health interventions via the Internet: Actualizing their potential. *Annual Reviews in. Public Health, 30*, 273–292.

Boulos, M. N., Wheeler, S., Tavares, C., & Jones, R. (2011). How smartphones are changing the face of mobile and participatory healthcare: An overview, with example from eCAALYX. *Biomedical Engineering Online, 10*, 24–37.

Brenner, J. (2013). *PEW Internet: Mobile.* PEW Internet and American Life. Retrieved from http://pewinternet.org/Commentary/2012/February/Pew-Internet-Mobile.aspx

Bull, S., Levine, D., Black, S., Schmiege, S., & Santelli, J. (2012). Social media delivered sexual health intervention: A cluster-randomized trial. *American Journal of Preventive Medicine, 43*, 467–474.

Bull, S., Walker, T., & Levine, D. (2012). Communities and technology: Enhancements in HIV Prevention research and practice among youth and young adults. In S. Rhodes & R. Aronson (Eds.), *Innovations in HIV prevention research and practice through community engagement* (1st ed., pp. 183–214). Springer-Verlag, New York.

Caldas de Castro, M., Sawyer, D. O., & Singer, B. H. (2007). Spatial patterns of malaria in the Amazon: Implications for surveillance and targeted interventions. *Health & Place, 13*, 368–380.

Car, J., Gurol-Urganci, I., de Jongh, T., Vodopivec-Jamsek, V., & Atun, R. (2012). Mobile phone messaging reminders for attendance at healthcare appointments. *Cochrane Database Systematic Reviews, 7*, CD007458.

Cole-Lewis, H., & Kershaw, T. (2010). Text messaging as a tool for behavior change in disease prevention and management. *Epidemiologic Reviews, 32*(1), 56–69.

Chen, Z., Fang, L., Chen, L., & Dai, H. (2008). Comparison of an SMS text messaging and phone reminder to improve attendance at a health promotion center. A randomized controlled trial. *Journal of Zhejiang University Science, 9*(1), 34–38.

Choudhri, A. F., & Radvany, M. G. (2011). Initial experiences with a handheld device digital imaging and communications in medicine viewer: OsiriX Mobile on the iPhone. *Journal of Digital Imaging, 24*(2), 184–189.

Christakis, N. A., & Fowler, J. H. (2007). Change to obesity: The spread of obesity in a large social network over 32 years. *New England Journal of Medicine, 357*, 370–379.

Comber, A. J., Brunsdon, C., & Radburn, R. (2011). A spatial analysis of variations in health access: Linking geography, socio-economic status and access perceptions. *International Journal of Health Geographics, 10*, 44.

Cromley, E. K. (2003). GIS and disease. *Annual Reviews in Public Health, 24*, 7–24.

Curran, K., Nichols, E., Xie, E., & Harper, R. (2010). An intensive insulin therapy mobile phone application built on artificial intelligence techniques. *Journal of Diabetes Science and Technology, 4*(1), 209–220.

Dala-Ali, B. M., Lloyd, M. A., & Al-Abed, Y. (2011). The uses of the iPhone for surgeons. *Surgeon, 9*(1), 44–48.

De Bourdeaudhuij, I., Maes, L., De Henauw, S., De Vriendt, T., Moreno, L. A., Kersting, M., ... HELENA Study Group. (2010). Evaluation of a computer-tailored physical activity intervention in adolescents in six European countries: The Activ-O-Meter in the HELENA intervention study. *Journal of Adolescent Health, 46*, 458–466.

De Bourdeaudhuij, I., Stevens, V., Vandelanotte, C., & Brug, J. (2007). Evaluation of an interactive computer-tailored nutrition intervention in a real-life setting. *Annals of Behavioral Medicine, 33*, 39–48.

De, V. H. & Brug, J. (1999). Computer-tailored interventions motivating people to adopt health promoting behaviours: introduction to a new approach. *Patient Education and Counseling, 36*, 99–105.

Déglise, C., Suggs, L. S., & Odermatt, P. (2012). Short message service (SMS) applications for disease prevention in developing countries. *Journal of Medical Internet Research, 14*(1), e3.

Emch, M., Ali, M., Root, E. D., & Yunus, M. (2009). Spatial and environmental connectivity analysis in a cholera vaccine trial. *Social Science and Medicine, 68*(4), 631–637.

Fjeldsoe, B. S., Marshall, A. L., & Miller, Y. D. (2009). Behavior change interventions delivered by mobile telephone short-message service. *American Journal of Preventive Medicine, 36*(2), 165–173.

Forestier, E., Grace, J., & Kenny, C. (2002). Can information and communication technologies be pro-poor? *Telecommunications Policy, 26*, 623–646.

Franklin, V., Walker, A., Pagliari, C., & Greene, A. (2006). A randomized controlled trial of SweetTalk, a text-messaging system to support young people with diabetes. *Diabetes Medicine, 23*, 1332–1338.

Franko, O. I. (2011). Smartphone apps for orthopaedic surgeons. *Clinical Orthopaedic Related Research, 469*, 2042–2048.

Franko, O. I., & Tirrell, T. F. (2012). Smartphone app use among medical providers in ACGME training programs. *Journal Medical Systems, 36*, 3135–3139.

Friedman, S. R., Mateu-Gelabert, P., Curtis, R., Maslow, C., Bolyard, M., Sandoval, M., Flom, P. (2007). Social capital or networks, negotiations, and norms? A neighborhood case study. *American Journal of Preventive Medicine, 32*, 160–170.

Gold, J., Pedrana, A., Stoove, M., Chang, S., Howard, S., Asselin, J., ... Hllard, M. (2013). Developing health promotion interventions on social networking sites: Recommendations from the FaceSpace Project. *Journal of Medical Internet Research, 14*, epub. http://www.jmir.org/2012/1/e30/

Google.org. (n.d.). *Google.org flu trends*. Retrieved from http://www.google.org/flutrends/

Gurman, T. A., Rubin, S. E., & Roess, A. A. (2012). Effectiveness of mHealth behavior change communication interventions in developing countries: A systematic review of the literature. *Journal of Health Communication, 17*(Suppl. 1), 82–104.

Gustafson, D. H., Hawkins, R. P., Boberg, E. W., McTavish, F., Owens, B., Wise, M., ... Pingree, S. (2002). CHESS: 10 years of research and development in consumer health informatics for broad populations, including the underserved. *International Journal of Medical Informatics, 65*, 169–77.

Gustafson, D. H., McTavish, F. M., Stengle, W., Ballard, D., Hawkins, R., Shaw, B. R., ... Landucci, G. (2005). Use and impact of eHealth system by low-income women with breast cancer. *Journal of Health Communication, 10*(Suppl. 1), 195–218.

Hamilton, A. D., & Brady, R. R. (2012). Medical professional involvement in smartphone apps in dermatology. *British Journal of Dermatology, 167*, 220–221.

Hicks, J. (2012, January 3). Smartphone app diagnoses malaria from drop of blood. *Forbes.com*. Retrieved from http://www.forbes.com/sites/jenniferhicks/2012/01/03/smartphone-app-diagnoses-malaria-from-drop-of-blood/.

Houghland, L. (2013). Cell phone use spreads faster than expected in Latin America. *Infosurhoy*. Retrieved from http://infosurhoy.com/cocoon/saii/xhtml/en_GB/features/saii/features/economy/2012/01/18/feature-02

Hsieh, C. H., Tsai, H. H., Yin, J. W., Chen, C. Y., Yang, J. C., & Jeng, S. F. (2004). Teleconsultation with the mobile camera-phone in digital soft-tissue injury: A feasibility study. *Plastic and Reconstructive Surgery, 114*(7), 1776–1182.

Hurling, R., Catt, M., De Boni, M., Fairley, B., Hurst, T., Murray, P., ... Sodhi, J. (2007). Using Internet and mobile phone technology to deliver an automated physical activity program: Randomized controlled trial. *Journal of Medical Internet Research, 9*(2), e7.

Jones, C., Wasunna, B., Sudoi, R., Githinji, S., Snow, R. W., & Zurovac, D. (2012). "Even if you know everything you can forget": Health worker perceptions of mobile phone text-messaging to improve malaria case-management in Kenya. *PLoS ONE, 7*(6), e38636.

Kelly, J. A. (2004). Popular opinion leaders and HIV prevention peer education: Resolving discrepant findings, and implications for the development of effective community programmes. *AIDS Care, 16*, 139–50.

Kelly, G. C., Tanner, M., Vallely, A., & Clements, A. (2012). Malaria elimination: Moving forward with spatial decision support systems. *Trends in Parasitology, 28*(7), 297–304.

Khokhar, A. (2009). Short text messages (SMS) as a reminder system for making working women from Delhi breast aware. *Asian Pacific Journal of Cancer Prevention, 10*, 319–321.

Korda, H., & Itani, Z. (2011). Harnessing social media for health promotion and behavior change. *Health Promotion Practice*. [Epub ahead of print] http://hpp.sagepub.com/content/14/1/15.long.

Kraidin, J., Ginsberg, S. H., & Solina, A. (2012). Anesthesia apps: Overview of current technology and intelligent search techniques. *Journal of Cardiothoracic and Vascular Anesthesiology, 26*, 322–326.

Kreatsoulas, J. (2010). Progress in ROP management through tele-ophthalmology. *Retina Today* (November/December), 18–20.

Kreuter, M., Farrell, D., Olevitch, L., & Brennan, L. (2000). *Tailoring health messages: Customizing communication with computer technology*. Mahwah, NJ: Erlbaum.

Krishna, S., Boren, S. A., & Balas, E. A. (2009). Healthcare via cell phones: A systematic review. *Telemedicine Journal of E-Health, 15*(3), 231–240.

Kroemer, S., Fruhauf, J., Campbell, T. M., Massone, C., Schwantzer, G., Soyer, H. P., & Hofmann-Wellenhof, R. (2011). Mobile teledermatology for skin tumour screening: Diagnostic accuracy of clinical and dermoscopic image tele-evaluation using cellular phones. *British Journal of Dermatology, 164*, 973–979.

Kubben, P. L. (2010). Neurosurgical apps for iPhone, iPod Touch, iPad and Android. *Surgery Neurology International, 1*, 89.

Kukafka, R., Lussier, Y. A., Eng, P., Patel, V. L., & Cimino, J. J. (2002). Web-based tailoring and its effect on self-efficacy: Results from the MI-HEART randomized controlled trial. *Proceedings of the American Medical Informatics Association Symposium*, 410–414.

Lenhart, A., Madden, M., Rankin Macgill, A., & Smith, A. (2007). *Teens and social media: The use of social media gains a greater foothold in teen life as they embrace the conversational nature of interactive online media*. PEW Internet and American Life. Retrieved from http://www.pewinternet.org

Lester, R. T., Ritvo, P., Mills, E. J., Kariri, A., Karanja, S., Chung, M. H., ... Plummer, F. A. (2010). Effects of a mobile phone short message service on antiretroviral treatment adherence in Kenya (WelTel Kenya1): A randomised trial. *Lancet, 376*, 1838–1845.

Levine, D., Madsen, A., Wright, E. C., Barar, R., Santelli, J., & Bull, S. (2011). Formative research on MySpace: Online methods to engage hard-to-reach populations. *Journal of Health Communication, 16*, 448–454.

Lund, S., Hemed, M., Nielsen, B. B., Said, A., Said, K., Makungu, M. H., & Rasch, V. (2012). Mobile phones as a health communication tool to improve skilled attendance at delivery in Zanzibar: A cluster-randomized controlled trial. *BJOG, 119*, 1256–1264.

McLafferty, S. L. (2003). GIS and health care. *Annual Reviews of Public Health, 24*, 25–42.

Merrell, R. C., & Doarn, C. R. (2011). Medical applications, mobility, and regulations. *Telemedicine Journal of E-Health, 17*(4), 235–236.

Mohan, A. T., & Branford, O. A. (2012). iGuide to plastic surgery: iPhone apps, the plastic surgeon, and the health care environment. *Aesthetic Surgery Journal, 32*(5), 653–658.

Moreira, M. T., Smith, L., & Foxcroft, D. (2010). Social norms interventions to reduce alcohol misuse in University or College students. The Cochrane Library. DOI: 10.1002/14651858.CD006748.pub2.

Moreno, M. A., Swanson, M. J., Royer, H., & Roberts, L. J. (2011). Sexpectations: Male college students' views about displayed sexual references on females' social networking web sites. *Journal of Pediatric & Adolescent Gynecology, 24*, 85–89.

Nations, D. (2012). What is Web 3.0? *Webtrends*. Retrieved from http://webtrends.about.com/od/web20/a/what-is-web-30.htm

Neiger, B., Thackeray, R., Van Wagenen, S., Hansen, C., West, J., Barnes, M., & Fagen, M. (2013). Use of social media in health promotion: Purposes, key performance indicators, and evaluation metrics. *Health Promotion Practice., 13*, 159–164.

Noar, S. M., Black, H. G., & Pierce, L. B. (2009). Efficacy of computer technology-based HIV prevention interventions: a meta-analysis. *AIDS, 23*, 107–115.

Oehler, R. L., Smith, K., & Toney, J. F. (2010). Infectious diseases resources for the iPhone. *Clinical Infectious Disease, 50*(9), 1268–1274.

O'Neill, S., & Brady, R.R.W. (2012). Colorectal smartphone apps: Opportunities and risks. *Colorectal Disease, 14*(9), e530–534.

Ostojic, V., Cvorisecec, B., Ostojic, S. B., Reznikoff, D., Stipic-Markovic, A., & Tudjman, Z. (2005). Improving asthma control through telemedicine: A study of short-message service. *Telemedicine Journal of E-Health, 11*(1), 28–35.

Patrick, K., Raab, F., Adams, M., Dillon, L., Zabinski, M., Rock, C., ... Norman, G. (2009). A text message-based intervention for weight loss: Randomized controlled trial. *Journal of Medical Internet Research, 11*(1), e1.

Pope, L., Silva, P., & Almeyda, R. (2010). I-Phone applications for the modern day otolaryngologist. *Clinical Otolaryngology, 35*, 350–354.

Radwanick, S. (2013). Facebook blasts into top position in Brazilian social networking market following year of tremendous growth. *Comscore*. Retrieved from http://www.comscore.com/Insights/Press_Releases/2012/1/Facebook_Blasts_into_Top_Position_in_Brazilian_Social_Networking_Market

Rajput, Z. A., Mbugua, S., Amadi, D., Chepngeno, V., Saleem, J. J., Anokwa, Y., ... Were, M. C. (2012). Evaluation of an android-based mhealth system for population surveillance in developing countries. *Journal of the American Medical Informatic Association, 19*(4), 655–659.

Rambaldi, G., Kyem, P.A.K., McCall, M., & Weiner, D. (2006). Participatory spatial information management and communications in developing countries. *Electronic Journal on Information Systems in Developing Countries, 25*, 1–9.

Rodgers, A., Corbett, T., Bramley, D., Riddell, T., Wills, M., Lin, R. B., & Jones, M. (2005). Do u smoke after txt? Results of a randomised trial of smoking cessation using mobile phone test messaging. *Tobacco Control, 14*, 255–261.

Rosser, B. A., & Eccleston, C. (2011). Smartphone applications for pain management. *J Telemed Telecare, 17*(6), 308–312.

Sanders, A. E., Lim, S., & Sohn, W. (2008). Resilience to urban poverty: theoretical and empirical considerations for population health. *American Journal of Public Health, 98*, 1101–1106.

Stockwell, M. S., Kharbanda, E. O., Martinez, R. A., Vargas, C. Y., Lara, M., Vawdrey, D., & Rickert, V. (2012a). Text4Health: Impact of text message reminder-recalls for pediatric and adolescent immunizations. *American Journal of Public Health, 102*, e15–21.

Stockwell, M. S., Kharbanda, E. O., Martinez, R. A., Vargas, C. Y., Vawdry, D. K., & Carmargo, S. (2012b). Effect of a text messaging intervention on influenza vaccination in an urban, low-income pediatric and adolescent population. *Journal of the American Medical Association, 307*, 1702–1708.

Sueur, D., & Tanser, F. C. (2002). The application of geographic information systems to important public health in Africa. *International Journal of Health Geographics, 1*, 4.

Tate, D. F., Wing, R. R., & Winett, R. A. (2001). Using Internet technology to deliver a behavioral weight loss program. *Journal of the American Medical Association, 285*, 1172–7.

Torugsa, K., Anderson, S., Thongsen, N., Sirisopana, N., Jugudee, A., Junlananto, P., ... Brown, A. E. (2003). HIV epidemic among young Thai men, 1991–2000. *Emerging Infectious Disease, 9*(7), 881–883.

Tsai, H. H., Pong, Y. P., Liang, C. C., Lin, P. Y., & Hsieh, C. H. (2004). Teleconsultation by using the mobile camera phone for remote management of the extremity wound: A pilot study. *Annals of Plastic Surgery, 53*(6), 584–587.

US Food and Drug Administration. (2011, July 20). *Draft guidance for industry and Food and Drug Administration staff—mobile medical applications*. Center for Devices and Radiological Health. Retrieved from http://www.fda.gov/medicaldevices/deviceregulationandguidance/guidancedocuments/ucm263280.htm.

US Food and Drug Administration. (2015, September 25). *Mobile medical applications: Guidance for industry and Food and Drug Administration staff*. Center for Devices and Radiological Health. Retrieved from http://www.fda.gov/downloads/MedicalDevices/DeviceRegulationandGuidance/GuidanceDocuments/UCM263366.pdf

Ushahidi. n.d. Retrieved from http://www.ushahidi.com/

Väänänen, A., Kouvonen, A., Kivimaki, M., Pentti, J., & Vahtera, J. (2008). Social support, network heterogeneity, and smoking behavior in women: the 10-town study. *American Journal of Health Promotion, 22*, 246–255.

Vilella, A., Bayas, J. M., Diaz, M. T., Guinovart, C., Diewz, V., Simo, D., ... Cerezo, J. (2004). The role of mobile phones in improving vaccination rates in travelers. *Preventive Medicine, 38*, 503–509.

Visser, B. J., & Buijink, A.W.G. (2012). Need to peer-review medical applications for smart phones. *Journal of Telemedicine and Telecare, 18*(2), 124.

Wand, H., Whitaker, C., & Ramje, G. (2011). Geoadditive models to assess spatial variation of HIV infections among women in local communities of Durban, South Africa. *International Journal of Health Geographics, 10*, 28.

Wantland, D. J., Portillo, C. J., Holzemer, W. L., Slaughter, R., & McGhee, E. M. (2004). The effectiveness of Web-based vs. non-Web-based interventions: A meta-analysis of behavioral change outcomes. *Journal of Medical Internet Research, 10*, 4–e40.

Wei, J., Hollin, I., & Kachnowski, S. (2011). A review of the use of mobile phone text messaging in clinical and healthy behavior interventions. *Journal of Telemedicine and Telecare, 17*(1), 41–48.

Whittaker, R., McRobbie, H., Bullen, C., Borland, R., Rodgers, A., & Gu, Y. (2012). Mobile phone-based interventions for smoking cessation. *Cochrane Database Systematic Reviews, 11*, CD006611.

Wikipedia. (2012). *What is social media*. Retrieved from http://en.wikipedia.org/wiki/Social_media

Wiltfong, J. (2013). Socialogue: Have a mobile phone, will access Internet. Maybe. *ipsos.com* Retrieved from http://www.ipsos-na.com/news-polls/pressrelease.aspx?id=5900

World Health Organization. (n.d.). *Global Health Atlas*. Retrieved from http://apps.who.int/globalatlas/

Ybarra, M., Bull, S., Prescott, T., Biringi, R., Bangsberg, D., & Kiwanuka, J. (2013). Adolescent abstinence and unprotected sex in CyberSenga, an Internet-based HIV prevention program: Randomized clinical trial of efficacy. *PLoS.ONE.*, DOI: 10.1371/journal.pone.0070083

Zurovac, D., Sudoi, R. K., Akhwale, W. S., Ndiritu, M., Hamer, D. H., Rowe, A. K., & Snow, R. W. (2011). The effect of mobile phone text-message reminders on Kenyan health workers' adherence to malaria treatment guidelines: A cluster randomised trial. *Lancet, 378*, 795–803.

CHAPTER 8

REDUCING MATERNAL AND INFANT MORTALITY

Meeting a Global Challenge

Padmini Murthy

Maternal, neonatal, and infant mortality rates remain excessively high in lower-income countries around the world. The science needed to simply and inexpensively reduce these rates is already known. What is needed is to get on with the task. Health promotion focuses on both providers and clients. A fundamental principle of primary health care is to provide service at the lowest, least expensive level of facility and provider. This chapter focuses on successes and continuing challenges in the areas of prenatal care, birth and delivery, postpartum care for mother and baby, and early child care, nutrition, and preventive health practices. As the target date of 2015 has passed for reaching the Millennium Development Goals (MDGs) approaches, a wide range of activities have been undertaken by various stakeholders, namely the member states of the United Nations; the UN system, which includes special agencies such as World Health Organization (WHO), UN Women, United Nations Population Fund (UNFPA), and United Nations Children's Fund (UNICEF); civil society organizations, academia, research institutions, and foundations to identify the shape and priorities of a post-2015 development agenda.

LEARNING OBJECTIVES

By the end of this chapter, the reader should be able to:

- **Appreciate the challenges and successes associated with MDG 4—that is, to reduce child mortality, and MDG 5—that is to improve maternal health**
- **Understand the importance of health education and promotion and using cost-effective strategies in providing service delivery to improve MDGs 4 and 5 in low- and middle-income countries**
- **Discuss the link between health and human rights with special reference to those of women and children**
- **Explain the relationship and interdependence among the eight MDGs in the context of maternal and child health in a global context**

The Millennium Development Goals

These were crafted in 2000 at the United Nations headquarters in New York, where leaders from 191 countries agreed to work to reduce poverty, promote universal primary education, improve the environment, prevent the spread of infectious diseases such as malaria and HIV, and improve maternal health and reduce **infant mortality rates** by the year 2015.

Following is a list of the eight Millennium Development Goals that were established in 2000 during the MDG Summit:

1. Eradicating extreme poverty and hunger,
2. Achieving universal primary education,
3. Promoting gender equality and empowering women,
4. Reducing child mortality rates,
5. Improving maternal health,
6. Combating HIV/AIDS, malaria, and other diseases,
7. Ensuring environmental sustainability, and
8. Developing a global partnership for development (United Nations, 2000).

Current Picture of MDG 4

Unfortunately, as the MDG target date of 2015 has now passed, maternal infant and under-five mortality rates remain disproportionately high in many developing countries. According to the 2012 MDG report, the two regions that contribute to the high rates of under-five mortality are sub-Saharan Africa and Southern Asia. In 2010 there were 6.2 million deaths in these regions, which corresponded to 82% of the deaths worldwide. Reasons for these persistently high rates of under-five mortality in these areas are

- Children born into poorer families have a much higher risk of dying before their fifth birthday when compared to their peers from wealthier families, highlighting the relationship between socioeconomic factors and child mortality.

- Malnutrition remains a major challenge among children under five, and it is alarming that at present one out of five children is underweight in the developing world. Poverty and low socioeconomic status are both directly and indirectly responsible for the wide discrepancies among children aged five years and lower in their nutritional status worldwide. An example is that children from low-income households in Southern Asia are 2.8 times more likely to be underweight than their peers from wealthier households. The rates of child mortality and morbidity tend to be higher among children who are underweight and stunted. According to data released by the United Nations in 2010, worldwide there was a reduction in the proportion of underweight children (aged under five) from 29% in 1990 to 18% in 2010—a span of 20 years. Although these results are encouraging, these milestones did not enable us to reach the global targets by 2015 (Department of Economic and Social Affairs [DESA], 2012).

- Gender disparity and gender inequality have resulted in the girl child facing discrimination and neglect. This translates into an increased risk for infant mortality and morbidity for the girls in many developing countries. Young girls are often not given the opportunity to attend secondary school because of sociocultural barriers and societal norms. Many families believe that educating their daughters is not financially viable and they will not get returns on their investment. Lack of security for girls attending secondary schools because of distance is another source of concern for parents. Many societies in Asia, Africa, and Latin America favor early marriage for young adolescent girls; this practice results in increased risk for maternal and infant mortality.

- Low birth weight, infection, lack of regular antenatal care and skilled birth attendants, and preterm birth are major contributors to neonatal mortality. According to the World Health organization neonatal deaths contribute to 40% of the under-five mortality rates worldwide (Jehan et al., 2009).

- Child immunization status is determined by many factors, such as at the individual, family environment, and community level, as well as by the existing health systems or patterns of service delivery issues. Barriers for vaccination may affect the demand for services (e.g., whether the parent or guardian takes the child for immunizations as per the recommended schedule), as well as the supply of these vaccines (e.g., how vaccination is made available and whether it is stored under optimum conditions). Lack of proper storage conditions often can compromise the safety and efficacy of these vaccines (Hilber et al., 2010).

- Childhood immunization rates vary globally and are influenced by geographic location, socioeconomic status, and level of education of mothers and access to health care facilities.

A study conducted by WHO and the Global Alliance for Immunization and Vaccines (GAVI) in 2010 examined the rates of childhood immunization globally. For example, in India the number of boys immunized was greater than the number of girls in poor rural areas. At the same time, in Madagascar and Tanzania, according to 2004 data, and in Haiti based on 2006 data, the immunization rates for girls were on par with that of boys (Hilber et al., 2010). Figure 8.1 shows a Haitian boy receiving a dose of oral vaccine.

In spite of the tremendous efforts made by GAVI and its partners to increase immunization rates globally, it has been a challenging task.

Box 8.1 lists the factors influencing global immunization rates and illustrates the influence of sociocultural and economic factors on the rate of immunization.

BOX 8.1 SOCIOCULTURAL FACTORS AND THEIR INFLUENCE ON GLOBAL IMMUNIZATION PREVALENCE

- Education level of mothers
- Women who have not been immunized (especially low doses of tetanus toxoid)
- Young mothers (teenage pregnancies)
- Low socioeconomic status
- Communities in rural areas
- Households that did not have access to radio or TV

- Male-dominated households in which the women did not have any decision-making power
- Lack of financial independence for women
- Lack of women's empowerment
- Myths about the dangers of vaccines
- Gender bias
- Geographic distance for access to health care

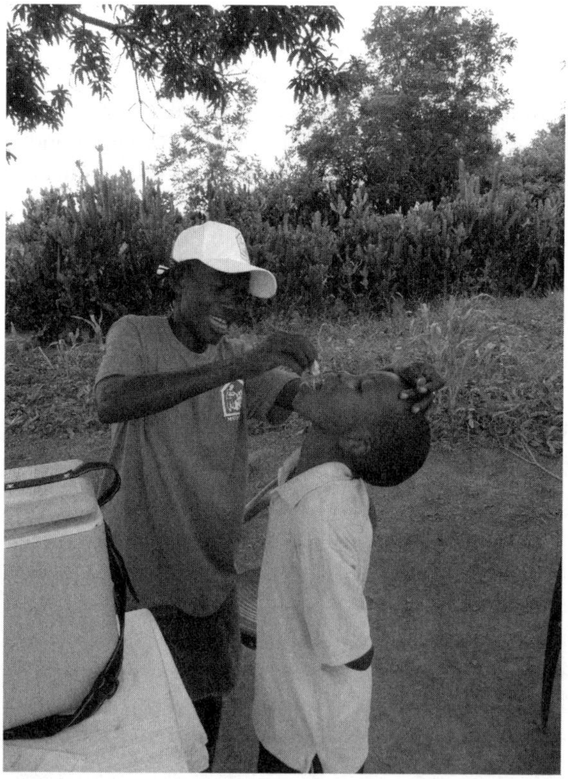

Figure 8.1 A public health field worker in Haiti administers a dose of oral cholera vaccine to a willing young boy, who tilts his head back to accept the drops of vaccine solution

Source: CDC Image Library.

Current Picture of MDG 5

Maternal mortality unfortunately remains a major public health challenge worldwide. The global socioeconomic burden resulting from maternal mortality is very high and amounts to a loss of US$15 billion every year. At the same time, the costs associated with improving access and health care systems in 49 of the least economically developed nations are estimated to be US$ 2.5 billion by the year 2015 (Hilton, Murray & Thomas, 2010).

These financial estimates demonstrate the importance and the economic benefits for investing in maternal health and promoting safe motherhood practices.

The incidence of maternal mortality and morbidity still remained high in 2012. In a report released by *Lancet* after a 10-year study on the incidence and factors contributing maternal mortality in 181 countries from 1998 to 2008, the authors estimated that there was a reduction of worldwide maternal deaths from an estimated 526,300 in 1980 to 342,900 in 2008 (Hogan, Freeman et al., 2010).

The progress toward achieving MDG 5 has often been inconstant and the indicators have not been uniform; for example, according to the authors, "More than 50% of all maternal deaths were in only six countries in 2008 India, Nigeria, Pakistan, Afghanistan, Ethiopia, and the Democratic Republic of the Congo" (Hogan et al., 2008). In addition, of the 181 countries included in the study, only 23 countries are on track to achieve a 75% decrease in **maternal mortality ratio** (MMR) by 2015. Egypt, China, Ecuador, and Bolivia have made remarkable progress in reducing maternal mortality rates in their countries.

In order to understand the current picture of MDG 5 globally, it is crucial that the readers are aware of the different terminology used in maternal and child health literature, which is included in Box 8.2.

Some of the causes of maternal mortality and morbidity are presented in Table 8.1.

BOX 8.2 DEFINITION OF MATERNAL MORTALITY ACCORDING TO ICD 10

Maternal death: The death of a woman while pregnant or within 42 days of termination of pregnancy, irrespective of the duration and site of the pregnancy, from any cause related to or aggravated by the pregnancy or its management but not from accidental or incidental causes

Pregnancy-related death: The death of a woman while pregnant or within 42 days of termination of pregnancy, irrespective of the cause of death

Late maternal death: The death of a woman from direct or indirect obstetric causes, more than 42 days but less than1 year after termination of pregnancy

Table 8.1 Causes of Maternal Mortality and Morbidity

1.	Abortion (including unsafe)
2.	Anemia
3.	Cardiovascular disease complicating pregnancy
4.	Depression/psychosis
5.	Ectopic pregnancy
6.	Embolism
7.	Hemorrhage (intrapartum and postpartum)
8.	HIV/AIDS
9.	Hypertension (including complications such as preeclampsia and eclampsia)
10.	Infection
11.	Lack of access to skilled birth attendants
12.	Malaria
13.	Obstructed labor
14.	Renal disease complicating pregnancy
15.	Sepsis
16.	Unmet need for contraception
17.	Teen pregnancy
18.	Tetanus
19.	Uterine rupture
20.	Violence

Source: Modified from WHO and Centers for Disease Control.

In addition to these mentioned factors, socioeconomic determinants such as low socioeconomic status, lack of education, and cultural norms have contributed to the high rates of maternal morbidity and mortality and **infant morbidity and mortality** worldwide.

According to the MDG report of 2012, sub-Saharan Africa has the highest birth rate among adolescents (120 births per 1,000), and progress has been minimal since 1990. Some of the major contributing factors to this has been the low levels of contraceptive use and lack of access to contraceptives. Sociocultural factors as mentioned above continue to be major barriers for unmet need of contraception. Indeed, it is alarming that the rate of contraceptive use has decreased by 25% from 1990 to 2010 (DESA, 2012).

As mentioned in Table 8.1 the lack of access to trained personnel or skilled birth attendants has contributed to the high rates of maternal mortality and morbidity. According to a report released by the UNFPA in many low- and middle-income countries only 58% of the deliveries are conducted by skilled birth attendants, that is, a midwife, nurse, or physician. In another alarming trend, sometimes only 10–12 % of deliveries in these countries are conducted by health care providers (UNFPA, n.d.). In addition, there is seldom access to or emergency obstetric care, and often the outcome is disastrous for the mother and the newborn. Lack of access to life-saving drugs and blood transfusions are major obstacles faced by women in many communities. The lack of access to magnesium sulphate, a drug used to treat eclampsia in pregnant women in the country of Chad, illustrates the dire need to strengthen health care systems that can deliver emergency obstetric care. A study conducted to estimate the **maternal mortality rates** by UNFPA and the World Bank from 1990 to 2010 highlighted the extremely high rates of maternal mortality in the countries of Chad and Somalia. The rates were 1,000 or greater than 1,000 per 100,000 live births (World Health Organization, The United Nations Children's Fund, World Bank, 2011). These numbers illustrate the devastating conditions that result in maternal morbidity or deaths and can be linked directly or indirectly to all or some of the causes mentioned in Table 8.1.

According to the 2010 estimates of trends in maternal mortality, one of the main challenges that this study (WHO, UNICEF, & World Bank 2011) could clearly identify was the lack of civil registration in many countries that did not record the cause of maternal death. This was a barrier to measuring the progress made toward reducing maternal mortality globally. The Maternal Mortality Estimation Inter-Agency group (MMEIG) has been working to streamline the data collection in these countries. The group members are the World Health Organization, the United Nations Children's Fund, the United Nations Population Fund, the United Nations Population Division, and the World Bank. Their academic partner is the University of California-Berkeley (WHO, UNICEF, & World Bank, 2011).

Unfortunately, the lack of prioritization of women's health, especially maternal health in national health policies in many countries, has been considered a major obstacle to achieving MDG 5. For example, in Uganda, which is a developing country, insufficient funding has been one of the key factors leading to failure in implementing policies and practices that promote safe motherhood made during the Abuja Declaration of committing 15% of the national income for the health sector. This has resulted in shortages in health care personnel, hospital supplies, and lack of a system that can cater to the needs of pregnant women in the community. Corruption and shortage of health care workers who leave the country in search of better financial opportunities (the so-called brain drain phenomenon) are also major contributors to the current dismal picture of MDGs in countries like Uganda (Walker, 2012).

Acts of violence against pregnant women can both directly and indirectly in increased rates of maternal and infant morbidity and mortality. Globally 1 in 4 women may experience physical, mental, or sexual violence directed against her. According to a report released by UN Women (2012), between 23 and 53% of pregnant women suffer abdominal trauma during pregnancy, which can lead to an increased incidence of abortion, infant death, and severe bleeding due to trauma that can result in maternal and infant deaths. One of the indirect consequences of violence is the increasing maternal mortality and morbidity of women. In addition, denying a woman access to contraception has been shown to be a major deterrent to her health, since the practice of spacing of births which is the result of access to contraception and education for women has demonstrated a positive outcome on the health of the mother and her infant. Unfortunately, some of the culturally accepted practices such as early marriage and female genital mutilation have increased the risk of complications such as obstructed labor, which, if prolonged, can lead to the formation of obstetric fistula. Violence against women has been a major contributor to their contracting HIV/AIDS. According to data released by UN Women (2012), young women represent 60% of those infected by HIV/AIDS. Unfortunately, these women are not aware that they have contracted HIV/AIDS and thereby the risk of maternal-to-child transmission is increased. It is alarming that 14.6% of women in sub-Saharan Africa and Southeast Asia reported that when they disclosed their HIV status, they were subject to violence and discrimination by their partners and their families. This prevented them from seeking health care services. In most cases these unfortunate women contacted HIV from their partners and were often blamed if they were known to be HIV-positive (UN Women, 2012).

Thus violence is a vicious cycle; it leads to increased maternal and infant morbidity and places an enormous socioeconomic burden on the communities these women live in. In many instances these women are blamed for the death of an infant or secondary infertility and are subject to more violence. These barriers to safe motherhood are summarized in Box 8.3.

The lack of trained health care workers is another major challenge to improving health care systems and access to pregnant women. According to a report released by the World Health Organization in 2010, the lack of

BOX 8.3 BARRIERS TO SAFE MOTHERHOOD

- Access to health care
- Lack of transportation/mobility
- Lack of autonomy and financial decision-making power
- Societal norms that do not favor health facilities for delivery
- Discrimination
- Gender-based violence
- Geographic barriers
- Lack of data/registries for recording births and maternal deaths
- Lack of female health professionals
- Lack of supplies and equipment
- Low socioeconomic status/poverty
- Control by male partners and family members
- Lack of education
- Lack of policies that address women's health

trained health care workers and their geographic distribution in many African countries is a major public health challenge. The ratio of trained health workers to the population is very low in Africa, and on average on average there are only 13.8 nursing and midwifery personnel for every 10,000 people. To further illustrate this dismal situation, a study conducted in Malawi found that only 12% of the health care clinics in the country had midwives available throughout 24 hours, a barrier to maternal and child health. The health staff shortage is grave in 57 developing countries of the world, and according to WHO (2010), a minimum of 2.4 million health workers (including physicians, midwives, and nurses) are required in these countries.

Improving MDG 4 and MDG 5

There is no cure for maternal and infant death, but these deaths are largely preventable and some of the measures and strategies that will help the global community to achieve the targets set forth in MDG 4 and 5 are cost-effective. Strengthening service delivery under the umbrella of primary care is an efficient and economically viable strategy that can be made use of even in resource-poor settings. Some examples of cost-effective interventions are discussed in the next sections.

Communication and Antenatal Care

According to a study conducted by Jennings, Yebadokpo, and Affo (2010) in Benin, which is one of the countries with a low GDP and high rates of maternal and infant mortality, communication between health care providers and pregnant women facilitated better outcomes in pregnancy. In order to expand antenatal coverage in resource-poor settings the World Health Organization has focused on antenatal models that have incorporated the strategies of providing information and counseling to pregnant women. The recommended areas for information and counseling are birth and emergency care, nutrition and preventive practices at home and in the community, and most important recognizing signs of danger during pregnancy. According to Moran et al. (2006), communication provided during the antenatal period to women has been an effective strategy in improving maternal health and pregnancy outcomes.

This has also been shown to reduce the mistrust of the health care providers who practice "Western medicine" and are viewed with suspicion. In many low- and middle-income countries effective communication is lacking, and the population served does not have the ability to make decisions that have a positive impact on their health status. Another pitfall is that less information is shared with pregnant women than what is recommended, which has resulted in patient dissatisfaction and noncompliance.

Based on these findings, Jennings et al. (2010) used a series of 11 flash cards with pictures and prioritized messages to cover the three trimesters of pregnancy. Their objective was to ensure that women would have access to the necessary information multiple times during their pregnancies. These cards were organized into modules based on the information context. For example, Module A included five cards to target women in their first trimester and included information on general pregnancy care, birth and emergency preparedness, how to recognize maternal danger signs, and the importance of a clean delivery. Module B included four cards for women in their second trimester of pregnancy, with information on newborn care, such as the need for immediate and duration breastfeeding, need for delayed bathing, and protection for the newborn. Module C consisted of two cards for women in the last trimester that reinforced key aspects of maternal and newborn care, some of which had been covered in the earlier modules. The rationale used by the authors was to introduce and pilot this intervention antenatally; traditionally in Benin counseling about the importance of newborn care was performed postnatally, and sometimes there was a gap in this information sharing that resulted in women not being educated in the practice of newborn care. In order to pilot this project, there were three interventional components that were followed: training, organizational changes, and field support. Before the pilot project was started, the health care workers had to receive mandatory three-day training in the areas of the content and use of the counselling cards, importance of optimal interpersonal communication, and quality improvement in the delivery of the services. In addition, the component of monitoring and probable performance evaluation on a simple basis was introduced by including role playing and didactic instruction. This simple exercise measured three important goals associated with improving maternal and infant health:

1. to measure the quality of counseling received by the pregnant women in the target population where the study was piloted;
2. the perceptions and feedback received from the health care workers with regard to using these cards, which were referred to as job aids;
3. to assess women's knowledge relating to crucial components of maternal and newborn care.

The messages that the health care providers used to educate women in this pilot project were categorized as follows (Jennings et al., 2010):

- *General Prenatal Care:* Under this category women were educated on the importance of prevention and treatment of malaria, especially the use of an insecticide-treated net and the use of malarial prophylaxis under medical supervision. They were also counseled on the importance of good nutrition and supplementing their diet with iron and folate and the importance of having four antenatal check-ups during their pregnancy.

- *Birth Preparedness:* This category included information about the importance of identifying a safe environment for delivery and to seek the services of a skilled birth attendant. In addition, these women were made aware of the importance of organizing safe transportation, budgeting money needed for delivery, and discussing these important issues with a family member. Identifying a blood donor was another key issue; there have been instances when women have bled to death because they did not have access to a blood transfusion when needed.

- *Danger Signs:* Under this category women were educated on nine symptoms that required immediate medical attention. These were vaginal bleeding during any trimester of pregnancy, convulsions, fever and chills, loss of fluid through the vagina, abdominal cramps or pain, headache, blurred vision, and swelling of feet and hands. Women were taught to count their fetal movements and note whether they observed diminished or loss of fetal movements.

- *Clean Delivery:* This category consisted of two messages about providing a clean, plastic cloth for delivery and clean, dry towels for the mother and newborn. These women were also made aware of the importance of cleanliness because it would help to reduce the incidence of maternal and newborn sepsis.

- *Newborn Care:* The six messages that women were made aware of under this category included skin-to-skin contact, early breastfeeding, exclusive breastfeeding, delayed bathing, clean cord care, and thermal protection, which is vital for a newborn.

This strategy has been shown to be cost-effective and can be replicated in other resource-poor settings.

Systems and Partnering to Improve Maternal and Infant Health

The partnership of maternal and child health has advocated the importance of improving maternal health in resource-poor settings by using three key interventions:

1. health systems interventions: health workers;
2. efficient financing mechanisms; and
3. political partnerships.

As an illustration, providing bicycles and cell phones and delivery to community health care workers or CHWs have shown to be highly beneficial. For example, CHWs who are an integral part of the health care system in many countries have facilitated the reduction of maternal mortality in countries such as Nepal and Ethiopia. The so-called skills gap that exists in resource-poor settings needs to be addressed; the health care workers need to be trained on a regular basis, get paid a decent wage, and have access to and support from a health care system that provides them the necessary tools and supplies to work (in order to retain them and prevent their migration to other areas in search of better opportunities). Other recommendations for implementation of comprehensive strategies include reducing costs incurred by the clients, reducing gender inequalities, and empowering women so that they are aware of the services available and utilize them, and improving and expanding existing facilities.

Some examples of the success stories of improvement in the MDG 5 indictors are in Tunisia, where, according to the UN, there was an 80% reduction in maternal deaths. This has been attributed largely to the country's emphasis on skilled birth attendants at delivery.

Another example is Nepal, where there has been marked improvement in the rates of maternal mortality between 1990 and 2008 from 471 per 100,000 live births to 240 per 100,000 live births. This has resulted in 5,000 fewer maternal deaths per year in this 10-year period. One of the main contributors to this has been the training and recruitment of female community health volunteers (FCHVs) who have made a great impact in the community. These women have been readily accepted by the community members; they can be trusted and are permitted to visit the rural women at home and give them counseling on the importance of family planning and antenatal and newborn care. They also visit women after delivery and treat the newborn infants if the need arises. In summary, these workers are the first line of health care professionals the rural women come into contact with.

In Tanzania, when women were provided with access to a sterile delivery kit during childbirth the outcome was dramatic. The risk of developing sepsis or infections was reduced by two-thirds when compared to their peers who did not have similar access (World Health Organization, 2010).

Role of Mobile Health (mHealth)

Mobile health, or mHealth as it is also known, refers to the use of technology in the form of portable devices (such as smartphones) with applications that provide health care services and collect data and manage patient medical records or collect information. At present, globally there are around 5 billion cell phone users, and many of them are in low- and middle-income countries.

At present cell phone technology is being harnessed to improve maternal health globally by providing information and health reminders to women. In addition this technology is a valuable tool that supports the work of health care workers in rural and underserved communities because it enables them to deliver integrated community case management to mothers and also their children (Källander et al., 2013).

Another example of innovative use of cell phone technology has been in Senegal in the region of Kedougou. Where the main contributors to the high rate of maternal and infant mortality and morbidity are limited availability and poor quality of obstetric services in the region. To address these challenges, a project has been set up in the region by Women and Health Alliance International (WAHA), an international nonprofit, nongovernmental organization based in France. An initiative of improving communication between the villagers and health centers was started in 2011; residents received prepaid cell phones that enabled them to contact the nearest health center in case of an emergency. WAHA has also designed an ambulance on a motorbike that can transport pregnant women once the message is received to the nearest health center or district hospital (Royal Tropical institute, 2013).

The United Nations Population Fund has been using mobile devices to improve maternal health in resource-poor settings. They have set up a project that is using cell phone technology in Tanzania to help women who have obstetric fistula—and do not have the funds to get the services they so desperately need—get treated by transferring money to them through mobile banking. This enables the women to travel to the clinic.

One of the reasons for the use of mobile devices is the widespread access to cell phones and their reliability when compared to Internet service and computer access. In Rwanda, health care workers use cell phones to receive and send alerts in the case of a maternal emergency such as obstructed labor or bleeding. Between March and May 2010 around 500 community health workers in the country received cell phones and were trained through the Rapid SMS project that was funded by UNICEF and WHO.

This enables service providers and other stakeholders to get a picture of the health care status of communities in the country. This project had a positive outcome because women needed emergency obstetric care in a timely manner, and it also led to increased health care access for pregnant women.

"I sent a text and after that they gave me feedback; in 15 minutes the ambulance came," said a community health worker in Musanze, Northern Rwanda. "It saved the life of a woman and her newborn son. She needed emergency obstetric care at the time of delivery; if it had not been for the availability of the mobile phone system, she would have had to be carried to the nearest health facility, a journey that could take more than one hour in the most precarious conditions"(One World Asia, 2011). The Rapid SMS project in Rwanda has been successful because about 75% of all pregnancies in a pilot district were registered through SMS and any relevant information related to the number of successful deliveries, complications during pregnancy, and maternal and neonatal deaths were reported from remote areas through mobile technology.

In Mali, mobile technology is being used to collect health data, including information about maternal morbidity and mortality rates, and these data are being compiled into a national database. In addition, these phones will be utilized to monitor unmet needs for contraception and provide an inventory of the available drugs in the health centers (One World Asia, 2011). (Also see Chapter 7 which focuses on mHealth more generally).

Other Strategies

Health care providers have been trained to administer tetanus immunizations during pregnancy to women in developing countries. With the help of GAVI, UN agencies, and donors, effective monitoring systems are in place to ensure that pregnant women and children are on target to receive their immunizations. Pregnant women who come in for their antenatal checkups receive their medical records and a personal immunization card that gives information about their health and immunization status, and how to identify maternal emergencies such as obstructed labor or bleeding (GAVI, 2013).

Summary

As discussed in this chapter women's health, especially maternal health, is a human rights issue. In many societies even today in the global north and south, women suffer because they are denied the opportunity to enjoy their rights and freedoms. The year 2015 marked the allocated time for the MDGs to be implemented by the 191 nations who signed the declaration in 2000 at the United Nations. It is a tragedy that indicators for MDGs 4 and 5 are lagging behind in many regions of the world. The contributing factors to this are gender-based discrimination and societal norms that treat women and girl children as chattel (movable property) with no decision-making power. The indicators for MDGs 4 and 5 are also closely linked to the indicators of the remaining six MDGs. To illustrate, often girls and women are denied the chance to receive education because they need to fulfill the role of caretaker in their families. As we are aware, young girls are often forced to walk two or three hours each way to fetch water for their families' needs; this reflects the lack of environmental sustainability—that is, MDG 7. Forced child marriages, especially when girls as young as 13 or 14 from low socioeconomic status are married to men who are in their late 30s or early 40s, highlight that these young girls are not educated, are not gender empowered, and have an increased risk for maternal mortality; their infants also have an increased risk of morbidity and mortality. This illustrates that the indicators for MDGs 1, 2, 3, 4, and 5 are lagging behind in communities where these young girls live.

In addition, women and girls living in poverty who may be forced into prostitution or trafficked face a higher risk of contracting HIV/AIDS and getting pregnant. Thus the progress made to achieve MDGs 4 and 5 is dependent on ensuring lack of gender discrimination, freedom from violence, and the opportunity for women and girls to enjoy their human rights to the fullest. Maternal and infant health is just not a women's issue, but an important contributor to the health and wealth of global societies.

The member states of the United Nations have now defined the Sustainable Development Goals (SDGs) as part of a new agenda to finish the job of the MDGs and leave no one behind. This agenda of the SDGs, indicated in Box 8.4, was adopted by member states at the Sustainable Development Summit in September 2015. As a global community there is still much work to be done in addressing the health of women and female infants.

BOX 8.4 SUSTAINABLE DEVELOPMENT GOALS

Goal 1. End poverty in all its forms everywhere

Goal 2. End hunger, achieve food security and improved nutrition, and promote sustainable agriculture

Goal 3. Ensure healthy lives and promote well-being for all at all ages

Goal 4. Ensure inclusive and equitable quality education and promote lifelong learning opportunities for all

Goal 5. Achieve gender equality and empower all women and girls

Goal 6. Ensure availability and sustainable management of water and sanitation for all

Goal 7. Ensure access to affordable, reliable, sustainable, and modern energy for all

Goal 8. Promote sustained, inclusive, and sustainable economic growth, full and productive employment, and decent work for all

Goal 9. Build resilient infrastructure, promote inclusive and sustainable industrialization, and foster innovation

Goal 10. Reduce inequality within and among countries

Goal 11. Make cities and human settlements inclusive, safe, resilient, and sustainable

Goal 12. Ensure sustainable consumption and production patterns

Goal 13. Take urgent action to combat climate change and its impacts*

Goal 14. Conserve and sustainably use the oceans, seas, and marine resources for sustainable development

Goal 15. Protect, restore, and promote sustainable use of terrestrial ecosystems, sustainably manage forests, combat desertification, and halt and reverse land degradation and halt biodiversity loss

Goal 16. Promote peaceful and inclusive societies for sustainable development, provide access to justice for all and build effective, accountable, and inclusive institutions at all levels

Goal 17. Strengthen the means of implementation and revitalize the global partnership for sustainable development.

Source: United Nations Department of Economic and Social Affairs, 2015.

KEY TERMS

1. **Infant morbidity:** Like infant mortality, conditions resulting from prematurity and low birth weight are strongly associated with infant morbidity. Infant morbidity can be measured by the presence of diagnosed conditions, such as respiratory distress and hyperbilirubinemia (or jaundice), as well as by service utilization indicators, including admission to a neonatal intensive care unit (NICU) and length of hospital stay
2. **Infant mortality rate:** Probability of dying between birth and exactly one year of age, expressed per 1,000 live births
3. **Maternal mortality rate:** The number of resident maternal deaths within 42 days of pregnancy termination due to complications of pregnancy, childbirth, and the puerperium in a specified geographic area (country, state, county, etc.) divided by total resident live births for the same geographic area for a specified time period, usually a calendar year, multiplied by 100,000
4. **Maternal mortality ratio (MMR):** The ratio of the number of maternal deaths during a given time period per 100,000 live births during the same time period

REVIEW QUESTIONS

1. What are the main factors contributing to the high rates of maternal and infant mortality in developing countries? What are cost-effective strategies that can aid in their improvement?
2. What is the relationship between maternal health and human rights? How can the issue of human rights be included when designing strategies to improve maternal health globally?
3. Describe how the targets specific to MDGs 4 and 5 are dependent on the remaining MDGs. What are specific examples to illustrate this interdependence?
4. Will the post-2015 agenda/Sustainable Development Goals keep up momentum so that the gains made with reference to MDGs 4 and 5 continue?

References

Department of Economic and Social Affairs. (2012). *DESA millennium development goals report.* Retrieved from http://www.un.org/en/development/desa/publications/mdg-report-2012.html

Global Alliance for Vaccines and Immunization. (2013). Retrieved from http://www.gavialliance.org

Hilber, A. M., Bosch-Capblanch, X., Schindler, C., Beck L., Secula F., McKenzie, O., … Merten, S. (2010). *Summary report for SAGE.* World Health Organization. Retrieved from http://www.who.int/immunization/sage/1_immunization_gender_reports_without_graphics.pdf

Hilton, L., Murray, S., & Thomas, D. (2010). The evidence towards MDG 5: A working paper. *Report of UK Government.* Retrieved from http://www.dfid.gov.uk/Documents/prd/Options-Evidence-Towards-MDG5.pdf

Hogan, C. M., Forman, K., Naghavi, M., Ahn, S., Wang, M., Makels, M. S., … Murray, C. (2010). Maternal mortality for 181 countries, 1980–2008: A systematic analysis of progress towards Millennium Development Goal 5. *Lancet, 375*(9726), 1609–1623.

Källander, K., Tibenderana, J., Akpogheneta, O., Strachan, D., Hill, Z., Asbroek, H. A., … Meek, R. S. (2013). Mobile health (mHealth) approaches and lessons for increased performance and retention of community health workers in low- and middle-income countries: A review. *Journal of Medical Internet Research 15*, 1. Retrieved from http://www.jmir.org/2013/1/e17/

Jehan, I., Harris, H., Solat, S., Zeb, A., Mobeen, N., Pasha, O., … Goldenberg, R. (2009). Neonatal mortality, risk factors and causes: A prospective population-based cohort study in urban Pakistan. *World Health Organization Bulletin,*

87, 2. Retrieved from http://www.scielosp.org/scielo.php?pid=S0042-96862009000200015&script=sci_arttext

Jennings, J., Yebadokpo, A., and Affo, J. (2010). Antenatal counseling in maternal and newborn care: Use of job aids to improve health worker performance and maternal understanding in Benin. *BMC Pregnancy and Child Birth* doi:10.1186/1471-2393-10-75. Retrieved from http://www.biomedcentral.com/1471-2393/10/75

Moran, A., Sangli, G., Dineen, R., Rawlins, B., Yameogo, M., Baya, B. (2006). Birth-preparedness for maternal health: findings from Koupela District, Burkina Faso. *Journal of Health, Population, and Nutrition, 24*(4), 489–497.

One World Asia. (2011). *m-Health projects cutting maternal mortality.* Retrieved from http://southasia.oneworld.net/archive/ictsfordevelopment/m-health-projects-cutting-maternal-mortality#.UTJ9p1dShoM

Royal Tropical Institute. (2013). *Mobile technology to reduce maternal death.* Retrieved from http://mhealthinfo.org/project/mobile-technology-reduce-maternal-death

United Nations. (2000). *Millennium Development Goals and beyond.* Retrieved from http://www.un.org/millenniumgoals/

United Nations Department of Economic and Social Affairs. (2015). *Time for global action for people and planet.* Retrieved from https://sustainabledevelopment.un.org/post2015/summit

United Nations Population Fund. (n.d.). *Skilled attendance at birth.* Retrieved from http://www.unfpa.org/public/mothers/pid/4383

United Nations Women. (2012). *The consequences and costs.* Retrieved from http://www.endvawnow.org/en/articles/301-consequences-and-costs-.html

Walker, A. (2012). *Challenges facing the reduction of Uganda's maternal mortality.* African Portal. Retrieved from Rateshttp://www.africaportal.org/articles/2012/10/12/challenges-facing-reduction-uganda%E2%80%99s-maternal-mortality-rates

World Health Organization. (2010). Maternal health investing. In *Lifeline of Healthy Societies and Economies.* Retrieved from http://www.who.int/pmnch/topics/maternal/app_maternal_health_english.pdf

World Health Organization, the United Nations Children's Fund and World Bank. (2011). *Trends in maternal mortality.* Retrieved from http://www.unfpa.org/webdav/site/global/shared/documents/publications/2012/Trends_in_maternal_mortality_A4-1.pdf

CHAPTER 9

MALARIA PREVENTION AND CONTROL

Fouzia Farooq and Elke S. Bergmann-Leitner

LEARNING OBJECTIVES

By the end of this chapter, the reader should be able to:

- Understand the impact of malaria on global health
- Understand the various layers of countermeasures to prevent malaria disease
- Develop an understanding for which factors are involved in the persistence of malaria
- Understand the effectiveness (or lack thereof) of various malaria elimination programs
- Identify the various funding organizations that are sponsoring and prioritizing the elimination of malaria

In 2012, there were an estimated 207 million cases of malaria, and 627,000 malaria deaths globally (World Health Organization [WHO], 2013). Estimates show that approximately 80% of cases and 90% of deaths occur in Africa, with children under five years of age and pregnant women most severely affected (Centers for Disease Control [CDC], 2014; WHO, 2013). Controlling malaria is part of the Millennium Development Goals (MDGs), specifically MDG 6, that aims to halt malaria by 2015 and begin to reverse the incidence of malaria along with other major diseases. These goals are to be reevaluated in the near future (United Nations Millennium Development Goals, 2014). In addition, the Roll Back Malaria Partnership has outlined a specific strategy to reduce malaria morbidity and mortality, namely, the Action and Investment to defeat Malaria 2016–2030 (AIM). has set a target of reducing malaria deaths to near zero by 2015.

Millennium Development Goals

1. Eradicate extreme poverty and hunger
2. Achieve universal primary education
3. Promote gender equality and empower women
4. Reduce child mortality
5. Improve maternal health
6. Combat HIV/AIDS, malaria, and other diseases
7. Ensure environmental sustainability
8. Develop a global partnership for development

In addition to the severe health outcomes, malaria places a heavy **economic burden of disease** on the affected countries, contributing immensely to poverty and limiting economic

Disclaimer: Material has been reviewed by the Walter Reed Army Institute of Research. There is no objection to its presentation and/or publication. The opinions or assertions contained herein are the private views of the authors, and are not to be construed as official, or as reflecting the position of the Department of the Army and Navy or the Department of Defense.

BOX 9.1 HUMAN RIGHTS

Having access to treatment and access to antimalarial countermeasures should be considered a human right as it affects the quality of life and life itself depends on it.

Despite this fact, most regions that are affected by malaria are highly impoverished, and people either simply do not have access to medical care, it may be several hours until they reach the next clinic, or they cannot afford the drugs. Even more disconcerting is the fact that in some African countries antimalarial drugs are either substandard (diluted down to a point where they are no longer effective) or that they are counterfeit such that there is no biological activity; in addition, wide use of substandard drugs also leads to drug resistance. The government inspectors often turn a blind eye toward this fact because they are involved in bribes that allow the counterfeit drugs to pass through border security. National regulatory agencies are also flooded with corruption, and a lack of sufficient manpower further convolutes the issue.

Bednets have proven to be highly effective for the management of malaria in many regions; however, it is appealing for people living in destitution to trade the cost of a bednet (roughly US$6) for food or other essentials. Global funding organizations have a responsibility to step in and saturate the communities with bednets in order to ensure compliance and make resale of bednets financially unattractive.

Some of the measures that are necessary to take in an attempt to eradicate malaria will infringe on human rights. Participating in drug treatment and surveillance programs may overwrite the individual's right to decide what may or may not be useful to them. Treatment courses are often prolonged, and individuals may not realize the intensity of the treatment course; those who are malnourished, as the case is in sub-Saharan Africa, are unable to handle the effects of harsh treatment drugs.

growth. Malaria is estimated to cost Africa about $12 billion per year in lost gross domestic product (GDP); this in turn can cause a drop in the GDP growth by as much as 1.3% a year (World Bank, 2013). Having access to treatment and at least some prophylactic measures, should be considered a human right (see Box 9.1) as this often decides over life and death.

Malaria Surveillance

Malaria occurs in more than 100 countries and territories, and more than 40% of the people in the world are at risk. Large areas of Central and South America, Hispaniola (Haiti and the Dominican Republic), Africa, the Indian subcontinent, Southeast Asia, the Middle East, and Oceania are considered malaria-endemic areas (Organisation for Economic Development and Co-operation [OECD], 2012). Effective **malaria surveillance** systems are fundamental to controlling malaria, but they currently detect only 10% of cases that occur worldwide and are weakest in countries with the highest numbers.

Surveillance measures depend on the level of malaria transmission and the available resources that compare high transmission areas to low/ no transmission areas (Harris et al., 2010). According to the World Health Organization, a reliable assessment of trends can be made in 58 countries out of 99 with current ongoing transmission; it is estimated that only 10% of all cases that occur each year are detected using national surveillance programs mainly because of a lack of resources (WHO, 2013). There is currently no reliable rapid diagnostic test (RDT) that can be used by individual physicians or community health care workers (CHWs) or even patients, and the sensitivity is not high enough that alternate testing is not needed. The Centers for Disease Control and Prevention (CDC) published the guidance to still perform examination of thick blood smears, in addition to performing the BinaxNOW® test, a substandard assay, in order to ensure that the diagnosis of a malaria infection is properly identified. Examining blood smears requires well-trained, qualified staff that are continuously being certified, as they are not available in every clinical setting. The need for medical **intervention**, along with limited access to diagnostic testing or delayed results, often leads to the overuse of malaria drugs, which in turn favors the development of resistance to the drugs similarly observed in the overuse of antibiotics and multi-drug resistance bacteria.

Impact of Malaria

Malaria is a classic example of the fact that the social standing of an individual often decides his and his family's fate. People with economic resources are able to buy full-strength medications (in contrast to cheaper counterfeit or diluted drugs) as well as ensure that other countermeasures are regularly employed. Malaria has social and economic impacts, and because of climate change, it is likely that more and more people in the world will be affected by these problems.

Fatalities

Despite the fact that malaria is a highly preventable and mostly curable disease, WHO estimates that about 207 million people suffered from malaria and an estimated 627,000 died of the disease in 2012 (WHO, 2013) because of lack of access to care and drugs. Children under the age of five are among the most vulnerable, and approximately 16% of fatalities among children in Africa are due to malaria (World Bank, 2013). The Pacific Asian regions carry the second-highest burden of malaria globally, accounting for approximately 30 million cases and 42,000 deaths each year ("Roll Back Malaria," 2014). However, there has been a huge expansion in financing malaria control programs, and WHO estimates that child mortality rates have fallen by 51% since 2000. This represents considerable progress toward fulfilling MDG 6 goals (United Nations Millennium Development Goals, 2014).

Loss in Gross Domestic Product

Malaria affects especially the poor in remote rural areas who cannot afford treatment or have limited access to health care. Malaria causes significant economic loss; more than 1% of GDP in countries with high levels of transmission; In heavy-burden countries, the disease may account for up to 40% of public health expenditures (OECD, 2012).

Malaria is endemic in many countries in the Asia/Pacific region; 89% of those cases occur in countries that include India, Indonesia, Pakistan, Myanmar, and Papua New Guinea and bear the largest burden of disease in the region. Malaria is heavily associated with specific ecological zones, such as forests in tropical and subtropical Southeast Asia, but it is also found in more temperate areas of the region (Cui et al., 2012). Similar to the situation in Africa, mobile and migrant populations, as well as infants, young children, and pregnant women are especially affected (Cui et al., 2012; WHO IRS List, 2013). The emergence of resistance to the most effective **antimalarials** on the market—artemisinin-based combination therapies (ACTs)—in areas of the Greater Mekong subregion, threatens to reverse the global progress (Gupta & Guin, 2010).

The WHO estimates that 1,200 cases of malaria are diagnosed in the United States each year. Most of those cases are in immigrants and travelers returning from malaria-endemic areas, including sub-Saharan Africa and Pacific Asia. A few cases of malaria result from blood transfusions, passage from mother to fetus during pregnancy, or transmission by locally infected mosquitoes (Mathai et al., 2010). Historically, the United States has been very effective at combating malaria; every U.S. state except Alaska was once malaria endemic. The first cases of malaria in the United States were noticed in 1906 during the construction of the Panama Canal, where 21,000 of the 26,000 workers involved in construction of the canal were hospitalized; the Centers for Disease Control and Prevention was actually established to combat malaria. The combined efforts of the CDC and malaria intervention programs allowed a complete elimination of the disease by 1951 (CDC, 2014).

Still, the U.S. battle with malaria was not over; the risk of contracting infectious diseases such as malaria is a major concern in endemic territories; such was the case during World War II (WWII). American soldiers were deployed to malaria-endemic areas such as Vietnam, where close to 24,606 cases were reported (Beadle & Hoffman, 1993); it was imperative for the military to fight malaria in such an instance. In 1946, the United States and Great Britain adopted the use of the antimalarial drug choloroquine, and by the end of the WWII, various militaries used dichloro-diphenyl-trichloroethane (DDT) for **insecticide** control against diseases such as malaria and typhus (Hong, 2007). The U.S. Army and Navy continue their commitment to malaria research and development (R&D), particularly through the Walter Reed Army Institute of Research (WRAIR) and the Naval Medical Research Center (NMRC), to protect the American military from this disease.

Growing Threat of Climate Change

There is an increasing number of mathematical predictive models that are trying to predict the impact of global warming, changes in rainfall, and season lengths on the vitality and expansion of mosquito populations and the transmission of insect-**vectored** diseases (IVDs). Many of the models agree that if the global temperature continues to rise and seasons become milder in the colder geographic areas, it will have a major impact on the expansion of tropical diseases. This will likely become an increasing **global health** issue with not just malaria reemerging, but many other diseases also.

Control Measures

The mosquito is the deadliest insect known to man. The objective of **control measures** is to reduce the number of mosquitoes in an effort to reduce the transmission and spread of malaria. The countermeasures range from high-impact actions such as reduction of standing waters and spraying standing waters to focused actions such as indoor residual spraying (IRS).

Environmental Changes on Malaria Burden

The earliest recommendation to stop malaria by draining swamps came from Giovanni Lancisi in 1717, as he associated malaria with insects (Cook & Webb, 2000). Historically, draining large bodies of water has successfully eradicated malaria from various geographic regions; for example, construction of the Panama Canal initially appeared futile because of the large numbers of workers' lives lost and the significant impact on productivity. Colonel William C. Gorgas, an Army physician during the construction of the canal who ordered the draining of swamp areas and treatment of water surfaces with the chemical Paris Green (Le Prince & Orenstein, 1916); as a result, Panama has a much lower disease burden than other countries in Central America. Another example is the successful **eradication** of malaria from southern Europe. During World War I malaria was a crucial factor in the battles where many more soldiers died of malaria rather than combat-related injuries (Beadle & Hoffman, 1993). The Pontine Marshes were drained by constructing an extensive channel system in an effort to eliminate breeding grounds for the mosquitoes.

Measures to Reduce the Mosquito Burden

Malaria control and reduction efforts have been ongoing for years and have predominantly been focused on improving vector control mechanisms such as insecticide-treated mosquito nets (ITNs) and indoor residual spraying (Tusting et al., 2013). Long-lasting insecticide-treated bednets (LLINs) and IRS reduce malaria transmission by killing the mosquito and play a key role in malaria control programs; mosquito nets work by creating a physical barrier between the mosquito and the individual. (See Box 9.2.)

Reduction in the number of mosquitoes appears to be an attractive approach because it will affect the transmission of any mosquito-borne illness. . It is not clear, however, how this will affect the ecosystem.

Environmental Spraying

Environmental spraying can be applied either on a large scale (treating entire biotopes such as swamps and standing waters) or on a small scale (residual

BOX 9.2 CONTINUOUS DISTRIBUTION OF LLINS FOR MALARIA CONTROL (MODEL)

Use of long-lasting insecticidal nets (LLINs) contributes immensely to the reduction of malaria transmission. It is also a highly cost-effective strategy and is a fundamental goal of most national malaria control programs. Improving the utilization of LLINs in malaria-endemic countries has been effective at reducing malaria incidence. Parts of countries like Ghana, Botswana, and Kenya have been successful at driving the LLIN Continuous Distribution Model of the long-lasting insecticide nets throughout their countries. Roll Back Malaria's (RBM) Continuous Distribution Framework brings together different distribution channels such as schools, community volunteers, and health facilities for a common purpose of providing LLINs. The sustenance of LLIN access and retention is key to a successful campaign and is not solely dependent on the subsidization of the LLINs. Mass distribution campaigns are effective methods of rapidly scaling up coverage, whether it is LLINs or an effective **vaccine**. The LLINs that are distributed generally have a time limit that begins soon after the distribution campaign; in order to maintain universal coverage, a complementary mechanism must ensure a continuous supply in order to replace the nets that have passed their fixed life span.

indoor spraying of households). This approach has resulted in liberating the South of the United States, as well as Central American countries such as Panama from the scourge of malaria.

Controlling Mosquitoes at the Larval Stage An effective method of controlling breeding grounds is the use of oils and films that disperse as a thin layer on the surface of the water, ultimately causing larvae and pupae to drown. This method is referred to as larval source management (LSM) that targets the mosquito in the larvae stage as they mature to adult mosquitoes on aquatic breeding grounds. The procedure is conducted by habitat manipulation with the addition of toxic substances to standing water that kills or inhibits the development of larvae on the breeding grounds (Tusting et al., 2013). In effect, LSM also works to reduce malaria burden by targeting the immature mosquito stage. A more permanent solution is the removal of the standing water, either by draining water reservoirs or filling land. Addition of chemical or biological larvicides can also disrupt the breeding cycle of the mosquito, and therefore it works as an effective mechanism (Tusting et al., 2013).

Several randomized controlled trials (RCTs) have been conducted to assess the efficiency of the LSM method in countries such as Sri Lanka, India, Kenya, Greece, the Philippines, and Tanzania (Okwundu et al., 1996). LSM is another effective policy option, alongside LLINs and IRS, for reducing malaria cases in areas where larval habitats can be effectively targeted. The feasibility of this method is yet to be evaluated in rural parts of Asia, where larval habitats such as swamps or riverbeds are part of the landscape (Okwundu et al., 1996).

When considering chemical or biological "weapons" to eliminate insects, one has to decide whether to target the larvae or the adult insect. Targeting the larvae may be logistically easier as one can either reduce the availability of breeding grounds and/or treat water surfaces with larvicides (e.g., Paris Green or the biological larvicide *Bacillus thuringiensis var. israelensis* [Bti] or *Bacillus spaericus* [BS, Vectolex]) (Fillinger, Knols, & Becker, 2003). Targeting the adult mosquito can reduce the burden by preventing reproduction. Larvicides have been used in many countries with a proven success record and they appear to be safe when mixed with drinking water. Larvicides were used until the cheaper and more efficacious DDT was developed. DDT is one of the 12 insecticides historically recommended by the WHO (US Environmental Protection Agency [EPA], 2014). It was used for outdoor as well as indoor spraying. However, vegetation and hiding of the insects in resting places that are not easily reached by chemicals allows the adult insects to evade poisoning.

Recently, a massive effort by a community-based program (Urban Malaria Control Program–UMCP) in Dar-es-Salaam, Tanzania has demonstrated promising results in population control of the mosquitos: 70% of the larval habitats have been generated with the expansion of agriculture. Restoring the original drains and maintaining a certain velocity of aquatic bodies, lead to a 40% reduction in larvae of insects that are vectors for a variety of tropical diseases (Castro et al., 2010). The ultimate efficacy of larval source management has been assessed in a large meta-analysis that included data from Tusting et al., 2013. The conclusion indicates that changes in various geographic regions can have additive or even synergistic effects leading to dramatically reduced larval burden.

Unfortunately, not all mosquitoes will be killed, leading to selective pressure to develop insecticide-resistant insects. It is likely that the chemicals do not affect just mosquitoes and that beneficial insects will also die, thus increasing the collateral damage and possibly have agricultural consequences. The price may be too high for poorer countries such as Tanzania, and thus these countries in particular focus on ITNs. The widespread use of insecticides has been received with worries since the days of DDT. DDT had a massive impact on global health and the environment. How far the distribution of DDT went became apparent when DDT was found in the eggshells and body fat of penguins living in Antarctica. Like other organochlorine pesticides, DDT bioaccumulates and is fat soluble. When an animal ingests DDT by eating contaminated vegetation, the chemical gets processed and concentrates in fat cells instead of getting excreted by the body (Inomata et al., 1996). Consequently, when that animal is eaten by either a predator or a scavenger, the chemical will be absorbed by digestion of the prey. This process leads to an increased and widespread concentration of DDT into the higher links of the food chain. Because DDT has a high chronic toxicity, long-term exposure is likely to cause physiological abnormalities and further leads to profound implications for both ecological and human health (Inomata et al., 1996). Recently, three neonicotinoids have been banned by the European Union because of their effects on developing brain cells as well as environmental damages (e.g., killing bees that leads to a tremendous agricultural impact) (Cressey, 2013).

Lack of Compliance and Overuse of Insecticides on Global Health and Global Economy Malaria also impedes the flow of trade, foreign investments, and commerce, thereby affecting a country's entire population and its GDP. Tourism and global investment opportunities are often affected by a high malaria burden and low economic development (Kim, Fedak, & Kramer, 2012). In addition to the political unrest, the fact that the center of Africa is rich in natural resources but the lack of economic development attributes partly to the fact that a high disease burden dampens development (United Nations Development Programme [UNDP], 2014).

Indoor Residual Spraying

Use of insecticides for malaria control has seen a revival in recent years, in part because of the technique of indoor residual spraying (IRS). Indoor residual spraying involves careful controlled spraying of insecticides along the inside walls of a home or community building in order to kill adult mosquitoes that enter during the day and wait for the night to fall in order to feed on the residents. The insecticide-treated walls kill mosquitoes and other insects that come in contact with it. Depending on the type of insecticide, the residual efficacy can range from two months to close to a year. WHO has a list of recommended insecticides for IRS (WHO IRS List, 2013). The list of approved insecticides constitutes 12 chemicals that range from a class of capsule suspensions to pyrethroids. The duration of the chemical's effectiveness varies from three months, to greater than six months, depending on its mode of action (WHO IRS List, 2013). The purpose of IRS is to kill the female mosquito before it becomes infective and is able to further the infection through subsequent bites (USAID, 2012). Since 2006, the WHO encouraged a scale-up in IRS methods for vector-borne disease control and concurrently endorsed DDT for this technique (WHO IRS List, 2013). According to Kim et al. (2012), there are 11 other chemicals currently recommended by the WHO for use in IRS.

Under the major classes of chemicals, there are different compounds sold by different manufacturers using different trade names, and a product may be registered under different trade names in different countries (Ranson et al., 2011; USAID, 2012). These chemicals include bendiocarb, malathion, lambda-cyhalothrin, and alphacypermethrin (WHO IRS List, 2013).

When applied correctly, IRS can be very effective in eliminating the malaria vector as follows:

- *Reduces vector–host contact.* The insecticide is absorbed by the mosquito when it lands on the treated surface either before it takes a blood meal, or after a blood meal, in order to digest the ingested blood. The insecticide may also simply repel mosquitoes from the treated room, which in turn reduces vector–human contact (USAID 2012).
- *Reduces disease transmission.* The reduced vector–host contact reduces disease transmission as an infected mosquito is killed before its next meal, preventing transmission (USAID 2012).

- *Lowers the disease burden.* If a high number of populations at risk are covered under IRS, the burden of disease may be reduced within population. When combined with good epidemic predictions and timely deployment, IRS has been shown to effectively disrupt the outbreak of malaria epidemics (USAID 2012).

There are potential negative environmental and health impacts of the IRS intervention; spray operators, along with the household beneficiaries of the treatment, are at an increased risk of insecticide exposure (CDC, 2014). At the same time, it also affects the general environment, including water, soils, and vegetation. Environmental impacts can include an effect on fish, aquatic invertebrates, and insects such as bees, and mitigation measures must be sought afterward in order to decrease these risks. Substantial training of all individuals involved in implementation, community education, utilization of personal protective equipment, and best practices of reuse or disposal of contaminated water from the operation must be provided (CDC, 2014).

How Effective Is the IRS Program?

There is a wide range of factors that are critical to the effectiveness of IRS. These range from policy, legislation, and institutional frameworks; program management, operations and monitoring capacities; technical skills and competencies; trained periphery providers; as well as educated and compliant targeted populations and households (USAID, 2012).

In order to prevent unauthorized use of insecticides, an effective legislative framework and policy is recommended, as well as an effective enforcement capacity. Countries implementing IRS are encouraged to have an effective legislation that covers the whole life cycle of insecticides. It must also regulate handling and use of these insecticides so that the adverse impact on both the environment and human health is reduced (USAID, 2012).

The ability of IRS to disrupt malaria transmission is usually linked to the timing of the spraying versus the onset of the local rainy seasons. Local malaria transmission normally peaks with the onset of raining season; the onset of rain creates more conducive breeding environments (temporary water reservoirs) that allow the mosquito population to flourish (USAID, 2012). The length of residual action of the selected insecticide is critical, and it is most efficacious if it covers the whole period of peak transmission time (USAID, 2012).

A major challenge to IRS implementation is the difficulty in accessing targeted areas, especially because transmission mainly occurs in rural parts of the country with minimal resources. Lack of accessible roads and transportation infrastructure or expense of transporting equipment and supplies over long distances hinders the efforts of a timely response. This is especially difficult because policies and planning are often performed in cities that are far removed from the impacted areas. It is therefore desirable to develop strategies to implement resources within the region that will conduct the IRS operations (USAID, 2012). Comprehensive planning and training must be required in order for the IRS operation to be effective throughout the region, and a plan for developing country capacity would be required (USAID, 2012). IRS, when applied properly, is a powerful malaria vector control intervention, rapidly reducing vector transmission capacity and malaria incidence.

Bednets

Insecticide-treated bednets have been shown to reduce malaria illness, severe disease, and death from malaria in endemic regions. In community-wide trials in several African settings, ITNs have been shown to reduce the death of children younger than five years from all causes by about 20% (President's Malarial Initiative [PMI], 2010). ITNs are nets designed to block mosquitoes physically from reaching people under the bednets; a long-lasting insecticide-treated bednet is an ITN designed to remain effective for multiple years without treatment. The WHO recommends that LLINs be distributed free of charge to achieve universal coverage (1 LLIN for every 1.8 people in the target community) of those at risk for malaria (Gates Foundation, 1999). Randomized controlled trials have been conducted to prove the efficacy of the LLINs.

Currently, 88 countries, including 39 in Africa, distribute ITNs free of charge. Due to the fact that ITNs remain effective for up to three years, the WHO estimates that 150 million ITNs each year are needed to protect 450 million people over three years. So far, 136 million ITNs were delivered in 2013 (WHO, 2013), and 214 million were delivered in 2014 (WHO, 2014). The percentage of the population in sub-Saharan Africa sleeping under an ITN was 55% in 2015 (WHO, 2015). However, significant resources are still required to ensure coverage approaching 100% (WHO, 2015).

Measures to Lower the Transmission Rate

Herbal remedies to treat malaria or alleviate the symptoms of the disease (in many cases without affecting outcome) are as old as the disease itself. Artemisia had been used for thousands of years in Chinese medicine to remedy a whole spectrum of diseases including fever episodes. The Quechua Indians in Peru processed the bark of *Cinchona Succirubra* to generate a powder that was applied when individuals suffered from fever chills (Butler, Khan, & Ferguson, 2010). This powder contained the potent quinine that later found a wide range of applications, including antimalaria effects. Artemisia, which had been first used as an herbal remedy by the Chinese physician Ge Hong (340 BC), was "rediscovered" in 1970s, by Chinese scientists who derived the class of artemesinin antimalaria drugs.

Drugs Targeting Blood Stage

Quinine and chloroquine block the development and multiplication of the blood stage parasite. Although quinine is an organic substance derived from the Cinchona tree, chloroquine was initially synthesized in the 1930s and it was a highly effective drug against malaria. However, the development of chloroquine-resistant malaria in Southeast Asia that rapidly spread to most malaria-endemic areas has led to new therapeutic regiments based on two or more drugs used in combination. The combination of the artemesinin drugs, Artemether with Lumefantrine, is being marketed as Coartem. All artemisinin combination therapies (ACT) are highly efficacious, fast acting and are also effective for the treatment of cerebral malaria. The relatively high cost of the treatment, however, is responsible for the fact that in malaria-endemic areas only a fraction of individuals that would need this treatment will actually receive it. Unfortunately, resistance to artemesinin drugs has recently been reported in Cambodia, giving rise to anxieties about further spread (White, 2008).

Drugs Targeting Liver Stage

There is an urgent need for drugs that can eliminate the liver stage parasites by targeting hypnozoites of *P. vivax* from which relapses occur. Currently, only Primaquine and Tafenoquine are known to affect this stage of the life cycle. Individuals with a deficiency of an enzyme called glucose-6-phosphate-dehydrogenase (G6PD) cannot be given these drugs because the drugs induce hemolysis. Therefore, these drugs can only be administered after testing individuals for this genetic trait. Moreover, a recent study identified a genetic point mutation in the cytochrome P-450 protein of two individuals as reason for Primaquine failure to clear liver infection of *P. vivax* (Bennett et al., 2013).

Vaccines

The advantage of vaccines over drug treatment is that successful establishment of immunity provides the vaccinee with long-term protection against disease and without side effects. In contrast, drugs can only be dispensed after the onset of symptoms, and may not always be effective especially in cases of severe malaria, and are required whenever symptoms arise.

The availability of an efficacious malaria vaccine would complement antimalaria control programs using insecticides and drugs. Vaccine research in the course of the past 50 years has demonstrated that:

- naturally acquired immunity is short-lived, suggesting that vaccines will have to induce protection over longer periods of time;
- immunity may be strain specific, suggesting that a multivalent vaccine formulation would be required that contains antigens from the most prevalent parasite strains in the area where the vaccine will be deployed. Such formulations are common for other diseases such as influenza (tri- or quadrivalent flu vaccine) and human papillomavirus.
- Immunity is stage specific, that is, antibodies targeting antigens expressed on the sporozoite will only result in neutralizing the sporozoite and will not provide immunity against liver and blood stage infection; different strategies to target more than one stage of the life cycle are also being developed. (See Box 9.3.)

BOX 9.3 TECHNOLOGY

Vaccine research and development can address a serious public health need that no amount of bednets or insecticide spraying can provide. A safe and effective vaccine is one of the most significant advancements because of current technological advances. WHO visions a minimum 75% protective efficacy of a suitable vaccine by year 2030. Vaccines that reduce the transmission of the parasite that manifests into clinical symptoms would effectively reduce the incidence of infections.

Development of malaria vaccines follows one of two principles:

- Screen sera from malaria-immune individuals for their reactivity toward molecules expressed by the malaria parasite and identify molecules that are recognized. These molecules are then tested as vaccine candidates. Caveat of this approach is the fact that the malaria parasite favors the induction of immune responses against molecules that are not essential for its survival, which in turn, renders the immune response useless.
- Profiling expression of proteins through gene chip arrays are essential for the function and viability of the parasite; these proteins are then tested as a vaccine candidate. The caveat of this approach is that many proteins identified by this approach are difficult or impossible to manufacture and therefore vaccine development is hampered or impossible.

The earliest and, to this day, the most efficacious vaccine approach was reported half a century ago. It is an attenuated pathogen-based vaccine and involves the use of irradiated sporozoites (Nussenzweig et al., 1967). Whether this approach is useful outside the laboratory setting still remains to be seen because it may not provide protection against other parasite strains than the one used in the vaccine. RTS,S, a recombinant malaria vaccine jointly developed by GlaxoSmithKline and WRAIR, has been tested in several Phase III field trials and has been licensed for Europe and Africa in 2016 (The RTS,S Clinical Trials Partnership, 2012). It has been the most efficacious malaria vaccine to date, able to prevent mortality in small children, and reduce morbidity in 30% of pediatric vaccinees. Although this may represent a glimpse of hope for parents in malaria endemic areas, there is a dire need for a highly efficacious vaccine that can prevent at least 80% of infections in all vaccinees (including travelers, pregnant women, and military service members).

Interventions

A complex mixture of biological, political, and economic interactions influences malaria transmission. Malaria control programs should be adapted to specific local ecological, epidemiological, economic, and social conditions. Even the goals of malaria interventions should be place specific (Kim et al., 2012).

The landscape of global malaria control has changed dramatically, especially in the past decade. There are several major initiatives that have been established to control malaria and some are discussed in the following sections.

The U.S. President's Malaria Initiative (PMI)

In June 2005, the United States announced a five-year initiative worth $1.2 billion in order to increase efforts for malaria prevention and treatment interventions across 15 sub-Saharan countries. The initiative is led by the US Agency for International Development (USAID) and implemented together with Department of Health and Human Services' (DHHS) and the CDC. The purpose of this initiative is to reduce malaria-related deaths by 50% across the 15 countries through a rapid scale-up of four proven malaria prevention and treatment measures (PMI, 2010): ITNs, IRS, ACTs, and Intermittent Prevention Treatment of pregnant women (IPTp).

Selection of the initial 15 focus countries was based on their malaria burden, the presence of technically sound national malaria control policies, willingness to partner with the United States, and a global fund (to fight AIDS, tuberculosis, and malaria) malaria grant. The initiative began in 2006, and now covers a population of 270 million residents in the 15 focus countries. Table 9.1 list the the current 15 focus countries (PMI, 2010).

In 2008, the Lantos/Hyde Act authorized another $5 billion in US government (USG) funding for malaria prevention and control. This act provides for the continuation of support to the 15 PMI focus countries with a target to expand help to other malaria-endemic countries (PMI, 2010).

The vision of the PMI 2009–2014 emphasizes the role it will play in reducing preventable malaria deaths to near-zero by 2015 (PMI, 2010).

Bill & Melinda Gates Foundation

The Bill & Melinda Gates Foundation has made control and eradication of malaria one of its top priorities. The Gates Foundation especially focuses its resources in areas where existing funds are limited and its support can have major impacts. The foundation heavily supports R&D for more effective

Table 9.1 President's Malaria Initiative Focus Countries

Fiscal Year (FY)	Focus Countries
2006	Angola, Tanzania, Uganda
2007	Malawi, Mozambique, Rwanda, Senegal (in addition to the 2006 selection)
2008	Benin, Ethiopia, Ghana, Kenya, Liberia, Madagascar, Mali, and Zambia (in addition to the 2006 and 2007 selection)
2009	All 15 PMI focus countries
2010	All 15 PMI focus countries ($1.265 billion spent)

treatments, diagnostics, mosquito control measures, and a safe and effective malaria vaccine ("Malaria No More," 2014).

The Global Fund to Fight AIDS, Tuberculosis, and Malaria

The Global Fund to Fight AIDS, Tuberculosis, and Malaria (GFAMT) was created in 2002, in order to drastically increase efforts and resources to fight the three pandemics, HIV/AIDS, tuberculosis, and malaria (PMI, 2010). GFAMT is a multibillion-dollar international financing portal whose goal is to increase the availability of funds to areas of health in their greatest need. This organization works as a partnership among governments, civil society, private sector, and affected communities in order to fight against HIV/AIDS, tuberculosis, and malaria and allocates funding through grant programs (PMI, 2010).

World Bank Malaria Booster Program

In 1998, the Roll Back Malaria (RBM) Partnership was launched with the World Bank at the core of its foundation. RBM was launched in response to the demands of the endemic countries for assistance in scaling up new and cost effective interventions for malaria control, especially in Africa (Roll Back Malaria, 2014). In 2005, the bank launched the Booster Program for Malaria Control in Africa as a 10-year effort to help countries achieve the Millennium Development Goals for child survival, maternal and malaria (Roll Back Malaria, 2014). Since its inception, the bank has committed more than US$772.8 million in combating malaria through 22 projects across 20 countries in sub-Saharan Africa. The bank particularly emphasizes effective partnerships in order to leverage resources and optimizing monitoring strategies and program evaluations (Roll Back Malaria, 2014).

Malaria No More

Malaria No More, established in 2006 is a nonprofit organization whose mission is to end deaths caused by malaria and by working, to raise the malaria awareness among the public, policymakers, and businesses. Malaria No More plays a major part in engaging the private sector in providing ITNs and other critical interventions to countries in Africa (Malaria No More, 2014).

Progress has been remarkable: between 2000 and 2010, 43 of the 99 countries with ongoing malaria transmission have reduced malaria incidence by more than 50%. Global incidence has decreased 17% since 2000. Programs focusing on malaria prevention and treatment have proven to have a profound impact on childhood mortality, particularly in sub-Saharan Africa. Tanzania serves as an exemplar for this metric: between 1999 and 2010, under-five mortality rates were slashed by 45%, a measurement that was concurrent with vast malaria control efforts by the Tanzanian government. Similarly, as malaria control and treatment increased in Senegal and Rwanda between 2002 and 2011, under-five mortality decreased 40% and 50%, respectively (CDC, 2014).

Summary

The global picture of malaria is widespread and exists in tropical and subtropical regions around the globe. It is a disease that debilitates the financial status of a country and keeps households in poverty. The morbidity and mortality due to malaria also have enormous social and cultural costs associated with it, as it is a geographically specific disease. The distribution and intensity of the disease is affected by the ecological conditions. Over the years, tackling malaria has been a prominent issue with an increase in resources that have led to drastic malaria control and reduction programs. The spread of the disease can be reduced by either, preventing or eliminating the mosquito vector from progressing in its life cycle, or by developing vaccines that gear up the human immune system against disease progression.

KEY TERMS

1. **Antimalarials:** Medication designed to prevent or cure malaria
2. **Control measures:** Interventions that are undertaken to reduce or delay the occurrence of disease or to reduce further transmission or exposure to disease
3. **Economic burden of disease:** Financial impact of ill health related to microeconomic level of households, firms, or government and the macroeconomic level of a country's gross domestic product
4. **Eradication:** The process of removing something permanently
5. **Global health:** Area of study, research, and practice that places a priority on improving health and achieving equity in health for all people worldwide
6. **Insecticide:** A type of chemical used for killing insects
7. **Intervention:** Action taken to improve a situation, especially a medical disorder
8. **Malaria surveillance:** The monitoring of malaria cases and deaths that helps ministries of health determine which areas and/or population groups are most affected by malaria
9. **Transmission rate:** Rate at which a communicable disease passes from an infected host to a noninfected host
10. **Vaccine:** A biological substance used to stimulate the production of immune system and provide immunity against a disease
11. **Vector:** An organism that spreads infection by conveying pathogens from one host to another but does not cause disease itself

REVIEW QUESTIONS

1. What is the impact of malaria on global health?
2. How does malaria affect the economy in malaria-endemic areas?
3. What are the preventive measures to reduce the **transmission rate** of malaria?
4. What are the caveats of antimalarial drugs?
5. What impact has overuse of insecticides and antimalarial drugs had on malaria prevalence?

References

Beadle, C., & Hoffman, S. L. (1993). History of malaria in the United States naval forces at war: World War I through the Vietnam conflict. *Clinical Infectious Diseases: An Official Publication of the Infectious Diseases Society of America, 16*(2), 320–329.

Bennett, J. W., Pybus, B. S., Yadava, A., Tosh, D., Sousa, J. C., McCarthy , … Ockenhouse, C. F. (2013). Primaquine failure and Cytochrome P-450 2D6 in Plasmodium Vivax Malaria. *New England Journal of Medicine, 369*(14), 1381–1382. doi:10.1056/NEJMc1301936

Butler, A. R., Khan, S., & Ferguson, E. (2010). A brief history of malaria chemotherapy. *Journal of the Royal College of Physicians of Edinburgh, 40*(2), 172–177.

Castro, M. C., Kanamori, S., Kannady, K., Mkude, S., Killeen, G. F., & Fillinger, U. (2010). The importance of drains for the larval development of lymphatic filariasis and malaria vectors in Dar Es Salaam, United Republic of Tanzania. *Public Library of Scicence Neglected Tropical Diseases, 4*(5), e693. doi:10.1371/journal.pntd.0000693

Centers for Disease Control and Prevention. (2014). *Centers for Disease Control and Prevention—Malaria*. Retrieved from http://www.cdc.gov/malaria/

Cook, G., & Webb, A. (2000). Perceptions of malaria transmission before Ross' discovery in 1897. *Postgraduate Medical Journal, 76*(901), 738–740. doi:10.1136/pmj.76.901.738

Cressey, D. (2013). Europe debates risk to bees. *Nature, 496*(7446), 408–408. doi:10.1038/496408a

Cui, L., Yan, G., Sattabongkot, J., Cao, Y., Chen, B., Chen, X., … Zhou, G. (2012). Malaria in the greater Mekong subregion, heterogeneity and complexity. *Acta Tropica, 121*(3), 227–239. doi:10.1016/j.actatropica.2011.02.016

Fillinger, U., Knols, B.G.J., & Becker. N. (2003). Efficacy and efficiency of new bacillus T*huringiensis Var. Israelensis* and bacillus *Sphaericus* formulations against Afrotropical anophelines in Western Kenya. *Tropical Medicine and International Health, 8*(1), 37–47. doi:10.1046/j.1365–3156.2003.00979.x

Gates Foundation. (1999). *Malaria strategy overview*. Bill & Melinda Gates Foundation. Retrieved from http://www.gatesfoundation.org/What-We-Do/Global-Health/Malaria.

Gupta, I., & Guin, P. (2010). Communicable diseases in the South-East Asia Region of the World Health Organization: Towards a more effective response. *Bulletin of the World Health Organization, 88*(3), 199–205. doi:10.2471/BLT.09.065540

Harris, I., Sharrock, W., Bain, L. M., Gray, K.-A., Bobogare, A., Boaz, L., … Cheng, Q. (2010). A large proportion of asymptomatic plasmodium infections with low and sub-microscopic parasite densities in the low transmission setting of Temotu Province, Solomon Islands: Challenges for malaria diagnostics in an elimination setting. *Malaria Journal, 9*(1), 254. doi:10.1186/1475–2875–9–254

Hong, S. C.. (2007). The burden of early exposure to malaria in the United States, 1850–1860: Malnutrition and immune disorders. *Journal of Economic History, 67*(4), 1001–1035. doi:10.1017/S0022050707000472

Inomata, O.N.K., Montone, R. C., Lara, W. H., Weber, R. R., & Toledo, H.H.B. (1996). Tissue distribution of organochlorine residues in Antarctic penguins. *Antarctic Science, 8*(3), 253–255. doi:10.1017/S0954102096000351

Kim, D., Fedak, K., & Kramer, R. (2012). Reduction of malaria prevalence by indoor residual spraying: A meta-regression analysis. *American Journal of Tropical Medicine and Hygiene, 87*(1), 117–124. doi:10.4269/ajtmh.2012.11–0620

Le Prince, J. A, & Orenstein, A. J. (1916). *Mosquito control in Panama: The eradication of malaria and yellow fever in Cuba and Panama*. New York, NY, and London: Putnam.

Malaria No More. (2014). Retrieved from http://www.malarianomore.org/

Mathai, S., Bishburg, E., Slim, J., & Nalmas, S. (2010). Severe malaria in immigrant population: A retrospective review. *Journal of Immigrant and Minority Health/Center for Minority Public Health, 12*(6), 921–924. doi:10.1007/s10903–009–9256–5

Nussenzweig, R. S., Vanderberg, J., Most, H., & Orton. C. (1967). Protective immunity produced by the injection of X-irradiated sporozoites of plasmodium berghei. *Nature, 216*(5111), 160–162. doi:10.1038/216160a0

Organisation for Economic Development and Co-operation. (2012). Malaria. In *Health at a Glance: Asia/Pacific*. Organisation for Economic Co-operation and Development. Retrieved from http://www.oecd-ilibrary.org/content/chapter/9789264183902-14-en

Okwundu, C. I., Nagpal, S., Musekiwa, A., & Sinclair, D. (1996). Home- or community-based programmes for treating malaria. *Cochrane Database of Systematic Reviews*. New York, NY: Wiley. Retrieved from http://onlinelibrary.wiley.com/doi/10.1002/14651858.CD009527.pub2/abstract

President's Malaria Initiative. (2010). *Lantos-Hyde U.S. government malaria strategy 2009–2014*. United StatesAgency for International Development. http://www.cdc.gov/malaria/malaria_worldwide/cdc_activities/pmi.html

Ranson, H., N'guessan, R., Lines, J., Moiroux, N., Nkuni, Z., & Corbel, V. (2011). Pyrethroid resistance in African anopheline mosquitoes: What are the implications for malaria control? *Trends in Parasitology, 27*(2), 91–98. doi:10.1016/j.pt.2010.08.004

Roll Back Malaria. (2014). *Roll back malaria: The global partnership for a malaria-free world.* Retrieved from http://www.rbm.who.int/keyfacts.html

RTS,S Clinical Trials Partnership. (2012). A phase 3 trial of RTS,S/AS01 malaria vaccine in African infants. *New England Journal of Medicine, 367*(24), 2284–2295. doi: 10.1056/NEJMoa1208394

Tusting, L. S., Thwing, J., Sinclair, D., Fillinger, U., Gimnig, J., Bonner, K. E., … Lindsay, S. W. (2013). Mosquito larval source management for controlling malaria. *Cochrane Database of Systematic Reviews, 8.* CD008923. doi:10.1002/14651858.CD008923.pub2

United Nations Development Programme. (2014). *African economic outlook 2014* (13th ed.). Retrieved from http://www.africaneconomicoutlook.org/en

United Nations Millennium Development Goals. (2014). Retrieved from http://www.un.org/millenniumgoals/aids.shtml

US Agency for International Development. (2012). *USAID: Integrated vector management programs for malaria vector control* (2012 Update). USAID. Retrieved from http://www.pmi.gov/docs/default-source/default-document-library/implementing-partner-reports/integrated-vector-management-programs-for-malaria-vector-control-programmatic-environmental-assessment--volume-1-of-2-main-document.pdf?sfvrsn=4

US Environmental Protection Agency. (2014). Controlling mosquitoes at the larval stage. Overviews and Factsheets. Retrieved from http://www2.epa.gov/mosquitocontrol/controlling-mosquitoes-larval-stage

White, N. J. (2008). Qinghaosu (artemisinin): The price of success. *Science, 320*(5874), 330–334. doi:10.1126/science.1155165

World Bank. (2013). *The World Bank: Malaria overview.* Retrieved from http://go.worldbank.org/S4X0AZMLS0

World Health Organization. (2013). *WHO—World Malaria Report 2013.* Retrieved from http://www.who.int/malaria/publications/world_malaria_report_2013/en/

World Health Organization. (2014, December). *WHO—fact sheet on the World Malaria Report 2014.* Retrieved from http://www.who.int/malaria/media/world_malaria_report_2014/en/

World Health Organization. (2015). *WHO—World Malaria Report 2015: Key points.* Retrieved from http://www.who.int/malaria/publications/world-malaria-report-2015/wmr2015-keypoints_eng.pdf?ua=1

World Health Organization IRS List. (2013). *WHO—indoor residual spraying: An operational manual for IRS for malaria transmission, control and elimination.* Retrieved from http://www.who.int/malaria/publications/atoz/9789241505123/en/

CHAPTER 10

GLOBAL IMMUNIZATION INITIATIVES FROM A HEALTH PROMOTION PERSPECTIVE

Marilyn E. Rice, Jon K. Andrus, Virginia Swezy, and Rick S. Zimmerman

LEARNING OBJECTIVES

By the end of this chapter, the reader should be able to:

- Identify advantages and disadvantages to Immunization Weeks and World Health Days
- Describe the advantages and application of social marketing techniques to immunization and other health issues
- Explain how immunization campaign strategies can be expanded in scope to improve the health and well-being of children and the population at large
- Identify and describe the four pillars of polio eradication
- Explain how lessons from polio eradication in Asia can be applied to other diseases and health issues
- Describe both progress in and barriers to HPV vaccination globally
- Identify advantages to pentavalent vaccine as compared to other vaccines

This chapter covers the history and pros and cons of several kinds of international initiatives to promote increased child immunizations. Two initiatives are discussed in detail as case studies: Global Immunization Week and the polio eradication program in Southeast Asia. Then, several other initiatives that have been undertaken internationally to increase the uptake of childhood immunizations are described: efforts to increase coverage of the pentavalent vaccine, HPV vaccination, and child immunization cards. The reader is challenged to identify ways that these types of public health approaches can best be applied in his or her own context and how policies and programs can be strengthened to provide continual support to these initiatives.

Immunization is arguably the most cost-effective public health intervention that medical science has to offer. Perhaps only safe water and sanitation and breast feeding may be more cost-effective. It is also arguably a basic human right and should be viewed as child protection under the Convention on the Rights of the Child. (See Box 10.1.)

However, immunization is not a one-time activity. A fully vaccinated child requires a massive volume of work that involves all sectors of society. A fully vaccinated child must undergo several medical visits and injections to provide the full protection against a host of killer diseases, such as pertussis, diphtheria, tetanus, measles, meningitis, and diarrhea. The parents and family must be fully engaged, and it helps if the community is as well.

The system that provides the vaccination services is complex. For example, the vaccine trail from factory to arm requires a **cold chain** to ensure the vaccine retains its potency at the point of service, often thousands of miles away from where the vaccine was manufactured. To fully vaccinate a child requires proper management and coordination of

BOX 10.1 CHILD RIGHTS

Immunization might be considered a basic human and child right. Countries should consider immunization services in that light; and as a result provision of such services should be an integral part of all health services. The Convention on the Rights of the Child was ratified by the UN General Assembly on the 30th anniversary of the Declaration of the Rights of the Child, and it came into force on September 2, 1990. Currently, 194 countries are party to it. It is a human rights treaty that sets out the civil, political, economic, social, health, and cultural rights of children, defining a child as any human being under the age of 18. It changed the way children were viewed and treated—that is, as human beings with a distinct set of rights instead of as passive objects of care and charity. The unprecedented acceptance of the Convention clearly shows a wide global commitment to advancing children's rights. The Convention applies to all children, whatever their race, religion, or abilities; whatever they think or say; whatever type of family they come from. It doesn't matter where children live, what language they speak, what their parents do, whether they are boys or girls, what their culture is, whether they have a disability, or whether they are rich or poor. No child should be treated unfairly on any basis. Governments have a responsibility to take all available measures to make sure children's rights are respected, protected, and fulfilled. The Convention clearly states that children have the right to live and that governments should ensure that children survive and develop healthily. Children have the right to good-quality health care—the best health care possible—to safe drinking water, nutritious food, a clean and safe environment, and information to help them stay healthy. Rich countries should help poorer countries achieve this (UNICEF, 2015).

human resources, multiple aspects of logistics and operations along the vaccine trail, as well as policy development, financing, surveillance to monitor impact, and most importantly public acceptance and engagement. Well-coordinated health promotion programs can help ensure and sustain the massive volume and complexity of work required to fully vaccinate the nation's children with adequate support. Such efforts need to have sustained essential political commitment and public support for this service.

Addressing Reluctance to Immunize

Figure 10.1 shows rates of key immunizations in the six World Health Organization (WHO) regions (Africa, the Americas, Europe, Eastern Mediterranean, Southeast Asia, and Western Pacific). As can be seen there, although much progress has been made in the past 25 years, there is still a lot of work to do. There are many reasons why populations are reluctant to receive immunizations. Often they are related to preconceived ideas that immunizations can cause illnesses, sterilization, and even death. These ideas come from the local folklore, messages that have been passed down through the generations from

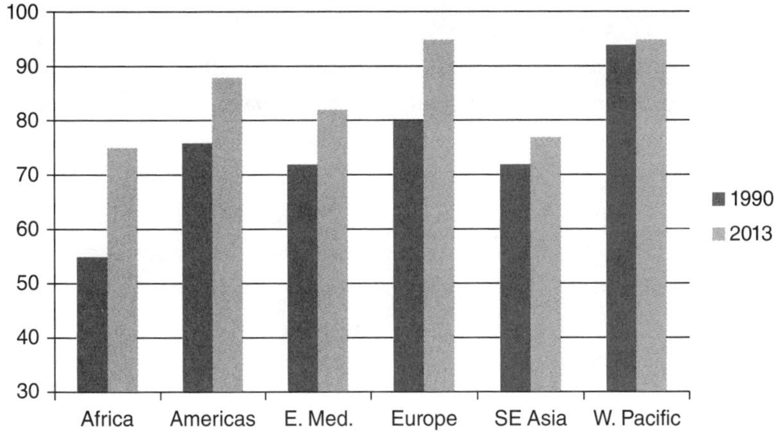

Figure 10.1 Immunization Rates, 1990 and 2013

one family or community member to another, or the wrong association between someone getting an immunization and then shortly afterward getting very sick or dying. In order to effectively immunize populations, it is important to first identify the overarching beliefs and practices, so that misconceptions can be effectively addressed by people the community knows, respects, and trusts.

Basic research may help to describe what a given population is currently doing or thinking and help shape realistic goals for promoting specific behaviors. Community-based research helps to identify specific target audience segments within a larger population, what they believe, who they trust to transmit health messages, and who they will consult when they have health concerns; all this information will be most useful in creating interventions that will influence or support the promotion of desired behaviors. Through **social marketing** techniques, benefits can be described in the most appealing and attractive manner. Social marketing planning requires incorporation of the "The Four Ps of Marketing" (see Box 10.2) into program planning. Social marketing is critical because it looks at the four Ps and the provision of health services from the viewpoint of the consumer (Centers for Disease Control [CDC], 2007). It is also important to use many different means of communication (interpersonal, social, and mass media); the more types often the better.

BOX 10.2 THE FOUR Ps OF SOCIAL MARKETING

Product represents the desired behavior you are asking your audience to carry out, and the associated benefits, tangible objects, and/or services that support behavior change.

Price is the cost (financial, emotional, psychological, or time related) of overcoming the barriers the audience faces in making the desired behavior change.

Place is where the audience will perform the desired behavior, where they will access the program, products, and services, or where they are thinking about your issue.

Promotion stands for communication messages, materials, channels, and activities that will effectively reach your audience.

Sometimes there is a fifth P: Policy. *Policies* are the laws and regulations that influence the desired behavior, such as requiring schools to admit only children who have been fully immunized, or establishing regulations to ensure adequate control of the cold chain.

Additionally, in many communities, the local population is very suspicious of the government and of outsiders who are unknown to them. For this reason it is important to organize mass campaigns by mobilizing the local stakeholders. It means getting them on board first so that they, together with the local leaders and role models, are the ones who are promoting the events. Unless the community feels that the initiative is its own, it will not be as willing to participate, facilitate, and get its children and its neighbor's children to come out for the immunization events.

The Healthy Settings Approach

One approach that can be very effective in creating local ownership for mass campaigns is to build on the **healthy settings initiatives** that might already exist in the communities. WHO as well as its regional offices (PAHO [Pan American Health Organization] for the Americas, etc.) have been very successful in helping countries to establish these types of initiatives. Examples of these initiatives include Healthy Municipalities, Cities and Communities; Health Promoting Schools; Health Promoting Universities; Healthy Markets; Healthy Workplaces; Eco Clubs; and Healthy Housing, among others. These initiatives are based upon having local commitment by many sectors and stakeholders (usually, a commitment is backed by a written policy or legislation with assigned resources); a long-term vision of what will make and sustain a healthy community and environment; active and representative social participation from all walks of life in the community; and effective monitoring and evaluation to measure outcomes, make note of successes, and highlight areas for improvement. Involvement and commitment of local policy and decision makers is another critical factor in ensuring success.

One way of massively mobilizing populations to take collective action simultaneously is to declare a local, national, or international day for a specific issue, policy, or program. The World Health Organization has taken the initiative to create worldwide health topic days. Mass media and community mobilization campaigns are then organized around these themes on their designated days. It started with the celebration of the anniversary of the formation of the Organization itself through worldwide celebrations of **World Health Day**. Each year the governing bodies of the Organization pick a topic to be the focus of this celebration; there are massive mobilization and country- and worldwide campaigns organized to carry out activities in relation to that issue. Promotion materials are produced to support the enticement of people to participate, and many groups are mobilized internationally, nationally, and locally for planned events. In addition to the topics selected each year for World Health Day, there are many other "health days" so designated to promote important public health issues, most of which are supported by the World Health Organization and its partners. A variety of such annually recurring official WHO health days mandated by the World Health Assembly now include World TB Day, World Malaria Day, World No Tobacco Day, World Blood Donor Day, World Hepatitis Day, and World AIDS Day (WHO, 2013a).

The Pros and Cons of Issue-Specific Campaigns

A major drawback to this approach is that it focuses a great deal of time and resources on the campaign while it is underway, taking personnel and other resources away from the regular and ongoing services that are otherwise provided. This means that leading up to, during, and immediately following mass campaigns, prevention, care, and rehabilitation services may not be available when they are needed by the entire population. Additionally, these campaigns are not sustainable over time, which is why they tend to be scheduled for just one day in the year, or in the case of childhood immunizations, two to three days in the year, spaced about a month apart to provide the opportunity for children to have their immunization schedules completed. For most prevention and promotion initiatives, focusing just one day on an issue does not create sustainable behaviors. Attention needs to be given to what kind of support can be generated in a more continuous way over time, in between the annual events.

However, in the case of immunizations, long-term sustainability is not an issue, as long as disease-specific campaigns are conducted at least annually and often enough for people to return periodically for boosters and follow-up. That is why this issue lends itself so well to producing positive results from mass campaigns, and why the most effective of mass campaign initiatives have been immunization campaigns to protect populations against the types of diseases for which protection can be ensured through a series of vaccinations that take place nationwide, regionwide, and today worldwide on predetermined days. Additionally, the increased attention provided to initiatives such as **Vaccination Week** in the Americas (see Case Study 10.1) creates a benefit of political commitment and public acceptance and engagement for week-long efforts that in turn help to sustain the daily work required over time. Immunization campaigns are therefore a good example of how a mass campaign strategy has been used for many years throughout the world to effectively immunize populations against specific diseases. Social media plays a key role in helping these campaigns to be successful.

CASE STUDY 10.1 VACCINE WEEK IN THE AMERICAS/WORLD IMMUNIZATION WEEK

Of various kinds of health/illness weeks, most relevant to this chapter, of course, is Global Immunization Week, which began in 2013. It was patterned after the original Vaccination Week in the Americas (VWA) begun in 2003 (PAHO, 2009a). Annually, the PAHO member countries and territories mobilize to promote equal access to immunization by all citizens (Ropero-Alvarez et al., 2012). VWA was initially adopted as a strategy in April 2002 following a measles outbreak in Venezuela and Colombia (PAHO, 2009a). The overarching objectives of VWA are to promote equity and access to immunization and strengthen immunization programs in the Region of the Americas by "reaching the unreached"—populations with otherwise limited access to regular health services and at heightened risk of contracting vaccine-preventable diseases. In the Americas, such populations can be found in areas such as urban fringes, low-coverage municipalities, indigenous communities, and rural and/or border zones (PAHO, 2009b). The participation of countries and territories in Vaccination Week is flexible, and goals and activities for the initiative are chosen in accordance with national health objectives (PAHO, 2009b). VWA has been used to conduct large-scale vaccination campaigns, introduce new vaccines, carry out communication and social mobilization campaigns, and to integrate other preventative measures (PAHO, 2008; Ropero-Alvarez et al., 2012). Since its inception in 2003, more than 519 million individuals of all ages have been vaccinated during campaigns conducted under the framework of VWA (PAHO, 2015a). The initiative also provides a platform from which to raise population awareness regarding the importance of immunization and to keep the topic on the forefront of political agendas (PAHO, 2013). The potential benefits of integrating other health interventions with immunization delivery have been widely discussed (PAHO, 2008). The 13th annual VWA was celebrated between April 25 and May 2, 2015, reaching more than 44 million children and adults. Vaccination Week in the Americas has been included as one of the five memorable moments in public health by the Global Development Professionals Network of the *Guardian* newspaper (UK) (PAHO, 2015a).

In addition to vaccination-related services such as tracking of unvaccinated people and implementing large-scale vaccination campaigns, the Vaccination Week in the Americas has begun to use the occasion as **Child Health Days** to deliver an integrated package of life-saving health interventions. These health interventions include vitamin A supplementation to boost children's immune systems, deworming medicine administration, child growth and development monitoring, and insecticide-treated nets distribution to prevent malaria. Throughout its 13-year history, Vaccination Week in the Americas has promoted expanded access to immunization, particularly for vulnerable groups and remote communities that traditionally lack access to health services. The initiative also promotes communication and cooperation among countries and helps keep immunization high on the regional and national political agendas.

The success of Vaccination Week in the Americas has served as a model for other regions of the WHO in the implementation of successful sister initiatives. It is a good example of how acting locally can have implications nationally and internationally and how good and effective approaches can go viral given enough time. In 2005, the European Region of WHO launched European Immunization Week (EIW) (WHO, 2014). The Eastern Mediterranean Region of the WHO launched their first Vaccination Week (VWEM) in 2010, with the participation of all member states. In 2011, the African and Western Pacific regions launched their first annual Vaccination Weeks. The Southeast Asian Region member states confirmed their commitment to implement an annual regional immunization week in 2012. As of April 2012, all six WHO regions joined together to celebrate World Immunization Week (PAHO, 2012). An increasing number of countries use VWA to integrate other preventative health interventions with vaccination campaigns (WHO, April 2012). Table 10.1 provides brief highlights of events and activities related to Global Immunization Week since the inception of Vaccination Week in the Americas in 2002. In 2012, 17 countries and territories reported plans to integrate activities such as deworming, vitamin A supplements, growth monitoring, cancer screening, distribution of water filters, body mass index screening, and foot care demonstrations for diabetics as part of the 10th anniversary of VWA. In the last week of April 2013, more than 180 countries, WHO, and partners marked World Immunization Week (WHO, 2013b). During Vaccination Week 2014, more than 63 million people of all ages were vaccinated in the Americas, and more than 100 million in other parts of the world. In the 2015 World Health Assembly, countries from around the world approved a resolution to improve access to sustainable supplies of affordable vaccines—a key issue for low- and middle-income countries aiming to extend immunization to the entire population, urging member states to increase transparency around vaccine pricing and exploring pooling for the procurement of vaccines (PAHO, 2015b).

Table 10.1 Chronology of Vaccination Week in the Americas/World Immunization Week

2002	Prompted by a measles outbreak in Venezuela and Colombia, the health ministers of countries in the Andean Region proposed an annual Vaccination Week in the Americas.
2003	In September, Vaccination Week in the Americas was accepted as an annual, hemispheric initiative, by the directing council of the Pan American Health Organization. The principles underlying Vaccination Week in the Americas are equity, access, and Pan-Americanism. The primary objectives of the new initiative were to strengthen the regular immunization programs in the Americas and to identify and reach populations who were most at risk of contracting vaccine-preventable diseases because of their lack of access to immunization services. Nineteen countries participated in the first VWA, the primary focus of which was measles elimination.
2004, April 24–30	The focus of the second regionwide VWA consisted of follow-up campaigns against measles, elimination of rubella and CRS, and the vaccination of older adults.
2005, April 24–30	The third VWA emphasized the vaccination of indigenous peoples and older adults, rubella elimination campaigns, the strengthening of regular immunization programs, and the introduction of new vaccines. Drawing inspiration from the activities in the Americas, European Immunization Week (EIW) was launched in October 2005 and focused primarily on social communication activities.

(*continued*)

Table 10.1 (*Continued*)

2006, April 22–29	In its fourth year, VWA activities highlighted the transition from child to family immunization programs, the strengthening of regular immunization programs, influenza, rubella elimination, and the introduction of new vaccines. In June 2006, PAHO confirmed its commitment to VWA by urging member states to continue to support and expand vaccination efforts, including the yearly celebration of Vaccination Week in the Americas.
2007, April 21–28	In 2007, 45 countries and territories participated in Vaccination Week in the Americas, the highest total thus far in the history of the initiative. More than 47 million individuals were vaccinated as a result of the week's initiatives that worked to strengthen border coordination, reach isolated populations, strengthen routine programs and advance the control of yellow fever and hepatitis B, among other goals.
2008, April 19–26	The sixth annual VWA took place with the participation of 45 countries and territories in the region. Multiple VWA launching events took place along binational and trinational borders throughout the region under the framework of a Health Caravan and with the participation of high-ranking authorities. Diverse arrays of vaccination campaigns took place as part of the week, including multiple measles/rubella elimination campaigns focused primarily in Central America. More than 59 million individuals were vaccinated through such efforts.
2009 April 25—May 2	The seventh annual VWA took place with themes that emphasized the importance of family vaccination as well as the vaccination of health workers. Multiple launching events took place throughout the region, including a series of events in the South American Chaco, the border area shared by Argentina, Bolivia, and Paraguay and one of the transnational priority areas as identified by the Pan American Alliance for Nutrition and Development.
2010, April 24– May 1	The eighth annual VWA took place under the theme of "reaching everyone." The Eastern Mediterranean (EMRO) Region of WHO celebrated its first-ever Vaccination Week (VWEM); it counted on 100% participation of the countries in that region.
2011, April 23–20	The ninth annual VWA was celebrated across the countries and territories of the Americas under the slogan "Vaccinate your family, protect your community." Regional launching events were organized throughout the Amazon subregion, and between Peru and Bolivia in the Altiplano. The African and Western Pacific WHO regions celebrated their first ever vaccination week initiatives, joining in this growing global effort.
2012, April 21–28	The 10th annual VWA was celebrated in conjunction with the first-ever World Immunization Week (WIW), under the respective themes of "For you, for me, for everyone. Get vaccinated" and "Protect your world, get vaccinated." One hundred and eighty countries participated. (See logo in Figure 10.2.)
2013, April 20–27	VWA continued as part of the second World Immunization Week, again with 180 countries participating worldwide. It highlighted the importance of governments, health workers, communities, and families doing their part to support immunization.
2014, April 20–30	The Third World Immunization Week had various themes across the six regions, including "Are you up to date? Vaccination: Your best shot. Vaccinate at birth." And "Vaccination: A shared responsibility". The overall international theme was "Immunization for a healthy future. Know, Check, Protect." Focus was placed on the use of new technologies. (See Figure 10.3.)
2015, April 24–30	The fourth World Immunization Week had as its theme "Close the Immunization Gap," with a focus on three steps to close that gap: (1) integrate immunization with other health services; (2) strengthen health systems to improve vaccine delivery to reach every last child; and (3) ensure vaccines are both accessible and affordable to all.

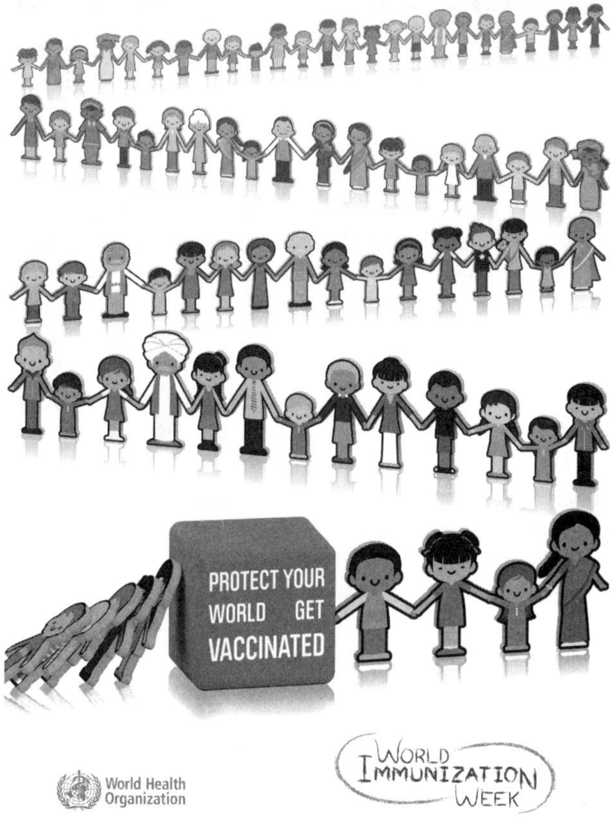

Figure 10.2 World Immunization Week Logo
Source: World Health Organization.

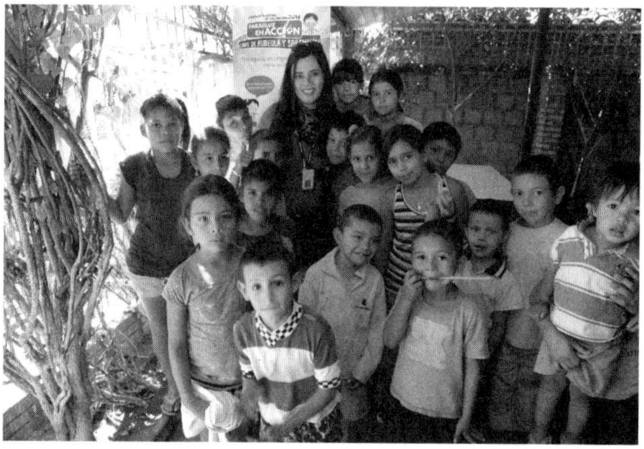

Figure 10.3 *Semana de Vacunación*
Source: Pan American Health Organizatio-PAHO/World Health Organization-WHO. From *Semana de Vacunación en las Americas 2014—Paraguay* on Flickr: https://www.flickr.com/photos/pahowho/14074736923/in/album-72157644447904163/ material. Licensed under Attribution-NoDerivs 2.0 Generic; https://creativecommons.org/licenses/by-nd/2.0/

Examples of Special Initiatives Connected to VWA

PAHO/WHO actively supported the ministry of health of Saint Maarten on the Open House Health Day that took place on May 19, 2012, in its capital, Philipsburg. This activity was organized within the Vaccination Week in the Americas, celebrated with millions of children vaccinated all over the region. Since the dissolution of the Netherlands Antilles in 2010, Saint Maarten is one of the constituent countries of the kingdom of the Netherlands located in the Caribbean. Nongovernmental organizations (NGOs) and ministry of health staff participated in the event. Not only were there nearly 200 children checked and 75 vaccinated, but the community benefited from a wide range of health information and promotion initiatives covering nutrition, HIV/AIDS, Alzheimer's disease, and diabetes, among others. A workout session, to the rhythm of Zumba, put the participants on the move by emphasizing the importance of exercise as a good intervention to help fight against obesity and nurture healthy behavior among the youth and the community as a whole. This is a nice example of how a VWA can be expanded and capitalized upon to incorporate more comprehensive health promotion activities.

In 2011, Bolivia initiated a measles-rubella follow-up campaign as part of its strategy to maintain measles and rubella elimination in the Region of the Americas and in response to the risk of virus reintroduction because of large outbreaks in Europe and Africa. Bolivia set a goal to vaccinate 917,546 children between the ages of two and five; all women ages 22–44 who were not vaccinated during the "speed-up campaign" of 2006 because of pregnancy; health care workers; and personnel in contact with tourists and travelers (airports, hotels, and transportation terminals).

After it was established that vaccination coverage had not reached >75% at the end of 2011, an innovative strategy called **VACUNATON**, was designed to achieve the vaccination goals. The VACUNATON was a mass campaign conducted on April 15, 2012, in 48 of 323 municipalities, selected because of their risk for measles and rubella. The goal was to vaccinate up to 200,000 children, ages two to five, who were not vaccinated during the follow-up campaign conducted between October and November 2011. The most important media strategy featured a live television broadcast that covered the national launches in all the main cities of the country.

The initiative is a good example of the health promotion principle of building partnerships and developing intersectoral collaboration. The main partners involved in the VACUNATON initiative were Bolivia's Expanded Program on Immunization (EPI) of the Ministry of Health, PAHO/WHO, the Bolivian Network for Communication in Risk (REBCOR), the Catholic University, armed forces and national police, nongovernmental organizations, television channels, and every EPI team responsible for immunization and social communication at the departmental level. The EPI staff mobilized personnel and funds to purchase all vaccines and supplies as well as logistics, transport, and cold chain expenses. A nationwide health sector strike that lasted from March 15 to May 15, 2012, threatened VACUNATON. However, a compromise was reached between the conflicting parties that allowed resumption of the organization and implementation of VACUNATON. This is an effective demonstration of how the health promotion principles of multiple stakeholders working together for a mutually beneficial cause can overcome barriers that might otherwise seem insurmountable. During VACUNATON, Bolivia vaccinated 177,976 children ages two to five years old. As of November 2012, Bolivia achieved > 95% coverage against measles and rubella nationwide (WHO, 2013, January).

Social Mobilization and the Role of Social Media

The increased attention provided to initiatives such as Vaccination Week in the Americas and now World Immunization Week creates a benefit of political commitment and public acceptance and engagement for weeklong efforts that in turn help to sustain the daily work required over time. Immunization campaigns are therefore a good example of how a mass campaign strategy has been used for many years throughout the world to effectively immunize populations against specific diseases. Increasingly, social media plays a key role in helping these campaigns to be successful. (See Box 10.3.)

BOX 10.3 SOCIAL MEDIA

Social media make use of electronic tools to help create, share, or exchange information, ideas, and pictures or videos. It uses virtual communities and networks that rely on Internet-based applications. Social media help to create highly interactive platforms through which individuals and communities share, co-create, discuss, and modify user-generated content.

Radio, television, and the press are forms of mass media that have traditionally been used to massively and simultaneously transmit messages that promote healthy ideas, programs, events, activities, and behaviors. However, in today's technological world, the range of tools to mass communicate with the public has greatly expanded to include avenues such as Facebook, Twitter, Flickr, blogs, professional networks, forums, photo sharing, social gaming, social networks, and video sharing.

Some social media sites have greater virality—defined as a greater likelihood that users will reshare content posted (by another user) to their social network, such as retweeting on Twitter.

The use of social media has greatly enhanced the reach, visibility, and involvement of the general population along with key stakeholders in mobilizing for immunization initiatives as well as other health- and well-being-related activities. It has served to share stories, strategies, and pictures of successful events that have taken place. In this way, immunization campaigns and vaccination week events have become more widely publicized, more popular, more accepted, and more transparent in their objectives, procedures, and outcomes.

Parents undergo a complex process when deciding whether or not to immunize their children. Parents make vaccination decisions largely based on their social networks. With so much confusing and even misleading information about vaccine safety available on the

Internet, it's no surprise that parents are influenced by their friends' attitudes when immunizing their kids. Social exposure to medical information raises people's perceptions of the benefits of immunization. Although the provider–parent conversation about vaccines may be the most influential to parent decision making, these conversations can be difficult to navigate, especially during the increasingly time-limited provider–parent encounter. Public health interventions aimed at shaping the social milieu of immunization decision making outside the examination room can complement providers' efforts to achieve the full benefit of immunizations.

As with other health promotion and education promotional materials, to develop effective social media programs that promote immunization uptake while simultaneously overcoming some of the fears and misperceptions about the true effect and impact of the vaccines, basic research must first be conducted that will identify why people might accept or refuse vaccines and who might influence these decisions. Arguments for and against are often intricately associated with existing cultural and religious beliefs and values. Use of popular celebrities and role models can help to bolster belief in the messages being transmitted, so identifying who these people or institutions are needs to be part of the initial research. Front-end research serves to tease out all of these arguments while identifying which terms, phrases, and social media sites the target population uses.

Partnerships for Polio Eradication in Southeast Asia

In March 2014, the WHO Southeast Asia Region (SEARO) achieved a major public health milestone that was years in the making. They became the fourth region in the world to be certified as polio-free, after the regions of the Americas, Europe, and Western Pacific. With the 11 countries in the region, including Bangladesh, Bhutan, Democratic People's Republic of Korea, India, Indonesia, Maldives, Myanmar, Nepal, Sri Lanka, Thailand, and Timor Leste added to the list of polio-free countries, the proportion of the world's population living in polio-free regions increased to 80% (MMWR, Center for Disease Control and Prevention's Morbidity and Mortality Weekly Report CDC, 2014). This battle was won after more than two decades of concerted effort, and involved tremendous support of national governments, global partners, countless families and frontline community volunteers, social mobilizers, health workers, and vaccinators. The polio eradication program in the Southeast Asia context has demonstrated a number of lessons about eradication in the immunization context and what it takes to get the job done. The SE Asia milestone is part of a larger initiative that began in 1988 when the World Health Assembly passed the resolution to eradicate polio globally. At that time, the global burden was estimated at more than 350,000 cases per year, with more than 70% of those believed to be from the Southeast Asia Region of

WHO (Polioeradication.org, 2013). Given the assumption that there was gross under-reporting in 1988 because of the nature of the surveillance network at the time, the number of cases was likely much higher. The resolution passed that year was the start of a massive effort that would go on to include more than 200 countries, millions of volunteers and take an international investment of approximately US$10 billion. As of 2013, it would also mean that more than 2.5 billion children would be immunized against polio (WHO, 2003). As of 2015, that massive effort has reduced the number of cases globally by 99% from the time when the initiative began.

The global polio eradication partnership provided advocacy, financial and technical advice to countries, and was instrumental in providing strategic policy and planning that spanned global, national, regional, and local levels. This partnership developed what came to be known as "the four pillars of polio eradication" (WHO, 2003). These four pillars of polio eradication were the cornerstones by which the national governments operated, and consisted of (1) strengthening routine immunization, (2) delivering mass polio immunization drives (supplemental immunization activities), (3) surveillance to detect the virus, and (d) providing "mop-up" immunization campaigns to target areas where the virus still circulated. In addition to the implementation of the "pillars of eradication" by national authorities, a number of key components were factors in achieving this milestone in the Southeast Asia region and are summarized in the following categories: partnerships, strategic policy and planning, sustained political commitment, oversight and independent monitoring, and flexibility and innovation (CDC, 2014).

Partnerships

The Global Polio Eradication Initiative (GPEI) partnership was established in 1988 and was spearheaded by Rotary International, the World Health Organization (WHO), UNICEF, and the US Centers for Disease Control and Prevention. Countless other global partners have also contributed to the program by way of financial support, advocacy, technical assistance, human resources, vaccines, know-how, program delivery, and more. The partnership would also initially include the US Agency for International Development (USAID), the Bill & Melinda Gates Foundation, and government support from Norway, Denmark, Japan, the United Kingdom, and the United States, in addition to the long-term dedication and commitments made by all national governments of the 11 countries in the region. As time went on and the initiative gained momentum, other partners and governments joined the effort, and the GPEI raised and donated nearly US$10 billion toward polio eradication. What can be said of this initiative is that a powerful global coalition was to come about which provided support at the international, national, subnational, and local levels.

In addition to the unprecedented global partnership, a remarkable partnership was demonstrated at the country and community levels. National immunization programs relied heavily on local leaders, women's groups, NGOs, community mobilizers, religious leaders, and other community influencers to access communities and deliver vaccines. The global partnership worked hand in hand with the countries' local and community-based partnerships to reach the common goal.

Strategic Policy and Planning

After years of application of the four polio pillars, many countries in the region were successful with interrupting poliovirus transmission within their borders. However, in very diverse and complex settings such as India, there was the realization that repetitive implementation of some strategies would not help them reach their goal, and thus a number of countries conducted operational research to better understand issues related to the efficacy of polio vaccines and population immunity. The findings of those studies allowed countries to identify pockets of high-risk areas, and further develop focused plans, tailored to the local circumstances and contexts. Examples of strategic policy and planning that came about from the findings are the development of annual plans that address the epidemiology of poliovirus transmission, conducting additional research to generate evidence when needed, putting in place national advisory groups, and local task forces to guide implementation and make recommendations.

Sustained Political Commitment

Without the sustained commitment of respective national governments, polio eradication could not have succeeded in the region. This includes commitment at the local and national levels by key stakeholders beyond the health care sector, such as parents, community groups, and local religious and traditional leaders. Although global partners played a key role in mobilizing resources and providing policy advice and technical assistance, national governments were responsible for enhancing health systems to enable the acute flaccid paralysis (AFP) laboratory network to function, thereby detecting virus circulation. This role included setting up or enhancing laboratory capacity, training front-line health workers and community members to detect, report, or investigate cases, as well as planning and implementing nationwide mass immunization campaigns. Such national support was sustained over years, and in many cases the governments in the region maintained this high level of both political and resource support years after their last case, to prevent to the extent possible the importation of cases from neighboring countries. This level of commitment was critical and challenging in the face of other public health priorities that also demanded and needed political attention and resource allocation.

Oversight and Independent Monitoring

As the countries tackled the countless challenges associated with chasing down a virus that moved fast, in high-population-density settings, with sanitation conditions that were conducive to the spread of the disease, and where routine immunization systems were weak, it was understood that in order to succeed, a strong oversight framework that would provide feedback on what was working and where there were gaps in program performance was required. This oversight framework included monitoring and management of this collaborative process, as well as the credibility and authority to give guidance to the governments.

The role of oversight and independent monitoring was played primarily by the Regional Immunization Technical Advisory Group and respective national immunization advisory groups at the country level. For polio, there was the Regional Certification Commission and the respective National Certification Committees that monitored performance indicators and constantly provided feedback and advice to national governments on areas to address or strengthen. These bodies were viewed by the respective governments as independent and credible, which was important to ensuring that recommendations were carried out.

Flexibility and Innovation

The countries in the region worked vigorously within their own national borders and across the region to address challenges as they emerged. This commitment included continuously monitoring, evaluating, and assessing program gaps. Flexibility and innovation were critical to reach all children—especially high-risk groups such as migrant children, children residing in brick kiln communities, children of seasonal workers, children in transit (e.g., on trains), and those hard-to-reach, access-compromised, and underserved areas. Special strategies were needed to capture those high-risk and hard-to-reach groups. For example, in India, the "Kosi River Operational Plan" was launched in 2008 when the surveillance network detected that the source of the virus continued to originate from the flooded plains of the Kosi River in Bihar (SEARO, 2009). The program concluded that the only way to interrupt this source of transmission was to reach all children in the flooded plain area, and thus the "stay points" were established. These "stay points" were simple building structures with supplies put in strategic locations where WHO medical officers could stay and work for several days at a time, for the amount of time needed to reach these challenging geographic areas. This allowed access to the river and plain areas that were flooded much of the year, but that were home to millions of people who lived on and around this constantly shifting river area.

Final Comments Lessons Learned from Southeast Asia Polio Eradication Efforts

When the goal of global polio eradication was set in 1988, more than 500,000 cases of polio were occurring annually. By the beginning of 2015, there was more than a 99% reduction in annual cases globally since the start of the program (Hagan et al., 2015). In addition to the number of lives saved, the increase in quality of life for countless children and adults is significant. In many countries, the stigma associated with paralysis (even partial paralysis) may commit one to a life of poverty and marginalization from society. The prevention of hundreds and thousands of such cases is an achievement to be celebrated.

In addition to the absence of a debilitating disease from the 11 countries in the region, the polio eradication program showcased how the countries in the region worked in solidarity to reach a common goal, ensuring that supplemental immunization activities were coordinated, that surveillance data were shared, and that staff remained engaged in regular technical forums over the years to asses gaps in program delivery to understand what further activities could be undertaken. This cohesive multicountry approach can be applied to other high-priority diseases in this region. Furthermore, the polio eradication program is helping to revitalize immunization systems, by garnering visibility and attention in many countries. The polio momentum is now being redirected to other vaccine-preventable disease initiatives as well as the shift to strengthening routine immunization systems. A major impact is seen on strengthening immunization services, delivery of other health services, enhancing disease surveillance and laboratory networks, and advancing the research agenda.

Large and complex network of assets (e.g., human resources, surveillance networks, etc.) spans across countries and includes a wide range of asset types and capabilities, from which other public health and development programs can potentially benefit. A number of countries are now taking assets established through polio eradication and mainstreaming those critical functions into other priority health programs.

What began as the AFP surveillance infrastructure is now the foundation of expansion of surveillance work for measles, rubella, neonatal tetanus, diphtheria, and pertussis surveillance in many of the countries of the Southeast Asia region. The same could be said about the laboratory networks that are now the model used to set up measles and rubella laboratory networks across South Asia. The outbreak response for immunization is also a model that is being replicated for other disease outbreaks in countries.

Moving forward, the eradication of polio offers a new opportunity to transition the capacities, processes, and assets created by the program to support other vaccine-preventable diseases and health priorities. Components that can be applied to other priority public health initiatives include:

- campaign delivery formats of polio to deliver other vaccines;
- techniques of social mobilization to raise awareness to address other health and development priorities;
- surveillance networks;
- how mobilization efforts of large groups of people could be valuable structures for public health priorities;
- how supply chains, labs, and data effectiveness and monitoring played a role in ensuring successful program delivery.

Leveraging these assets for other health priorities will require a planned, coordinated approach, and, done well, is likely to result in public health benefits for communities.

Other International Initiatives to Increase Childhood Immunizations

National childhood immunization programs in developing countries have now expanded into "family" immunization programs. This is illustrated by the experience of HPV vaccination, wherein innovative strategies have been used to introduce a new vaccine to protect females from contracting cervical cancer.

HPV Vaccine: A Leap Forward for Girls' and Women's Health

Cervical cancer is reported as the most common cancer in women worldwide (WHO, 2013, June), and indeed in many developing countries it is the leading cause of cancer (Andrus et al., 2008). Because of poor access to screening and treatment services, more than 85% of the 275,000 deaths annually from cervical cancer are in low- and middle-income countries (Hopkins & Wood, 2013). With the recent advent of the **HPV vaccine**, the incidence of cervical cancer could be greatly reduced. HPV vaccine has a number of special characteristics, however, that make it potentially more difficult to administer than most of the other vaccines administered, especially in lower income countries:

- The infrastructure is generally developed for reaching newborns who receive the vast majority of vaccinations, and HPV vaccine is targeted at 9- to 14-year-olds.
- Most childhood vaccines target both boys and girls, but especially in lower-income countries with high cervical cancer rates, it makes most sense to target girls for HPV vaccination.
- Because HPV vaccine relates to a sexually transmissible disease, parents may be a bit more reluctant to have their early adolescents vaccinated for this; this has been a larger problem in some high-income countries than lower income countries so far (Ferrer et al., 2014).

A fairly recent review of performance of 21 HPV vaccination programs implemented in 14 low- and middle-income countries between 2009–2013 (3 countries were in Southeast Asia, 3 in the Americas, 3 in Europe, and 5 in Africa) (Ladner et al., 2014) found an overall vaccine uptake rate of 88.7%. The high uptake in these countries is likely related to the free supply of the (otherwise very expensive) Gardasil vaccine in these countries by the manufacturer Merck. Because of the small sample size (21 programs), only 3 of 14 differences between various contexts were conditions found to be significantly related to vaccine uptake: those that used a message about the vaccine safety and efficacy had higher rates than those that did not; those where implementation was managed by a NGO had greater uptake than those managed by the ministry of health; and those where the community participated in following up with girls had higher uptake.

Another review of the international uptake of HPV vaccination, this one including all countries that had included HPV vaccine in their national immunization program as of 2011, found that 22 European countries, 6 countries in the Americas (including 4 low- or middle-income countries), 1 low-income country in Southeast Asia (Bhutan), 1 high-income country in the Eastern Mediterranean (Abu Dhabi), 10 high-income countries in the Western Pacific, and 1 low-income country in Africa—had done so. Their review among these countries indicated that school-based programs had greater success than community- or clinic-based programs, though the impact on potentially vulnerable, out-of-school youth being missed was a concern of this approach. They also found, not surprisingly, that publicly financed programs had greater uptake than those that required financing by parents and/or patients (Markowitz et al., 2012). Other factors that appear to be related to levels of coverage include good communication strategies, organized outreach, and medical profession and public acceptance (Widgren et al., 2011). Another important and fairly recent promising event for HPV vaccination in low- and middle-income countries was the decision in 2012 by the Global Alliance for Vaccines and Immunizations (GAVI) to agree to begin to add HPV vaccine to its list of funded vaccines. In 2013 GAVI negotiated a very low price of US$4.50 (as compared to more than the $100 cost in high-income countries) for the vaccine, and hopes to vaccinate 30 million girls in 40 countries by 2020 (GAVI, 2015). Having reviewed what is happening around the world with HPV vaccine uptake, the next three case studies are presented of countries' experiences with HPV vaccination: Argentina, Uganda, and India, to understand some of the types of campaigns and approaches that have been successful and the lessons being learned.

CASE STUDY 10.2 ARGENTINA

In Argentina, the WHO-recommended human papillomavirus vaccine is given to all girls at 11 years of age to prevent cervical cancer later in life. In Argentina, whether or not a child gets vaccinated has nothing to do with socio-economic status. Health centers across the country provide all children free and compulsory vaccines against 15 diseases. For girls there is a 16th—the WHO-recommended vaccine against HPV, which can cause cervical cancer. Argentina is one of the first countries in the Region of the Americas to provide the HPV vaccine. PAHO's Revolving Fund supports the program for the procurement of vaccines, syringes, and related supplies for participating Member States. It ensures that immunization programs have a continuous supply of high-quality products for a low price. HPV currently causes more than 3,000 new cases of cervical cancer and some 1,800 deaths in Argentina every year, especially among the most vulnerable populations, such as those who are mobile or rural.

Since the HPV vaccine was included in Argentina's national schedule in 2011, the first dose has reached more than 80% of girls in the target age group, nearly 60% have received the second dose, and 50% have had the final third dose. The Argentinean authorities decided to vaccinate 11-year-olds to ensure that they are protected before they are most likely to come into contact with the virus (WHO recommends vaccination against HPV in girls 9 to 13 years old); by vaccinating in early adolescence, girls who are going to become sexually active later in life are already protected by the vaccine. Educational and promotional activities are an essential part of mobilizing girls and their families to make use of this important service (WHO, 2013, May).

Even so, many girls and women may be timid or ashamed to go to the health centers to receive this type of vaccination. It is important to find ways of maintaining their privacy and confidentiality, as well as ways to ensure that they are appropriately tested. Along those lines, Argentina is also promoting a groundbreaking HPV self-testing project in the northern province of Jujuy. The Self-Sampling Modality Evaluation Project was implemented in 2011 with the collaboration of the provincial health ministry and WHO's International Agency for Research on Cancer (Arrossi et al., 2015). The objective of this research project is to evaluate the efficiency of the self-test, which could be a fundamental tool in overcoming some of the barriers women face in being able to access HPV testing. This is linked to geographical inaccessibility of the health centers, the lack of human resources to implement the measures, and women's shyness in coming forward for this test.

CASE STUDY 10.3 UGANDA

Uganda has hosted a pilot/demonstration project conducted by the Program for Appropriate Technology in Health (PATH), funded in part by the Bill & Melinda Gates Foundation. It also has been approved as one of the first three countries in Africa for support for national introduction of the HPV vaccine by GAVI, funded by the Bill & Melinda Gates Foundation, UNICEF, pharmaceutical companies, and Western countries. Cervical cancer accounts for 40% of all cancers in Uganda, as compared to around 1% in high-income countries (Global Burden of Disease Cancer Collaboration Group, 2015). HPV vaccine was made available through the PATH pilot project to more than 10,000 girls in Uganda in 2008–2009.

Formative work conducted before the implementation of the PATH pilot project suggested that two strategies should be implemented for recruitment of adolescent girls for HPV vaccination: a school-based grade-based recruitment plan, as well as an age-based recruitment program in schools with follow-up in communities. The first strategy recruited girls in primary grade 5 as well as those 10 years old not enrolled in or attending school. The second strategy delivered the first and third doses of HPV vaccines to girls 10 years old at the same time as vitamin A and albendazole (a medication to treat parasitic worm infestations) were distributed, two times per year in another district in Uganda; the second dose was delivered at an additional outreach session developed specifically for HPV vaccination. Uptake was 85% for all three doses in the district using the school-/grade-based strategy, and 50% in the district using the age-based strategy. Acceptability was very high (more than 80%) in both districts. Main reasons for partial or non-vaccination were absences from school or difficulty in determining girls' ages. The cold chain was improved, but increased workload and disruption of other activities resulted from the introduction of HPV vaccination. Incremental cost was significantly lower with the school-based strategy, because health workers were already at the school for the administration of the other drugs with the age-based strategy (PATH, 2011).

Other lessons learned from the PATH pilot project included the importance of close coordination between education and health sectors; greater effectiveness of separate trainings for teachers and health workers; importance of endorsement by national and district government; and community education messages providing information about cervical cancer, HPV vaccination, and the need for three doses (PATH, 2011).

The GAVI pilot project in Uganda, in which Gardasil was contributed by Merck, targeted 985 girls at a total of 10 health clinics, implemented by a NGO. The uptake rate was 95% and the adherence rate for three doses among those who received the first dose, was 88% (Ladner et al., 2014). Community involvement in outreach to girls was a significant predictor of vaccine uptake, especially with involvement of community opinion leaders in presentations to parents. Such involvement was less important for adherence to all doses (Ladner et al., 2014).

CASE STUDY 10.4 INDIA

India is another country that also implemented a PATH-HPV vaccination pilot project, though the outcomes have been quite different from those of other countries. The current estimates indicate approximately 132,000 new cases of cervical cancer are diagnosed and 74,000 deaths occur annually in India, representing nearly one-third of all cervical cancer deaths in the world (Kaarthigeyan, 2012). The pilot or demonstration project began in 2009. As in the other pilot/demonstration countries (e.g., Uganda, Vietnam, and Haiti), both school- and community- and age-based recruitment strategies were attempted for girls. 13,791 girls (95% via administrative report, 77%–88% by population-based survey) (LaMontagne et al., 2011; Tsu, Cernuschi, & LaMontagne, 2014) received three doses of the HPV vaccine using campaign-style delivery with outreach, and 9,864 (78% per administrative report, 68%–83% by population survey) received three doses of the vaccine using routine delivery at schools. Clearly here, as elsewhere in these pilot projects, the implementation with campaign-style messages and outreach for follow-up was more successful than the traditional school-only delivery method.

Conservative politics, disempowerment of women, and safety concerns have all been suggested as reasons why routine HPV vaccination has not been maintained as the norm in India. Out of approximately 23,000 girls vaccinated for HPV, seven died fairly soon after receiving the vaccine. A commission appointed by the ICMR concluded that while there may have been some irregularities related to parental signatures for tribal girls under the custody of the state, 4 of the causes of death were definitely not due to the vaccine (poisoning, suicide, or drowning) and none of the other three could be linked to the vaccine (Indian Council of Medical Research [IMCR], 2011). According to Dr. Purnima Madhivanan, "The cause of HPV vaccination in India has been set back" by these results. She also suggests that until HPV is "defined as a serious issue for both sexes … It stands little chance of gaining support and resources in a country with many other urgent problems" (Kabat, 2013). Indeed, the Indian Supreme Court case continues, with a final hearing scheduled for April 4, 2015 (Chamberlin, 2015). Our most recent online search in September 2015 did not reveal any updates to the trial.

Thus, despite the high rate of cervical cancer deaths in India and large, multicountry safety and efficacy trials of HPV vaccines, including in India, physicians and government officials in India continue to argue that "the implementation of the vaccination as a routine in India is still controversial" because of concerns related to safety, efficacy, cost, and its presumed impact on reducing the uptake of routine Pap test screening in India (Nigam et al., 2014), despite the fact that only 2.5%–5% of women in India are estimated to receive routine Pap tests (Aswawthy et al., 2012).

Summary Points on HPV Vaccination

We can see that when a national government includes HPV vaccination as a mandatory and routine part of services provided in all of its health centers and/or when the vaccination is paid for by the government or outside donors, then many more young girls are vaccinated and protected against cervical cancer. Working through schools and community outreach are also effective strategies in reaching 10- and 11-year-old girls, and schools appear to be important partners. When public messages are used to promote the importance of completing the three-dose series, or are about safety and efficacy, uptake can be greatly improved. Additionally, assessing local cultural norms and community-based needs and then tailoring implementation strategies accordingly helps to encourage more acceptance and response by the general population. National mores and political considerations also need to be taken into account for a sustainable HPV vaccination program.

Five-in-One (Pentavalent) Vaccine

The **"five-in-one" pentavalent vaccine** protects children from diphtheria, tetanus, whooping cough, hepatitis B, and *Haemophilus influenzae* type b (Hib) which causes pneumonia and meningitis. Essentially it adds hepatitis B and Hib vaccines to the traditional DPT (diphtheria-pertussis/whooping cough-tetanus) combination vaccine. Especially in lower-income countries, these "combination vaccines" reduce costs, personnel needs, and the number of required visits for children and their parents to complete their immunizations. The WHO and GAVI have been working with poorer countries around the world to integrate the new vaccine into national immunization programs.

By combining more vaccines into one, initiatives were developed to more comprehensively achieve vaccine coverage. Fewer shots had to be given and the number of visits to health facilities were reduced.

Haiti

PAHO has been working with Haiti's Ministry of Health and Population to integrate the new vaccine into the national immunization program—putting Haiti on par with the rest of the Americas.

Haiti is among the countries in the Americas with the highest child mortality rates. The main causes are acute respiratory infections like pneumonia, diarrheal diseases, anaemia, and chronic malnutrition (WHO, 2013, June). Vaccines are an effective way of preventing many of these diseases.

Haitian health workers and ministry of health officials have been promoting the pentavalent vaccine since it was introduced in November 2012. Since then, growing numbers of children have been showing up to get vaccinated in health centers. Estimates suggest that some 3,000 children under the age of five will be saved over the next four years as a result of the adoption of the new vaccine. Although it is too soon to measure the impact, early results show that communication and social mobilization have been effective; many parents are interested in a vaccine that was previously available only in the private sector. Now it is available free of charge for everyone. The ministry's goal is to administer three doses of the vaccine to 288,000 children younger than one year of age. To reach the goal, WHO recruited and trained a team of 12 Haitian doctors, educated in Cuba and the Dominican Republic, to in turn train health workers to use the pentavalent vaccine throughout the country's 10 departments. Haiti's introduction of the new vaccine was supported by WHO, GAVI, and the US Centers for Disease Control and Prevention, which also helped to ensure that the vaccines were bought at affordable prices and distributed appropriately. This mutual collaboration extended to partnering with local communities so that good health education and health promotion tradition services could be tailored to and be made appropriate for the local populations, thereby increasing their acceptability and accessibility.

The African Continent

GAVI began its introduction of pentavalent vaccine into poorer countries in 2001, in Guyana. In 2014, South Sudan was the 73rd and final GAVI-supported country to implement pentavalent vaccinations. The focus here is placed on African countries, because 34 of the 69 countries supported for pentavalent vaccine by GAVI are in Africa.

Table 10.2 Pentavalent VACCINE COMPONENTS UPTAKE, Selected African Countries

Country	Population	Infant Mortality Rate, 2000	Infant Mortality Rate, 2013	GNI	DTP3 Uptake, 2000	DPT3 Uptake, 2013	HepB3 Uptake, 2010	Hep B Uptake, 2013	Hib3 Uptake, 2010	Hib3 Uptake, 2013
Angola	22 mill	128	102	5300	44	93	91	93	91	93
Cameroon	22 mill	93	61	1350	62	89	84	89	84	89
Chad	13 mill	97	92	1010	36	48	39	48	39	48
Cote d'Ivoire	21 mill	100	71	1550	65	80	85	80	85	80
Ethiopia	97 mill	90	44	550	30	72	62	72	62	72
Ghana	26 mill	65	52	1620	88	90	94	90	94	90
Kenya	46 mill	69	48	1280	82	76	83	82	83	82
Lesotho	2 mill	81	73	1350	82	96	93	96	94	96
Liberia	4 mill	119	54	400	46	76	47	76	47	76
Namibia	2 mill	49	35	5820	79	89	83	89	83	89
Niger	18 mill	101	60	430	34	67	70	67	70	67
Nigeria	178 mill	112	74	2950	29	63	29	32	—	49
Sierra Leone	6 mill	141	107	720	44	92	86	92	86	92
Zambia	15 mill	100	56	1760	85	79	83	79	83	79
Zimbabwe	15 mill	61	55	860	78	95	79	93	89	93
Sub-Saharan Africa	1.2 bill	95	61	860*	56	70	69	68	60	63
Global	7.3 bill	53	34	5820*	73	83	74	79	42	45

*Median.

Table 10.2 presents results of the introduction of the pentavalent vaccine in selected African countries, including estimated uptake rates of three doses of the DPT vaccine components, the hepatitis B vaccine, and the Haemophilus influenza B vaccine. Especially impressive increases in DPT3 (receipt of three doses of the DPT vaccine) vaccine uptake can be seen in many of the countries. Rates at least doubled in Angola, Ethiopia, Niger, Nigeria, and Sierra Leone; they increased by 25% or more in Cameroon, Chad, Liberia, Niger, and for the continent as a whole. Rates of HepB3 and Hib3 generally remained fairly constant for the shorter available reporting period (2010–2013). Chad, Liberia, Zambia, and Zimbabwe all showed at least a 20% increase in the rate for one or both of these vaccine components (changes were nearly identical in all countries because they were both introduced in almost every case as part of the pentavalent vaccine). Almost certainly owing to the introduction of the pentavalent vaccine, it is evident that the African continent as a whole and many of the selected African countries shown in Table 10.2 had higher rates of Hib3 vaccine uptake than even the global average of 42% and 45% respectively. Clearly, for this relatively new vaccine, the GAVI-supported countries had received a huge boost.

Data in the Hands of Families: Vaccination Cards

Home-based child health records (called in many places *vaccination cards*) are an inexpensive yet effective instrument for systematically recording the vaccines received by an individual (WHO, 2013, June). Home-based health records can enhance health professionals' ability to make clinical decisions, empower parents and caregivers in the health care of their children, and support public health monitoring. Child health records serve at least five functions in a health system by providing:

1. a unique identifier that is intimately connected to the child;
2. a source of critical information for health workers about the child's health and vaccination status, and what the child needs at each point of contact with the health system;
3. a source of critical information for families, such as date of next visit for vaccination;
4. a source of critical information for household surveys, which many countries and policymakers rely on to validate coverage levels obtained from administrative data systems;
5. an educational tool for families to learn more about health interventions.

By giving families cards that record vaccines received, both families and health care professionals were able to monitor child health and vaccination status.

However, child health records may fail to serve these functions for a variety of reasons. They are too often underutilized or inappropriately used by parents and health care workers and therefore do not always fulfill their intended purpose. Many families never receive health records for their children, or, if they do receive them, they can be easily lost. In many cases, records are not accurately filled out because they are designed in a way that confuses the health workers and information is not correctly recorded by type of vaccine or age of the child. Accurate and accessible records are needed to maintain accurate health histories for children, identify those who need to be immunized and those who have missed immunizations or are off schedule. When the record is unclear, inaccessible or unused, it's harder to reach children with life-saving vaccines.

Two websites were recently developed to help better understand the current state of child health records. The first site is a repository for home-based child health or vaccination cards (http://www.immunizationcards.org/). The purpose of the site is to support the free and open exchange of information related to card content and design, perhaps of particular interest to national EPI programs that are considering a redesign of their cards due to the introduction of a new vaccine. A second site provides a summary of the prevalence of home-based vaccination cards observed in UNICEF-supported Multiple Indicator Cluster Surveys and USAID-supported

Demographic and Health Surveys conducted since 2000 (http://data.unicef.org/resources/home-based-record-prevalence-among-children-aged-12-23-months-from-180-demographic-and-health-surveys). It will be important to improve the child health record, thereby improving information systems and empowering health workers and families to protect children from vaccine-preventable diseases.

Summary

This chapter focused on a variety of strategies for increasing immunization rates in a population, including media campaigns, community mobilization, and the building of partnerships and infrastructure for improving the health and well-being of the population, children in particular, but also the overall population in general. It emphasized the benefits and drawbacks to these approaches to public health overall and then specifically to protecting the population against communicable diseases. Emphasis was placed on how different aspects of this approach can be more effective than others, with country examples to illustrate real-life experiences.

Successful experiences included strategies such as:

- creating single-issue-focused campaigns, such as annual Vaccination Week in the Americas (becoming World Immunization Week) and focused annual health days;
- using communication and social mobilization strategies to encourage families to go to health centers or schools for a new vaccination or to add a dose to regular vaccinations already in place;
- creating new partnerships among international, national, and local organizations within the health sector, as well as across sectors (especially including education), and involving community leaders to ensure the success of the polio eradication program in Southeast Asia;
- using key stakeholder analysis to glean information about the factors that influence decision making among key stakeholders that can be incorporated into targeted message formulation;
- introducing a new vaccine (pentavalent vaccine) to reduce the number of shots and visits required by children and their families;
- providing numerous examples (with varying levels of success) of how the new HPV vaccine has been successfully introduced into countries in an effort to prevent cervical cancer.

The reader is challenged to identify ways that these types of public health approaches can best be applied in his or her own context and how policies and programs can be strengthened to provide continual support to these initiatives outside the context of the specific days and weeks of campaigns or the particular vaccine or disease being prevented.

KEY TERMS

1. **Child Health Days:** Incorporation into VWA interventions that include vitamin A supplementation, deworming medicine, growth monitoring, and insecticide-treated nets
2. **Cold chain:** A system that ensures vaccine potency by maintaining proper vaccine temperatures from factory to place of administration, requiring coordination of human resources, logistics, and operational management
3. **"Five-in-one" pentavalent vaccine:** A combined vaccine that protects children from diphtheria, tetanus, whooping cough, hepatitis B, and Haemophilus influenzae type b (Hib)
4. **Healthy settings initiatives:** Initiatives based upon local commitment by key stakeholders and local decision makers, active and representative social participation, and effective monitoring and evaluation
5. **Home-based child health records:** Child- and family-specific cards to systematically record vaccines received
6. **HPV vaccine:** A three-dose human papillomavirus vaccine given to all girls at the time of puberty and before they become sexually active to prevent cervical cancer later in life
7. **Social marketing:** Commercial marketing principles that influence ideas, attitudes, and behaviors to benefit the population's health and well-being; primary focus is on the consumer
8. **Vaccination Week:** An annual, national one-week mobilization by countries to promote equal access to immunization by all citizens, and especially the most vulnerable populations
9. **VACUNATON:** A one-day intensive vaccination strategy used in Bolivia to reach measles and rubella vaccination targets
10. **World Health Day:** An annual worldwide celebration of the formation of WHO focusing on a health promotion theme that changes every year

REVIEW QUESTIONS

1. List two advantages and two disadvantages of Immunization Weeks and World Health Days.
2. What are the four Ps of social marketing?
3. Give at least one example of how a Vaccination Week in the Americas can be expanded to incorporate other health promotion activities.

4. What are essential strategies and what types of key stakeholders should be included in all immunization campaigns?
5. How do immunizations relate to the Convention on the Rights of the Child?

References

Andrus, J. K., Lewis, M. J., Goldieb, S. J., Garcíac, P. J., Winklerd, J. L., Ruiz-Matusa, C., & de Quadrose, C. A. (2008). Human papillomavirus vaccine policy and delivery in Latin America and the Caribbean. *Vaccine, 26S*, L80–L87.

Arrossi, S., Thouyaret, L., Herrero, R., Campanera, A., Magdaleno, A., Buberli, M., ... Orellana, L. (2015). Effect of self-collection of HPV DNA offered by community health works at home visits on uptake of screening for cervical cancer (the EMA study): A population-based cluster-randomised trial. *Lancet Global Health, 3*(2), e85–e94.

Aswathy, S., Quereshi, M. A., Kurian, B., & Leelamoni, K. (2012). Cervical cancer screening: Current knowledge and practice among women in a rural population of Kerala, India. *Indian Journal of Medical Research, 136*(2), 205–210.

Bahl, S., Kumar, R., Menabde, N., Thapa, A., McFarland, J., Swezy, V., ... Cochi, S. (2014). Polio-free certification and lessons learned: South-East Asia Region. *Morbidity and Mortality Weekly Report, 6*(42), 941–946.

Centers for Disease Control and Prevention. (2007, March). *CDC cynergy: Social marketing edition.* Retrieved from http://www.orau.gov/cdcynergy/soc2web/

Centers for Disease Control and Prevention (2014). *CDC's Morbidity and Mortality Weekly Report - MMWR.*

Chamberlain, G. (2015, January 13). Judges demand answers after children die in controversial cancer vaccine trial in India. *Dailymail.com.* Retrieved from http://www.dailymail.co.uk/news/article-2908963/Judges-demand-answers-children-die-controversial-cancer-vaccine-trial-India.html

Ferrer, H. B., Trotter, C., Hickman, M., & Audrey, S. (2014). Barriers and facilitators to HPV vaccination of young women in high-income countries: A qualitative systematic review and evidence synthesis. *BioMed Central Public Health, 14*, 700.

Global Alliance for Vaccines and Immunizations. (2015). *Every child counts: The Vaccine Alliance Progress Report 2014.* New York, NY: Author.

Global Burden of Disease Cancer Collaboration Group. (2015). The global burden of cancer 2013. *Journal of the American Medical Association Oncology, 1*(4), 505–527.

Hagan, J. E., Wassilak, S.G.F., Craig, A. S., Tangermann, R. H., Diop, O. M., Burns, C. C., & Quddus, A. (2015). Progress toward polio eradication–Worldwide, 2014–2015. *Morbidity and Mortality Weekly Report, 64*(19), 527–531.

Hopkins, T. G., & Wood, N. (2013). Female human papillomavirus (HPV) vaccination: Global uptake and the impact of attitudes. *Vaccine, 31*, 1673–1679.

Indian Council of Medical Research. (2011, February 15). *Final report of the committee appointed by the govt. of India, to enquire into alleged irregularities in the conduct of studies using human papilloma virus (HPV) vaccine by PATH in India.* New Delhi, India: Author.

Kaarthigeyan, K. (2012). Cervical cancer in India and HPV vaccination. *Indian Journal of Medical Paediatric Oncology, 33*(1), 7–12.

Kabat, G. (2013, June 28). HPV vaccination in India: An historic opportunity and a daunting challenge. *Forbes* 2013. Retrieved from http://www.forbes.com/sites/geoffreykabat/2013/06/28/hpv-vaccination-in-india-an-historic-opportunity-and-a-daunting-challenge/print/

Ladner, J., Besson, M., Rodrigues, M., Audureau, E., & Saba, J. (2014). Performance of 21 HPV vaccination programs implemented in low-income countries, 2009–2013. *BioMed Central Public Health, 14*(670). doi: 10.1186/1471-2458-14-670

LaMontagne, D. S., Barge, S., Le, N. T., Mugisha, E., Penny, M. E., Gandhi, S., … Jumaan, A. O. (2011). Human papillomavirus vaccine delivery strategies that achieved high coverage in low- and middle-income countries. *Bulletin of the World Health Organization, 89*(11), 821–830B.

Markowitz, L. E., Tsu, V., Deeks, S. L., Cubie, H., Wang, S. A., Vicari, A. S., & Brotherton, J.M.O. (2012). Human papillomavirus vaccine introduction: The first five years. *Vaccine, 30*(Suppl. 2), F139–F148.

Nigam, A., Saxena, P., Acharya, A. S., Mishra, A., & Batra, S. (2014). HPV vaccination in India: Critical appraisal. *ISRN Obstetrics and Gynecology*, Article ID 394595.

Pan American Health Organization. (2008). *Vaccination Week in the Americas:* 2008. Retrieved from http://www1.paho.org/English/DD/PIN/vw2008_final.pdf

Pan American Health Organization. (2009a). *History of Vaccination Week in the Americas.* Retrieved from http://new.paho.org/hq/index.php?option=com_content&view=article&id=940%3Avwa_history&lang=en

Pan American Health Organization. (2009b). *Vaccination Week in the Americas.* Retrieved from http://new.paho.org/hq/index.php?option=com_content&view=article&id=750&Itemid=1

Pan American Health Organization. (2012). *World Immunization Week.* Retrieved from http://www.paho.org/vwa/?p=1312

Pan American Health Organization. (2013). *Comprehensive family immunization.* Retrieved from http://new.paho.org/hq/index.php?option=com_content&view=category&layout=blog&id=956&Itemid=358&lang=en.

Pan American Health Organization. (2015a). *Vaccination Week in the Americas.* Retrieved from http://www.paho.org/vwa/

Pan American Health Organization. (2015b). *Immunization.* Retrieved from http://www.paho.org/hq/index.php?option=com_content&view=category&layout=blog&id=956&Itemid=358&lang=en

Polioeradication.org. (2013). *The history of polio.* Retrieved from http://www.polioeradication.org/Polioandprevention/history of polio

Program for Appropriate Technology in Health (PATH). (2011). *HPV vaccination in Africa: Lessons learned from a pilot program in Uganda.* Seattle, WA: Author.

Program for Appropriate Technology in Health. (2013). *Statement from PATH: Cervical cancer demonstration project in India.* Retrieved from http://www.path.org/news/press-room/642/

Ropero-Alvarez, A.M., Kurtis, H. J., Danovaro-Holliday, M. C., Ruiz-Matus, C., & Tambini, G. (2012). Vaccination Week in the Americas: An opportunity to integrate other health services with immunization. *Journal of Infectious Diseases, 205* (March, Suppl. 1), S210–S215. Retrieved from: http://www.ncbi.nlm.nih.gov/pubmed/22315379

SEARO. (2009). *Kosi operational plan Bihar, India, updated June, 2009.* Delhi, India: Southeast Asian Regional Office, World Health Organization.

Tsu, V. D., Cernuschi, T., & LaMontagne, D. S. (2014). Lessons learned from HPV vaccine delivery in low-resource settings and opportunities for HIV prevention, treatment, and care among adolescents. *Journal of Acquired Immune Deficiency Syndrome, 66*(Suppl. 2), 209–216.

WHO Southeast Asia Region, World Health Organization (2009). *Kosi Operational Plan Bihar, India: Revised for 2009–2012.* New Delhi, India: Author.

UNICEF (2015). *Fact sheet: A summary of the rights under the Convention on the Rights of the Child.* Retrieved from http://www.unicef.org/crc/files/Rights_overview.pdf

Widgren, K., Simonsen, J., Valentiner-Branth, P., & Molbak, K. (2011). Uptake of the human papillomavirus-vaccination within the free-of-charge childhood vaccination programme in Denmark. *Vaccine, 29,* 9663.

World Health Organization (2003). Global polio eradication initiative: Strategic plan 2004–2008. *Weekly Epidemiological Record, 78,* 138–144.

World Health Organization. (2012, April). *Global immunization news.* Retrieved from http://www.who.int/immunization/GIN_April_2012.pdf

World Health Organization. (2012, May). *Global immunization news.* Retrieved from http://www.who.int/immunization/GIN_May_2012.pdf

World Health Organization. (2013a). *Official WHO Health Days.* Retrieved from http://www.who.int/mediacentre/events/official_days/en/

World Health Organization. (2013b). *Country stories on vaccination.* Retrieved from http://www.who.int/campaigns/immunization-week/2013/en/index.html

World Health Organization. (2013, January). *Global immunization news.* Retrieved from http://www.who.int/immunization/GIN_January_2013.pdf

World Health Organization. (2013, June). *Global immunization news.* Retrieved from http://www.who.int/immunization/GIN_June_2013.pdf

World Health Organization. (2013, May). *Global immunization news.* Retrieved from http://www.who.int/immunization/GIN_May_2013.pdf

World Health Organization. (2014, March). *European Immunization Week.* Retrieved from http://eiw.euro.who.int/page/what-is-eiw.

CHAPTER 11

THE EVOLVING GLOBAL HIV PANDEMIC

Epidemiology, Prevention, and Future Priorities

Ralph J. DiClemente, Puja Seth, and Purnima Mehrotra

LEARNING OBJECTIVES

By the end of this chapter, the reader should be able to:

- Identify regional trends in the HIV epidemic
- Summarize the reasons for the current trends in HIV epidemiology in different regions
- Understand the primary HIV prevention strategies for the general population and populations at high risk
- Describe the comprehensive approaches to HIV prevention being adopted
- Summarize the importance of the dissemination of best practices and potential implementation approaches
- Analyze the importance of cost evaluation of HIV prevention interventions

Globally, HIV continues to exact a substantial toll on the health and well-being of millions of people, causing considerable suffering, morbidity, and death. The pandemic insidiously exploits and amplifies existing social and economic disparities, particularly in sub-Saharan Africa, where productivity has been adversely affected and national revenues have consequently declined. Early death and prolonged illness is incapacitating social systems, including governance. The net effect is reduced state capacity, creating an environment that further exacerbates the pandemic.

The prospect of HIV infection remains one of the most significant public health risks. Though the disease is caused by a pathogen, the epidemic is driven by a number of social, behavioral, societal, and cultural forces. HIV is actually a syndemic, fueled by the concurrent epidemics of poverty, internecine conflict, deeply embedded cultural practices, and of course, other prevalent diseases. Understanding the full spectrum of issues and subsequently creating efficacious HIV risk-reduction interventions is a public health priority.

Understanding the evolving HIV pandemic is critical for allocating constrained human and fiscal resources. Additionally, understanding programmatic successes in reducing the burden of HIV and the remaining challenges is also important as societies strategize the development of new and innovative programs to curtail HIV. Of course, no single factor accounts for such a massive epidemic. There are myriad factors and influences that affect not only the likelihood of acquiring HIV but, likewise, the likelihood of being identified as HIV-positive through testing programs, of entering into effective clinical care, of adhering to antiretroviral therapy, of adopting risk-reduction practices, and of being retained in care.

This chapter describes the magnitude and temporal trends in HIV by geographic region. Additionally, the chapter describes effective programmatic efforts to control HIV, including individual-, community-, and structural-level interventions. We also describe advances in biomedical technology, such as treatment as prevention (TasP) and pre-exposure prophylaxis, and the implications of these biomedical strategies for HIV prevention. Finally, the chapter highlights the importance of cost evaluation of prevention interventions and the need for a coordinated and systematic dissemination and scale-up of effective prevention interventions to have a broad and sustained impact on the HIV epidemic.

Background and Epidemiology

At the end of 2014, 36.9 million persons were living with HIV worldwide; the HIV prevalence for adults ages 15–49 was approximately 0.8%. Of these, 4 million were ages 15–24, 29% of whom were adolescents ages 15–19 years. Approximately 3.2 million children younger than 15 years were living with HIV. Globally, new HIV infections peaked in 1997 but have been declining since the mid-2000s (by 35% from 2000 to 2014), with the greatest declines observed in sub-Saharan Africa (39% decline between 2000 and 2014) and the Caribbean (52% between 2000 and 2014). The exceptions to the declining trend in HIV incidence are the Middle East, North Africa, Eastern Europe, and Central Asia regions. AIDS-related deaths also have been declining (42% between 2004 and 2014), attributable to wider availability of **antiretroviral treatments** (ART) and the continuing decline in HIV incidence. Although variable by region, in 2014, women accounted for half (51%) of the adults (15 years and older) living with HIV, and this proportion has remained stable over the past 15 years. The most significant gains in reversing the HIV epidemic have been made among children under the age of 15 years, with new infections declining by 58% since 2000 (UNAIDS, 2015). However, despite gains made in the past decade, much needs to be done to achieve the UNAIDS goals of zero new HIV infections, discrimination, and AIDS-related deaths. Statistics from the end of 2011 are shown in Table 11.1. The maps in Figures 11.1 and 11.2 show prevalence of and change in HIV.

Reasons for the Current Trends in HIV Epidemiology

The HIV epidemic continues to evolve. However, this evolution has not been uniform across geographic regions. Next we describe trends in HIV epidemiology by region.

Sub-Saharan Africa

Sub-Saharan Africa remains disproportionately affected by the HIV epidemic; in 2014, 25.8 million persons were living with HIV (PLHIV). Southern Africa remains the worst affected subregion in the world, accounting for nearly 70% of PLHIV worldwide in 2014 (UNAIDS, 2015). The HIV epidemic may be stabilizing in Eastern Africa, and there are smaller proportions of PLHIV in Western and Central Africa. The number of AIDS-related deaths fell by 48% between

Table 11.1 Regional HIV/AIDS Statistics and Features, End of 2011

Region	Adults and Children Living With HIV	Adults and Children Newly Infected in 2011	Trend in Diagnosis of New Infections	Percentage of HIV-Positive Adults Who Are Women	Main Model(s) of Transmission (Number) for Adults Living With HIV
Sub-Saharan Africa	23.5 million	1.8 million	↓	59%	Hetero
Asia	4.37 million	369,000	↓	35%	Hetero, IDU, MSM
Eastern Europe and Central Asia	1.4 million	140,000	↑	35%	IDU
Caribbean	230,000	13,000	↓	53%	Hetero, MSM
Latin America	1.4 million	83,000	↓	36%	MSM, IDU, Hetero
North America and Western and Central Europe	2.3 million	81,000	↓	26%	MSM, IDU, Hetero
Middle East and North Africa	300,000	37,000	↑	41%	Hetero, IDU
Oceania	53,000	2,900	↓	44%	MSM

Note: Hetero (heterosexual transmission), IDU (transmission through injecting drug use), MSM (sexual transmission among men who have sex with men).
Source: UNAIDS, 2012a.

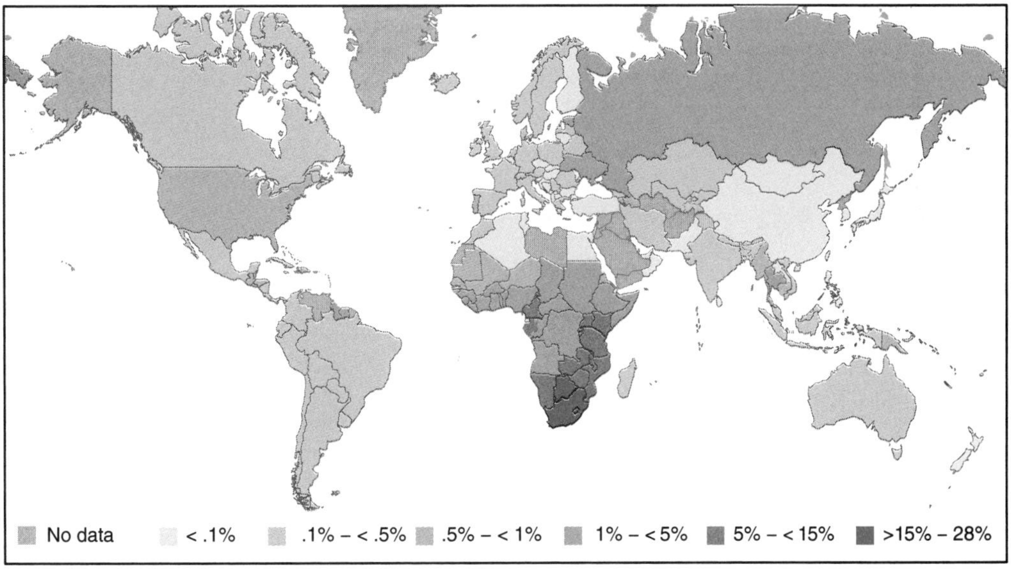

Figure 11.1 Global Prevalence of HIV, 2009
Source: UNAIDS (2012).

2005 and 2014, and 41% of PLHIV were accessing antiretroviral treatment in 2014 (UNAIDS, 2015). Overall, more than half of PLHIV in sub-Saharan Africa were women in 2014 (UNAIDS, 2015). Condomless heterosexual intercourse and mother-to-child transmission are the primary means of HIV transmission (UNAIDS, 2011).

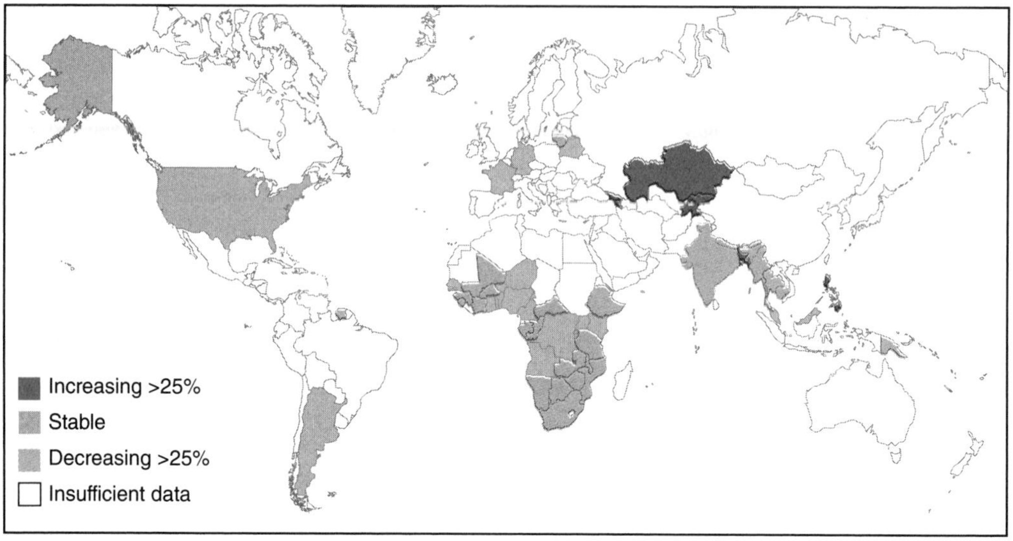

Figure 11.2 Changes in the Incidence of HIV Infection, 2001–2009
Note: To assess changes in incidence, the estimated national incidence rate was compared between 2009 and 2001. Countries with a change (decrease or increase) in the incidence rate of 25% or more during this period were identified. In most cases, the assessment was based on EPP/Spectrum modeling results (1, 2). For selected countries, published analyses of country-level incidence were also used. The EPP/Spectrum criteria for including countries in this analysis were as follows: EPP files were available and trends in EPP were not derived from workbook prevalence estimate, prevalence data were available up to at least 2007, there were at least four time points between 2001 and 2009 for which prevalence data were available for concentrated epidemics and at least three data points in the same period for generalized epidemics, for the majority of epidemic curves for a given country, EPP did not produce an artificial increase in HIV prevalence in recent years due to scarcity of prevalence data points, data were representative of the country; the EPP/Spectrum-derived incidence trend was not in conflict with the trend in case reports of new HIV diagnoses; and the EPP/Spectrum-derived incidence trend was not in conflict with modelled incidence trends derived from age-specific prevalence in national survey results.
Source: UNAIDS (2012).

Asia and the Pacific

In Asia and the Pacific, there were 5 million PLHIV in 2014. The HIV epidemic generally is declining in this region, registering a 32% decline between 2000 and 2014 (UNAIDS, 2015). Countries with older epidemics are witnessing a decrease in HIV incidence, but there are larger numbers of PLHIV attributable to expanded ART access. Over the past decade AIDS-related deaths have remained stable. However, in 2010, the number of AIDS-related deaths was the largest after sub-Saharan Africa, and in East Asia, the death toll doubled in the past decade. India, China, and Indonesia account for 78% of PLHIV in this region. The number of AIDS-related deaths increased by 11% between 2000 and 2014 (UNAIDS, 2015). Fewer women (35%) than men are living with HIV (UNAIDS, 2011), and there has been a 27% decline in new HIV infections among children in this region between 2000 and 2014. Treatment coverage is estimated at 36%. The majority acquired HIV through condomless sex with their spouses or regular male partners. Condomless **heterosexual sex,** especially paid sex, is the main driver of the mature epidemics. **Injection drug use** (IDU) is also a major route of HIV transmission in many Asian countries (UNAIDS, 2011). Also, the HIV epidemic among **men who have sex with men** (MSM) is growing (Brahmam et al., 2008; Chow et al., 2011; Morineau et al., 2011) and the HIV prevalence among male **sex workers** (MSWs) and

transgendered (TG) persons is high in certain regions (Guadamuz et al., 2011; Yu et al., 2011).

Outside of Asia, in 2010, there were an estimated 53,000 PLHIV. The largest number of PLHIV was in Papua New Guinea (Secretariat of the Pacific Community, 2010), which has a generalized epidemic, followed by Australia (National Centre in HIV Epidemiology and Clinical Research, 2010). In Papua New Guinea, the primary mode of HIV transmission is condomless heterosexual intercourse, while condomless sex among MSM is the major mode of transmission in Micronesia, Polynesia, Australia, and New Zealand (UNAIDS, 2011).

Eastern Europe and Central Asia

In 2014, there were approximately 1.5 million PLHIV in Eastern Europe and Central Asia. Since 2000, this region has witnessed a steep increase (40%) in the number of PLHIV, and the number of AIDS-related deaths has more than trebled between 2000 and 2014 (UNAIDS, 2015). The proportion of women (35%) living with HIV has remained stable in the past decade (UNAIDS, 2011). In 2009, the highest prevalence rates were in the Russian Federation (1%) and Ukraine (1.1%). Unlike the rest of the world, the number of AIDS-related deaths continues to increase in this region, and treatment coverage is estimated at 18% (UNAIDS, 2015). Injection drug use and risky sexual behaviors practiced by IDUs have been the main drivers of the epidemic since the late 1990s (UNAIDS, 2011). Although condomless sex between men is considered a minor route of HIV transmission, small-scale surveys have shown a high HIV prevalence among MSM in Georgia (5%) and the Russian Federation (6%) (van Griensven et al., 2009) and among MSWs in Moscow (16%) (Baral et al., 2010), Kyiv (4%) and Ukraine (23%) (Kruglov et al., 2008).

Caribbean

In 2014, there were approximately 280,000 PLHIV in the Caribbean. The epidemic has been declining since 2001, and overall there has been a decline of 52% in new HIV infections between 2000 and 2014. In the same time period, the number of AIDS-related deaths fell by more than half, with Haiti accounting for half of these deaths. Treatment coverage is estimated at 44% among adults (UNAIDS, 2015). There are more women (53%) than men living with HIV (UNAIDS, 2011). Sexual intercourse, both heterosexual and among MSM, is the main route of transmission (CareC, 2007). MSM are still criminalized in many Caribbean countries and as a result, this mode of transmission is considerably under-represented in official reports (Tomlinson, 2010). Injection drug use also is a major route of HIV transmission in Bermuda and Puerto Rico (Centers for Disease Control and Prevention [CDC], 2009).

Latin America

In 2014, there were 1.7 million PLHIV in Latin America and the epidemic has stabilized, with an estimated 13% decline in new infections between 2000 and 2014 and a 29% reduction in AIDS-related deaths between 2005 and 2014.

Treatment coverage is estimated at 47% among adults (UNAIDS, 2015). In 2010, 36% of adults living with HIV were women. Brazil accounts for approximately 33% of PLHIV in Latin America (UNAIDS, 2011). However, the HIV epidemic in Brazil is controlled, largely attributable to an early well-coordinated response, protection of human rights, and a focus on HIV prevention among MSM, female sex workers (FSWs), and IDUs (Beyrer, 2011). Sexual intercourse among MSM is the main route of HIV transmission, but there is a major gap in the data for HIV trends among MSWs and TG sex workers (UNAIDS, 2011).

North America and Western and Central Europe

In 2014, the HIV epidemic has stabilized in these regions, with an estimated 2.4 million PLHIV. More than half (~1.2 million) of PLHIV in this region live in the United States, where African Americans and Hispanics/Latinos are disproportionately affected (UNAIDS, 2015). The proportion of HIV-positive women (26%) has remained stable since the late 1990s. However, there are variations at the subregional level, with the number of new HIV cases doubling between 2001 and 2009 in Bulgaria, Czech Republic, Hungary, Lithuania, Slovakia, and Slovenia and a 50% increase in the United Kingdom. During the same period, the number of new HIV cases decreased by more than 20% in Latvia, Portugal, and Romania (European Centre for Disease Prevention and Control & WHO Regional Office for Europe, 2010). Condomless sex among MSM continues to be the main driver of transmission (European Centre for Disease Prevention and Control & WHO Regional Office for Europe, 2010; UNAIDS, 2011), with IDU and paid sex playing less of a role.

Middle East and North Africa

In 2014, the Middle East and North Africa had approximately 240,000 PLHIV. Evidence shows continuing increases in the number of newly infected persons (22% increase between 2000 and 2014), and AIDS-related deaths (trebled between 2000 and 2014), while treatment coverage was estimated at 14% among adults (UNAIDS, 2015). With the exception of Djibouti and South Sudan, HIV prevalence is low. However, the number of PLHIV almost doubled between 2001 and 2010, with women comprising approximately 41% of PLHIV (UNAIDS, 2011). Condomless sex (including MSM) and sharing needles are the main modes of HIV transmission (Abu-Raddad, 2010). Sex between men is still criminalized in many countries, and this, in combination with risky sexual behaviors, low levels of condom use, and lack of HIV knowledge, contributes to the growing epidemic (Beyrer, 2011).

HIV Prevention Strategies

Given current economic conditions, with fiscal resources severely constrained, HIV prevention efforts need to focus on the adaptation, translation, and scale-up of evidence-based interventions. Within resource-limited settings, when scaling-up prevention interventions, it is particularly important to be strategic when allocating resources to address the drivers of the HIV epidemic.

Strategic planning and a better understanding of each country's epidemic within specific populations and cultural contexts will have the highest impact on sexual attitudes, risky sexual behavior, and HIV incidence rates. Previous research findings have identified several behavioral, biomedical, and structural interventions with demonstrated efficacy to avert new HIV infections.

Behavioral Interventions

Behavioral interventions primarily focus on strategies to decrease risk behaviors and to support biomedical interventions through demand creation, improving ART and condom use adherence, and providing overall psychosocial services to improve the uptake of essential HIV services.

Community-Level Interventions

Community mobilization efforts provide the opportunity to increase the uptake of essential HIV prevention services (Sweat et al., 2011; Tan et al., 2012; Townsend, Mathews, & Zembe, 2013). Previous research has indicated that these efforts can help increase the uptake of **HIV testing** and counseling (HTC) services, regardless of infrastructure, epidemic, and culture (Sweat et al., 2011). This is particularly important when targeting rural areas or key populations, such as sex workers, MSM, or truck drivers. Community-based organizations are in an optimal position to better understand the unique contextual factors that drive the HIV epidemic within communities they serve (Chillag et al., 2002). Community-level activities can be beneficial when targeting community norms and discrimination or stigma that may perpetuate risk behaviors directly or indirectly affecting the likelihood of HIV acquisition and transmission (Khumalo-Sakutukwa et al., 2008). Mass media campaigns also can complement **community-based interventions** to create awareness and demand for services, as they are able to reach a large number of persons (Abroms & Maibach, 2008).

Biomedical Interventions

Biomedical intervention strategies directly affect the biological systems by utilizing medical and public health approaches to block infection, to decrease degree of infectiousness, and to reduce susceptibility.

HIV Testing and Counseling and Linkage to Care

As a standalone intervention, the impact of HTC on HIV incidence is mixed (Ross, 2010). However, HTC serves as a gateway to relevant prevention, care, and treatment services for both high-risk HIV-negative and HIV-positive persons. Partner or couples HTC help identify serodiscordant couples and support safe sexual behaviors and disclosure of HIV status (Burton, Darbes, & Operario, 2010; Dunkle et al., 2008). Linking and enrolling HIV-positive persons in care and treatment services is the first step in the continuum of HIV care (Kilmarx & Mutasa-Apollo, 2013; Rosen & Fox, 2011). However, a recent review from resource-limited settings has indicated that approximately 40% of persons testing HIV-positive never enroll in HIV care and treatment services (Rosen & Fox, 2011).

Health care settings provide opportunities to offer HTC, identify HIV-positive persons, and address HIV prevention. However, HTC has not been widely implemented (Nakanjako et al., 2007; Sanders et al., 2010). The health-care provider is well-positioned to offer optimal outpatient care if HIV status is determined. Due to limited staff in many settings as well as cost-effectiveness measures, task-shifting responsibility of these services to nurses or counselors may improve implementation (Callaghan, Ford, & Schneider, 2010; Sanders et al., 2010). In addition to health care settings, scale-up of community-based and mobile HTC is also an advantageous strategy depending on the cultural context and environment.

In the United States, the Centers for Disease Control and Prevention recommends routine HIV screening in health care settings for clients ages 13 to 64 years, where prevalence is $\geq 0.1\%$ (Branson et al., 2006). Additionally, targeted testing in non-health care settings may more effectively facilitate access to at-risk populations who are unaware of their status and do not routinely seek care (CDC, 2001). A study examining CDC-funded testing programs in the United States indicated that although testing in non–health care settings identified a higher percentage of new positives, it is often more expensive per test than health care settings and may not target all hard to reach populations. However, health care settings, which offer more efficient methods of testing and linkage, may miss undiagnosed HIV-positive persons who do not access health care (Seth et al., 2015).

Male and Female Condoms

Sexual intercourse is the primary mode of HIV infection worldwide. When used consistently and correctly, the effectiveness of male latex condoms can be as high as 95% in preventing the transmission of HIV and other sexually transmitted infections (STIs) (Foss et al., 2007; Pinkerton & Abramson, 1997) and may result in an 80% reduction in HIV incidence (Weller & Davis-Beaty, 2002). However, the effectiveness of condoms at the population-level is less known (Padian et al., 2008).

In contrast to male condoms, which require men's willingness to use them, female condoms allow women to have power in their sexual decision making without having to engage in condom negotiation with their male partners. Female condoms also are an effective method for prevention against HIV and may provide similar levels of protection as male condoms; although further research is needed (French et al., 2003; Gallo, Kilbourne-Brook, & Coffey, 2012; Padian et al., 2008). Findings on the acceptability of the female condom have been mixed, and they are not used as widely as male condoms because of several barriers (French et al., 2003; Gallo et al., 2012).

Challenges with both male and female condoms include that they must be used correctly and consistently. Persons also may use condoms only with certain sexual partners, placing themselves or their partners at risk for HIV transmission. However, the increased availability, education, promotion campaigns, and demand creation has increased the uptake of condoms (Padian et al., 2008).

A review of behavioral intervention programs for heterosexual men in low- to middle-income countries indicated that several interventions increased condom use among men. Various intervention strategies were used, including **information-motivational-behavioral (IMB) principals,** peer education, and community-based interventions (Townsend et al., 2013). Additionally, reviews of HIV prevention programs in the United States for women have suggested that the most efficacious interventions (a) are guided by social psychological theories, (b) include only women, (c) emphasize gender-related influences, such as gender-based power imbalances, and sexual assertiveness, and (d) are led by peers (Exner, Seal, & Ehrhardt, 1997; Wingood & DiClemente, 1996; Wingood, Reddy et al., 2013). Multiple HIV behavioral interventions for women in the United States also have been shown to be effective in reducing risky sexual behavior and increasing condom use (Lyles et al., 2007). Additionally, interventions among diverse populations that addressed sociocultural barriers were more effective at increasing condom use (Scott-Sheldon et al., 2011). However, despite the strong evidence for behavioral interventions and increased condom use, a recent review indicated that there is limited effectiveness for behavioral interventions improving condom use for dual protection (Lopez et al., 2013). Therefore, further research and programmatic efforts are needed for dual protection condom use. A large number of HIV prevention behavioral interventions have been theory based and several reviews and meta-analyses have examined the frameworks and models which have been used most often, resulting in effective behavior change (see Box 11.1).

BOX 11.1 THEORIES/MODELS OF BEHAVIOR CHANGE AND HIV PREVENTION (CONTRIBUTED BY RICK S. ZIMMERMAN)

Theories or models can be used in a variety of ways related to understand behavior change in an area like HIV prevention: 1) see how well one theory/model explains or predicts risk behavior (e.g., frequency of unprotected intercourse), 2) compare how two or more theories/models explain or predict risk behavior, 3) see how effective interventions based on various theories/models are at changing behavior, and 4) see what components of interventions were most important in leading to behavior change. As we have said elsewhere (Noar & Zimmerman, 2005), we strongly believe that there is too much research both in HIV prevention and other areas that tests only one theory and finds it adequate, rather than comparing it to results for other theories or models. So where possible in this box we will focus on research that has compared theories or reviewed the literature across multiple theories as most useful.

- Study 1: In a large meta-analysis (statistical analysis and review of many already-published research articles), Albarracin and her colleagues (2005) found that behavioral HIV preventive interventions that included content related to condom attitudes (components of the Theory of Planned Behavior, barriers and benefits from the Health Belief Model, the Information-Motivation-Behavioral Skills Model, and the Extended Parallel Process Model) and behavioral skills (components of self-efficacy theory, IMB, and EPPM models) were most effective and that interventions that attempted to increase fear (perceived susceptibility and/or seriousness of the Health Belief Model) were least effective.

- Study 2: In a review of 44 longitudinal studies where model variables at one time predicted sexual behavior outcomes at a later time, Huebner & Perry (2015) found that of the traditional health-behavior model variables, only behavioral skills (most related to self-efficacy and skills from the IMB) was consistently related to subsequent sexual behavior, with inconsistent or weak results for condom attitudes, condom use norms, self-efficacy and perceived risk. They also found that the vast majority of experimental studies rarely assessed which components of the intervention (i.e., which variables in the theoretical model(s) on which the intervention was based) resulted in positive intervention effects, and those rare results were generally quite mixed.
- Study 3: An interesting and informative recent study designed and implemented two interventions based on the Health Belief Model and the Theory of Planned Behavior (Montanaro & Bryan, 2014) with sexually experienced college students. Results indicated that both interventions had effects on intentions and preparatory behaviors (purchasing condoms, talking to a boyfriend/girlfriend about condoms, and carrying condoms). The TPB variables were much better predictors of behavior before the intervention, and attitudes (from the TPB) and self-efficacy (from the HBM), were the better predictors of changes in intentions and preparatory behaviors. They conclude that the TPB may be generally more useful, but that the "constructs that appear most useful in explaining behavior may not be the same constructs that can be manipulated to produce behavior change."

Please also see our discussion in Chapter 4 about attempts to increase the scope of health behavior change theories to include interpersonal, ecological, and/or structural components beyond those of the individual.

Pre-exposure Prophylaxis

Pre-exposure prophylaxis (PrEP) is an HIV prevention method in which persons who are not HIV-positive take medication to reduce their risk of acquiring HIV. PrEP substantially reduces the risk of HIV acquisition in heterosexual men, women, discordant couples, MSM, and injection drug users (Baeten et al., 2012; Choopanya et al., 2013; Grant et al., 2010; Paltiel et al., 2009; Thigpen et al., 2012). Studies have found that when taking a pill (Truvada) containing tenofovir plus emtricitabine consistently, MSM were 44% less likely to acquire HIV than those who were given a placebo, and their risk of HIV infection was reduced by up to 92% (Grant et al., 2010); heterosexually active men and women were 62% less likely (Thigpen et al., 2012); discordant couples were 75% less likely, and their risk of infection was reduced by up to 90% (Baeten et al., 2012); injection drug users were 49% less likely, and their risk of infection was reduced by up to 74% (Choopanya et al., 2013).

The World Health Organization (WHO) and the US Public Health Service have released clinical guidelines for PrEP (US Public Health Service, 2014; WHO, 2014). Challenges to PrEP have included the cost, potential drug toxicity, viral resistance, and behavioral disinhibition leading to increased risk taking (Paltiel et al., 2009). Additionally, some trials have not found favorable results; varying adherence rates, biological determinants, integrity of the vaginal epithelium, and acute stage of HIV infection for the index partner serve as potential explanations (van der Straten et al., 2012). PrEP-based prevention is most appealing when used with high-risk populations, particularly with those that have t with HTC and **linkage to care and treatment services** if HIV-positive. PrEP could significantly reduce the lifetime risk of HIV infection (Paltiel et al., 2009), but it requires strict adherence and repeat HIV testing. PrEP should not be implemented as a sole intervention but instead should be combined and integrated with other HIV prevention methods (CDC, 2012).

Treatment as Prevention

Although efforts in the global response to the HIV epidemic primarily focused on the prevention of transmission (Ford, Calmy, & Mills, 2011), the focus has shifted to the scale-up of HIV treatment as costs for treatment have decreased. Combined antiretroviral (ARV) therapy decreases the morbidity and mortality rate among HIV-positive persons (Ray et al., 2010). ARV treatment for the HIV-positive partner has been associated with up to 92% reduced risk of HIV transmission. The test-and-treat approach has been seen as an opportunity to potentially transform the face of the HIV epidemic (Attia et al., 2009; Dieffenbach & Fauci, 2009; Donnell et al., 2010). The findings from HPTN 052, the first randomized clinical trial, indicated that early initiation of ARV treatment reduced transmission rates of HIV-1 among serodiscordant couples by 96% (M. S. Cohen et al., 2011). A multi-country, randomized controlled trial, Strategic Timing of AntiRetroviral Treatment (START), found that HIV-positive persons have a significantly lower risk of developing AIDS or other illnesses if they begin ARV treatment when their CD4+ T-cell count is higher. These findings support initiation of treatment for all HIV-positive persons, rather than waiting until CD4 count drops to a certain level (National Institutes of Health, 2015).

Treatment as prevention (TasP) provides an opportunity to improve prevention and clinical services along the continuum. This includes scale-up of HTC, strengthening linkages and retention in care and treatment, and adherence to treatment. However, with these benefits, there also are challenges, because each step along the continuum is critical in the success of TasP (McNairy, Cohen, & El-Sadr, 2013). It is important to take a strategic approach with the implementation and scale-up of TasP in order to have the largest impact (Smith et al., 2011).

Prevention of Mother-to-Child Transmission

At the end of 2011, approximately 3.4 million children were living with HIV worldwide, with 91% in sub-Saharan Africa (WHO, UNICEF, & UNAIDS, 2011). Most children acquire HIV during labor and delivery or breastfeeding; therefore prevention of mother to child transmission (PMTCT) is a key intervention toward ending pediatric HIV epidemic and achieving an AIDS-free generation. According to the Global Report from UNAIDS (2013), ARV coverage among pregnant women living with HIV reached 62% in 2012, and there was a 35% reduction in the number of children newly infected from 2009 to 2012.

In 2013, the World Health Organization updated their 2010 PMTCT guidelines. The 2010 guidelines recommended "Option A" or "Option B" treatment regimens, where the ARVs given are different and initiation of treatment is based on CD4 count for Option A, whereas treatment is initiated regardless of CD4 count for Option B. However, treatment is stopped after breastfeeding for women with CD4 counts >350 cells/mm^3 (WHO, 2010). This has now been updated to CD4counts >500 cells/mm^3 (WHO, 2013).

The advent of treatment as prevention (M. S. Cohen et al., 2011) and Malawi's option B+ approach (Schouten et al., 2011) has the potential to change the face of PMTCT. Option B+ involves placing all HIV-positive pregnant women on lifelong treatment, regardless of CD4 count or clinical stages (WHO, 2012). The benefits of Option B+ include lower mortality for the mother and the reduction and potential elimination of pediatric HIV (Schouten et al., 2011). It also leads to the next steps of scaling-up treatment and **combination prevention** strategies (Goosby, 2013). Therefore, the 2013 consolidated guidelines no longer recommend Option A and strongly recommend providing ART to all pregnant and breastfeeding women regardless of CD4 count (Option B). They also recommend that countries who are transitioning to or implementing Option B should weigh the advantages and disadvantages of lifelong ART for programmatic and operational reasons (WHO, 2013).

Voluntary Medical Male Circumcision

Voluntary medical male circumcision (VMMC) performed by trained medical professionals can reduce men's risk of acquiring HIV through sexual intercourse with female partners by 60% (Bailey et al., 2007; Gray et al., 2007; Weiss et al., 2008). Mathematical models have indicated that rapid scale-up of VMMC has the potential to avert new infections in countries with a high HIV prevalence but low rate of VMMC (UNAIDS/WHO/SACEMA, 2009; Njeuhmeli et al., 2011). Other benefits have included decreased risk of HSV-2, human papillomavirus (HPV), and cervical cancer in men (Castellsague et al., 2002; Sobngwi-Tambekou et al., 2009; Tobian et al., 2009). Additionally, a systematic review identified an estimated 20% reduction of HIV incidence among female sexual partners of men who had been circumcised (Weiss, Hankins, & Dickson, 2009). There has been some evidence that VMMC also has been associated with a decrease in STIs in women (Gray et al., 2009; UNAIDS/WHO/SACEMA, 2009; Wawer et al., 2009).

The greatest public health benefit is derived by scaling-up VMMC in generalized, high-HIV-prevalence settings. In sub-Saharan Africa alone, universal access of VMMC could prevent 5.7 million new HIV infections and 3 million deaths over 20 years (Williams et al., 2006). Although the realization of the benefits of VMMC on HIV incidence will be in the future, the efficacy of VMMC is significant. Since VMMC provides partial protection, a comprehensive HIV prevention approach with messaging on condoms, STI management, and risk reduction should also be offered (Weiss et al., 2010).

Structural Interventions

Structural approaches to HIV prevention address pervasive social, cultural, economic, and political factors, such as stigma, discrimination, gender inequality, and income disparities (i.e., **social determinants of health**) (Gupta et al., 2008). **Structural interventions,** in combination with other individual-level interventions, can lead to greater demand generation for HIV prevention, treatment, and care services (J. Cohen, 2004). Thus, structural approaches, whether they are government policies to address discriminatory practices (e.g., those directed at MSM) or transformational processes (e.g., empowerment of marginalized communities) seek to change the "structures" or contextual factors associated with HIV vulnerability. This approach to HIV prevention is reflected in the human rights based Sustainable Development Goals (SDGs) which seek to end the HIV epidemic by 2030 (see Box 11.2).

School-based interventions in Kenya (Cho et al., 2011) and Zimbabwe (Hallfors et al., 2011) have found that after approximately one year, comprehensive school support (i.e., school fees, uniforms, and a "community visitor" who monitored school attendance and helped resolve problems that would lead to absence or dropout) decreased school dropout, delayed sexual debut, and reduced risk factors (e.g., attitudes supporting early sexual debut) associated with HIV.

Poverty and gender inequality also exacerbate the spread of HIV and economic empowerment may be an important prevention strategy, particularly for women. Some examples of microfinance programs, such as JEWEL (Sherman et al., 2006) for sex workers using drugs in Baltimore, and the IMAGE Program in South Africa (Kim et al., 2007; Pronyk et al., 2006; Pronyk, Kim, et al., 2008), have shown promising results including increased HIV testing, increased condom use, reduction in number of sexual partners, reduced drug use, and increased ability to refuse sex and women's empowerment. Although much work remains to be done to understand the role and impact of microfinance on HIV prevention, this increase in social capital shapes women's ability to fight issues related to gender inequality, such as violence (Pronyk, Harpham, et al., 2008).

Finally, there also have been strong correlations between improved housing status and reduced HIV risk behaviors (e.g., drug use, needle use, or sex exchange), improved access to health care for PLHIV, and overall better health outcomes. This approach presents a complex but effective tool for HIV prevention (Aidala et al., 2005).

BOX 11.2 A HUMAN RIGHTS BASED APPROACH TO ENDING HIV/AIDS

SDG (Sustainable Development Goal) 3 seeks to ensure healthy lives and promote well-being for all. Target 3.3 is specifically focused on ending the epidemic of AIDS and several other infectious diseases by 2030 (UN, 2015). SGDs 1-5, 8, 10, 11, 16, and 17 taken together with SDG 3.3 address the human rights-based approach to ending AIDS by 2030. These SDGs address the issues of poverty and hunger, quality healthcare and education, gender inequality, economic growth and decent work, unsafe cities, discriminatory norms, behaviors and laws in societies, and war, all of which have been found to be underlying factors that leave people vulnerable to HIV infection (Maleche, 2015).

According to UNAIDS, many of the MDG 6 (which had two key HIV targets: halting and beginning to reverse the spread of HIV by 2015; and to achieve, by 2010, universal access to treatment for HIV & AIDS) targets have been achieved. UNAIDS attributes this achievement to increased funding, empowering communities, and adopting evidence-informed human rights-based approaches (HRBAs) to programs and policies (UNAIDS, 2015).

A paper published by UNAIDS and the Lancet Commission (2015) highlights the importance of upholding human rights among its seven recommendations for achieving SDG 3.3. The paper asserts that it is important to address criminalization, stigma, and discrimination related to HIV, using practical approaches to change laws, policies, and public attitudes that violate human rights. Despite overwhelming evidence to support this approach, very few countries' national AIDS plans have a clearly delineated human-rights approach (UNAIDS, 2012b).

The Global Commission on HIV and the Law in its July 2012 report, Risks, Rights and Health emphasizes that enabling legal environments is essential to addressing AIDS (Global Commission on HIV and the Law, 2012) with reports claiming that a conducive legal environment could halve new HIV infections globally.

Government-led interventions and grassroots community-led movements, rather than top-down policy-level approaches, are critical (Evans & Lambert, 2008; Swendeman et al., 2009). Programs at the national level (Bernard, Kippax, & Baxter, 2008; Okware et al., 2001) have been instrumental in reducing and containing the epidemic. A variety of programs and activities that promote partnerships between government, communities, and research organizations should be encouraged.

Developing Comprehensive Approaches to HIV Prevention

The HIV pandemic continues to exact a heavy toll in human suffering, mortality, and government resources. The HIV pandemic also continues to evolve.

Although prevention efforts have been effective, to accelerate the end of the HIV pandemic, we need to redouble our efforts. There is no "magic bullet." A vaccine is not in the foreseeable future, and even if it were available, it may require multiple doses, may not be 100% effective, and some who should be vaccinated may not adopt the vaccine. Thus, intensifying prevention efforts tailored for persons who are HIV-negative but engaging in HIV-associated behaviors and for persons who are living with HIV but engaging in transmission behaviors, represents a pragmatic strategy to reduce HIV.

The Advent of Treatment as Prevention

The past few years have witnessed remarkable advances in biomedical prevention. The advent of treatment as prevention (TasP) for HIV-positive persons and chemoprophylaxis (pre-exposure prophylaxis or PrEP) has added new strategies to our armamentarium to combat HIV. HIV testing and linkage to care also remains a critical component of any prevention strategy. Although the degree of efficacy varies, particularly by level of regimen adherence, it is clear that biomedical prevention is an emerging and important component in the HIV prevention toolkit.

To maximize prevention, the field of HIV prevention may benefit from focusing on the development of complementary strategies, employing where appropriate a combination of biomedical and behavioral interventions. As a result of rapid advances in biomedical and behavioral HIV prevention technology, scientists have suggested that the integration of biomedical and behavioral interventions can be guided by a systematic approach that optimizes program effectiveness, in essence, creating "prevention synergy" (Wingood et al., 2013). Without a comprehensive framework, combined interventions may inadvertently produce scattered, redundant, or mutually opposing effects. This perspective also provides a compelling approach for the scale-up of combination interventions across different levels of influence to facilitate their reach, impact, and sustainability.

The Need for Implementation Science

No HIV prevention is perfect. It should be axiomatic that not every person exposed to a behavioral or biomedical intervention will adopt the appropriate preventive behaviors and avoid becoming infected. Currently, given the state of the science, such a goal is unrealistic and unnecessary for affecting the HIV trajectory at a population level. Striving for this goal may even be counterproductive, creating inertia among policy experts, practitioners, and other consumers while they search for the "magic bullet" that protects everyone exposed.

However, this does not mean that we lower the standard for determining effective HIV prevention programs. Quite to the contrary, failure to adopt and maintain rigorous standards for identifying effective interventions comes with the cost of wasting scarce resources on ineffective programs. It does mean, however, that while the continued efforts of scientists and practitioners need to be directed at developing more effective interventions, existing interventions, both behavioral and biomedical, that have demonstrated programmatic efficacy need to be widely disseminated, adopted by consumers, and scaled up to have optimal impact at a population level. Ultimately, reducing HIV does not only depend on the development and evaluation of innovative interventions but on how effectively these interventions can be translated into clinical practice, school curricula, or community programs.

One area, ripe for research, is to focus squarely on identifying strategies, processes, and mechanisms for the timely translation of effective interventions into sustainable programs (DiClemente et al., 2013). The development of sustainable programs is, however, contingent on a myriad of factors. Foremost is the need for an infrastructure responsible for collecting and collating new information, as well as organizing, managing, and coordinating the active transfer of new prevention information to practitioners and other consumers (policy analysts, elected officials, health department officials, clinical and social service providers, and program managers in community-based organizations). For efficient program transfer, investing in the development of an infrastructure to design and continually monitor systems and processes needed to promote rapid and widespread adoption and deployment of evidence-based preventions interventions is critical and could yield a significant return on investment.

It should be noted that there is a clear distinction between the passive transfer of prevention programs and the actions required to encourage, facilitate, and enable adoption, uptake, and maintenance of these programs. The transfer of HIV prevention must be an active and purposive application of skills, systems, and resources dedicated to supporting the adoption and uptake of newly identified HIV prevention programs. Gaps and inadequacies in the infrastructure responsible for supporting the transfer and uptake of new HIV prevention programs limits how efficiently systems and processes can be designed, implemented, maintained, and evaluated. Without a competent and fully operational infrastructure for prevention program **dissemination**, it is doubtful that advances in HIV prevention will achieve their potential and fulfill their promise of reducing HIV. Thus, one recommendation is to support the adoption of these programs, to invest in training, the provision of relevant materials and medications, and to establish an ongoing program of technical assistance designed to sustain program utilization. To this end, we will need to foster more **implementation science** approaches to facilitate adaptation of evidence-based prevention programs, improve their dissemination, enhance their uptake, and promote their sustainability at the community level (Brown et al., 2013; Glasgow, Eckstein, & Eizarrad, 2013).

The Need for a Broader Social Ecological Paradigm

A discrete but related area of importance is the need to reconceptualize the HIV epidemic as a function of multiple co-occurring psychological, behavioral, sociological, cultural, and economic influences. Thus, a broader theoretical perspective, such as **social ecological** models (Ewart, 2009; Flay, Snyder, & Petraitis, 2009; Hovell, Wahlgren, & Adams, 2009; McLeroy et al., 1988), may be more sensitive to the diversity of influences that affect HIV risk and how these multiple influences coalesce and affect the likelihood of HIV acquisition

(DiClemente, Salazar, & Crosby, 2007; Salazar et al., 2010). The central principle of the ecological paradigm is that the risk of acquiring and/or transmitting HIV arises from a complex interaction of multiple determinants corresponding to different "levels of influence." The ecological paradigm emphasizes interdependence among levels of influence. Thus, interventions at one level may influence interventions at another level. Hence, interdependence emerges as a central mechanism for integrating prevention interventions at multiple levels. This paradigm argues for multilevel intervention approaches, strategies that transcend the person and acknowledge the importance of extrapersonal influences. Increasing research on newly developed community mobilization approaches such as community-based participatory research (Blumenthal et al., 2013), use of innovative social technologies as behavior change modalities (e.g., social media, Twitter, Internet, Facebook—see Box 11.3) (Sullivan, Grey, & Rosser, 2013) and expanding the potential array of implementation sites to include nontraditional intervention venues (e.g., incarceration facilities) (Rich et al., 2013), social networks (Latkin et al., 2013), community-based organizations (Rhodes et al., 2013; Wingood, Reddy, et al., 2013), and faith institutions (Wingood, Robinson, & Braxton, 2013), offer promise of engaging those populations that are often "hidden" or difficult to access.

BOX 11.3 TECHNOLOGY AND HIV PREVENTION

There is a gap between new research knowledge, innovations (intervention development), and their translation into practice, particularly with behavioral interventions that may also impact the success of biomedical interventions. Compounding this problem in translation, adopted new knowledge is often applied unevenly and ineffectually. Thus, the temporal chasm between research and prevention practice means we have invested substantial fiscal resources in developing evidence-based programs that are inappropriately utilized, underutilized, or not utilized.

Efficacious, group-delivered interventions often require significant fiscal and personnel resources to train staff and implement the intervention; thus, they may not be feasible in resource-constrained settings. To reduce the cost and related personnel constraints, newer implementation modalities may permit accessing a larger proportion of the at-risk population in resource limited settings. Social media, text messaging, computer-based, and web-based intervention may provide an innovative, less costly, and more readily implementable modality to translate and disseminate evidence-based HIV risk-reduction interventions.

Given the reach of the Internet and smartphones, these modalities provide an avenue to implement interventions to reach diverse populations at a large scale. As an example, use of mobile, social networking or online platforms may provide for more flexible intervention delivery. However, there is an important caveat for implementation science. Even when interventions are translated into a less costly delivery modality, are less personnel-intensive, and offered with ongoing technical assistance, there is no assurance that this will result in the successful implementation of interventions. To overcome obstacles to effective intervention implementation may require a more thorough understanding of the complexity and diversity of barriers that may adversely affect optimal implementation. Additional strategies to incorporate HIV interventions into the existing flow of clinical services for HIV-positive and HIV-negative persons are needed. Furthermore, enhancing public health clinic staff's "buy-in" to such interventions is essential for the effective dissemination among all clinic attendees. Implementation of HIV interventions could also be fostered by policies supporting their use. Ultimately, dissemination of evidence-based HIV interventions via technology modalities offers great promise to reach those most at-risk. However, realizing the promise and potential of new technology-delivered HIV risk-reduction interventions will require further detailed study to optimize implementation.

A summary of a study implementing a computer-based intervention for African American adolescent females is provided below.

Although group-delivered HIV/STD risk-reduction interventions for African American adolescent females have proven efficacious, they require significant financial and staffing resources to implement and may not be feasible in personnel- and resource-constrained public health clinics. We conducted a study assessing adoption and implementation of an evidence-based HIV/STD risk-reduction intervention that was translated from a group-delivered modality to a computer-delivered modality to facilitate use in county public health departments. Usage of the computer-delivered intervention was low across eight participating public health clinics. Further investigation is needed to optimize implementation by identifying, understanding, and surmounting barriers that hamper timely and efficient implementation of technology-delivered HIV/STD risk-reduction interventions in county public health clinics (DiClemente, Bradley, & Davis, 2013).

The Need for Cost Evaluation

The increasing emphasis on cost containment, the emergence of the managed care environment and the disproportionate increase in the cost of health care versus other expenditures, has prompted **cost evaluation** as one criterion for evaluating HIV prevention programs. In a constrained fiscal environment, it becomes imperative that we not only evaluate program efficacy in terms of impact (e.g., changes in behavior, attitudes, norms, knowledge) and outcomes (e.g., changes in morbidity, mortality, and quality of life) but also assess cost. Such information is vitally important to program planners, policymakers, practitioners, and other persons involved in the design and implementation of HIV prevention programs.

Arguably, one might question whether HIV prevention programs should be held accountable to the standard that a program's economic benefit to society outweighs its financial costs. However, whether or not one accepts that standard, the application of economic evaluation techniques is as appropriate to HIV prevention as they are to other health programs. For example, if two programs, using rigorous evaluation methodology, yielded similar impact (e.g., reduction in HIV incidence), but one program cost $2 per participant to avert an incident HIV infection while the other program cost $10 per participant, the cost differential would favor the former program. Indeed, the former program could be markedly expanded to reach many more persons and still cost less than the latter program, yielding substantial population-level benefit.

Unable to sidestep the issue of cost, HIV prevention researchers, health care providers, policy analysts, and program planners need to become familiar with the theory and methods used to conduct cost evaluation studies (AIDS2031, 2010). This methodology represents an entirely different perspective for many researchers and practitioners. Most often, HIV prevention researchers and practitioners have had their philosophical, theoretical, and methodological roots in their own particular discipline rather than economics.

Given the human suffering, economic costs, lost productivity, and medical care resources associated with morbidity and mortality, interventions that demonstrate programmatic efficacy will be an important component in any public health strategy to accelerate the eradication of HIV. Further, given the monetary expenditure involved in developing and evaluating behavioral and biomedical HIV prevention programs, it is critical that these studies be adequately designed, conducted, analyzed, and reported. Although HIV prevention programs, adequately funded and innovative in design, offer great potential to effectively reduce risk behaviors and HIV infections, this progress will not be rapid. Behavior change, both by end users and practitioners, on a scale large enough to affect population level health will require a comprehensive and sustained effort. New opportunities and new challenges lie ahead for HIV prevention research. How we, as a field, leverage these opportunities and resolve challenges will be critical to maximize prevention efforts to end the HIV pandemic.

Summary

Globally, considerable changes in the epidemiology of HIV have been observed within and across geographic regions. However, these changes have not been uniform. Some regions have demonstrated greater effectiveness in combating HIV through the use of diverse prevention, testing, and treatment strategies.

Although new and innovative strategies are critical, the efficient and effective dissemination of current evidence-based prevention, testing, treatment programs, and policies is also critical. Using implementation science we can design, evaluate, and identify the most cost-effective strategies to enhance the uptake, adoption, use, and sustainment of effective programs and policies. Thus, we do not have to "re-invent the wheel" to reduce the burden of HIV: we have the arrows in our quiver. However, we need the support and cooperation of state governments to release those arrows. Changes of the magnitude needed to effectively curtail the HIV epidemic will not be swift or easily attained. However, through a sustained, systematic, and coordinated global effort we can hope to eradicate HIV.

KEY TERMS

1. **Antiretroviral treatment:** The use of HIV medication to treat HIV infection
2. **Behavioral interventions:** Interventions that primarily focus on strategies to decrease risk behaviors and to support biomedical interventions through demand creation, improving antiretroviral treatment and condom use adherence, and providing overall psychosocial services to improve the uptake of essential HIV services
3. **Biomedical interventions:** Medical, clinical, and public health approaches designed to directly affect the biological systems by utilizing medical and public health approaches to block infection, to decrease degree of infectiousness, and to reduce susceptibility
4. **Combination prevention:** Approaches that seek an optimal mix of mutually reinforcing biomedical, behavioral, and structural interventions to meet the needs of different groups
5. **Community-based testing:** HIV testing that takes place in non–health care settings, such as through community-based organizations, mobile HIV testing, home-based testing, schools, workplace, testing events or campaigns, and outreach activities
6. **Community-based interventions:** HIV interventions that are targeted at levels higher than the individual (e.g., neighborhood, large subgroups of the community), often using media, schools, and/or community organizations with significant reach within a community, and often involving the community in the development of the interventions
7. **Cost evaluation:** A comparison of the costs and health effects of an intervention to assess the extent to which it can be regarded as providing value for money; informs decision makers who have to determine where to allocate limited health care resources
8. **Dissemination:** The targeted distribution of information and intervention materials to a specific public health or clinical practice audience to spread knowledge and the associated evidence-based interventions
9. **Heterosexual sex:** The practice of engaging in anal, oral, or vaginal intercourse with persons of the opposite gender.
10. **HIV testing:** A test that determines whether a persons is infected with HIV; some HIV tests check for antibodies that your immune system produces in reaction to HIV infection, other HIV tests look for evidence of the virus itself
11. **Implementation science:** The study of methods to promote the integration of research findings and evidence into health care policy and practice; seeks to understand the behavior of health care professionals and other stakeholders as a key variable in the sustainable uptake, adoption, and implementation of evidence-based interventions
12. **Information-motivational-behavioral (IMB) principals:** Model that incorporate and address three components: information targets the cognitive domain by offering

knowledge to support the behavior change; motivation addresses the affective domain, providing the opening to develop a favorable attitude toward the new behavior, and tapping into existing support systems to enhance motivation; behavior addresses the psychomotor domain, with return demonstrations and practice

13. **Injection drug use (IDU):** Dermic needle and syringe; also called intravenous drug use
14. **Linkage to care and treatment services:** Attendance at first medical appointment with a health care provider within 90 days of diagnosis
15. **Men who have sex with men (MSM):** Men who engage in anal or oral intercourse with persons of the same gender, regardless of how they identify themselves (gay, bisexual, homosexual)
16. **Pre-exposure prophylaxis (PrEP):** The prevention of acquisition of HIV through use of antiretroviral (ARV) agents before potential exposure to HIV by taking a pill every day
17. **Prevention of mother-to-child transmission (PMTCT):** Interventions to prevent transmission of HIV from a mother living with HIV to her infant during pregnancy, labor, and delivery, or during breastfeeding
18. **Sex worker:** A person who engages in the use of sexual activity for income or employment or for nonmonetary items such as food, drugs, or shelter
19. **Social determinants:** The conditions in which people are born, grow, work, live, and age, and the wider set of forces and systems shaping the conditions of daily life, including economic policies and systems, development agendas, social norms, social policies, and political systems
20. **Social ecological:** A model that considers the complex interplay between individual, relationship, community, and societal factors, allowing us to understand the range of factors that put persons at risk for HIV, for example, or protect them from acquiring HIV
21. **Structural interventions:** Interventions that address pervasive social, cultural, economic, and political factors, such as stigma, discrimination, gender inequality, and income disparities
22. **Transgendered:** Persons whose gender identity does not conform to a binary classification of gender based on biological sex, external genitalia, or sex assigned at birth; includes gender-nonconforming people with identities beyond the gender binary who self-identify as male-to-female or transgender women; female-to-male or transgender men; two-spirit; and people who self-identify simply as women or men
23. **Treatment as prevention (TasP):** HIV prevention methods that use antiretroviral treatment (ART) to decrease the risk of HIV transmission
24. **Voluntary medical male circumcision (VMMC):** Surgical removal of the foreskin—the retractable fold of tissue that covers the head of the penis—in order to reduce susceptibility to HIV infection

REVIEW QUESTIONS

1. Explain why HIV is witnessing a spike in some geographies. What are the primary drivers of this increasing prevalence?
2. Which HIV prevention approaches or combination of approaches have been found effective for a generalized epidemic? A concentrated epidemic?
3. Which HIV prevention approaches have been effective for various populations: general population, men who have sex with men, injection drug users, HIV-positive persons?
4. Analyze the different prevention approaches in terms of dissemination and implementation. Consider uptake among different populations and regions and technical capacity, settings with limited resources, and cost effectiveness.
5. Why does HIV prevention and care merit continued significant resource allocation in light of other infectious diseases competing for resources?

References

Abroms, L. C., & Maibach, E. W. (2008). The effectiveness of mass communication to change public behavior. *Annual Review of Public Health, 29*, 219–234. doi: 10.1146/annurev.publhealth.29.020907.090824

Abu-Raddad, L. J. (2010). *Characterizing the HIV/AIDS epidemic in the Middle East and North Africa: Time for strategic action.* Washington, DC: World Bank.

Aidala, A., Cross, J. E., Stall, R., Harre, D., & Sumartojo, E. (2005). Housing status and HIV risk behaviors: Implications for prevention and policy. *AIDS and Behavior, 9*, 251–265. doi: DOI 10.1007/s10461–005–9000–7

AIDS2031 Costs and Financing Working Group (2010). *Costs and choices: Fighting the long-term fight against AIDS.* Washington, DC: Results for Development Institute.

Albarracin, D., Gillette, J. C., Earl, A. N., Glasman, L. R., Durantini, M. R., & Ho, M-H. (2005). A text of major assumptions about behavior change: A comprehensive look at the effects of passive and active HIV-prevention interventions since the beginning of the epidemic. *Psychological Bulletin, 131 (6),* 857-897.

Attia, S., Egger, M., Muller, M., Zwahlen, M., & Low, N. (2009). Sexual transmission of HIV according to viral load and antiretroviral therapy: Systematic review and meta-analysis. *AIDS, 23*, 1397–1404. doi: 10.1097/Qad.0b013e32832b7dca

Baeten, J. M., Donnell, D., Ndase, P., Mugo, N. R., Campbell, J. D., Wangisi, J., … Celum, C.; Partners PrEP Study Team. (2012). Antiretroviral prophylaxis for HIV prevention in heterosexual men and women. *New England Journal of Medicine, 367*(5), 399–410. doi: 10.1056/NEJMoa1108524

Bailey, R. C., Moses, S., Parker, C. B., Agot, K., Maclean, I., Krieger, J. N., ... Ninya-Achola, J. O. (2007). Male circumcision for HIV prevention in young men in Kisumu, Kenya: A randomised controlled trial. *Lancet, 369,* 643–656. doi: 10.1016/S0140–6736(07)60312–2

Baral, S., Kizub, D., Masenior, N. F., Peryskina, A., Stachowiak, J., Stibich, M., ... Beyrer, C. (2010). Male sex workers in Moscow, Russia: A pilot study of demographics, substance use patterns, and prevalence of HIV-1 and sexually transmitted infections. *AIDS Care, 22,* 112–118. doi: 10.1080/09540120903012551

Bernard, D., Kippax, S., & Baxter, D. (2008). Effective partnership and adequate investment underpin a successful response: key factors in dealing with HIV increases. *Sexual Health, 5,* 193–201. doi: 10.1071/Sh07078

Beyrer, C. (2011). *The global HIV epidemics among men who have sex with men.* Washington, DC: World Bank. Retrieved from http://siteresources.worldbank.org/INTHIVAIDS/Resources/375798-1103037153392/MSMReport.pdf

Blumenthal, D., DiClemente, R. J., Braithwaite, R. L., & Smith, S. (2013). *Community-based participatory health research: Issues, methods, and translation to practice.* New York, NY: Springer.

Brahmam, G. N. V., Kodavallaa, V., Rajkumar, H., Rachakulla, H. K., Kallam, S., Myakala, S. P., ... Paranjape, R. S.; IBBA Study Team. (2008). Sexual practices, HIV and sexually transmitted infections among self-identified men who have sex with men in four high HIV prevalence states of India. *AIDS, 22,* S45–S57. doi: 10.1097/01.aids.0000343763.54831.15

Branson, B. M., Handsfield, H. H., Lampe, M. A., Janssen, R. S., Taylor, A. W., Lyss, S. B., & Clark, J. E. (2006). Revised recommendations for HIV testing of adults, adolescents, and pregnant women in health-care settings. *Morbidity and Mortality Weekly Report: Recommendations and Reports, 55*(RR–14), 1–17.

Brown, C. H., Mohr, D. C., Gallo, C. G., Mader, C., Palinkas, L., Wingood, G., ... Jacobs, C. (2013). A computational future for preventing HIV in minority communities: How advanced technology can improve implementation of effective programs. *Journal of Acquired Immune Deficiency Syndromes, 63*(Suppl. 1), S72–S84. doi: 10.1097/QAI.0b013e31829372bd

Burton, J., Darbes, L. A., & Operario, D. (2010). Couples-focused behavioral interventions for prevention of HIV: Systematic review of the state of evidence. *AIDS and Behavior, 14,* 1–10. doi: 10.1007/s10461–008–9471–4

Callaghan, M., Ford, N., & Schneider, H. (2010). A systematic review of task-shifting for HIV treatment and care in Africa. *Human Resources for Health, 8,* 8. doi: 10.1186/1478–4491–8–8

Care C. (2007). *CAREC annual report 2007.* Port of Spain: Caribbean Epidemiology Centre.

Castellsague, X., Bosch, F. X., Munoz, N., Meijer, C. J. L., Shah, K. V., de Sanjose, S., ... Eluf-Neto, J.; IARCM. (2002). Male circumcision, penile human papillomavirus infection, and cervical cancer in female partners. *New England Journal of Medicine, 346,* 1105–1112. doi: 10.1056/Nejmoa011688

Centers for Disease Control and Prevention. (2001). Revised guidelines for HIV counseling, testing, and referral. *Morbidity and Mortality Weekly Report: Recommendations and Reports, 50*(RR–19), 1–58.

Centers for Disease Control and Prevention. (2009). Incidence and diagnoses of HIV infection–Puerto Rico, 2006. *Morbidity and Mortality Weekly Report, 58*, 589–591.

Centers for Disease Control and Prevention. (2012). *PrEP: A new tool for HIV prevention.* Retrieved from http://www.cdc.gov/hiv/prep/pdf/PrEPfactsheet.pdf

Chillag, K., Bartholow, K., Cordeiro, J., Swanson, S., Patterson, J., Stebbins, S., … Sy, F. (2002). Factors affecting the delivery of HIV/AIDS prevention programs by community-based organizations. *AIDS Education and Prevention, 14*, 27–37. doi: 10.1521/aeap.14.4.27.23886

Cho, H., Hallfors, D. D., Mbai, I. I., Itindi, J., Milimo, B. W., Halpern, C. T., & Iritani, B. J. (2011). Keeping adolescent orphans in school to prevent human immunodeficiency virus infection: Evidence from a randomized controlled trial in Kenya. *Journal of Adolescent Health, 48*, 523–526. doi: 10.1016/j.jadohealth.2010.08.007

Choopanya, K., Martin, M., Suntharasamai, P., Sangkum, U., Mock, P. A., Leethochawalit, M., … Vanichseni, S.; Bangkok Tenofovir Study Group. (2013). Antiretroviral prophylaxis for HIV infection in injecting drug users in Bangkok, Thailand (the Bangkok Tenofovir Study): A randomised, double-blind, placebo-controlled phase 3 trial. *Lancet, 381*, 2083–2090. doi: 10.1016/S0140–6736(13)61127–7

Chow, E.P.F., Wilson, D. P., Zhang, J., Jing, J., & Zhang, L. (2011). Human immunodeficiency virus prevalence is increasing among men who have sex with men in China: Findings from a review and meta-analysis. *Sexually Transmitted Diseases, 38*(9), 845–857. doi: 10.1097/Olq.0b013e31821a4f43

Cohen, J. (2004). HIV/AIDS in India: Sonagachi sex workers stymie HIV. *Science, 304*, 506. doi: 10.1126/science.304.5670.506

Cohen, M. S., Chen, Y. Q., McCauley, M., Gamble, T., Hosseinipour, M. C., Kumarasamy, N., … Flemin, T. R.; Hptn 052 Study Team. (2011). Prevention of HIV-1 Infection with early antiretroviral therapy. *New England Journal of Medicine, 365*, 493–505. doi: 10.1056/Nejmoa1105243

DiClemente, R. J., Bradley, E., Davis, T. L., Brown, J. L., Ukuku, M., Sales, J. M., … Vanichseni, S.; Wingood, G. M. (2013). Adoption and implementation of a computer-delivered HIV/STD risk-reduction intervention for African American adolescent females seeking services at county health departments: Implementation optimization is urgently needed. *Journal of Acquired Immune Deficiency Syndromes, 63*(Suppl. 1), S66–S71. doi: 10.1097/QAI.0b013e318292014f

DiClemente, R. J., Salazar, L. F., & Crosby, R. A. (2007). A review of STD/HIV prevention interventions for adolescents: Sustaining effects using an ecological approach. *Journal of Pediatric Psychology, 32*, 888–906. doi: 10.1093/ipepsy/jsm056

Dieffenbach, C. W., & Fauci, A. S. (2009). Universal voluntary testing and treatment for prevention of HIV transmission. *Journal of the American Medical Association, 301*, 2380–2382. doi: 10.1001/jama.2009.828

Donnell, D., Baeten, J. M., Kiarie, J., Thomas, K. K., Stevens, W., Cohen, C. R., ... Transm, P. P. H. H. (2010). Heterosexual HIV-1 transmission after initiation of antiretroviral therapy: A prospective cohort analysis. *Lancet, 375*, 2092–2098. doi: 10.1016/S0140–6736(10)60705–2

Dunkle, K. L., Stephenson, R., Karita, E., Chomba, E., Kayitenkore, K., Vwalika, C., ... Allen, S. (2008). New heterosexually transmitted HIV infections in married or cohabiting couples in urban Zambia and Rwanda: an analysis of survey and clinical data. *Lancet, 371*, 2183–2191. doi: 10.1016/S0140–6736(08)60953–8

European Centre for Disease Prevention and Control & WHO Regional Office for Europe. (2010). *HIV/AIDS surveillance in Europe, 2009.* Stockholm: Author. Retrieved from http://ecdc.europa.eu/en/publications/Publications/101129_SUR_HIV_2009.pdf

Evans, C., & Lambert, H. (2008). Implementing community interventions for HIV prevention: Insights from project ethnography. *Social Science and Medicine, 66*(2), 467–478. doi: 10.1016/j.socscimed.2007.08.030

Ewart, C. K. (2009). Changing our unhealthy ways: Emerging perspectives from social action theory. In R. J. DiClemente, R. A. Crosby & M. Kegler (Eds.), *Emerging theories in health promotion research and practice: Strategies for enhancing public health* (2nd ed., pp. 359–392). San Francisco, CA: Jossey-Bass.

Exner, T. M., Seal, D. W., & Ehrhardt, A. A. (1997). A review of HIV interventions for at-risk women. *AIDS and Behavior, 1*, 93–124. doi: 10.1023/b:aibe.0000002972.61606.99

Flay, B. R., Snyder, F. J., & Petraitis, J. (2009). The theory of triadic influences. In R. J. DiClemente, R. A. Crosby, & M. Kegler (Eds.), *Emerging theories in health promotion research and practice: Strategies for enhancing public health* (2nd ed., pp. 451–510). San Francisco, CA: Jossey-Bass.

Ford, N., Calmy, A., & Mills, E. J. (2011). The first decade of antiretroviral therapy in Africa. *Globalization and Health, 7*, 33. doi: 10.1186/1744–8603–7–33

Foss, A. M., Hossain, M., Vickerman, P. T., & Watts, C. H. (2007). A systematic review of published evidence on intervention impact on condom use in sub-Saharan Africa and Asia. *Sexually Transmitted Infections, 83*, 510–516. doi: 10.1136/sti.2007.027144

French, P. P., Latka, M., Gollub, E. L., Rogers, C., Hoover, D. R., & Stein, Z. A. (2003). Use-effectiveness of the female versus male condom in preventing sexually transmitted disease in women. *Sexually Transmitted Diseases, 30*, 433–439. doi: 10.1097/00007435–200305000–00010

Gallo, M. F., Kilbourne-Brook, M., & Coffey, P. S. (2012). A review of the effectiveness and acceptability of the female condom for dual protection. *Sexual Health, 9*, 18–26. doi: 10.1071/Sh11037

Glasgow, R. E., Eckstein, E. T., & Eizarrad, M. K. (2013). Implementation science perspectives and opportunities for HIV/AIDS research: Integrating science, practice and policy. *Journal of Acquired Immune Deficiency Syndromes, 63*(Suppl. 1), S26–S31. doi: 10.1097/QAI.0b013e3182920286

Global Commission on HIV and the Law (2012). *Risks, rights, and health.* UN: New York.

Goosby, E. P. (2013). Is option B+ the best choice? *Lancet, 381,* 1272. doi: 10.1016/S0140-6736(13)60832-6

Grant, R. M., Lama, J. R., Anderson, P. L., McMahan, V., Liu, A. Y., Vargas, L., ... Glidden, D. V.; iPrEx Study Team. (2010). Preexposure chemoprophylaxis for HIV prevention in men who have sex with men. *New England Journal of Medicine, 363,* 2587–2599. doi: 10.1056/Nejmoa1011205

Gray, R. H., Kigozi, G., Serwadda, D., Makumbi, F., Nalugoda, F., Watya, S., ... Wawer, M. J. (2009). The effects of male circumcision on female partners' genital tract symptoms and vaginal infections in a randomized trial in Rakai, Uganda. *American Journal of Obstetrics and Gynecology, 200,* e41–e47. doi: 10.1016/j.ajog.2008.07.069

Gray, R. H., Kigozi, G., Serwadda, D., Makumbi, F., Watya, S., Nalugoda, F., ... Wawer, M. J. (2007). Male circumcision for HIV prevention in men in Rakai, Uganda: A randomised trial. *Lancet, 369,* 657–666. doi: 10.1016/S0140-6736(07)60313-4

Guadamuz, T. E., Wimonsate, W., Varangrat, A., Phanuphak, P., Jommaroeng, R., McNicholl, J. M., ... van Griensven, F. (2011). HIV prevalence, risk behavior, hormone use and surgical history among transgender persons in Thailand. *AIDS and Behavior, 15,* 650–658. doi: 10.1007/s10461-010-9850-5

Gupta, G. R., Parkhurst, J. O., Ogden, J. A., Aggleton, P., & Mahal, A. (2008). HIV prevention 4: Structural approaches to HIV prevention. *Lancet, 372,* 764–775. doi: 10.1016/S0140-6736(08)60887-9

Hallfors, D., Cho, H., Rusakaniko, S., Iritani, B., Mapfumo, J., & Halpern, C. (2011). Supporting adolescent orphan girls to stay in school as HIV risk prevention: Evidence from a randomized controlled trial in Zimbabwe. *American Journal of Public Health, 101,* 1082–1088. doi: 10.2105/Ajph.2010.300042

Huebner, D. M., & Perry, N. S. (2015). Do behavioral scientists really understand HIV-related sexual risk behavior? A systematic review of longitudinal and experimental studies predicting sexual behavior. *Archies of Sexual Behavior, 44,* 1915–1936.

Hovell, M., Wahlgren, D., & Adams, M. (2009). The logical and empirical basis for the behavioral ecological model. In R. J. DiClemente, R. A. Crosby, & M. Kegler (Eds.), *Emerging theories in health promotion research and practice: Strategies for enhancing public health* (2nd ed., pp. 414–450). San Francisco, CA: Jossey-Bass.

Khumalo-Sakutukwa, G., Morin, S. F., Fritz, K., Charlebois, E. D., van Rooyen, H., Chingono, A., ... Coates, T. J.; NIMS Project Accept Study Team. (2008). Project Accept (HPTN 043): A community-based intervention to reduce HIV incidence in populations at risk for HIV in sub-Saharan Africa and Thailand. *Journal of Acquired Immune Deficiency Syndromes, 49,* 422–431. doi: 10.1097/Qai.0b013e31818a6cb5

Kilmarx, P. H., & Mutasa-Apollo, T. (2013). Patching a leaky pipe: The cascade of HIV care. *Current Opinion in HIV and AIDS, 8,* 59–64. doi: 10.1097/Coh.0b013e32835b806e

Kim, J. C., Watts, C. H., Hargreaves, J. R., Ndhlovu, L. X., Phetla, G., Morison, L. A., … Pronyk, P. (2007). Understanding the impact of a microfinance-based intervention on women's empowerment and the reduction of intimate partner violence in South Africa. *American Journal of Public Health, 97*, 1794–1802. doi: 10.2105/Ajph.2006.095521

Kruglov, Y. V., Kobyshcha, Y. V., Salyuk, T., Varetska, O., Shakarishvili, A., & Saldanha, V. P. (2008). The most severe HIV epidemic in Europe: Ukraine's national HIV prevalence estimates for 2007. *Sexually Transmitted Infections, 84*, 137–141. Doi: 10.1136/sti.2008.031195

Latkin, C. A., Davey-Rothwell, M. A., Knowlton, A. R., Alexander, K. A., Williams, C. T., & Boodram, B. (2013). Social network approaches to recruitment, HIV prevention, medical care, and medication adherence. *Journal of Acquired Immune Deficiency Syndromes, 63*(Suppl. 1), S54–S58. Doi: 10.1097/QAI.0b013e3182928e2a

Lopez, L. M., Otterness, C., Chen, M., Steiner, M., & Gallo, M. F. (2013). Behavioral interventions for improving condom use for dual protection. *Cochrane Database of Systematic Reviews* (*10*), CD010662.pub2. Doi: 10.1002/14651858.

Lyles, C. M., Kay, L. S., Crepaz, N., Herbst, J. H., Passin, W. F., Kim, A. S., … Mullins, M. M. (2007). Best-evidence interventions: Findings from a systematic review of HIV behavioral interventions for US populations at high risk, 2000–2004. *American Journal of Public Health, 97*, 133–143. doi: 10.2105/Ajph.2005.076182

Maleche, A. (2015). SDG Series: Are SDGs the vehicle to end AIDS by 2030? Only if driven by human rights. *Health and Human Rights Journal*, September 17, 2015. Available at: http://www.hhrjournal.org/2015/09/sdg-series-are-sdgs-the-vehicle-to-end-aids-by-2030-only-if-driven-by-human-rights/

McLeroy, K. R., Bibeau, D., Steckler, A., & Glanz, K. (1988). An ecological perspective on health promotion programs. *Health Education and Behavior, 15*, 351–377.

McNairy, M. L., Cohen, M., & El-Sadr, W. M. (2013, January 13). Antiretroviral therapy for prevention is a combination strategy. *Current HIV/AIDS Reports*. [E-pub ahead of print]. doi: 10.1007/s11904–013–0152–1

Montanaro, E. A., & Bryan, A. D. (2014). Comparing theory-based condom interventions: Health Belief Model versus Theory of Planned Behavior. *Health Psychology, 33*(10), 1251-1260.

Morineau, G., Nugrahini, N., Riono, P., Nurhayati, Girault, P., Mustikawati, D. E., & Magnani, R. (2011). Sexual risk taking, STI and HIV prevalence among men who have sex with men in six Indonesian cities. *AIDS and Behavior, 15*, 1033–1044. doi: 10.1007/s10461–009–9590–6

Nakanjako, D., Kamya, M., Daniel, K., Mayanja-Kizza, H., Freers, J., Whalen, C., & Katabira, E. (2007). Acceptance of routine testing for HIV among adult patients at the medical emergency unit at a National Referral Hospital in Kampala, Uganda. *AIDS and Behavior, 11*, 753–758. doi: 10.1007/s10461–006–9180–9

National Centre in HIV Epidemiology and Clinical Research. (2010). *HIV/AIDS, viral hepatitis and sexually transmissible infections in Australia annual surveillance report, 2010.* Sydney: University of New South Wales. Retrieved from http://www.med.unsw.edu.au/nchecrweb.nsf/resources/SurvRep07/$file/ASR2010-rev1.pdf

National Institutes of Health. (2015). *Starting antiretroviral treatment early improves outcomes for HIV-infected individuals.* Retrieved from http://www.niaid.nih.gov/news/newsreleases/2015/Pages/START.aspx

Njeuhmeli, E., Forsythe, S., Reed, J., Opuni, M., Bollinger, L., Heard, N., … Hankins, C. (2011). Voluntary medical male circumcision: Modeling the impact and cost of expanding male circumcision for HIV prevention in Eastern and Southern Africa. *Plos Medicine, 8*(e1001132). doi: 10.1371/journal.pmed.1001132

Noar, S. M., & Zimmerman, R. S. (2005). Health behavior theory and cumulative knowledge regarding health behaviors: Are we moving in the right direction? *Health Education Research: Theory & Practice, 20(3),* 275-290.

Okware, S., Opio, A., Musinguzi, J., & Waibale, P. (2001). Fighting HIV/AIDS: Is success possible? *Bulletin of the World Health Organization, 79,* 1113–1120.

Padian, N. S., Buve, A., Balkus, J., Serwadda, D., & Cates, W. (2008). HIV prevention 2: Biomedical interventions to prevent HIV infection: Evidence, challenges, and way forward. *Lancet, 372,* 585–599. doi: 10.1016/S0140–6736(08)60885–5

Paltiel, A. D., Freedberg, K. A., Scott, C. A., Schackman, B. R., Losina, E., Wang, B. X., … Walensky, R. P. (2009). HIV preexposure prophylaxis in the United States: Impact on lifetime infection risk, clinical outcomes, and cost-effectiveness. *Clinical Infectious Diseases, 48,* 806–815. doi: 10.1086/597095

Pinkerton, S. D., & Abramson, P. R. (1997). Effectiveness of condoms in preventing HIV transmission. *Social Science and Medicine, 44* (9), 1303–1312. doi: 10.1016/S0277–9536(96)00258–4

Pronyk, P. M., Hargreaves, J. R., Kim, J. C., Morison, L. A., Phetla, G., Watts, C., … Porter, J. D. H. (2006). Effect of a structural intervention for the prevention of intimate-partner violence and HIV in rural South Africa: A cluster randomised trial. *Lancet, 368,* 1973–1983. doi: 10.1016/S0140–6736(06)69744–4

Pronyk, P. M., Harpham, T., Morison, L. A., Hargreaves, J. R., Kim, J. C., Phetla, G., … Porter, J. D. (2008). Is social capital associated with HIV risk in rural South Africa? *Social Science and Medicine, 66,* 1999–2010. doi: 10.1016/j.socscimed.2008.01.023

Pronyk, P. M., Kim, J. C., Abramsk, T., Phetla, G., Hargreaves, J. R., Morison, L. A., … Porter, J. D. H. (2008). A combined microfinance and training intervention can reduce HIV risk behaviour in young female participants. AIDS, *22,* 1659–1665. doi: 10.1097/qad.0b013e328307a040

Ray, M., Logan, R., Sterne, J. A. C., Hernandez-Diaz, S., Robins, J. M., Sabin, C., … Collaboration, H.-C. (2010). The effect of combined antiretroviral therapy on the overall mortality of HIV-infected individuals. *AIDS, 24,* 123–137. doi: 10.1097/Qad.0b013e3283324283

Rhodes, S. D., Duck, S., Alonzo, J., Ulloa, J. D., & Aronson, R. E. (2013). Using community-based participatory research to prevent HIV disparities:

Assumptions and opportunities identified by the Latino Partnership. *Journal of Acquired Immune Deficiency Syndromes, 63*(Suppl. 1), S32–S35. doi: 10.1097/QAI.0b013e3182920015

Rich, J. D., DiClemente, R. J., Levy, J., Lyda, K., Ruiz, M. S., Rosen, D. L., & Dumont, D.; Collaboration on HIV in Corrections Working Group. (2013). Correctional facilities as partners in reducing HIV disparities. *Journal of Acquired Immune Deficiency Syndromes, 63*(Suppl. 1), S49–S53. Doi: 10.1097/QAI.0b013e318292fe4c

Rosen, S., & Fox, M. P. (2011). Retention in HIV care between testing and treatment in sub-Saharan Africa: A systematic review. *Plos Medicine, 8.* doi: 10.1371/journal.pmed.1001056

Ross, D. A. (2010). Behavioural interventions to reduce HIV risk: What works? *Aids, 24,* S4–S14. doi: 10.1097/01.aids.0000390703.35642.89

Salazar, L. F., Bradley, E. L. P., Younge, S. N., Daluga, N. A., Crosby, R. A., Lang, D. L., & DiClemente, R. J. (2010). Applying ecological perspectives to adolescent sexual health in the United States: Rhetoric or reality? *Health Education Research, 25,* 552–562. doi: 10.1093/Her/Cyp065

Sanders, G. D., Anaya, H. D., Asch, S., Hoang, T., Golden, J. F., Bayoumi, A. M., & Owens, D. K. (2010). Cost-effectiveness of strategies to improve HIV testing and receipt of results: Economic analysis of a randomized controlled trial. *Journal of General Internal Medicine, 25,* 556–563. doi: 10.1007/s11606-010-1265-5

Schouten, E. J., Jahn, A., Midiani, D., Makombe, S. D., Mnthambala, A., Chirwa, Z., … Chimbwandira, F. (2011). Prevention of mother-to-child transmission of HIV and the health-related Millennium Development Goals: Time for a public health approach. *Lancet, 378,* 282–284. doi: 10.1016/S0140-6736(10)62303-3

Scott-Sheldon, L. A. J., Huedo-Medina, T. B., Warren, M. R., Johnson, B. T., & Carey, M. P. (2011). Efficacy of behavioral interventions to increase condom use and reduce sexually transmitted infections: A meta-analysis, 1991 to 2010. *Journal of Acquired Immune Deficiency Syndromes, 58,* 489–498. doi: 10.1097/Qai.0b013e31823554d7

Secretariat of the Pacific Community. (2010). *HIV epidemiological update for Pacific Island countries 2008 and 2009.* Retrieved from http://www.spc.int/hiv/index2.php?option=com_docman&task=doc_view&gid=399&Itemid=148

Seth, P., Wang, G., Collins, N. T., & Belcher, L. (2015). Identifying new positives and linkage to HIV medical care: 23 testing site types, United States, 2013. *MMWR Morbidity and Mortality Weekly Report, 64*(24), 663–667.

Sherman, S. G., German, D., Cheng, Y., Marks, M., & Bailey-Kloche, M. (2006). The evaluation of the JEWEL project: An innovative economic enhancement and HIV prevention intervention study targeting drug using women involved in prostitution. *AIDS Care, 18,* 1–11. doi: 10.1080/09540120500101625

Smith, K., Powers, K. A., Kashuba, A.D.M., & Cohen, M. S. (2011). HIV-1 treatment as prevention: The good, the bad, and the challenges. *Current Opinion in HIV and AIDS, 6,* 315–325. doi: 10.1097/Coh.0b013e32834788e7

Sobngwi-Tambekou, J., Taljaard, D., Lissouba, P., Zarca, K., Puren, A., Lagarde, E., & Auvert, B. (2009). Effect of HSV-2 serostatus on acquisition of HIV by young men: Results of a longitudinal study in Orange Farm, South Africa. *Journal of Infectious Diseases, 199,* 958–964. doi: 10.1086/597208

Sullivan, P. S., Grey, J. A., & Rosser, B. R. S. (2013). Emerging technologies for HIV prevention for MSM: What we've learned, and ways forward. *Journal of Acquired Immune Deficiency Syndromes, 63* (Suppl. 1), S102–S107. DOI: 10.1097/QAI.0b013e3182949e85

Sweat, M., Morin, S., Celentano, D., Mulawa, M., Singh, B., Mbwambo, J., ... Coates, T.; Project Accept Study Team. (2011). Community-based intervention to increase HIV testing and case detection in people aged 16–32 years in Tanzania, Zimbabwe, and Thailand (NIMH Project Accept, HPTN 043): A randomised study. *Lancet Infectious Diseases, 11,* 525–532. doi: 10.1016/S1473–3099(11)70060–3

Swendeman, D., Basu, I., Das, S., Jana, S., & Rotheram-Borus, M. J. (2009). Empowering sex workers in India to reduce vulnerability to HIV and sexually transmitted diseases. *Social Science and Medicine, 69,* 1157–1166. doi: 10.1016/j.socscimed.2009.07.035

Tan, J. Y., Huedo-Medina, T. B., Warren, M. R., Carey, M. P., & Johnson, B. T. (2012). A meta-analysis of the efficacy of HIV/AIDS prevention interventions in Asia, 1995–2009. *Social Science and Medicine, 75,* 676–687. doi: 10.1016/j.socscimed.2011.08.038

Thigpen, M. C., Kebaabetswe, P. M., Paxton, L. A., Smith, D. K., Rose, C. E., Segolodi, T. M., ... Grp, T. S. (2012). Antiretroviral preexposure prophylaxis for heterosexual HIV transmission in Botswana. *New England Journal of Medicine, 367,* 423–434. doi: 10.1056/Nejmoa1110711

Tobian, A.A.R., Serwadda, D., Quinn, T. C., Kigozi, G., Gravitt, P. E., Laeyendecker, O., ... Gray, R. H. (2009). Male circumcision for the prevention of HSV-2 and HPV infections and syphilis. *New England Journal of Medicine, 360,* 1298–1309. doi: 10.1056/Nejmoa0802556

Tomlinson, R. (2010). *Resolving to save lives: HIV/AIDS prevalence among MSM in the anglophone Caribbean and OAS Resolutions 2435 and 2504.* Paper presented at the AIDS 2010XVIII International AIDS Conference, Vienna, Austria.

Townsend, L., Mathews, C., & Zembe, Y. (2013). A systematic review of behavioral interventions to prevent HIV infection and transmission among heterosexual, adult men in low-and middle-income countries. *Prevention Science, 14,* 88–105. doi: 10.1007/s11121–012–0300–7

UN. (2015). Transforming Our World: *The 2030 Agenda for Global Action.* New York, NY: UN. Available at: https://sustainabledevelopment.un.org/content/documents/7891Transforming%20Our%20World.pdf;

UNAIDS. (2011). *Global HIV/AIDS response: Epidemic update and health sector progress towards universal access.* Retrieved from http://www.unaids.org/en/media/unaids/contentassets/documents/unaidspublication/2011/20111130_ua_report_en.pdf

UNAIDS. (2012a). *UNAIDS report on the global AIDS epidemic.* Retrieved from http://www.unaids.org/en/media/unaids/contentassets/documents/epidemiology/2012/gr2012/20121120_UNAIDS_Global_Report_2012_with_annexes_en.pdf

UNAIDS. (2012b). *Key programmes to reduce stigma and discrimination and increase access to justice in national HIV responses.* Available at: http://www.unaids.org/en/resources/documents/2012/Key_Human_Rights_Programmes

UNAIDS. (2013). *Global report: UNAIDS report on the global AIDS epidemic 2013.* Retrieved from http://www.unaids.org/sites/default/files/media_asset/UNAIDS_Global_Report_2013_en_1.pdf

UNAIDS. (2015). *How AIDS changed everything.* Retrieved from http://www.unaids.org/sites/default/files/media_asset/MDG6Report_en.pdf

UNAIDS and Lancet Commission. (2015). *Defeating AIDS, advancing global health.* London, UK: *The Lancet.* Available: http://www.thelancet.com/journals/lancet/article/PIIS0140-6736%2815%2960658-4/abstract

UNAIDS/WHO/SACEMA Expert Group on Modelling the Impact and Cost of Male Circumcision for HIV Prevention (2009). Male circumcision for HIV prevention in high HIV prevalence settings: What can mathematical modelling contribute to informed decision making? *Plos Medicine, 6,* e1000109. doi: 10.1371/journal.pmed.1000109

US Public Health Service. (2014). *Preexposure prophylaxis for the prevention of HIV infection in the United States—2014 clinical practice guideline.* Retrieved from http://www.cdc.gov/hiv/pdf/PrEPguidelines2014.pdf

van der Straten, A., Van Damme, L., Haberer, J. E., & Bangsberg, D. R. (2012). Unraveling the divergent results of pre-exposure prophylaxis trials for HIV prevention. *Aids, 26,* F13–F19. doi: 10.1097/Qad.0b013e3283522272

van Griensven, F., van Wijngaarden, J.W.D., Baral, S., & Grulich, A. (2009). The global epidemic of HIV infection among men who have sex with men. *Current Opinion in HIV and AIDS, 4,* 300–307. doi: 10.1097/Coh.0b013e32832c3bb3

Wawer, M. J., Makumbi, F., Kigozi, G., Serwadda, D., Watya, S., Nalugoda, F., … Gray, R. H. (2009). Circumcision in HIV-infected men and its effect on HIV transmission to female partners in Rakai, Uganda: A randomised controlled trial. *Lancet, 374,* 229–237. doi: 10.1016/S0140–6736(09)60998–3

Weiss, H. A., Dickson, K. E., Agot, K., & Hankins, C. A. (2010). Male circumcision for HIV prevention: Current research and programmatic issues. *AIDS, 24,* S61–S69. doi: 10.1097/01.aids.0000390708.66136.f4

Weiss, H. A., Halperin, D., Bailey, R. C., Hayes, R. J., Schmid, G., & Hankins, C. A. (2008). Male circumcision for HIV prevention: from evidence to action? *AIDS, 22,* 567–574. doi: 10.1097/QAD.0b013e3282f3f406

Weiss, H. A., Hankins, C. A., & Dickson, K. (2009). Male circumcision and risk of HIV infection in women: A systematic review and meta-analysis. *Lancet Infectious Diseases, 9,* 669–677.

Weller, S. C., & Davis-Beaty, K. (2002). Condom effectiveness in reducing heterosexual HIV transmission (review). *Cochrane Database of Systematic Reviews (1),* CD003255. doi: 10.1002/14651858.CD003255

Williams, B. G., Lloyd-Smith, J. O., Gouws, E., Hankins, C., Getz, W. M., Hargrove, J., ... Auvert, B. (2006). The potential impact of male circumcision on HIV in sub-Saharan Africa. *Plos Medicine, 3,* 1032–1040. doi: 10.1371/journal.pmed.0030262

Wingood, G. M., & DiClemente, R. J. (1996). HIV sexual risk reduction interventions for women: A review. *American Journal of Preventive Medicine, 12,* 209–217.

Wingood, G. M., Reddy, P., Lang, D. L., Saleh-Onoya, D., Braxton, N., Sifunda, S., & DiClemente, R. J. (2013). Efficacy of SISTA South Africa on sexual behavior, HIV stigma and relationship control among isiXhosa women in the Western Cape Province, South Africa: Results of a randomized controlled trial. *Journal of Acquired Immune Deficiency Syndromes, 63* (Suppl. 1), S59–S65.

Wingood, G. M., Robinson, L. S., & Braxton, N. D. (2013). Comparative effectiveness of a faith-based HIV intervention for African American women: Importance of enhancing religious social capital. *American Journal of Public Health.*

Wingood, G. M., Rubtsova, A., DiClemente, R. J., Metzger, D., & Blank, M. (2013). A new paradigm for optimizing HIV intervention synergy: The role of interdependence in integrating HIV prevention interventions. *Journal of Acquired Immune Deficiency Syndromes, 63* (Suppl. 1), S108–S113. doi: 10.1097/QAI.0b013e318291fff4

World Health Organization. (2010). *Antiretroviral drugs for treating pregnant women and preventing HIV infection in infants: Recommendations for a public health approach; 2010 version.* Retrieved from http://whqlibdoc.who.int/publications/2010/9789241599818_eng.pdf

World Health Organization. (2012). *Programmatic update: Use of antiretroviral drugs for treating pregnant women and preventing HIV infection in infants.* Retrieved from http://www.who.int/hiv/PMTCT_update.pdf

World Health Organization. (2013). *Consolidated guidelines on the use of antiretroviral drugs for treating and preventing HIV infection.* Retrieved from http://www.who.int/hiv/pub/guidelines/arv2013/download/en/

World Health Organization. (2014). *Consolidated guidelines on HIV prevention, diagnosis, treatment and care for key populations.* Retrieved from http://www.who.int/hiv/pub/guidelines/keypopulations/en/

World Health Organization, UNICEF, & UNAIDS. (2011). *Progress report 2011: Global HIV/AIDS response. Epidemic update and health sector progress towards universal access.* Retrieved from http://whqlibdoc.who.int/publications/2011/9789241502986_eng.pdf

Yu, B. N., Wang, X. A., Yu, F., Wang, J., & Blanchard, J. (2011). An exploratory survey of male sex workers and HIV risk in an urban area of southwest China. *Sexually Transmitted Infections, 87,* A67–A68. doi: 10.1136/sextrans-2011–050109.100

CHAPTER 12

COMMUNITY-BASED RISK COMMUNICATION IN EPIDEMICS AND EMERGING DISEASE SETTINGS

Renata Schiavo, Karen M. Hilyard, and Ewart C. Skinner

LEARNING OBJECTIVES

By the end of this chapter, the reader should be able to:

- **Define community-based risk communication interventions in epidemics and emerging disease settings**
- **Discuss theory, practice, and interrelationships with other risk communication areas**
- **Provide examples of effective community-based interventions, their impact on behavioral and social results, and ultimately, on public and patient health outcomes**
- **Describe strategic planning frameworks for health risk communication that support and allow the integration of community-based interventions with other communication areas and media**
- **Summarize trends in community-based interventions that seek to be inclusive of vulnerable, underserved, and other high-risk populations**

Never, as in our times, have we had both many new challenges as well as new lessons and tools to communicate about health risk within **epidemics** (a widespread occurrence of an infectious disease in a community at a specific time that exceeds what would be normally expected from the disease occurrence) and **emerging disease** (a disease that has "appeared in a population for the first time, or that may have existed previously but is rapidly increasing in incidence or geographic range," World Health Organization [WHO], 2013) settings. Recent public health emergencies—including the 2001 anthrax crisis in the United States, the SARS epidemic, the 2009 H1N1 influenza **pandemic**, and the 2014–2015 Ebola epidemic—have highlighted the importance of communication preparedness and response across different sectors, audiences, and stakeholders (Blanchard et al., 2005; Schiavo, 2009a, 2009b, 2013, 2014; Schiavo, Leung, & Brown, 2014).

Risk communication can be defined as "an interactive process of exchange of information and opinion among individual, groups, and institutions" (US Department of Health and Human Services [DHHS], 2002) that results in "the dissemination of individual and population health risk information" (US [DHHS], 2005, 11–13) and, ultimately, leads to short-term and long-term behavioral and social results that are critical to preventing and mitigating the impact of epidemics and emerging disease outbreaks. Communicating about health risk is grounded within key health communication principles, theories, and planning models (Schiavo, 2013) and is one of health communication's key focus areas in a variety of international settings. For example, Healthy People 2020, the US public health agenda for one decade, includes specific objectives for risk communication so that the public's health would be protected via the use of best practices in this field (DHHS, 2015). Similarly, the World Health Organization, UNICEF, and many other international organizations have compiled a number of resources and guidelines on health risk communication. In recent years, risk communication has emerged at the intersection of crisis, risk, and public health emergency communication (Centers for Disease Control and Prevention [CDC], 2009, 2011; Reynolds, 2005; Reynolds & Seeger, 2005).

Within this context, community mobilization and citizen engagement have emerged as key areas of research and practice and, ultimately, critical components of participatory communication processes that address cultural values, social norms, beliefs, attitudes, needs, preferences, and community-specific obstacles that influence the adoption and sustainability (or lack thereof) of disease mitigation measures among different groups and populations (Paek et al., 2010; Reynolds, 2005; Schiavo, 2009a, 2009b, 2013, 2014). Moreover, community mobilization and citizen engagement have been credited as a strategy for providing additional community and public services during epidemics and disease outbreaks and to secure the buy-in of key stakeholders and average citizens on key mitigation measures (Communication Initiative, 2008; Palen, Hilts, & Liu, 2007; Schiavo, 2009b, 2013, 2014; Schoch-Spana et al., 2006). Several fields of theory and practice as well as strategic planning frameworks that are used in health risk communication and/or public health emergency communication, also support a community-based focus in integration with other communication areas and media (Health Communication Partnership, 2003; Hosein, Parks, & Schiavo, 2009; UNICEF, 2013; WHO, 2004a, b, 2012; Schiavo, 2013, 2014; Gamhewage, 2015) This chapter provides an overview of community-based risk communication, including its theoretical and strategic foundation, lessons learned from past epidemics and disease outbreaks, planning frameworks, and future directions.

A Theory-Driven Participatory Approach

A **participatory approach to communication** includes two-way interaction with the community at every step of the risk mitigation process, even from the point of determining what health issues should be addressed, and why. Participation is both a goal and a tool. This approach differs from the typical **top-down approach** in which public health indicators and their economic implications drive resource allocation and programming decisions. For example, top-down decision-making in a developing country about an emerging disease being transmitted from livestock to humans might depend on surveillance by hospitals or health agencies at an institutional level. Government economists might recommend culling entire herds as the most cost-effective mitigation tool. Alternatively, a **bottom-up approach** might encourage community and stakeholder participation, and for example, consult caretakers of herds, which in some countries might include predominantly women and children. Not only might these less powerful players offer faster and more sensitive monitoring of the emerging disease situation than institutional agents, but they might also propose less disruptive policy recommendations, such as isolating or euthanizing sick animals, not culling whole herds (Tufte & Mefalopulos, 2009).

Participatory risk communication not only acknowledges the expertise and problem-solving ability of community members, but sees them in the context of a larger **social-ecological model** (see Bronfenbrenner, 1992, 1981) in which individuals, communities, institutions, and policies are interdependently linked and nested within each other.

Initial two-way communication with the community can and should include the evaluation of health statistics and data on knowledge, attitudes, behaviors, and intentions, but it should also include open-ended dialogue in which other issues, perhaps unknown to the researcher or practitioner, may surface. More traditional communication methods typically do not involve the audience again until the message-testing or pilot-testing phase of program development, but a participatory approach involves the community in each step of the communication planning process: from the situation analysis stage, to the generation of goals, objectives, strategies, and tactics, on to message development and content creation and testing, and finally, to the implementation and evaluation phases. In development work, this is referred to as the **community action cycle** (Baum, MacDougall, & Smith, 2006).

Social marketing is a communication-related approach to behavior change used widely in public health that begins with an in-depth understanding of individuals in the intended community and then applies corporate marketing principles to achieve pro-social objectives (Grier & Bryant, 2005). Although not explicitly participatory, social marketing shares two characteristics with other participatory communication techniques: (1) it is a grassroots approach informed by the needs of the people whose behavior it seeks to change, and (2) it is situated in a social ecological framework in which context is just as important as communication. Based on intensive formative research with the audience, social marketers often seek change at policy and organizational levels as well as among communities and individuals. Reconceptualizing the initial stage of audience analysis as audience dialogue can shift social marketing to a more participatory model. Especially in the environmental movement, there are many case studies of community-based social marketing campaigns fully created and implemented by members of intended audiences (McKenzie-Mohr, 2013) Similarly, **integrated marketing communication** theory ("a concept of marketing communications planning that recognizes the added value of a comprehensive plan that evaluates the strategic roles of a variety of communication disciplines," Belch & Belch, 2004) has been used within the context of participatory program planning (Hosein et al., 2009).

When lines of communication are open in a community and all voices are encouraged to express themselves with the expectation their ideas will be acknowledged and considered, more solutions, and more creative ones, can emerge (Osborn, 1953). **Ideation theory,** based on studies of group idea generation or brainstorming, contends that the more diverse a group is, the more innovative the ideas and linkages it will generate (Thornburg, 1991; Woodman, Sawyer, & Griffin, 1993). Getting the maximum benefit of diversity requires intentionally bringing together individuals from very different walks of life, including vulnerable and underserved populations who are at the most risk of severe consequences during epidemics and emerging disease outbreaks. To be effective, however, brainstorming sessions should first encourage the free flow of ideas, even outlandish ones, without criticism, and only later engage in critical discussion of idea merit and feasibility. Potential pitfalls in group brainstorming can include unequal participation by some members, ideas being lost or forgotten amid a flood of input, or a particular session simply reaching a point of saturation or fatigue (Briggs & Reinig, 2007). To protect against these problems and maximize creative problem solving, ideation sessions should be an iterative process, with multiple interactions between different combinations of stakeholders. Specialists in **development communication** suggest that this *participatory approach,* in which communication is "not a vertical process of information transmission from the knowledgeable to the less knowledgeable, but rather a horizontal process of information exchange and interaction" (Morris, 2003, p. 226) may lead to more sustainable development solutions compared to a more traditional top-down *diffusion approach* to communication.

Indeed, without open channels for community-based communication, the true nature of community attitudes, opinions, and values may be impossible to ascertain. If people with minority opinions fear retaliation or isolation, they may be reluctant to voice their opinions, and as minority opinions are voiced less and less, people may self-censor, creating a *spiral of silence* (Noelle-Neumann, 1974) in which less-popular opinions cease to be expressed. Likewise, without open communication, individuals may be subject to cognitive biases about the opinions of others. Community leaders or public health professionals, for example, may assume that most people share their beliefs (**false consensus effect**) and base decisions on this inaccurate assessment (Marks & Miller, 1987). At the other end of the continuum, without open dialogue, individuals may erroneously think their beliefs or values are in the minority and therefore fail to take action, when in reality most people would support change. Sociology research indicates such pluralistic ignorance may have prolonged the existence of segregation in the United States and totalitarian rule in the Soviet Union, even when a majority of individuals supported ending those policies of oppression. Engaging in dialogue is a first step in overcoming these biases. Even after initial information is gathered from the community, communicators have an obligation to widen the circle and gather information from a larger sample to determine whether public opinion is being distorted by a *vocal minority* or *silent majority* (Mustafaraj et al., 2011).

Public health professionals as well as all other professionals and community leaders who should be engaged in multisectoral approaches to global risk communication must pay particular attention to dialogue and discourse when addressing issues of health disparity in traditionally marginalized communities. As seen in Table 12.1, below, Ford and Airhihenbuwa's (2010) application of critical race theory to public health emphasizes the importance of "centering in the margins," or beginning the conversation from the perspective of the minority group rather than from the position of the majority. As part of this process of "public health critical race praxis," practitioners should strive to get below the surface and understand deeper meanings, beliefs, and biases in the community, while also remaining cognizant of the influence their own biases and experiences have on the dialogue. Using planning frameworks that recognize the multidisciplinary nature of health-risk communication and the importance of integrating community-based interventions with other

Table 12.1 Definitions of Public Health and Selected Concepts of Critical Race Theory

Concept	Definition
Public Health	The art (i.e., practice) and science (i.e., research) of protecting and improving the health of communities
Centering in the margins	Making the perspectives of socially marginalized groups, rather than those of people belonging to the dominant race or culture, the central axis around which discourse on a topic revolves
Critical consciousness	Digging beneath the surface of information to develop deeper understandings of concepts, relationships, and personal biases
Experiential knowledge	Ways of knowing that result from critical analysis of one's personal experiences
Ordinariness	The nature of racism in post-civil rights society: that is, integral and normal rather than aberrational
Praxis	Iterative process by which the knowledge gained from theory, research, personal experiences, and practice inform one another
Primacy	Prioritizing the study of racial influences on outcomes
Race consciousness	Explicit acknowledgment of the workings of race and racism in social contexts or in one's personal life
Social construction of race	The endowment of a group or concept with a delineation, name, or reality based on historical, contextual, political, or other social considerations

Table 12 from Ford & Airhihenbuwa, 2010.
Source: Critical race theory concepts adapted from Delgado and Stefancic (2012).

communication areas and media is key to fostering a truly participatory approach to risk communication (see other relevant sections in this chapter for an overview of different planning frameworks for strategic health communication in risk settings).

From Theory to Practice: Lessons Learned From the Past

The 21st century has been marked by several epidemics, disease outbreaks, and other kinds of public health emergencies that have propelled the field of health risk communication (and more generally, health communication) to the forefront of global health (Schiavo, 2013, 2014). In the wake of the 2001 anthrax bioterrorist attack in the United States, communication "emerged as one of the most important public health sciences of the 21st century" as highlighted by U.S. Surgeon General David Satcher (Schiavo, 2009a, 2009b). Another important turning point in the evolution of risk communication was the 2002–2003 SARS epidemic, which not only represented a "wake up call about global interdependence" and the need for "coordination of all efforts" but also supported "the central role communication plays in improving public understanding and support of recommended individual, community, and social behaviors" to mitigate the impact of disease outbreaks (Schiavo, 2009, p. 49). Similarly, the 2009–2010 H1N1 influenza **pandemic** (a pandemic is "an epidemic occurring worldwide, or over a very wide area, crossing international boundaries and usually affecting a large number of people"; European Centre for Disease Prevention and Control, 2013; Last, Spasoff, Harris, & Thuriaux, 2001) showcased the importance of risk communication preparedness, active coordination, and monitoring, which in some countries led to expert recommendations about the importance of establishing operational risk communication units within local ministry of health (MOPH) (Ungchusak et al., 2012), so that preparedness and strategic coordination could be enhanced.

As part of this renewed emphasis on health risk communication, one of the key lessons learned from recent and past disease outbreaks and epidemics is about the importance of community leaders' engagement and participation in the risk communication process as well as the role of community members and social mobilization strategies in preparing and responding to public health emergencies. For example, a study examining lessons learned from the 2001 anthrax attack in the United States revealed that those who were exposed to anthrax—primarily US Postal Service workers from vulnerable and underserved groups such as African Americans and the hearing impaired—regarded the close involvement of the affected community as a key element of communication effectiveness (Blanchard et al., 2005). In their own words, participants in the Blanchard et al. (2005, p. 494) study suggested that:

- Communication efforts should closely involve people within the community of exposed individuals, preferably someone who is widely recognized and trusted and who can provide input as well serve as a spokesperson.... Preparedness efforts in the workplace should involve identification and training of such potential leaders.
- The community of exposed individuals should be involved in helping to devise plans for intervention, treatment, and communication.

Issues of trust, transparency, and increased cultural competence and/or communication effectiveness as associated with community engagement and participation were also highlighted by the US postal workers who participated in the study (Blanchard et al., 2005). Such lessons also resonate with key learnings from other disease outbreaks and epidemics within the context of improved behavioral and social outcomes as the result of integrated and multicomponent communication interventions. For example, during the 2004 Ebola outbreak in South Sudan (see Case Study 12.1 for a more detailed discussion), social mobilization teams established by WHO using the Communication for Behavioral Impact (COMBI) planning framework included local pastors, teachers, and community development workers and were instrumental in communicating with local communities and countering misconceptions both about the outbreak and recommended mitigation measures (Schiavo, 2009a, 2013; WHO, 2004). Similarly, a UNICEF-led communication for development (C4D) intervention to control and mitigate the impact of avian flu in Egypt also included community- and school-based components, which were considered the "cornerstones of the communication strategy to reach an estimated 4.8 million households and more than 3.8 million primary schoolchildren with the protective messages" (Schiavo, 2013, p. 470).

CASE STUDY 12.1 EBOLA CONTROL IN YAMBIO, SOUTH SUDAN

Case Context

In April/May 2004 a highly contagious Ebola haemorrhagic fever outbreak occurred in South Sudan. It was discovered that a 23-year-old radio technician had been hunting, had shot two baboons, and probably consumed the meat. Two weeks later he developed a fever, subsequently a rash, vomited, and passed bloody stools, all symptoms of the virus. He was taken to the hospital, where he died. His father, who had washed his body, also died. The virus spread through the young man's family and the hospital care community following an incubation period of 21 days. No specific treatment or vaccine was yet available.

First Communication Outbreak Response

A WHO Early Warning Alert and Response Network (EWARN) was activated:

- A human network for information gathering and surveillance was set up within 24–48 hours.
- A crisis management committee oversaw the response, with four technical subcommittees: case management, surveillance, social mobilization, and logistics and security.
- Committee members: leaders in health, education, religious organizations, and local government were engaged in outbreak response.
- External key agencies: WHO, UNICEF, CDC, Medicine Sans Frontiers (MSF) worked together.
- Local social mobilizers: teachers, pastors, volunteers with past outbreak volunteer experience were trained to engage local communities.
- Public communication: One vehicle with a public address system was put in use to reach local communities.

Rapid Situation Analysis

Local social mobilization committee support: WHO's Global Outbreak and Response Network (GOARN).

- First Step: Listening exercises:
  - What people thought, felt, and understood about Ebola.
  - What people were doing and not doing (and why) to protect themselves during the crisis.
  - Communication design: Reliance on key informant interviews and focus group discussions with key players and stakeholders in the community.
- Result of First Step: Outbreak awareness was high but there were obstacles:

- First, communication infrastructure such as radio and newspapers was lacking.
- Second, people were not convinced the outbreak was Ebola because in previous Ebola outbreaks more people had died.
- Third, people feared the hospital's isolation ward because of local unfounded rumors and therefore they hid sick loved ones from the surveillance teams.

Focus on Key Behaviors Strategy

First Step: Identify a limited number of preventive behaviors people could embrace to protect themselves and their families. It was extremely difficult to frame the behaviors as positive actions, however:

- Sick individuals were asked to contact Ebola control team within 24 hours from symptoms onset.
- Caregivers were asked to self-protect, to avoid direct contact with the bodily fluids of sick individuals.
- Traditional practices of sleeping next to and touching dead bodies were to be avoided in outbreak.
- Individuals were urged to wash hands regularly, thoroughly cook food, and refrain from shaking hands, sharing utensils, or picking up dead animals.

The COMBI Blend of Communication Interventions

1. Public advocacy/mobilizing decision makers and administrative structures

   Support was intensified when the commissioner asked chiefs and church leaders to specifically focus on addressing distressing rumors to remind people of the key behaviors.

2. Community mobilization

   Meetings were held with chiefs and traditional healers in areas with high numbers of potential cases. Ebola survivors spoke at these sessions. People were encouraged to ask questions. Households, marketplaces, and schools were provided with mobilization materials.

3. Personal selling (mobilizing local networks and advocates)

   Social mobilizers, wearing distinct T-shirts, provided training in basic verbal and nonverbal communication techniques, how to answer difficult questions, and using public address system. Leaflets were produced and distributed in the local language, and pastoral counseling from the local bishop was provided to families with multiple deaths.

4. Promotional materials and advertising

   Banners were placed in local market places, health centers, and churches as triggers to remind people to be vigilant during the crisis period.

Results and Evaluation

- In August, 2004, WHO declared the Yambio outbreak over. Response and containment considered rapid.
- The Yambio experience proved the communication value of rapid outbreak detection, local response capacity building, active community involvement, and coordination of specialized international assistance to outbreak's containment. Listening, participation, networking, a strategic mix of media, and local capacity building were all important.

Lessons Learned

- Effective community and partner engagement were the foundation for developing successful social mobilization and communication strategies and outbreak control interventions, which took into account local culture and existing obstacles.
- Risk communication should be a process with a specific outcome (outbreak control).
- An official ceremony should be held after an outbreak to acknowledge participants' efforts and local social mobilization partners and personnel, so that everyone involved could be formally rewarded for their commitment and dedication (e.g., via official certificates or other culturally friendly formats).
- Those who died should be remembered to facilitate community healing, honor people's lives, and discuss ways to prevent additional deaths (and potential obstacles) in the case of future outbreaks.

Sources: Odugleh-Kolev, A., 2012; WHO, 2004a, b, c.

Moreover, the engagement of community health workers and/or other kinds of social mobilization partners has proven to be effective in improving provider–patient communication and patient outcomes in a TB (tuberculosis) outbreak setting in Thailand (Thiam et al., 2007) and/or providing essential services that neither the government nor the private sector could supply as in the case of SARS in Canada (Communication Initiative, 2008).

Although community mobilization and citizen engagement are only select action areas of well-designed health risk communication interventions and need to be strategically integrated with other communication areas and media (e.g., policy communication, interpersonal communication, mass media, and new media communication, etc.) (Schiavo, 2013), community participation in all phases of intervention planning, implementation, and evaluation is likely to have a positive impact on disease control and mitigation. Among others, community participation has already been credited to have contributed to (a) "the development of key constituency groups made of citizens and community members who are invested in the success of emergency response and related interventions, and work toward achieving positive outcomes and behavioral results in their communities," and (b) "increased outreach to and inclusion of vulnerable and hard-to-reach populations" (Communication Initiative, 2008; Schiavo, 2009a, b; Schiavo, 2013, p. 213; Schoch-Spana, 2006). Box 12.1 highlights sample reasons that support the inclusion of vulnerable and underserved populations in all phases of the risk communication planning, implementation, and evaluation process. Finally, community participation is also supported and integrated within many strategic planning frameworks for health communication (including risk communication), including those we briefly discuss in the next session of this chapter.

BOX 12.1 INCLUDING VULNERABLE AND UNDERSERVED POPULATIONS IN HEALTH RISK COMMUNICATION PROCESSES: WHY DOES IT MATTER?

- Higher and group–specific risk for severe consequences and death as an outcome of epidemic and disease outbreaks
- Inclusiveness is grounded within human rights principles
- Heightened understanding of key social determinants and barriers influencing implementation and adoption of recommended disease mitigation measures and behaviors
- Full integration of culture, race, ethnicity, social status, social norms, language, and other key factors in health risk communication interventions
- Increased opportunities for:
  - Improving access to services and information
  - Meeting specific health literacy needs
  - Bridging digital divide
- Improved focus on diversity
- Community empowerment and sustainable development of long-term solutions for health risk communication preparedness and response
- Development of social networks and resources that may improve outcomes among vulnerable and underserved populations
- Improved compliance with mitigation measures and behaviors

Sources: Andrulis, Siddiqui, & Gantner, 2007; Bouye et al., 2009; Carter-Pokras et al., 2007; Vaughan and Tinker, 2009; Schiavo, 2009a, 2009b, 2013, 2014; Schiavo, Leung, & Brown, 2014.

Integrating With Other Communication Areas and Media

Epidemics and emerging disease outbreaks have significant impact on health and social outcomes as well as the political context in which different populations find themselves at the time of an emergency. Other authors have highlighted the importance of health, social, and political consequences of communicable diseases as central issues for future interventions and challenges "because of the enormous unfulfilled potential to reduce morbidity and mortality globally" (Schiavo, Leung, & Brown, 2014; Schlipköter & Flahault, 2010).

Because of the multicomponent nature of epidemics and disease outbreaks, it's important that risk communication interventions address different intervention levels (individual, community, social, political) and integrate different communication action areas (including community-based risk communication) to mirror how people speak about health and illness and make health decisions within and outside health risk settings (Schiavo, 2013, 2014). The integration of different communication areas and media is a key feature of health communication in the 21st century (Schiavo, 2013) and is supported by the Socio-Ecological Model/Perspective (SME/SSE) of public health (Gregson, 2001, Oetzel et al., 2006). In fact, "in stark contrast with individual-level approaches," ecological approaches like the SME/SSE "target multiple influences of health behaviors" (Crosby, Salazar, & Di Clemente, 2011, p. 231) and therefore rely on multiple communication areas and media (community mobilization, mass media, and new media communication, interpersonal communication, policy communication, etc.). There are several reasons that support an integrated approach to health risk communication, including the increased likelihood of:

- mirroring how people talk about health and illness in real-life settings;
- creating a resonance effect: "I heard it from many places" among at-risk groups and different populations;
- engaging multiple groups and stakeholders in the health issue, its potential risk and solutions by using communication areas and media that reflect their cultural preferences;
- increasing cost-effectiveness of all interventions because of greater synergy among different components of the risk communication intervention;
- expanding reach among key groups and stakeholders, and most important, at-risk groups;
- heightening the intervention's ability to recruit and engage multiple partners that may be more familiar with specific action areas or may prefer specific media (Schiavo, 2013).

This section includes examples of strategic frameworks and models that support and facilitate the integration of community-based risk communication with other communication areas and media as well as an overview of strategies to use new media and the building of online communities to support offline and community-based efforts.

Using Theory-Based Models

Numerous theory-driven communication models and programs are available to practitioners engaged in the control and prevention of disease outbreaks and epidemics as globally diseases emerge and re-emerge with alarming frequency. In such an environment there is a great need for "evidence based public health" interventions (Haveman-Nies, et al., 2010, p. 83) as well as the use of communication frameworks (Schiavo, 2013) that rely on "sound principles in the design of programs and interventions", and ultimately enable "quick and informed action to health risks and public health emergencies" (DHHS, 2015).

Epidemiology and Public Health Communication Models

There is a common epidemiological interest at the core of strategic public health communication planning models (Haveman-Nies et al., 2010) that recognizes that communication interventions ultimately should improve people's overall quality of life and reduce disease burden. At the same time, understanding communication theory, concepts, and strategy is a core responsibility in epidemiology (Sandman, 1991, p. 1). Applied communication skills and planning are required for successful field epidemiology training programs ([Academy for Educational Development, AED], 2009; Haveman-Nieset al., 2010) and are also reflected in social epidemiology, a field of study that incorporates psychosocial and other disease-causation factors in integration to **epidemiological causes** (Krieger, 2001) of health conditions.

The models described here are all drawn from and embrace theoretical and fundamental principles stemming from a variety of disciplines, from communication and epidemiology to social and behavioral sciences, health sciences, anthropology, sociology, and marketing. They are all to some extent ecological models, are all used in global settings, engage in social mobilization, and are concerned at some level with empowerment and participation—which are measurable indicators of behavior and social change—and all possess a heightened consciousness regarding program monitoring, process evaluation, and intervention adjustment. Although similar in many ways, they also present with many unique features in the way they approach behavioral and/or social change objectives and outcomes within and outside the context of risk communication.

Within this context, modernization theory and national development have emerged as dominant paradigms for change in the developing world after World War II both in academic and United Nations circles (Melkote & Steeves, 2001). "Communication" and "Health" were indispensable components of these paradigms and gave rise to Communication for Development (C4D) and Public Health Communication (PHC) programs as solutions to some problems in development. For example, rapid worldwide spread of SARS, H1N1, HIV/AIDS, and other epidemics drew attention to infectious disease outbreaks as global threats in a closely interconnected and interdependent world (Hufnagel, Brockmann, & Geisel, 2004, p. 1; Ritzer, 2011, p. 233). Thus, global health emergencies inspired new ways of looking at development (Cambridge, 2007; Melkote & Steeves, 2001), and induced new and innovative frameworks for tackling disease outbreak interventions in terms of reach, timeliness, and effectiveness (Food and Agriculture Organization of the United Nations [FAO], 2007).

Planning models are conceptual and "exist at a macroscopic level" (Crosby & Noar, 2011, p. S7). Model designers are communication impact architects who create and often oversee behavioral and social change intervention programs based on carefully designed conceptual frameworks. These frameworks are blueprints for building and improving intervention programs in disease outbreaks and in other health campaigns (Crosby & Noar, 2011, p. S7).

Some models for communication are widely used: P-PROCESS, PRECEDE-PROCEED, COMBI, the Five-Stage Community Organizing Model, and others such as the TELL-ME (2013) model are emerging. Additional models for risk communication are being developed in the wake of the 2014–2015 Ebola epidemic (Gamhewage, 2015) to integrate different communication areas and media in epidemics and emerging disease outbreak settings. This section discusses four strategic frameworks or theoretical approaches in public health communication that have also been used in emerging disease settings: Communication for Development (C4D); the P-PROCESS Model; PRECEDE-PROCEED Model (PPM); and COMBI.

Communication for Development

C4D began as a set of human rights–based principles that focused on sustainability, human rights, and community development but has gradually become a systematic, strategic, and result-oriented framework and process by also integrating within its human rights–based framework some of the precepts of other disciplines and models including social and behavioral sciences, health promotion, the social ecological model of health, and marketing, which itself based its theory "on a mix of elements from … anthropology, social psychology, behavioral science, and communication theory" (Fraser & Restrepo-Estrada, 1998, pp. 53, 54). C4D is arguably a broader framework than other models because of its wide adoption by UN agencies globally as well as the breadth of behavioral, social, development, and human rights–driven objectives its interventions seek to achieve. Cornerstones of C4D are (a) communication for coordination, (b) communication for promotion, (c) communication for implementation, and (d) communication for empowerment (McCall, 2011). Development scholar Vibbert Cambridge describes communication for development as "the systematic use of a social system's communication resources to stimulate, promote, and support human development" (2007, p. 181). C4D integrates principles and interventions as they relate to behavior change communication, advocacy, participation, community dialogue, communication for social change, democracy, and human rights, as well as capacity-building efforts within communication systems and other vital societal structures in seven UN organizations (McCall, 2011, p. ix).

The importance of C4D in epidemics and emerging disease settings is that within these settings process-related models often draw and/or mirror much of their overall history, inspiration, and structure from communication for development philosophies, principles, and practices and from the emerging sensibilities of C4D theorists, which are informed by public health needs, experiences, strategies, and theory building.

C4D projects have been implemented in influenza epidemics in Asia and the Pacific since 2005 through globally funded UNICEF programs, particularly in Mongolia (2007), and in Cambodia, where "Avian influenza provided the impetus for public health preparedness interventions and the development of a National Comprehensive Avian and Human Influenza plan in 2007"; and in 2012, UNICEF commissioned "a review of its C4D programming in relation to … preparedness and communicable diseases in Cambodia, Lao People's Democratic Republic, and Mongolia" (UNICEF, 2013).

More recently, C4D has been widely implemented in the control of the 2014–2015 Ebola epidemic across different countries, including Sierra Leone and Liberia (UNICEF, 2015a). Within this context, C4D interventions have been focusing on strategies that supported "a shift in the rituals and activities of entire population" (UNICEF 2015a), via community engagement, social mobilization, collaborative efforts with the rapid response teams, and other systems-changing strategies (UNICEF, 2015a).

For example, in Sierra Leone, C4D interventions were designed by UNICEF, which worked with the local Ministry of Health and Sanitation, to establish "46 local EVD [Ebola Virus Disease] Community Care Centers (CCCs) for rapid isolation, diagnosis, protection, and care," as well as "to engage and encourage communities and families to take personal responsibility for the … response, improve health seeking behaviors of self and others, and increase utilization of the CCCs" (UNICEF, 2015b). In Liberia, C4D strategies focused on (a) formalizing engagement with traditional and religious leaders, so they could provide psychosocial support to families affected by Ebola and "ensure safe and dignified burials"; (b) reinforcing community networks as well as "empowering and building the capacity of community members by providing them with access to the same tools, materials and training guides about EVD"; (c) support "synergy among partners working in the communities" to ensure "thorough geographic coverage, and avoided duplication"; and (d) "identifying and designing the role of social mobilization in the Rapid Response Teams by working with front-line workers in communities" (UNICEF 2015c). Overall, the role of communities in being able to "fend for themselves" was instrumental in the control of the Ebola crisis (UNICEF, 2015c).

P-PROCESS

The Johns Hopkins Bloomberg School of Public Health/Center for Communication Programs (CCP) and its partners in the USAID-supported Population Communication Services (PCS) project developed the P-PROCESS in 1982 as a tool for planning strategic, evidence-based communication programs (Health Communication Capacity Collaborative [HCCC], 2103, p. 3; UNICEF, 2008, p. 8). The P-PROCESS is a template practitioners use to recognize a health problem and identify, implement, and evaluate theory-sourced behavior (HCCC, 2013, p. 4). Updated in 2013, the P-PROCESS anticipates the influence of new technologies on communication, social norms, and individual decision-making behavior. It draws from "many other disciplines, including design theory, behavioral economics, social psychology and anthropology" (HCCC, 2013, p. 3).

The P-PROCESS is a five-step strategic plan: (1) inquire, (2) design strategy, (3) create and test, (4) mobilize and monitor, and (5) evaluate and evolve. Three important concepts (theory, participation, and capacity) guide the model's key steps. Capacity focuses on the obstacles that "inhibit people ... and organizations from realizing their developmental goals while enhancing their abilities ... to achieve measurable and sustainable results" (Regional AIDS Training Network [RATN], 2014). The P-PROCESS model includes community-wide capacity building and provides users with "a communication campaign framework for strategy development, project implementation, technical assistance, institution building, and training" (Valente, 2002, p. 10). The P-Process model has been used by the Center for Communication Programs (CCP) to develop avian and pandemic influenza communication strategies, including the Avian and Pandemic Influenza Strategic Communication Action Planner (ASAP) project in Japan (JHUCCP, 2011), and the Uganda-based Mango Tree Program in HIV prevention materials (Mango Tree, 2012).

PRECEDE-PROCEED

The PRECEDE-PROCEED Model (PPM) was developed from key concepts from the disciplines of epidemiology, social, behavioral, and educational sciences, health administration, medical care, family planning, psychology, communication theories of diffusion, and behavior adoption and education (Ahmad, 2005, p. 45; Green, 2013). It was first developed by L. W. Green in 1974 as a health process model that "originated as a cost-benefit (CB) evaluation framework ... tested systematically in a series of clinical and field trials that confirmed its utility and predictive validity" (Green 2013). The CB, from welfare economics, measures both positive and negative consequences of an intervention program (CDC, n.d.).

It is designed to give a clear and detailed overview of the planning process with attention to the "assessment and evaluation stages at the beginning and at the end of the planning process" (Haveman-Nies et al., 2010, p. 90). The PRECEDE-PROCEED framework is built on nine steps:

1. social assessments,
2. epidemiological assessment,
3. behavioral and environmental assessment,
4. educational and ecological assessment,
5. administrative and policy assessment,
6. implementation,
7. process evaluations,
8. impact evaluation, and
9. outcome evaluation (Crosby & Noar, 2011, p. 58).

PRECEDE-PROCEED pays special attention to predisposing, enabling, and reinforcing factors that impact behavior change (Ahmad, 2005, p. 45). Phillips, Rolley, and Davidson underscore the effectiveness of the process in "targeted nursing-led chronic illness interventions" in Australia (2012, p. 1). The model has also been used in prevention campaigns on domestic violence against high school girls in Iran (Ekhtiari et al., 2013), HIV/AIDS prevention in India (Banerjee & Jones, 2006), and in other contexts globally. It has been recognized as being flexible, comprehensive, and scalable (adaptable to project size), participatory, and evidence-based (Green & Ottoson, 2006, p. 9).

Communication for Behavioral Impact

COMBI is a very comprehensive and extensively used model. Developed by Everold Hosein (Hosein, 2011; WHO 2006, 2012) in 1994 at a summer institute at New York University with input from leading advertising and public relations agencies (e.g., Young & Rubicam, and Burson Marsteller/NY) and international organizations (The World Health Organization [WHO], United Nations Children's Fund [UNICEF], United Nation Population Fund [UNFPA]). It was informed by integrated marketing communication theory, private sector experience, and sensibility to global health issues (Hosein, 2011). In 2000 COMBI was adopted by WHO, where "social mobilization and communication specialists drew on three core fields: Public Health Communication; Social Mobilization; and Integrated Marketing Communication (IMC) to refine the model (Renganathan et al., 2005, p. 306). More recently COMBI was integrated at UNICEF in its Communication for Development (C4D) program (Water Supply & Sanitation Collaborative Council, 2013). Today, COMBI "integrates health education, information-education-communication (EC), community and social mobilization, consumer communication techniques and market research. All directed ... to specific, precise behavioral outcomes in health" (WHO, 2006, p. 7).

Before the program is launched, COMBI practitioners and planners need to consider two principal mantras that guide the COMBI process: "First: Do nothing—Produce no T-shirts, no posters, no leaflets, no videos, until you have set out clear, precise, specific behavioral objectives. Second: Do nothing—Produce no T-shirts, no posters, no leaflets, no videos, until you have successfully undertaken a situational market analysis in relation to those preliminary behavioral objectives" (Renganathan et al., 2005, p. 306, 310; WHO, 2006, p. 9). COMBI's situation (market) analysis is "a consumer-oriented" exploration of the factors influencing the attainment of the behavioral objectives that will inform the strategy and the communication mix" (WHO, 2006, p. 20). Practitioners then implement a 10-step process from within the COMBI Plan of Action. Also included in the Plan are five communicative action areas: 1. Administrative Mobilization/Advocacy/Public Relations, 2. Community Mobilization, 3. Personal selling (interpersonal communication), 4. Media/Advertising, and 5. Point of Service Promotion. These are integrated according to the needs and preferences of key groups and stakeholders as assessed via a participatory approach.

COMBI programs have reached at least "100 million people worldwide, and have affected the health and/or social behavior of an average of 60 percent of those individuals" (Hosein et al., 2009, p. 536), and with WHO and its partners have trained public health officials in more than fifty countries" (Hosein et al., 2009, p. 536, 537). COMBI has been successfully applied in scores of disease outbreaks: Ebola haemorrhagic fever in Yambio, South Sudan (2004) (see Case Study 12.1), Marburg haemorrhagic fever in Angola (2005), Asian influenza in Cambodia (2004), a measles outbreak in Fiji (2006) (WHO, 2012, pp. 85–100), as well as in the adoption of insecticide-treated bednets (ITNs) in Sudan's Blue Nile state (2006) (Elsheikh, 2007, p. 7).

Building New Media-Based Communities to Enhance Offline Efforts

Evolving technology and the latest generation of new media—often referred to as "Web 2.0"—provides "potential opportunities to engage people in health-related issues, stimulate an active role in their own health care, connect them with others and evidence-based interventions, and create social action focused on the social determinants of health disparities" (Gibbons et al., 2011, p. 78). Web 2.0 has the potential to greatly enhance community-based participatory risk communication by democratizing the production and distribution of media content, as well as broadening and speeding access to information. Many emerging technology platforms are also free or low cost to use and can improve the dissemination of information even in locations with relatively poor communication infrastructure, enabling public health officials to stretch resources.

Several categories of technology or media are already in use by public health communicators:

- environmental monitoring and passive collection of community-generated Web content;
- social media;
- mHealth.

For almost as long as the Internet has existed, public health communicators have been able to use discussion forums and blogs as listening posts through which they can monitor the environment and tap into public discourse on health issues. In emergency situations, these platforms can provide informational and therapeutic benefits to users and even help rescuers locate people in need of evacuation or other services (Macias, Hilyard, & Freimuth, 2009). This environmental monitoring remains an important tool for communicators, but the addition of Web analytics can reveal even more information and make the resulting data more valuable. For example, Google Flu Trends tracks searches by Web users for flu-related topics and symptoms. This de-identified but geographically pinpointed information can provide an accurate early indicator of disease trends, typically several days in advance of other surveillance that tracks patients only when they seek medical treatment (Ginsberg et al., 2008).

Similar analytic information is available for other search engines, website traffic, and social media posts. If this information is used not only by public health officials, but is also made available to the community, it can provide a foundation for dialogue about risk and for both community and individual behavior and decision making.

In addition to analytics and passive listening, engagement in social media takes Web 2.0 one step further. Social media create and sustain relationships by involving users in the collaborative creation of shareable content. Although Facebook and Twitter are the social media platforms that immediately come to mind for many, communicators should consider the full range of media available and how it is used: from blogs such as Tumblr to special interest platforms such as Meetup or LinkedIn, from Flickr, Instagram, and Pinterest for photos to Vine, Vimeo, and YouTube for video, to social bookmarking like Reddit, StumbleUpon, and Del.icio.us, to geolocation services like FourSquare, Gowalla, and Google Places, to Amazon or Ebay for customer reviews, comments sections for online newspapers or media outlets, to multiplayer online games like Everquest or Words with Friends, to virtual worlds like Second Life. Around the globe, other networks such as Renren, Bebo, Wer-kennt-wen, and Tuenti predominate (Jain, 2012). In an emerging health crisis or disaster, users in the community may be able to provide the first and most accurate eyewitness accounts, uploading photos, videos or geolocation information that illustrate the extent of the problem. Via this user-generated information in official communication, public health officials create a "relationship of exchange" (Veil, Buehner, & Palenchar, 2011, p. 114) that builds relationships and goodwill and may enhance the collection of field data. Dialogue between the public and public officials may also encourage more timely reporting of new developments and help to control rumors. Most of all, trusted relationships built on social media can reduce uncertainty in a crisis.

Social media are also a ready venue for mass messaging in a crisis, but only if people and organizations are already connected. Just as a cardinal rule of emergency risk communication is to develop relationships with community partners ahead of a crisis, so must social media relationships be developed as part of pre-crisis planning (Veil et al., 2011). In addition to connecting with members of the public, communicators should actively use social media to engage journalists from traditional media outlets, who themselves may reach nonusers of social media.

mHealth uses wireless technology to make data and applications "easily accessible by health workers through mobile devices such as mobile phones, smart phones, PDAs, laptops and tablet PCs" (Li et al., 2010, p. 3). At its simplest, mHealth can use mobile phones without Internet connectivity to send and receive short message service (SMS) or text messages. Text messages can often be sent with much lower signal strength than is required for a voice call, making them ideal for less-developed areas or for emergency situations when communication infrastructure is weakened or in high demand.

Rural St. Gabriel's Hospital in western Malawi is an example of the successful implementation of a very basic mHealth program (Li et al., 2010). St. Gabriel's serves a radius of 100 miles with only two doctors, and it depends on volunteer community health workers (CHWs) to deliver health services in isolated villages. Previously these CHWs might need to walk, bicycle, or travel by oxcart as far as 100 miles to communicate with the hospital, significantly slowing the exchange of medical information that could save lives, and inhibiting surveillance of emerging disease outbreaks. In 2008, the nonprofit now known as Medic Mobile (formerly Frontline SMS Medic) set up a system using recycled mobile phones and a single donated laptop to link St. Gabriel's hospital with CHWs not only for instantaneous one-on-one communication, but also to enable aggregation of health statistics for a big-picture overview of emerging medical situations. More than 50 mHealth programs are currently operating in 26 countries (Vital Wave Consulting, 2009) and with the number of mobile phones predicted to exceed the global population in 2014 ("World to Have More Cellphone Accounts Than People by 2014," 2013), the success of the text messaging system in Malawi could be replicated in many nations, reaching beyond hospitals, physicians, and health care workers to include patients and community groups in the conversation.

Public health agencies and NGOs can also create their own mobile applications, or apps, that can be used in the absence of Internet connectivity to interactively provide information to health care workers or members of the public. With sufficient infrastructure in place, such apps can generate real-time information in the other direction as well, providing health monitoring or geolocation information in emergency situations (Milošević, Shrove, & Jovanov, 2011). For example, in a pandemic, an interactive app might provide highly tailored local information to patients about when and where to seek medical treatment. In turn, information about the prevalence of symptoms in specific geographic areas—based on queries entered by users—could be collected and used to make decisions about where to deploy public health resources. If such apps include community members in their design, content creation, and data analysis, they can foster a community participatory exchange. This would be quite innovative given that the participation of community members and stakeholders, and ideally, the community at large, in the design, implementation, and evaluation of new media-based interventions is still a relatively new and emerging concept (see Box 12.2).

BOX 12.2 CAN SOCIAL MEDIA FACILITATE MORE PARTICIPATORY COMMUNICATION?

With its shareable, collaboratively generated content, and the ability to reach people in real time during an emerging pandemic, social media seems born to facilitate community participatory risk communication (Merchant, Elmer, & Lurie, 2011). It can be used not only simply to share experiences, but combined with video, audio, and geolocation capabilities, can help both authorities and citizens react quickly to developing emergencies, changing policy and behavior as events warrant. However, examples from the United States and China during the 2009 H1N1 "swine flu" pandemic show that social media's full potential has not yet been realized (Ding & Zhang, 2010).

Although China has no Facebook, no Twitter, and no YouTube, its vibrant social media scene includes more than an estimated 400 million users who are more active than those in other nations such as Japan and the United States ("China's Massive Web Audience Turns to Social, Mobile, Video," 2012; Chiu, Ip, & Silverman, 2012). Social media's popularity has grown despite tight monitoring by government censors, who sometimes remove messages that are perceived as subversive, or seek retribution against bloggers and editors (Ding & Zhang, 2010). In the early days of the H1N1 pandemic, China's Ministry of Health attempted to capitalize on social media's popularity by departing from its usual focus on one-way risk communication via mainstream media. The health ministry's new strategy, which included online surveys, discussion forums, and video interviews, was quickly outpaced by users of social media sites such as http://www.renren.com and aggregators such as http://www.sina.com. These sites circumvented government restrictions to offer anecdotal reports from Chinese people all over the world that sometimes challenged official communications about the pandemic. The ability to post comments and interact with bloggers led to vigorous bottom-up risk communication, but there was little documented impact on authorities, except in one case: when student bloggers contradicted official reports about the H1N1 death of a student who had been part of a mandatory military exercise in Beijing. Overwhelming questions and criticism from students eventually snowballed and were picked up by mainstream media, leading to disciplinary action against the military base and the university several months later. However, this policy impact was the exception rather than the rule and there was little explicit interaction between Chinese health authorities and student bloggers or other social media users.

In contrast, risk communicators at the US Centers for Disease Control and Prevention, actively used numerous social media platforms, including Twitter, Flickr, Facebook, and YouTube, to interact with audiences during the H1N1 pandemic. Using specially created widgets, podcasts, buttons, and badges, the CDC issued updates, guidelines, and prevention tips. Interactivity was encouraged and audience numbers rose sharply, including an increase from 2,700 to more than 370,000 Twitter followers. But though the public was able to comment on and circulate top-down government risk messages, the CDC's limited two-way approach did not explicitly involve social media users as partners in risk assessment or policy-making decisions. Even with a freer and more open social media environment than China's, US public health officials fell short of a truly participatory approach to pandemic risk communication (Ding & Zhang, 2010).

Linking top-down and bottom-up social media messages into a true exchange in future pandemics could not only help people respond to risks more quickly and more effectively, but as Merchant et al. (2011) suggest, would also serve to build social capital and community resilience, leading to a more participatory process of both communication and policymaking.

Yet, in designing new media-based interventions it's important to take into account that new media may not always be the preferred channel for risk communication interventions intended to reach and engage vulnerable and underserved populations because of limited health literacy and media literacy skills among these groups. In the past few years, the digital divide that once separated people with access to technology from those without has closed considerably. Indeed, in many communities, minority, disadvantaged, or vulnerable populations may not only have access to the Internet via mobile phones at rates that are indistinguishable from others, but are often the heaviest users of social media and text messaging (Fox, 2013). Increasingly, the issue is no longer access to the Internet; such a digital divide occurs primarily "because of a combination of technology access and quality, costs of Internet connectivity—which in some African countries may be hundreds of times higher than in the United States or most European countries (WHO, 2007)—and most important, media and health literacy" (Schiavo, 2013, p. 135). Moreover, although Internet and mobile use is widespread, many groups may not use it yet for exchanging health-related information. For example, although "social network sites are popular, they are used only sparingly for health updates and queries" (Fox, 2011).

Yet, according to the Pew Research Center's Internet & the American Life Project, such personal communication can be "the most important source of information for people making a day-to-day health decision ... not a website, or even a clinician, but another person who shares the same condition. As mobile, social tools spread throughout the population, people are connecting with each other. Why not harness those tools for health?" (Fox, 2012). However, health communicators must exercise caution so that use of the Internet does not exacerbate health disparities. Overdependence on peer-to-peer health communication could isolate people from clinicians and public health resources. There are also cultural differences in the way people seek and use information on the Internet, and navigating digital health information requires health literacy skills and computer literacy skills that many disadvantaged populations may lack: the ability to discern credible sources of information, to navigate websites effectively, and to process information on medical websites that are typically written at an advanced reading level (Viswanath & Kreuter, 2007). Developing new media-based interventions and tools via a participatory and community-driven approach may also result in increased health literacy and media literacy among disadvantaged groups and therefore may emerge as an effective strategy to continue to close the digital divide as it relates to risk communication settings.

Summary

This chapter summarizes key theories, planning frameworks, and lessons learned in support of the integration of participatory community-based risk communication interventions with other communication areas and media. In doing so, it also points to potential future directions, research questions, and action areas that may be instrumental in implementing such approach on a larger scale. These include the importance of capacity building at the local, national, and international levels; the development of local community and organizational champions who believe in the importance of social mobilization and community empowerment as part of intervention design, implementation, and evaluation; the potential of new and emerging technologies to build communities in support of offline efforts; and the role of global coordination efforts that yet give priority to local cultures, issues, needs, and preferences in risk communication preparedness and response.

KEY TERMS

1. **Bottom-up approach:** A participatory approach that engages community members and stakeholders and encourages participation and ownership in all phases of intervention design, implementation, and evaluation
2. **Communication:** An interactive process of exchange of information and opinion among individual, groups, and institutions
3. **Community action cycle:** A participatory approach that involves the community in each step of the communication planning process: from the situation analysis stage, to the generation of goals, objectives, strategies, and tactics, on to message development and content creation as well as pilot testing, and finally, to the implementation and evaluation phases
4. **Development communication:** A participatory approach, in which communication is not a vertical process of information transmission but rather a horizontal process of information exchange and interaction
5. **Emerging disease:** A disease that has appeared in a population for the first time or that may have existed previously but is rapidly increasing in incidence or geographic range
6. **Epidemics:** A widespread occurrence of an infectious disease in a community at a specific time that exceeds what would be normally expected from the disease occurrence
7. **Epidemiological causes:** An agent or activity that causes a specific health outcome.
8. **False consensus effect:** A misconception about public opinion that occurs when community leaders or public health professionals, for example, assume that most people share their beliefs
9. **Ideation theory:** A theory that is based on studies of group idea generation or brainstorming and contends that the more diverse a group is, the more innovative the ideas and linkages it will generate
10. **Integrated marketing communication:** A concept of marketing communications planning that recognizes the added value of a comprehensive plan that evaluates the strategic roles of a variety of communication disciplines

11. **mHealth:** The use of mobile and wireless technology for health-related interventions; to share data, information, and applications
12. **Pandemic:** An epidemic occurring worldwide, or over a very wide area, crossing international boundaries and usually affecting a large number of people
13. **Participatory approach to communication:** Two-way interaction with the community at every step of the risk mitigation process, even from the point of determining what health issues should be addressed, and why
14. **Risk communication:** An interactive process of exchange of information and opinion among individual, groups, and institutions that leads to short-term and long-term behavioral and social results that are critical to preventing and mitigating the impact of epidemics and emerging disease outbreaks
15. **Social-ecological model:** A framework for intervention design in which individuals, communities, institutions, and policies are interdependently linked and nested within each other
16. **Social marketing:** A communication-related approach to behavior change used widely in public health that begins with an in-depth understanding of individuals in the intended community, and then applies corporate marketing principles to achieve pro-social objectives
17. **Top-down approach:** An approach in which public health indicators and their economic implications drive resource allocation and programming decisions

REVIEW QUESTIONS

1. If you were an administrator in the Yambio Ebola outbreak, how would you address problems of capacity building? *Hint:* First, define capacity building.
2. What are the main differences and similarities in the four public health communication frameworks discussed in this chapter? Focus on their ongoing and/or potential applications in epidemics and emerging disease settings.
3. If you were a public health communication theorist and were asked the question: What is the meaning of the term "communication" to you? How would you answer the question?
4. What is a recent real-world example of risk communication? Identify and research such a case. Discuss lessons learned and key success factors in achieving outbreak control and/or

sustainable behavioral and social results that may prevent future disease outbreaks and epidemics.

5. What kind of community-based strategies and specific activities could be used to involve vulnerable and underserved populations in the design of risk communication interventions, including new media-based interventions? Reflect on recent experiences, case studies, and propose suitable strategies and activities.

References

Academy for Educational Development (AED). (2009). *Field epidemiology training program: Applied communication skills.* Retrieved from http://avianflu.aed.org/docs/FETP_Curri.pdf

Ahmad, J. S. (2005). Push and pull factors in changing health behavior: A theoretical framework. In M. Haider (Ed.), *Global public health communication: Challenges, perspectives, and strategies* (pp. 39–58). Sudbury, MA: Jones & Barlett.

Andrulis D. P., Siddiqui, N. J., and Gantner, J. L. (2007). Preparing racially and ethnically diverse communities for public health emergencies. *Health Affairs, 26*(5), 1269–1279.

Banerjee, P., and Jones, C.M.C. (2006). *Utilizing* the *PRECEDE-PROCEED Model as a theoretical framework for HIV/AIDS prevention programs in India.* Poster session presented at the meeting of the APHA Annual Meeting and Exposition. Boston, November 4–8.

Baum, F., MacDougall, C., & Smith, D. (2006). Participatory action research. *Journal of Epidemiology and Community Health, 60*(10), 854.

Belch, G., & Belch, M. (2004). *Advertising and promotion: An integrated marketing communication perspective* (6th ed.). Boston, MA: McGraw Hill.

Blanchard, J.C. Haywood, Y., Stein, B. D., Tanielian, T. L., Stoto, M., & Lurie, N. (2005). In their own words: Lessons learned from those exposed to anthrax. *American Journal of Public Health, 95*(3), 489–495.

Bouye, K., Truman, B., Hutchins, S., Richard, R., Brown, C., Guillory, J. A., & Rashid, J. (2009). Pandemic influenzaa preparedness and response among public-housing residents, single-parent families, and low-income populations. *American Journal of Public Health, 99*(S2), S287–S293.

Briggs, R. O., & Reinig, B. A. (2007). *Bounded ideation theory: A new model of the relationship between idea quantity and idea-quality during ideation.* Paper presented at the 40th Annual Hawaii International Conference on the System Sciences. Waikoloa, HI, January.

Bronfenbrenner, U. (1992). Six theories of child development: Revised formulations and current issues. In R. Vasta (Ed.), *Ecological systems theory* (pp. 187–249). London and Philadelphia: PA: Jessica Kingsley.

Bronfenbrenner, U. (1981). *The ecology of human development: Experiments by nature and design.* Cambridge, MA: Harvard University Press. Retrieved from https://books.google.com/books?id=8cf0FYm0jW0

Cambridge, V. C. (2007). Milestones in communication and national development. In Y. R. Kamalipour (Ed.), *Global communication* (pp. 181–200). Belmont, CA: Thomson Wadsworth.

Carter-Pokras, O., Zambrana, R. E., Mora, S. E., & Aaby, K. A. (2007). Emergency preparedness: Knowledge and perceptions of Latin American immigrants. *Journal of Health Care for the Poor and Underserved, 18*(2), 465–481.

Centers for Disease Control and Prevention. (2009). *Emergency risk communication CDCynergy.* Retrieved from http://www.orau.gov/cdcynergy/erc/default.htm

Centers for Disease Control and Prevention. (2011). *Crisis and Risk Communication Course (CERC).* Retrieved from http://emergency.cdc.gov/cerc/overview.asp

Centers for Disease Control and Prevention (n.d.). *Cost benefit analysis.* Retrieved from http://www.cdc.gov/owcd/eet/cba/PrintAll.html

China's massive web audience turns to social, mobile, video. (2012). Retrieved from http://www.emarketer.com/Article/Chinas-Massive-Web-Audience-Turns-Social-Mobile-Video/1008882

Chiu, C., Ip, C., & Silverman, A. (2012). Understanding social media in China. *McKinsey Quarterly.* Retrieved fromhttp://www.mckinsey.com/insights/marketing_sales/understanding_social_media_in_china

Communication Initiative. (2008). *The Drum Beat Issue 427.* Emergency Communication. Retrieved from http://www.comminit.com/global/drum_beat_427.html

Crosby, R., and Noar, S. M. (2011). What is a planning model? An introduction to PRECEDE-PROCEED. *Journal of Public Health Dentistry, 71, Suppl. 1:* S7–11

Ding, H., & Zhang, J. (2010). Social media and participatory risk communication during the H1N1 flu epidemic: A comparative study. *China Media Research, 6,* 80–90.

Crosby, R. A., Salazar, L. F., & Di Clemente, R. J. (2011). Ecological approaches in the new public health. In R. A. Crosby, L. F. Salazar, & R. J. Di Clemente (Eds.), *Health behavior theory for public health: Principles, foundations, and applications* (pp. 231–251). Sudbury, MA: Jones & Bartlett.

Delgado, R., & Stefancic, J. (2012). *Critical race theory: An introduction* (2nd ed.) New York, NY: New York University Press.

Ekhtiari, Y. S., Shojaeizadeh, D., Foroushani, A. R., Ghofranipour, F., & Ahmadi, B. (2013). The effect of an intervention based on the PRECEDE-PROCEED model on preventive behaviors of domestic violence among Iranian high school girls. *Iranian Red Crescent Medical Journal, 15*(1), 21–28. doi: 10.5812/ircmj.3517

Elsheikh, I. E. (2007). Effectiveness of Communication for Behavioral Impact (COMBI) strategy in increasing utilization rate of insecticide treated bed nets (ITNs)—Blue Nile State, 2006. *Sudanese Journal of Public Health, 2*(2), 103–111. Retrieved from http://www.sjph.net.sd/files/vol2i2p103-111.pdf

European Centre for Disease Prevention and Control. (2013). *Definition of a pandemic.* Retrieved from http://ecdc.europa.eu/en/healthtopics/pandemic_preparedness/basic_facts/Pages/definition_of_pandemic.aspx

Food and Agriculture Organization of the United Nations and the World Bank. (2007). *World Congress on Communication and Development: Lessons, challenges, and the way forward.* The Communication Initiative. Washington DC. International Bank for Reconstruction and Development. ftp://ftp.fao.org/docrep/fao/010/ai143e/ai143e00.pdf.

Ford, C. L., & Airhihenbuwa, C. O. (2010). Critical race theory, race equity, and public health: toward antiracism praxis. *American Journal of Public Health, 100*(S1), S30–S35.

Fox, S. (2011). *Social media in context.* Washington DC: Pew Research Center. Retrieved from http://www.pewinternet.org/2011/05/12/social-media-in-context/

Fox, S. (2012). *Health, technology and communities of color.* Washington, DC: Pew Research Center's Internet & American Life Project.

Fox, S. (2013). *Mobile health in context: How information is woven into our lives.* Washington, DC: Pew Research Center's Internet & American Life Project.

Fraser, C., and Restrepo-Estrada, S. (1998). *Communicating for development: Human change for survival.* New York, NY: I.B. Taurus. Retrieved from http://www.cf-hst.net/unicef-temp/Doc-Repository/doc/doc478691.pdf

Gamhewage, G. M. (2015, July 28). Increasing risk communication publications from Africa, Latin America, and Asia. Webinar presentation at Increasing Publications from Developing Nations. *Journal of Communication in Healthcare: Strategies, Media, and Engagement in Global Health.* Retrieved from https://www.youtube.com/watch?v=t3C1FHz_axg

Gibbons, M. C., Fleisher, L., Slamon, R. E., Bass, S., Kandadai, V., & Beck, J. R. (2011). Exploring the potential of Web 2.0 to address health disparities. *Journal of Health Communication, 16*(Suppl. 1), 77–89.

Ginsberg, J., Mohebbi, M. H., Patel, R. S., Brammer, L., Smolinski, M. S., & Brilliant, L. (2008). Detecting influenza epidemics using search engine query data. *Nature, 457*(7232), 1012–1014.

Green, L. W. (1974). Toward cost-benefit evaluations of health education: Some concepts, methods and examples. *Health Education Monograph, 2*(1), 34–64. (1975). Reprinted in *Supplement to the Report of the President's Committee on Health Education.* New York, NY: National Health Council. Also: US Congress. (1975). *Disease control and health education and promotion.* Washington, DC: US Congress) (pp. 939–965).

Green, L. W. (2013). *PRECEDE-PROCEED.* http://www.lgreen.net/precede.htm

Green, L. W., & Ottoson, J. M. (2006, October). *A framework for planning and evaluation: PRECEDE-PROCEED evolution and application of the model.* Montreal, Quebec. Retrieved from http://www.eldis.org/vfile/upload/1/document/0803/ID2188.pdf

Gregson, J. (2001). System, environmental, and policy changes: Using the social-ecological model as a framework for evaluating nutrition education and social marketing programs with low-income audiences. *Journal of Nutrition Education, 33*(1), 4–15.

Grier, S., & Bryant, C. A. (2005). Social marketing in public health. *Annual Review of Public Health, 26*(1), 319–339. doi:10.1146/annurev.publhealth.26.021304.144610

Haveman-Nies, A., Jansen, S. C., van Oers, J. A. M. & van 't Veer, P. (2010). *Epidemiology in public health practice.* Wageningen, The Netherlands: Wageningen Academic Publishers.

Health Communication Capacity Collaborative. (2013). *The P-Process. Five steps to strategic communication.* Baltimore, MD: Johns Hopkins Bloomberg School of Public Health, Center for Communication Programs. Retrieved from http://www.thehealthcompass.org/sites/default/files/strengthening_tools/P%20Process%20Brochure.pdf

Health Communication Partnership. (2003, December). *The new P-Process: Steps in strategic communication.* Retrieved from http://www.jhuccp.org/resource_center/publications/ field_guides_tools/new-p-process-steps-strategic-communication-2003

Hosein, E. (2011). *Comment mesurer l'impact des campagnes de prévention?* [How to *Measure Impact Prevention Campaigns*?] In *Exemple d'évaluation de la méthode COMBI* [*Examples of Evaluation Methods of COMBI*]. Symposium conducted at the meeting of the World Health Organization, Geneva, Switzerland, December 9, 2011. Retrieved from http://www.inpes.sante.fr/30000/pdf/colloque-9dec/Hosein.pdf

Hosein, E., Parks, W., & Schiavo, R. (2009). Communication-for-Behavioral-Impact: An integrated model for health and social change. In R. J. DiClemente, R. A. Crosby, & M. C. Kegler (Eds.), *Emerging theories in health promotion practice and research: Strategies for improving public health* (2nd ed.). San Francisco, CA: Jossey-Bass.

Hufnagel, L., Brockmann, D., & Geisel, T. (2004). Forecast and control of epidemics in a globalized world. *Proceedings of the National Academy of Sciences of the United States of America, 101*(42), 15124–15129. doi: 10.1073/pnas.0308344101

Jain, S. (2012). 40 most popular social networking sites of the world. *Social Media Today.* Retrieved from http://socialmediatoday.com/soravjain/195917/40-most-popular-social-networking-sites-world

Johns Hopkins University Center for Communication Programs. (2011). *Global program on Avian and pandemic influenza.* Retrieved from http://www.jhuccp.org/whatwedo/globalhealthprograms/global-program-avian-and-pandemic-influenza

Last J. M., Spasoff, R. A., Harris, S., & Thuriaux, M. C. (2001). *A dictionary of epidemiology* (4th ed.). Oxford: Oxford University Press

Li, J., Moore, N., Akter, S., Bleisten, S., & Ray, P. (2010). *mHealth for influenza pandemic surveillance in developing countries.* Paper presented at the System Sciences (HICSS), 2010 43rd Hawaii International Conference on System Sciences, Waikoloa, HI, Jan. 5–Jan. 8, 2010.

Krieger, N. (2001). Theories for Social epidemiology in the 21st century: An ecosocial perspective. *International Journal of Epidemiology, 30*(4), 668–677. Retrieved from https://umdrive.memphis.edu/xyu2/public/pubh7140/ecosocialmodel.pdf

Marks, G., & Miller, N. (1987). Ten years of research on the false-consensus effect: An empirical and theoretical review. *Psychological Bulletin, 102*(1), 72.

McCall, E. (2011). *Communication for development: Strengthening the effectiveness of the United Nations.* Food and Agriculture Organization of the United Nations, the International Labour Organization, the Joint United Nations Programme on HIV/AIDS, the United Nations Children's Fund, the United Nations Development Programme, the United Nations Educational, Scientific, and Cultural Organization, and the World Health Organization, coordinated by the UNDP Oslo Governance Centre. Retrieved from http://www.unesco.org/new/fileadmin/MULTIMEDIA/HQ/CI/CI/pdf/communication_form_development_oslo_c4d_pda_en.pdf

Macias, W., Hilyard, K., & Freimuth, V. (2009). Blog functions as risk and crisis communication during Hurricane Katrina. *Journal of Computer-Mediated Communication, 15*(1), 1–31.

Mango Tree. (2012). *The Mango Tree P-PROCESS: Steps in strategic communication.* Retrieved from http://www.mangotreeuganda.org/pprocess.pdf

Melkote, S. R., & Steeves, H. L. (2001). *Communication for development in the third world: Theory and practice for empowerment.* New Delhi: Sage India Pvt Ltd.

Merchant, R. M., Elmer, S., & Lurie, N. (2011). Integrating social media into emergency-preparedness efforts. *New England Journal of Medicine, 365*(4), 289–291.

McKenzie-Mohr, D. (2013). *Fostering sustainable behavior: An introduction to community-based social marketing.* Gabriola, Canada: New Society Publishers.

Milošević, M., Shrove, M. T., & Jovanov, E. (2011). Applications of smartphones for ubiquitous health monitoring and wellbeing management. *Journal of Information Technology and Applications (Banja Luka)-APEIRON, 1*(1), 7–15.

Morris, N. (2003). A comparative analysis of the diffusion and participatory models in development communication. *Communication Theory, 13*(2), 225–248.

Mustafaraj, E., Finn, S., Whitlock, C., & Metaxas, P. T. (2011). *Vocal minority versus silent majority: Discovering the opinions of the long tail.* Paper presented at the Privacy, Security, Risk and Trust (PASSAT), 2011). IEEE Third International Conference on Social Computing (*socialcom*). Boston, October 9–11.

Noelle-Neumann, E. (1974). The spiral of silence a theory of public opinion. *Journal of Communication, 24*(2), 43–51.

Odugleh-Kolev, A. (2012, October 25). Applying COMBI Ebola Control in Yambio, Southern Sudan. *Communication Initiative Network* [Blog]. Retrieved from http://www.comminit.com/global/content/applying-combi-ebola-control-yambio-southern-sudan

Osborn, A. F. (1953). *Applied imagination*. New York, NY: Charles Scribner's Sons.

Oetzel, J. G., Ting-Toomey, S., Rinderle, S. (2006). Conflict communication in contexts: A social ecological perspective. In J. G. Oetzel & S. Ting-Toomey (Eds.), *The SAGE handbook of conflict communication*. Thousand Oaks, CA: Sage.

Paek, H. J., Hilyard, K., Freimuth, V., Barge, J. K., & Mindlin, M. (2010). Theory-based approaches to understanding public emergency preparedness: Implications for effective health and risk communication. *Journal of Health Communication, 15*,428–444.

Palen, L., Hiltz, S. R., & Liu, S. B. (2007). Online forums supporting grassroots participation in emergency preparedness and response. *Communications of the ACM, 50*(3). Pew Internet & American Life Project (2011).

Phillips, J. L., Rolley, J. X., & Davidson, P. M. (2012). Developing targeted health service interventions using the PRECEDE-PROCEED model: Two Australian case studies. *Nursing Research Practice*. Article ID 279431. doi.org/10.1155/2012/279431

Regional AIDS Training Network. (2014). *What is capacity building. Regional AIDS Training Network: Developing capacity in HIV and AIDS in eastern southern Africa*. Retrieved from http://www.ratn.org/index.php?option=com_content&view=article&id=228:what-we-do&catid=19:about-ratn1&Itemid=598

Renganathan, E., Hosein, E., Parks, W., Lloyd, L. Suhaili, M. R., & Odugleh, A. (2005). Communication-for-Behavior-Impact (Combi): A review of WHO's experiences with strategic social mobilization and communication in the prevention and control of communicable diseases. In M. Haider (Ed.), *Global health communication: Challenges, perspectives, and strategies* (pp. 305–320). Sudbury, MA: Jones & Barlett.

Reynolds, B. (2005). Crisis and emergency risk communication. *Applied Biosafety, 10*(1), 47–56. Retrieved from http://www.absa.org/abj/abj/051001reynolds.pdf

Reynolds, B., & Seeger, M. W. (2005). Crisis and emergency risk communication as an integrative model. *Journal of Health Communication, 10*, 43–55.

Ritzer, G. (2011). *Globalization: The essentials*. Oxford, England, and Malden, MA: Wiley-Blackwell.

Sandman, P. M. (1991). Emerging communication responsibilities of epidemiologists. *Journal of Clinical Epidemiology, 44*(1), 41S–50S. Retrieved from http://www.psandman.com/articles/sess-3.htm

Schiavo, R. (2009a). *Mapping and review of existing guidance and plans for community- and household-based communication to prepare and respond to pandemic flu. Research Report*. New York, NY: UNICEF. Retrieved from http://www.unicef.org/influenzaresources/index_1072.html

Schiavo, R. (2009b). *Public health communications: Conceptual frameworks and models relevant to public health emergencies.* Presented at a WHO consultation. Geneva, Switzerland, December.

Schiavo, R. (2013). *Health communication: From theory to practice* (2nd ed.). San Francisco CA: Jossey-Bass.

Schiavo, R. (2014). Risk communication: Ebola and beyond. *Journal of Communication in Healthcare: Strategies, Media, and Engagement in Global Health, 7*(4), 239–241.

Schiavo, R., Leung, M. M., & Brown, M. (2014). Communicating risk and promoting disease mitigation measures in epidemics and emerging disease settings. *Pathogens and Global Health, 108*(2), 76–94.

Schlipköter, U., & Flahault, A. (2010) Communicable diseases: Achievements and challenges for public health. *Public Health Reviews, 32,* 90–119.

Schoch-Spana, S., Chamberlain, A., Franco, C., Gross, J., Lam, C., Mulcahy, A., … Usenza, C. (2006). Disease, disaster, and democracy: The public's stake in health emergency planning, biosecurity and bioterrorism. *Biodefense Strategy, Practice, and Science, 4*(3), 313–319.

TELL-ME. (2013). *Minor infectious outbreaks are good tests for communication in case of pandemics. TELL-ME: Transparent communication in epidemics: Learning lessons from experience, delivering effective messages, providing evidence.* Retrieved from http://www.tellmeproject.eu/content/minor-infectious-outbreaks-are-good-tests-communication-case-pandemics

Thiam, S., LeFevre, A. M., Hane, F., Ndiaye, A., Ba, F., Fielding, K,.L., … Lienhardt, C. (2007). Effectiveness of a strategy to improve adherence to tuberculosis treatment in a resource-poor setting: A cluster randomized controlled trial. *Journal of the American Medical Association, 297*(4), 380–386. doi:10.1001/jama.297.4.380

Thornburg, T. H. (1991). Group size and member diversity influence on creative performance. *Journal of Creative Behavior, 25*(4), 324–333.

Tufte, T., & Mefalopulos, P. (2009). *Participatory communication: A practical guide:* Washington, DC: World Bank Publications.

Ungchusak, K., Sawanpanyalert, P., Hanchoworakul, W., Sawanpanyalert, N., Maloney, S. A., Brown, R. C., … Chusuttiwat, S. (2012). Lessons learned from influenza A(H1N1)pdm09 pandemic response in Thailand. *Emerging Infectious Diseases.* Retrieved from http://wwwnc.cdc.gov/eid/article/18/7/11-0976_article.htm

UNICEF Bangladesh. (2008). *The three communication components in writing a communication strategy for development programme: A guideline for programme managers and communication officers* (chapter 1). Retrieved from http://www.unicef.org/cbsc/files/Writing_a_Comm_Strategy_for_Dev_Progs.pdf

UNICEF. (2013). *UNICEF communication for development support to public health preparedness and disaster risk reduction in East Asia and the Pacific: A review.* Bangkok, Thailand: UNICEF East Asia and Pacific Regional Office. Retrieved from http://www.unicef.org/cbsc/files/Communicatiln_for_development_support_to_public_health_preparedness.pdf

UNICEF. (2014). *Communication for development: The big picture.* Retrieved from http://www.unicef.org/ cbsc/index.html

UNICEF. (2015a). *Ebola and C4D.* Retrieved from http://www.unicef.org/cbsc/index_73157.html

UNICEF. (2015b). *Community care centers, community dialogue and engagement: Key ingredients in Sierra Leone.* Retrieved from http://www.unicef.org/cbsc/files/UNICEF_Community_Care_Centers%281%29.pdf

UNICEF. (2015c). *Lofa County: Communities took the matter in their own hands.* Retrieved from http://www.unicef.org/cbsc/files/Communities_took_the_matter_in_their_own_hands-Lofa%284%29.pdf

US Department of Health and Human Services. (2002). *Communicating in a crisis: Risk communication guidelines for public officials.* Washington, DC: Author. Retrieved from http://www.hhs.gov/od/documents/RiskCommunication.pdf

US Department of Health and Human Services, Office of Disease Prevention and Health Promotion. (2005). *Healthy People 2010* (vols. 1 and 2). Retrieved from http://www.healthypeople.gov/2010/Document/tableofcontents.htm#parta

US Department of Health and Human Services, Office of Disease Prevention and Health Promotion. (2015). *Healthy People 2020.* Retrieved from http://www.healthypeople.gov/2020/topicsobjectives2020/overview.aspx?topicid=18

Valente, T. W. (2002). Frameworks, models, and rationales. In *Evaluating Health Promotion Programs* (pp. 3–18). New York, NY: Oxford University Press.

Vaughan, E., & Tinker, T. (2009). Effective health risk communication about pandemic influenza for vulnerable populations. *American Journal of Public Health, 99*(S2), S324–S332. doi: 10.2105

Vital Wave Consulting. (2009). *mHealth for development: The opportunity of mobile technology for healthcare in the developing world.* Washington & Berkshire: UN Foundation-Vodafone Foundation Partnership. Available at: http://www.vitalwaveconsulting.com/insights/articles/mHealth.htm

Veil, S. R., Buehner, T., & Palenchar, M. J. (2011). A work-in-process literature review: Incorporating social media in risk and crisis communication. *Journal of Contingencies and Crisis Management, 19*(2), 110–122.

Viswanath, K., & Kreuter, M. W. (2007). Health disparities, communication inequalities, and e-Health: A commentary. *American Journal of Preventive Medicine, 32*(Suppl. 5), S131.

Water Supply & Sanitation Collaborative Council. (2013). Dr. Everold Hosein. Global Forum on Sanitation and Hygiene. Retrieved from http://wsscc-global-forum.org/dr-everold-hosein.html

Woodman, R. W., Sawyer, J. E., & Griffin, R. W. (1993). Toward a theory of organizational creativity. *Academy of Management Review, 18*(2), 293–321.

World Health Organization. (2004a). *Ebola: Containing the outbreak in Sudan.* Retrieved from http://www.who.int/features/2004/ebola/en/index.html

World Health Organization. (2004b). *Social mobilization to fight Ebola in Yambio, Southern Sudan.* Action Against Infection. Retrieved from http://wmc.who.int/pdf/ Action_Against_Infection.pdf

World Health Organization. (2004c). *WHO announces end of Ebola outbreak in Southern Sudan*. Retrieved from www.who.int/csr/don/2004_08_07/en/

World Health Organization. (2007). Appropriate Information-Communications Technologies for Developing Countries. *Bulletin of the World Health Organization, 85*(4). www.who.int/bulletin/volumes/85/4/07-041475/en. Retrieved July 2013.

World Health Organization. (2012). *Communication for behavioural impact (COMBI): A toolkit for behavioural and social communication in outbreak response*. Retrieved from http://www.who.int/ihr/publications/combi_toolkit_outbreaks/en

World Health Organization's Communicable Diseases Division, WHO Mediterranean Centre for Vulnerability Reduction. (2006). *Manual for planning Communication-for-Behavioral-Impact (COMBI) programmes for health*. Retrieved from http://www.undg.org/docs/9555/COMBI-Manual-ENH-Jan-2006.pdf

CHAPTER 13

NONCOMMUNICABLE DISEASES (NCDs)

Moving Toward Health Promotion

C. James Hospedales, André Pascal Kengne, Branka Legetic, and Adriana Blanco Marquizo

Especially with the transition of an increasing number of countries from lower to middle income, noncommunicable diseases (NCDs, known as chronic diseases and major causes of morbidity and mortality in the wealthier countries of the world) have become serious health and development concerns in a larger and larger portion of the world (World Health Organization [WHO], 2010). In this chapter, fairly recent efforts at preventing NCDs in middle-income countries are chronicled, with an emphasis on cardiovascular diseases, diabetes and obesity, cancer and chronic respiratory diseases, tobacco use prevention and control, diet, and physical activity.

The efforts are described through the health promotion lenses of **healthy public policy**, creating supportive environments, community action, and reorienting health services. Partnership and alliances are a cross-cutting strategy, all anchored in good surveillance and data. The chapter focuses on the experiences of the mostly middle-income countries of the Americas and Africa, along with the role of regional offices of WHO in catalyzing the application of health promotion principles and strategies to the prevention and control of NCDs in the past 10 to 15 years. Within these two WHO regions, the use of health promotion as a cross cutting strategy is standing organizational policy (Pan American Health Organization [PAHO], 2013; Rice, 2011).

The Americas and the Caribbean countries in particular led the world to convening a UN high-level meeting (UNHLM) on NCDs in September 2011, only the second time in history that a UN general assembly considered a health problem (the first was HIV/AIDS in 2001). The resulting political declaration (United Nations [UN], 2011) and subsequent adoption in 2013 of a set of global targets and indicators by the World Health Assembly (WHA), including

LEARNING OBJECTIVES

By the end of this chapter, the reader should be able to:

- **Understand key definitions and concepts related to the application of health promotion strategies to the prevention and control of chronic noncommunicable diseases (NCDs)**
- **Understand that a complex issue like NCDs and related risk factors represent significant human and economic development challenges for the world**
- **Describe the major health promotion strategies and the tools and instruments employed in NCD prevention and control**
- **Appreciate that organizations like PAHO and WHO have leadership roles in global health promotion**
- **Identify similarities and differences between Latin America/Caribbean and Africa in distribution of NCDs and implementation of national policies for NCD control, surveillance, and prevention**

reducing premature mortality due to the four main NCDs 25% by 2025, represents a landmark in global consensus. The health promotion actions described herein, and the advocacy and collaboration between a broad range of actors in government, civil society and in international organizations, particularly WHO, contributed significantly to this global awakening to NCDs as a significant development threat, with links to several other challenges such as climate change and poverty.

Chronic noncommunicable diseases, principally cardiovascular diseases (CVD), cancer, diabetes, and chronic respiratory diseases, represent the leading cause of death and of avoidable health care costs worldwide, with nearly 80% of the burden occurring in low- and middle-income countries (LMICs) (WHO, 2011a). NCDs are largely caused by common risk factors, particularly tobacco use and exposure to secondhand smoke, unhealthy diet, physical inactivity, obesity, and harmful use of alcohol, among others.

NCDs are recognized to be both a cause and an effect of poverty, with people who are poorer and less educated having less access to quality health services and being more exposed to risk factors of poor diet, tobacco use, air pollution, etc. Globally, the economic impact of NCDs and mental health was estimated to be $47 trillion in direct and indirect costs from 2010 to 2030, of which NCDs was $30 trillion, in work by the World Economic Forum (Bloom, Cafiero, Jané-Llopis, Abrahams-Gessel, Bloom, & Fathima, S., 2011). Representing some 5% loss in GDP, most of which is avoidable, NCDs represent symptoms of the failure of our development paradigms.

The NCD epidemic is driven by globalization, urbanization, economic situations and demographic and lifestyle changes. It is also strongly influenced by the social determinants of health, such as income, education, employment and working conditions, ethnicity, and gender (WHO, 2012a). Private sector and cultural forces also play major roles. Thus, NCDs are both a complex public health matter and an economic development challenge, requiring interventions by the health sector as well as other sectors of government, civil society, and the private sector (UN, 2012), a fact repeated 15 times in a UNHLM report.

It has been estimated that by 2030, NCDs will be responsible globally for three times as many Disability Adjusted Life Years (DALYs) and nearly five times as many deaths as infectious diseases, maternal, perinatal, and nutritional conditions combined. Of great concern is the high level of premature death, which has major negative impacts on socioeconomic development (Bloom, Cafiero, Jané-Llopis, Abrahams-Gessel, Bloom, & Fathima, S., 2011). Worldwide, some 44% of deaths due to NCDs occur before 70 years of age. However, in LMICs, a high proportion (48%) of all NCD deaths are estimated to occur in people under the age of 70, versus 26% for high-income countries (WHO, 2012c). The burden of premature death disproportionately affects the poor. Worldwide, NCDs are estimated to account for 66.5% of all years lived with disability in low- and middle-income countries (WHO, 2011a).

Although the diseases themselves, and associated risk factors are reasonably clear, one also needs to consider how race, ethnicity and culture, and gender roles may affect male and female risks for NCD and how the various groups react to them. Tobacco and alcohol use have long been associated with masculine gender norms; however, the prevalence of these risks is growing among females, especially adolescent girls (Simons-Morton et al., 2009). Cultural habits of food preparation and consumption may also influence the occurrence and progression of chronic diseases. Gender biases may also determine the effectiveness of diagnosis. For example, women with a heart attack may seek emergency services later than do men, and may be misdiagnosed or treated inadequately (Mosca et al., 2013). Consequently, women may have higher rates of mortality due to heart attack compared with men.

Healthy Public Policy and NCDs

One of the gurus of the healthy public policy concept, Nancy Milio (1981, 1985a, 1988), states that the present and future of a population's health is mainly determined by public policies. In her view, these policies set parameters for the type and character of production (industrial, agricultural); for the environment; for communities including schools, workplaces, and cities; for business management; for consumption; as well as for individual behavior. She defines health as a "response of people to their environments" rather than a state of physical, mental, and social well-being or achievement that is final. When health is perceived in such a broad context for policy purposes, it also means that it goes beyond the absence of disease and viewpoints of medical practitioners. It encompasses the general population's opinion and dynamics, knowledge of social science and economy, and is applicable to the overall population, including its various segments.

Policy decisions today have to take into account sustainability issues, the future positive and negative impacts from economic, social, and environmental perspectives and to consider current as well as future generations. Building healthy public policy is a tough job today. The present is more complex than ever before, and is highly dynamic and highly interconnected thanks to the technologies of communication and transport, research and evidence that is rapidly growing and changing so policy making related to health, whether it addresses economic issues, or social or environmental, is done with significant levels of uncertainty.

The complexity of policy issues today is well illustrated through the processes of shaping policies related to NCD prevention and control at global, regional, subregional, and national levels. Although NCDs have been in the focus of public health in North America and Europe since the 1950s, they appeared for the first time in the global policy agenda in 2000 when the WHO Global Strategy for NCD prevention and control (WHA53.17) was endorsed at the World Health Assembly. Since then, several global policies and strategies have been developed, discussed, and endorsed by member states. These policies either address one risk factor like tobacco and its regulatory aspects (WHO Framework Convention on Tobacco Control (WHO 2003) or physical activity and nutrition recommendations, or policies to reduce the harmful use of alcohol (Global Strategy to Reduce the Harmful Use of Alcohol, WHO 2010b).

The main global breakthrough was in 2011 at the UN High Level Meeting on NCDs that moved the topic from the global health agenda to the global development agenda. This meeting was a result of strong advocacy activities started by the Caribbean and spread throughout other continents, based on high burden in the region and research and evidence published in a report by the Commission of Macroeconomics and Health (2001) that raised the profile of global health in the international arena and promoted the long-neglected link between health and wealth. The Oxford Health Alliance publication, *Chronic Disease: An Economic Perspective* (Suhrcke et al., 2006), highlights the economic rationale for prevention before the NCD burden strikes hardest. The WHO report, "Scaling Up Action Against NCDS: How Much Will It Cost?" (2011b), showed that implementing a set of "Best Buy" interventions in low-income, middle-income, and high-income countries will cost per person, per day, US$1, US$2, or US$3, respectively.

The Caribbean countries provided sterling leadership that was crucial to the global movement by having their Summit of Heads of Government of CARICOM in September 2007. This resulted in the landmark Declaration of Port-of-Spain, with 15 articles containing 26 actionable commitments. Progress has been monitored annually using a scorecard and results are shared with Caribbean Ministers of Health and Heads of Government (Samuels, Kirton, & Gueber, 2014). The lessons learned from this process have been analyzed and include the importance of champions at different levels; the importance of political process; packaging evidence speak to the head, heart, and pocket; and strong partnership and collaboration between agencies. Currently, an evaluation of the Port-of-Spain Declaration is underway with support from IDRC Canada.

The World Bank joined the preparatory process for the UNHLM by issuing the discussion paper called "Chronic Emergency: Why NCDs Matter" (World Bank, 2011) that made the case for elevating the challenge of NCDs as a priority item to be addressed on the agenda of decision makers. During the UNHLM, further support came from the World Economic Forum and Harvard School of Public Health, which launched a report to inform decisions of top economic leaders about allocation of resources to react to the enormous threat that NCDs pose. This shows a staggering projected cost of $30 trillion over the next 20 years. If mental health conditions are added, the cost rises to $47 trillion. These documents became advocacy tools for different actors of society and for voices of people and not only of government. Civil society international organizations like the International Diabetes Federation, the World Heart Federation, and the International Union for Cancer Control formed the NCD Alliance that strongly supported preparation of the UNHLM by preparing the joint statement (NCD Alliance, 2014).

Supportive Environments

There is continual interaction between people and their environments. Patterns of life, work, and free time have a significant impact on health, well-being, and disease experience. Health promotion seeks to generate living and working conditions that are safe, stimulating, satisfying, and enjoyable (WHO, 1986). Systematic assessment of the health impact of a rapidly changing environment, particularly in areas of technology, work, energy production, and urbanization, has shown that actions related to food and nutrition, such as the elimination of trans fats, reduction of dietary salt consumption and added sugar; with physical activity promotion using built environments; and reducing exposure to tobacco are key aspects of creating more supportive environments, which benefit prevention of NCDs and the physical and mental health of the population. These measures are all part of the "WHO Best Buys" (WEF, 2011) for NCD prevention and control, that is, the most cost-effective measures that can be implemented in low-resource settings.

In the rest of this chapter, we provide case studies of two World Health Organization regions: the Americas, served by the Pan American Health Organization (Case Study 13.1); and Africa, served by the World Health Organization African Regional Office (Case Study 13.2).

The Americas

NCDs account for two-thirds of all mortality in the Americas. As seen in Figure 13.1, of all deaths due to NCDs in the Americas, more than one-third (37%) were due to cardiovascular diseases, one-fifth (20%) were due to cancer, and smaller percentages were due to chronic respiratory disease (8%), diabetes (6%), and other NCDs (20%). Almost 90% of deaths were due to NCDs in North America; the percentage of all mortality ranged from under 50% in Haiti and the Dominican Republic to 52% in Guatemala, between 60% and 70% in Belize, El Salvador, Jamaica, Peru, Guyana, Ecuador, and Colombia, to 80% or greater in Argentina, Dominica, Costa Rica, Uruguay, and Chile (Population Reference Bureau, 2013).

CASE STUDY 13.1 PAHO AND THE AMERICAS

In the Americas, the PAHO Directing Council/Pan American Sanitary Conference endorsed in 2006 a Regional Strategy and Action Plan for Prevention and control of NCDs, with a corresponding resolution that provided a guide for the country work on prevention and control of NCDs, as well as a guide for international cooperation in health on the continent. In 2010, following five years of implementation, the progress report submitted to directing council indicated the progress being made by countries as well as the need for revision due to rapid changes in the capacities in the countries, emerging economic crises, multiple players in international and national arenas as well as a need for stronger engagement of other government sectors in the prevention of NCDs as well as organized engagement of civil society. To support the latter, the Pan American Health Organization has developed a platform for multistakeholder engagement called Pan American Forum for Action on NCDs as a space for dialogue between public and private sectors at the international level. Some countries followed and Trinidad and Tobago and Guatemala, and later central America has developed similar platforms to support the dialogue and coordination.

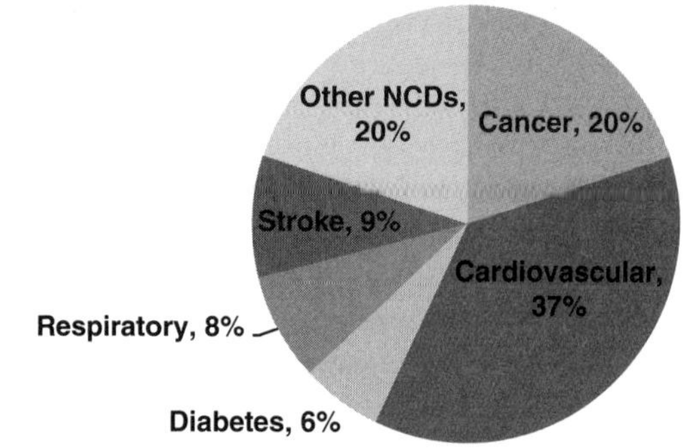

Figure 13.1 Proportion of Mortality Due to NCDs in the Americas, 2012

Against this background, the past 5 to 10 years in the region have witnessed major new policy developments and strategic initiatives on NCDs at the national, subregional, and regional levels, many with the active participation and support of PAHO/WHO. The most notable political declarations include: the Caribbean Community (CARICOM) Port-of-Spain Declaration on Non-Communicable Diseases (2007), the political declaration of the Regional High-Level Consultation of the Americas on Non-Communicable Diseases and Obesity (PAHO 2011), in addition to the Moscow Declaration on NCDs (WHO 2011c), and the UNHLM on the Prevention and Control of NCDs (United Nations 2011).

Strategic Initiatives

A range of strategic initiatives were implemented, taking account of evidence of burden or risk, feasibility, and opportunities for action in member states and with partners.

Reduced Trans Fats

The Trans Fat Free Americas (TFFA) initiative was launched in 2007 by PAHO calling together an expert advisory group. The initiative was based on evidence that, hydrogenated oils or industrially produced trans fatty acids (TFA) are deleterious to human health, while unsaturated fatty acids, such as those found in soybeans, sunflower, canola, and corn have a cardio-protective effect. This evidence is what led the US FDA in 2003 to require labeling of industrially produced TFA on the nutritional contents.

Because of their properties in improving taste and shelf life, TFAs are in widespread use commercially for baking and frying, and most people in LAC are not aware of their significance. In this situation, it's very difficult for an "individual choice" approach to succeed in reducing population levels of consumption of TFA; it is much more feasible to reduce or eliminate at the source, thereby creating a more supportive environment. People in low-income groups are often more exposed to food environments with high levels of TFAs, and reduction in the manufacturing process is also a pro-poor policy, as are many primary prevention measures.

PAHO's expert group estimated that in Latin America and the Caribbean, a daily reduction of 4.5 grams (g) of TFA intake would prevent in the range of 30,000 to 130,000 events of coronary heart disease, while a reduction of 9g a day would prevent from 62,000 to 225,000 events of coronary heart disease (PAHO, 2007).

Canada and the United States introduced regulations in 2005 and 2013, respectively, to eliminate industrially made trans fats and replace them with unsaturated fatty acids. In Latin America, regulations have been introduced in Argentina, Brazil, and Chile, and Costa Rica has employed nonregulatory health promotion strategies to reduce TFA content in foods. These initiatives were developed as part of the Regional Strategy and Plan of Action for an Integrated Approach to the Prevention and Control of Chronic Diseases, including Diet, Physical Activity, and Health 2006–2015 (PAHO Resolution CD47.R9).

The expert group issued Recommendations of the Task Force for a "Trans Fat Free Americas." The document advocates the replacement of industrially produced TFA with unsaturated fats, including omega-3 fatty acids, and promotes the development of regulations to this effect. The task force recommended the adoption of a $< 2\%$ limit of TFA-derived fat for vegetable oils and soft margarines and of $< 5\%$ for other foods, as well as the promotion of other normative measures such as nutritional labeling and standards to regulate claims regarding the health properties of foods and their fat and oil content, especially TFA. It also recommends restaurants and processed food manufacturers eliminate all or virtually all partially hydrogenated oil, the source of artificial TFA, and replace it with ingredients as low in saturated fat as possible.

On June 8–9, 2008, public health authorities, food industry representatives, and cooking oil companies convened by PAHO issued a jointly agreed Declaration of Rio de Janeiro on a Trans Fat Free Americas, as a pledge to jointly work on agreed action points. Reviews of the impact of recommendations and industry pledges to work on eliminating industrial TFAs from the food supply in LAC shows that there is still work to be done in low- and middle-income countries in the region. Still missing is a clear consensus on the definition of TFA across the region to facilitate regulation, and consumer education and monitoring and surveillance efforts. Thus different approaches were implemented by different countries, from banning and limiting TFA (Puerto Rico, Argentina, Brazil, Chile, Peru, Mexico), through mandatory labeling of TFA (Brazil, Peru, Ecuador, Chile, Puerto Rico), to voluntary regulations (Central America [COMISCA], Colombia, Jamaica, and Mexico).

Salt Reduction

The Pan American Health Organization in September 2009 convened a group of independent international experts from North, Central, and South America and the Caribbean on salt and health to guide the first two years of a regional initiative, "Cardiovascular Disease Prevention Through Dietary Salt Reduction," based on the evidence that reducing dietary salt at the population level is one of the most cost-effective public health measure available to lower blood pressure and related CVD mortality. It can save lives and health care dollars across low-, middle-, and high-income countries. The expert group included representatives from ministries of health, academia, WHO, and civil society groups such as Consumers International.

The internationally **recommended salt intake** level is less than 5 g/person/day (WHO, 2012b). Actual consumption levels are with few exceptions much higher worldwide, proven for the first time by the INTERSALT Study (WHO, 2006) that determined population sodium intake levels in 32 countries, based on 24-hour urine collections. Several recent dietary and urinary sodium data from observational and interventional studies continue to show excess intake (Brown et al., 2009).

In the Americas, recent studies confirm high daily per capita salt intake: Brazil: 11g/day (Sarno et al., 2009); Argentina: 12g/day (*Encuesta nacional de nutricion y salud,* 2004–2005); Chile: 9.8g/day (*Encuesta nacional de salud ENS Chile,* 2009–2010); United States: 8.7g/day (Committee on Strategies to Reduce Sodium Intake, 2010); and Canada: 7.7g/day (Sodium Working Group, Sodium Reduction Strategy for Canada, 2010). Sources of dietary sodium vary: in the United States (Committee on Strategies to Reduce Sodium Intake, 2010) and Canada (Sodium Working Group, Sodium Reduction Strategy for Canada, 2010), 75% and 77% respectively of sodium consumed comes from processed foods; in parts of Brazil, 70% is attributed to salt added in household cooking or at the table (Sarno et al., 2009). In places where most of the salt consumed is in processed foods, an individual choice approach is again very limited in potential, and creating a supportive environment is best done by reducing salt in the manufacturing process in collaboration with industry.

It is estimated that lowering blood pressure by reducing salt intake even a modest amount (15%) can prevent 8.5 million premature deaths in 10 years in low- and middle-economies and can deliver cost savings in high-income countries (Asaria et al., 2007; Bibbins-Domingo et al., 2010; Cobiac, Vos, & Veerman, 2010). As part of implementing the WHO Global Strategy for Diet, Physical Activity and Health, WHO set up a salt reduction strategy with three platforms: (1) creating enabling environments, (2) monitoring and evaluation, and (3) salt as a vehicle for fortification, particularly iodine. In 2010, WHO and the UK Food Safety Agency organized the first platform, creating enabling environments. It included an information exchange forum with the private sector and nongovernmental organizations (NGOs). Discussed were interventions for consumer education and reformulation of industrially produced foods to enable consumers to make appropriate choices to reduce the total sodium content of their diet (WHO, 2010).

Following global recommendations and the policy statement issued for the Americas, over the course of its two-year mandate, the expert group issued press releases and offered webinars through PAHO; published articles in peer reviewed journals; and made presentations at international conferences and meetings.

The policy statement for the Americas stimulated much action in Latin America and the Caribbean. For the governments of Uruguay and Costa Rica, their endorsement of the policy statement supported development of national initiatives. For civil society in Latin America, led by Consumers

International and the Inter-American Heart Foundation, the policy statement was the basis for organizing information exchanges for mobilizing action and providing support for the regional initiative. In 2008, the Healthy Caribbean Coalition (HCC) was launched with initial support from PAHO. The coalition developed culturally tailored material to raise awareness of high-salt diets and their harmful effects. The Heart Federation of Jamaica promoted "Drop the Salt—Protect Your Health" as the theme for Salt Awareness Week in 2011, which served as a foundation for launching national initiatives.

The Healthy Caribbean Coalition is one of very active members in the regional initiative and has been advocating for consumption of less salt in the Caribbean, widely disseminating the policy statement of the expert group. HCC used the Agrofest, a large agricultural fair in Barbados and attended by some 60,000 people in a country of 270,000 to highlight salt reduction in the Caribbean. HCC was a patron of and gave support for Agrofest 2011, "Healthy Living Through Agriculture." Activities included a workshop for food vendors and discussion with bakeries and food producers on reformulation. HCC also prepared a new "culturally specific" salt jingle for use on radio and at public events and via Facebook.

Consumers International performed a study in five countries of the Americas to explore attitudes toward salt consumption and labelling of salt on packaged foods. The results showed that 90% of participants associated high salt intake with occurrence of adverse health conditions, and 60% reported trying to reduce their salt intake. Only 47% claimed that they check the salt content on the label and 80% would like to have clear labels with high or low salt warnings (Claro et al., 2012).

PAHO and members of the expert group collaborated with the World Economic Forum on Latin America and representatives of the food industry, governments, regulatory agencies, and civil society to produce *Dietary Sodium/Salt Reduction in the Americas 2011 Statement of Rio de Janeiro* (WEF/PAHO, 2011). It is the first position document created jointly by governments, the food industry, and civil society that distills elements of the policy statement into a set of priorities and commitments regarding their respective roles and responsibilities in reducing the overconsumption of salt. In the statement of Rio de Janeiro, governments, the food industry, and civil society together strongly committed to the principle of sustainable food consumption; recognized that international organizations have a strong role to play in convening stakeholders; and encouraging stakeholders to act now to improve the health of the people of the Americas. This document, as well as work of the SaltSmart Consortium under the Pan American Forum for Action on NCDs (Hospedales & Jane-Llopis, 2011), has facilitated securing advances in supportive environments from the industry side, that is, Kraft Foods and Nestlé pledged a 10% reduction across their products globally and in the Americas.

The regional initiative and the activities of PAHO have had a positive impact. Countries reported that the f initiative:

- has helped advocacy to prioritize the issue as a national public health problem;
- helped with national plans and strategies through tools and resources;

- assisted with analysis of evidence and identification of effective interventions;
- has made available a network of accessible experts and updates on experiences across the Americas;
- provided the opportunity to explore the epidemiological situation and review of policies and interventions based on evidence;
- developed recommendations for standardized methodology to measure and monitor population salt intake allows results to be compared across LAC; and
- facilitated collaborations between countries and members of the LATINFOODS network.

The initiative showed that many experiences with industry engagement are also transferrable:

- In negotiations of targets and timelines, most important is information about what food companies have achieved elsewhere.
- Where regulation to limit salt content is pending, industry is particularly motivated.
- Some countries engage with the industry through national associations representing industry—for example, artisanal bread makers, meat producers, supermarkets, food and beverage associations, and others.
- Existing relationships between public health and industry, for example, in Chile and Argentina with associations of artisanal bread makers for flour fortification and facilitated national dietary salt reduction through bread products.
- A draft national action plan can be useful in engaging stakeholders as a template to secure concrete commitments from stakeholders through a participatory process.

Tobacco Control

Tobacco use and exposure to secondhand smoke are among the leading causes of preventable mortality, morbidity, and disability. They are common risk factors for all major NCDs. The tobacco epidemic is a global public health problem, driven by the aggressive marketing of the multinational tobacco industry. For this reason WHO envisioned that this global problem will also require a global solution. In 2003 the World Health Assembly adopted the WHO Framework Convention on Tobacco Control (WHO, 2003), the first public health treaty negotiated under the auspices of WHO—as a mechanism of promoting national public health action and multilateral cooperation. Its overarching objective is "to protect present and future generations from the devastating health, social, environmental and economic consequences of tobacco consumption and exposure to tobacco smoke." Toward this end, the treaty covers a broad range of scientifically based measures aimed at reducing both the demand for and the supply of tobacco products. Among others, the main measures are protection from secondhand smoke (SHS); health warnings in the packaging and labeling of tobacco products; total ban of tobacco advertising, promotion, and sponsorship; offering smokers help to quit tobacco; raise taxes; and eliminate illicit trade of tobacco products.

With more than 170 parties, this is one of the most rapidly embraced treaties, and at the moment of writing, 29 countries of the Americas are parties to it. Even so, in order to have effect at the country level, the requirements of the FCTC should be incorporated into national legislation. The Region of the Americas has seen great progress and has been a leader in the implementation of some of the measures; however, coverage of the region's population is far from complete. Seventeen countries have passed smoke-free legislation covering at least indoor public places and workplaces and public transportation, but this still represents fewer than half of the region's people. Almost half of the Americas population can see pictorial warnings in the packages of tobacco products. Five countries have a total ban on tobacco advertisement, promotion, and sponsorship, and in the area of taxation, there are only two countries where the percentage of the tobacco taxes reaches 75% of the final price as recommended by WHO (PAHO, 2013).

Community Action

Community action and development is an important strategy in health promotion, and there are many examples in the region where NGOs and communities have engaged. In 2011, the Healthy Caribbean Coalition, a 35-member non-governmental organization alliance dedicated to combating chronic diseases, conducted a unique GetTheMessage text campaign across 17 countries to support the UNHLM (see Box 13.1) (HCC 2011). In 2011, support was also provided to catalyze the formation of a Healthy Latin American coalition, which rapidly grew from 40 to more than 100 NGOs advocating for NCD and the UNHLM. The participation of civil society in issues such as food marketing to children and child obesity has also increased significantly over the past five years, notably in Brazil, Canada, Chile, Mexico, and the USA (see Box 13.2).

BOX 13.1 GETTHEMESSAGE

The GetTheMessage text campaign used state-of-the art technology to combat NCDs. The two mobile phone operators in the region, LIME and Digicel, with collaboration of regional insurance and media companies and ministries of health allowed subscribers to text for free a message of support for the United Nations High Level Meeting on NCDs in New York. Following an integrated promotional campaign including text blasts, traditional media promotion, and "textathons" using media personalities, more than 500,000 signatures of support were secured from 17 countries. This bottom-up support, leveraging new social media and text messaging across many national boundaries, a first for the region, led to a high level of representation of Caribbean policymakers attending the UNHLM and describes a good platform for leveraging technology for advocacy, education and information, and preventive care (Healthy Caribbean Coalition, https://www.facebook.com/GettheMessage).

BOX 13.2 MARKETING TO CHILDREN: A HUMAN RIGHTS ISSUE

Children in the Americas and most of the world are subject to continuous, pervasive marketing of nutrient-poor foods that are high in fats, salt, and sugar. This is contributing to rising rates of overweight and NCDs, stigma, mental health, and job issues for affected children and young people, and rising health costs. Such continuous advertising is a human rights issue because children are not yet rational economic decision makers. Children are very vulnerable to such marketing, and protection of children has universal acceptance. In 2010, WHO passed a resolution urging countries to undertake efforts to restrict marketing of poor-quality food to children (WHO, 2010). In 2011, PAHO published step-by-step guidance for implementing the WHO resolution within an 18-month time frame, helping to spur action throughout the Americas and the Caribbean. Further adoption of these guidelines would address an important health and human rights issue. However, it's an area where there is strong conflict of interest with many food companies, which profit greatly from products targeting children and adolescents. Leadership from policymakers and civil society will be needed, along with incentives to consume healthier foods, and recognition of the more progressive companies.

Increasing levels of physical activity is a key health-promoting action to reduce NCDs and improve mental health. *Ciclovias,* a Spanish term meaning "cycleway," is either a permanent bike path or the closing of certain streets to automotive vehicles for a few hours weekly for cyclists and pedestrians, sometimes called "open streets." Making use of built environment, *Ciclovias* were invented in Colombia, spread throughout the region and beyond, representing a very cost-effective way of promoting mass physical activity and environmental sensitivity. On any given weekend in LAC, more than 3 million people actively participate for an hour or more; this number is growing. Alternative transport such as biking and walking are good for health, good for climate change, and good for energy security, a so-called triple bottom line return.

As part of the 2007 CARICOM Heads of Government Declaration, *Uniting to Stop the Epidemic of NCDs* (Samuels et al., 2013), a Caribbean Wellness Day (CWD) was declared on the second Saturday of every year. Inaugurated in 2008, CWD aims to support public, private, and community participation and partnership and promote multisector, community-based activities across the region. Twenty countries and territories regularly celebrate the day with engagement of NGOs, health and other ministries such as education and local government, and the private sector such as banks, insurance companies, and media. Policymakers leading health walks, health fairs, healthy food promotion, music for dancing, and health screenings are among the major types of activities undertaken with organizational support from PAHO/WHO and CARICOM. CWD has been a catalyst in many instances to more sustained physical activity initiatives, for example, in Trinidad and Tobago's "Family and Fitness Sunday" in which streets are closed for four hours on a Sunday for physical activity, or in the British Virgin Islands yearlong walking initiative, "Walk Into It." Several countries have initiated and sustained ongoing physical activity in

BOX 13.3 BEHAVIOR CHANGE INITIATIVES

Throughout the PAHO region, many national and regional communications and initiatives have been conducted to raise awareness of the importance of physical activity. 5-pasos in Mexico is a nationwide campaign to raise awareness and promote healthy living, including messages about moving, measuring yourself, and drinking water. Private companies like Univision support the efforts of "Don Francisco," host of their popular Latin American TV show, *Sabado Gigante*, to educate its 100-million audience on diabetes, weight, and physical activity. Michelle Obama, US First Lady, leads the "Let's Move" campaign in response to the epidemic of childhood obesity, and has raised awareness greatly, resonating with PAHO's regional campaign, *A comer sano, a vivir bien y a moverse América* ("Eat healthy, live well, and get moving").

primary health care clinics, and in the case of Trinidad and Tobago, half of the 105 primary health care centers have been expanded to provide additional space for physical activity. (See Box 13.3.)

CWD was part of the inspiration for PAHO to launch a "Wellness Week" in the Americas in 2011 to help translate commitments of the UNHLM in the Americas. The purpose of Wellness Week is to mobilize multiple stakeholders, including local authorities, private sector, NGOs, and the general public to emphasize the importance of enabling environments that make healthy choices the easy choices. During the week, countries in the region showcase successful practices in health promotion and engage all sectors about underlying determinants of health, emphasizing vulnerable groups, and improving quality and coverage of health services.

Faith-based organizations (FBOs) play very important roles in most countries of the region, and in some countries have engaged strongly in NCD prevention. In Barbados, Jamaica, Suriname, and Trinidad and Tobago, churches and FBOs have been actively involved in educating their congregations and communities, conducting screening and health walks, and other initiatives, in collaboration with ministries of health. The Seventh-day Adventist Church has been a recognized leader in this regard.

The Reorientation of Health Services

The prevention and control of NCDs requires both a population approach, such as tobacco control, dietary salt reduction, or educational programs, and an individual approach in which patients with NCDs and those at high risk are detected in a timely manner and then managed in an integrated fashion to optimize quality of life and minimize complications like heart attacks and strokes, renal failure, and amputations. This requires a reorientation of health services from a traditional acute care model, in which patients are seen for episodic events like an infection or an injury, to a chronic care model, in which patients require ongoing care and lifelong follow-up, adherence to treatment, and lifestyle changes. Integral to chronic care is patient self-care.

PAHO promotes the organization of evidence-based, patient-centered care as established by the chronic care model and works closely with member states, professional associations, and other partners to support the development and implementation of evidence-based guidelines and protocols for the integrated management of NCD.

In 2010, 18 countries were working with PAHO in the implementation of integrated primary health care strategies to improve quality of care for persons living with chronic diseases such as diabetes, hypertension, and cancer. In 2009, a rapid assessment in 24 countries (PAHO, 2009) on the capacity of disease management showed the availability of guidelines or protocols for hypertension and diabetes in 23 countries (97%). Twenty countries (86%) had protocols for cancer, but very few had guidelines and protocols for weight control and physical activity. There were no policies for the access to some medications and services, particularly for low-income groups, though all countries had a list of essential medicines for NCD. The Central American region, through the support of the Spanish International Cooperation Development Agency, has developed a list of essential medicines, mainly for cancer, for consolidated procurement. NCDs are associated with catastrophic family expenditure, which sharpens and deepens poverty.

Access to treatment for low-income persons is hindered by 39% to 63% of the population having to pay the full cost of basic medications for diabetes and hypertension. Between 25% and 75% of basic procedures and tests, including blood glucose monitor, X-rays, mammography, cervical cancer smears, colonoscopy, lipid profile, and dialysis, are not mentioned in guidelines to address NCD. However, they are available in about 85% of the countries of the region. Dialysis services are accessible in 83% of countries. It is estimated that around 40% of the population have to pay from their pocket an average of $99 per dialysis session, or $15,500 a year.

To support the shifts needed, a chronic care training program was implemented with face-to-face, train-the-trainer courses, and virtual courses via the Organization of American States (OAS) and PAHO virtual campuses. Self-management involving patients and families is critical to success in managing NCDs and living with chronic health conditions.

PAHO also is actively championing universal health coverage,. To further support this, in 2012 PAHO opened a window for NCD-related medicines and diagnostics in its Strategic Fund for Essential Public Health Supplies, which benefits countries through bulk procurement and ensures quality of medicines. Another way in which reorientation of services is being supported is the promotion of an "all-risk" approach for cardiovascular disease (CVD), versus a single-risk approach, for example, focusing only on blood pressure or diabetes. Use of the total-risk approach focuses resources and effort on the percentage of the population most likely to have a CVD event.

Building Partnerships and Alliances

The cross-cutting strategy of building partnerships, networks, and alliances is well recognized in health promotion. Ranging from loose networks at the national or regional level, through alliances and coalitions, to more structured partnerships, these approaches have been critical success factors in many initiatives. Several partnership approaches were used in some of the foregoing examples in the chapter.

Within the Americas, a key network has been the CARMEN (Collaborative Action for Risk Factor Prevention & Effective Management of NCDs) network, which comprises heads and coordinators of national chronic disease programs, civil society organizations such as the Inter American Heart Foundation, and several WHO collaborating centers, for example, in the Public Health Agency of Canada and the US Centers for Disease Control (CDC). Established in 1999, the network grew from an initial three members (Canada, Chile, Cuba) to include all the countries in the region, and provides virtual and face-to-face biennial forums for exchanging information, sharing experiences and lessons learned, and joint planning and collaboration between the countries of the Americas to prevent and control NCDs, their risk factors, and social determinants. The CARMEN school is one of the collaborative areas, and regional courses have been conducted in collaboration with academic partners in evidence-based public health practice, social marketing, physical activity, and chronic disease care.

In 2009, PAHO established a Partners' Forum for Action on Chronic Diseases with the CARMEN network at its core (Hospedales & Jane-Llopis, 2011). It serves as a mechanism to bring together the private sector and the civil society with member states, because no one sector can solve the problem by itself. This instrument leverages unique roles and capacities of each sector to take joint action to accomplish policy and environmental change to promote health and prevent chronic disease. Early operationalization took place in 2010, and five initial regional working groups were established that focused on healthy workplace; access to health services; healthy diet/salt reduction; information, communication, and advocacy; and physical activity. Subsequently, Trinidad and Tobago launched a national partners' forum in March 2010, Mexico established a multisector National Council on Chronic Diseases in February 2010, and Brazil launched a national multisector forum in August 2011. In September 2011, to strengthen emphasis on action, the initiative was rebranded as the Pan American Forum for Action on NCD, and enhances the capacity of the member states to implement the UNHLM declaration in respect of multisector action. In May 2012, a landmark meeting was held in Brasilia in which 32 countries, 45 NGOs, and 26 companies participated. The SaltSmart consortium of countries, companies, NGOs, and academia emerged from this as a very active area of collaboration.

Africa

Africa is the only World Health Organization region in the world that still has fewer than 50% of deaths due to NCDs (indeed 28.6% of all deaths in 2012), but a number of countries (e.g., South Africa, Namibia, Ghana) have surpassed the 40% mark for percentage of mortality due to NCDs, and the region is likely to have a majority of deaths due to NCDs in the next few years. Figure 13.2 shows the proportions of mortality due to the various NCDs in Africa. As of 2011

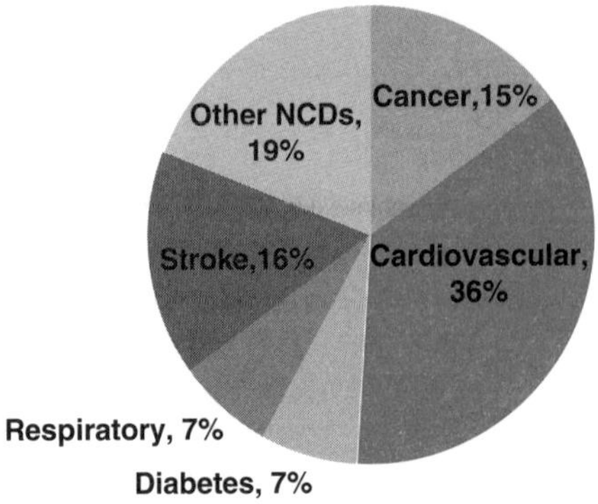

Figure 13.2 Proportion of Mortality Due to the NCDs in Africa, 2012

data, these are now fairly similar to those in the Americas, with proportionately more deaths due to stroke (16%) and fewer due to cancer (15%). Countries range from a low of 20% (Central African Republic, Chad, Democratic Republic of Congo, Angola, Zambia, Nigeria) to mid-30% (e.g., Benin, Gabon, Eritrea, Liberia, Senegal, Rwanda) to South Africa and Namibia at over 40%.

CASE STUDY 13.2 WHO STRATEGY ON NCDs FOR AFRICA

In Africa, the Strategy for the African Region on NCDs was adopted at the 50th session of the Regional Committee in 2000 in Ouagadougou. This strategy was updated in 2010 at the 60th session of the Regional Committee in Ouagadougou. The commitment of member states to this strategy was reiterated in the Brazzaville Declaration on NCDs, which was adopted in 2011, ahead of the high-level UN summit on NCDs. Through this declaration, member states committed to develop integrated national action plans and strengthen institutional capacities for NCD prevention and control. The rising burden of NCDs, in spite of these commitments, prompted the organization of the Regional Office of WHO for Africa, a regional multistakeholders' dialogue in Johannesburg in 2013, to share the lessons learned and shape the way going forward. Over the past 15 years local and regional actions have been initiated to promote the application of health promotion across Africa, including for NCDs. The extent of the implementation of the initiatives varies substantially. Some have remained at the stage of demonstration projects, while other have been scaled up to the national level, and at times across several countries.

The Strategy on Health Promotion of the Africa Region of WHO adopted in 2001 represents the first collective regional effort to embrace health promotion practices as effective components of strategies for preventing diseases and improving the general living conditions of populations in the region (WHO Regional Office for Africa, 2001). It was by then thought that health promotion action could significantly contribute to the achievement of the African Region's priority program objectives of which four (out of five) had direct relevance for NCDs, including:

1. prevention of priority NCDs such as mental illness, cardiovascular disease, diabetes, and cancers;
2. reducing risk factors for conditions and behaviors that expose people to HIV/STIs, tobacco use and other substance abuse, diabetes and other priority communicable diseases and NCDs;
3. fostering lifestyles and conditions that are conducive to physical, social, and emotional well-being, such as healthy dietary practices, active living, and use of life skills; and
4. increasing effective use of existing health services and stimulating demand for others.

The aims of the strategy were

- to advocate for increased awareness of and support for the use of health promotion across sectors;
- to develop national strategies incorporating policy frameworks and action plans;
- to plan, implement, and evaluate health promotion actions for intervening in disease-specific issues, population groups, or settings; and
- to mobilize resources by engaging new players such as civil society and public and private sectors (WHO Regional Office for Africa, 2001).

During the decade following the adoption of the strategy and with the assistance of WHO, some countries in the region developed their national health promotion policies and/or strategic plans. Guidelines for implementing health promotion interventions in the region were also developed. Training workshops were held in Benin, Uganda, and Zimbabwe between 2007 and 2010 to equip countries with knowledge on the use of health promotion tools and strategies to address the risk factors and determinants of NCDs. Moreover, to further support countries in their efforts to address disease risk factors and determinants, a health promotion cluster was established within the Regional Office of WHO in 2010. A progress report on the implementation of the Heath Promotion Strategy in the African Region published in 2011 concluded that between 2007 and 2010, 10 countries in the region developed national health promotion strategic action plans and 16 countries received technical support in developing national health promotion policies (WHO Regional Office for Africa, 2011). The report further identified the many gaps and challenges uncovered by the implementation of the strategy including:

- weak leadership and stewardship role of ministries of health;
- low level of involvement of various players including civil society and communities in advocacy actions;
- inadequate evidence regarding the effectiveness of health promotion;

- lack of sustainable financing mechanisms to support health promotion activities; and
- the need to build a critical mass of health promotion practitioners.

A key recommendation of the report was on the importance of updating the strategy to facilitate an effective application of health promotion actions commensurate with the priority public health challenges facing countries in the region (WHO Regional Office for Africa, 2011).

With lessons learned from the implementation of the initial strategy, an updated Strategy on Health Promotion in the African Region was adopted in 2012 (WHO Regional Office for Africa, 2012). The strategy covers a period of 10 years and aims to build on and scale up existing multisectoral health promotion interventions in order to contribute to reducing the leading causes of preventable deaths, disabilities, and major illnesses from communicable diseases and NCDs, violence and injuries, maternal and child health conditions, and new reemerging threats to health in the African Region. The strategy builds on key guiding principles:

- ownership of programs by individuals and communities;
- equity in health;
- human rights and gender equity;
- intersectorial collaboration and coordination of various players to promote health; and
- mutual accountability and shared responsibility among national governments, service providers, funding agencies, and intended beneficiaries.

The strategy further proposes eight key actions to address priority public health conditions:

1. strengthening the stewardship role of the ministries of health;
2. strengthening national technical and institutional capacity for health promotion;
3. sustaining institutional capacity for health promotion at national, regional, and local levels;
4. developing communication, social mobilization, and advocacy;
5. gathering and disseminating evidence on best practices and effective health promotion approaches;
6. establishing sustainable mechanisms for innovative financing of health promotion to ensure adequate funding of interventions across programs;
7. strengthening functional partnerships, alliances, and networks; and
8. strengthening community capacity for health promotion (WHO Regional Office for Africa, 2012).

Apart from WHO led initiatives, the African Health Strategy 2007–2015 of the African Union (African Union, 2007), has acknowledged the critical importance of community participation and empowerment, as well as strategic partnership with other stakeholders, as components of strategies for strengthening health systems in Africa.

Initiatives With Broad Applications

Preventing and controlling NCDs in Africa is a developing story and has gained importance only in the past two decades, in part as the local replication of global efforts to address NCDs but also in response to the accumulating evidence to support the harmful effects of NCDs on health and survival of the population within the region (WHO Regional Office for Africa, 2013). Successive regional initiatives targeting NCDs and risk factors in the African Region, mostly championed by the WHO, have integrated health promotion in their strategies. During the 48th (1998) and 49th (1999) sessions of the Regional Committee of the WHO for Africa, member states voiced their concern regarding the increasing importance of NCDs in the region, a concern that was further reiterated during the fourth meeting of health ministers of the Organization of African Unity held in Cairo in 1999. This concern was addressed at least in part at the 50th session of the Regional Committee in Ouagadougou, through the adoption of the Strategy for the African Region on NCDs (WHO Regional Office for Africa, 2000a). The strategy aimed to alleviate the burden of NCDs through the promotion of healthy lifestyles among populations of the African Region. The strategy further distinguished five key objectives, six guiding principles for achieving successful NCD prevention in the region, identified priority interventions to be addressed by member states, and suggested frameworks for implementation, monitoring, and evaluation (WHO Regional Office for Africa, 2000b). A decade later, another strategy with relevance for NCDs was adopted during the 60th session of the Regional Committee held in Malabo in 2010 (WHO Regional Office for Africa, 2010b). This strategy aimed to address the key determinants of health in the region, by assisting member states to promote actions to reduce health inequities through intersectorial policies and plans (WHO Regional Office for Africa, 2010b). The strategy strongly supported the notion that priority should be given to mainstreaming health promotion in all policies and programs to reduce the equity gap through community empowerment.

The commitment of member states to the African Strategy on NCDs was further reiterated in the Brazzaville Declaration on NCD prevention and control in the African Region, which was adopted in March 2011 at the regional consultation meeting of ministers of health, in preparation for the high level UN Summit on NCDs (WHO Regional Office for Africa, 2011b). Through the Brazzaville Declaration, member states further committed themselves to develop integrated national action plans and strengthen institutional capacities for NCD prevention and control. Actions proposed included strengthening and standardizing national health systems to generate disaggregated data on NCDs and using appropriate means including information and communication technology, to promote health awareness on NCD prevention and control strategies. Ministers of health further pledged to take action to protect their populations from unhealthy diets, harmful use of alcohol, and tobacco use including secondhand effects of smoking.

In spite of these commitments and efforts, NCDs continued to rise in the African Region, motivating the organization in March 2013 by The WHO Regional Office for Africa in Johannesburg, to convene a regional multistakeholders' dialogue to bring together all the key players to address the risk factors and effective interventions for NCDs in the region (WHO Regional Office for Africa, 2013). The dialogue was attended by delegates from 43 countries of the region, nonprofessional organizations and civil societies, and other partners. Specific objectives of the dialogue included (a) sharing information about the trends of NCD risk factors and burden of disease in the region; (b) identifying the challenges and opportunities for governments and relevant stakeholders in addressing risk factors for NCDs; (c) identifying priority actions and the roles and responsibilities of various stakeholders; and (d) proposing mechanisms for facilitating national dialogue and promoting public awareness on risk factors for NCDs. On the harmful use of alcohol, delegates strongly recommended the use of a more inclusive approach to involve communities and relevant stakeholders in policy development, and in relation to legislation, enforcement, and enactment. On tobacco use, delegates emphasized the urgency for countries to have clear action plans for the implementation of the Framework Convention on Tobacco Control (FCTC) and monitor its implementation.

Initiatives for Specific NCDs

Initiatives addressing specific NCDs have also been developed in Africa. Again, these developments have mostly occurred as part of the local or regional efforts to replicate or adapt international initiatives. Nevertheless, in some areas like tobacco control, Africa has at times led the global efforts.

Oral Health

Oral health, which also has an impact on the prevention and control of NCDs, is among the health problems to receive early attention at the regional level in Africa. The Conference of Heads of Dental Services in the African Region in 1969 and the Regional Expert Committee on Oral Health in 1978 recommended the establishment of dental services modelled on the public health approach. The resolution AFR/RC24/R9 of the Regional Committee of WHO in 1974 requested the regional director for Africa to provide for the establishment of dental advisory services within the regional office. The resolution AFR/RC30/R4 in 1980 called on member states of the region to integrate oral health into primary health care programs, while the resolution AFR/RC44/R13 in 1994 called on member states to formulate a comprehensive national oral health policy and plan based on primary health care. Finally, the first regional strategy on oral health was adopted at the 48th regional session in 1998. This strategy aimed at strengthening the capacity of countries to improve community oral health by effectively using proven interventions to address specific oral health needs. A progress report on the strategy was produced in 2008. By this time, the 10-year evaluation report showed significant progress by member states in implementing national oral health strategies, policies and programs (WHO Regional Office for Africa, 2008b). However, the effects of these efforts on the oral health of populations in the region have yet to be fully experienced (Thorpe, 2006).

Salt Reduction

Although policy and strategies on nutrition have been in place across Africa for years, the focus has been more on undernutrition and little on dietary risk factors for NCDs (Metta et al., 2014). Salt intake is perhaps the diet that has received the most attention so far in Africa. A related activity involved the technical workshops on "creating an enabling environment for population-based salt reduction strategies in the African Region" convened by the WHO in Mauritius in 2012 (Sookram et al., 2015). Participants at this meeting were from the health sectors, ministries of industry, and trade and academia. The meeting provided an opportunity to sensitize member states and other stakeholders on population-wide strategies for disease prevention through reduction of salt intake (Sookram et al., 2015). A year later another meeting on salt reduction brought together 15 countries from the West African Health Organization. The meeting focused on health benefits associated with reduction of salt intake and ended with the adoption by member states of a statement on salt reduction. The statement called on countries in the region to (a) develop and implement policies and plans to assist in the reduction of salt consumption by communities down to the levels recommended by the WHO; (b) increase awareness on the health benefits of dietary salt reduction; (c) work with industries to reduce the salt content of foods and beverages; and (d) set up an information system in order to monitor dietary salt intake (Sookram et al., 2015).

In practice, South Africa appears to be the only country in Africa with a national program to reduce dietary salt content. This program, however, builds on solid national evidence and strong advocacy, which are likely lacking in many other countries in the region (Hofman & Tollman, 2013). For instance, research conducted by the South African Medical Research Council (MRC) and universities in Cape Town has revealed that daily salt intake among adults in South Africa is on average 7.8 grams for black, 8.5 grams for mixed ancestry, and 9.5 grams for white persons; of which 45.5%, 32.8%, and 42.2% respectively are derived from processed food (Charlton et al., 2005a). These averages are higher than the 5 grams per day recommended by the World Health Organization. Bread and cereals have been consistently reported to be the major contributor to the daily salt intake from processed foods in South Africans, with other important sources being meat products, soup powder, and brick margarine (Charlton et al., 2005b). Furthermore, evidence to demonstrate that increased salt intake antedates the rise in blood pressure have been available from populations within Africa for more than two decades (Poulter et al., 1990), and the link between salt intake and rising blood pressure levels appear to be very consistent across populations and settings around the world. Beside the adverse effects on blood pressure levels, studies have also linked high salt intake with increased risk of stroke and cardiovascular diseases, including in African populations (Li et al., 2012; Strazzullo et al., 2009). In the global INTERHEART study, comprising participants from 52 countries including some within Africa, this risk of heart attack was 20 to 30% higher for patients who consumed more salty foods (Iqbal et al., 2008).

There is also compelling evidence that reducing salt intake will lower blood pressure levels, which in turn will result in significant health benefits among

South Africans. A collaborative study conducted by the South African MRC and universities in the Langa Township in Cape Town has reported a beneficial effect on blood pressure of food modification comprising 41% reduction in salt intake (Bertram et al., 2012). In this intervention study of eight weeks duration, modified food regimens reduced systolic blood pressure levels by 6.2 millimeter mercury. Moreover, study participants were unable to detect any taste differences between the experimental and regular bread (Charlton et al., 2008). This is interesting in the sense that local evidence has shown that by reducing by about half the sodium content of bread, it may be possible to prevent up to 6,400 deaths each year from stroke, ischemic heart disease, and hypertensive heart diseases. Further, more people may be prevented from developing the nonfatal forms of those conditions (Bertram et al., 2012). This research evidence accumulated over time, the continuous engagement of health policymakers in the course of gathering the various evidence, and the supportive global context led to the formulation and promulgation in March 2013 of the South African legislation on salt (Hofman & Tollman, 2013). These mandatory regulations, set to become effective in 2016, will affect the salt content of processed food, with expected benefits on health beyond South Africa considering the growing influence of the South African food industry on the entire African region.

Smoking

Tobacco control is perhaps the area that has received the most coordinated response from countries in Africa. Tobacco was introduced to Africa about five centuries ago (Mackey & Erikson, 2002), but tobacco use on the continent has remained low until about two decades ago when Africa became the prime target of multinational tobacco companies in the quest for new markets. This was followed by a shift in the uptake of smoking habits and prevalence on the continent, prompting gradual adoption of control policies by countries in the region. One of the earliest initiatives to promote a pan-African response to tobacco use was the maiden Inter-country Meeting on the Contribution of Parliamentarians to Tobacco Control in the African Region, which was held in Lome, Togo, in 1999. Parliamentarians at this meeting voiced their concern about tobacco use growing faster in Africa than in other developing economies and urged governments in the region to update or formulate their tobacco control laws and to "support WHO's effort for the preparation and adoption of the international Framework Convention on Tobacco Control (FCTC)" (WHO Regional Office for Africa, 1999). The policy focus of the African Region on tobacco control was clearly formulated a year later in Nairobi, at the Inter-country Meeting on Tobacco Control Policy and Programming in the African Region. The Nairobi meeting urged governments in the region to advocate and mobilize support for the negotiation and ratification of an evidence-based FCTC, and suggested some specific provisions for national tobacco control policies that included:

- increasing taxation above the inflation rate;
- banning advertising, sponsorship, and promotion;

- banning or restricting smoking in public places;
- requiring prominent health warnings and messages on tobacco packages;
- requiring constituent labels and additive levels and testing methods; and
- prohibiting sales and distribution of tobacco products to and by minors.

The common vision achieved at the regional level on issues relating to tobacco placed African countries in a comfortable situation to play a leading role during the FCTC negotiations. As such, African delegates were the first to negotiate the FCTC as a bloc with clear principles and to serve as a model for other WHO regions. As of July 2011, of the 46 countries in the WHO Africa Region, 41 were parties to the Framework Convention on Tobacco Control (Tumwine, 2011). Although countries in the region have implemented initiatives to control smoking, these countries also recognize the continued challenges in tobacco control, and particularly the negative impact on policy-planning of powerful tobacco industries at the country level (Tumwine, 2011; Valluri & Gaziano, 2013). There are also challenges in effectively contextualizing some of the FCTC articles. For instance, implementation of the packaging and labeling requirements of the FCTC may not be that effective in contexts where selling single cigarettes is by far more popular than selling the whole pack.

Diabetes Mellitus

A strategy for diabetes prevention and control in Africa was adopted at the 57th session of the Regional Committee for Africa of WHO in 2007 (WHO Regional Official for Africa, 2007a). The strategy's goal was to contribute to the reduction of the burden of diabetes-related morbidity and mortality and its associated risk factors. The strategy acknowledged the prime role of prevention, including primary, secondary, and tertiary prevention. Implementation of the strategy was to be guided by key principles including equity, a multisectorial approach and partnerships, and community participation (WHO Regional Office for Africa, 2007a) diseases in 2009, the Mauritius Call for Action was adopted. This call identified key strategies and commitment required for planning and implementing national diabetes, cardiovascular, and other NCD prevention and control programs in order to reduce their burden in the African Region (International Conference on Diabetes and Associated Diseases, 2009).

Other Initiatives

There have been other specific initiatives targeting NCDs in the African Region. The regional strategy for mental health 2000–2010 aimed to strengthen the capacity of member states to improve the quality of life of their populations by promoting healthy lifestyles and preventing and controlling mental, neurological, and psychological disorders (WHO Regional Office for Africa, 2000b). The 2010 regional strategy on the harmful use of alcohol aimed to contribute to the prevention of the harmful and related problems in the African Region. The adoption of this strategy followed the technical consultation on the harmful public health effects of alcohol use in the region organized in Brazzaville in

2006 (WHO Regional Office for Africa, 2010b). Delegates at this consultation unanimously agreed on the public health importance of the challenges posed by alcohol-related problems in the region (WHO Regional Office for Africa, 2007b). A regional strategy on cancer adopted in 2008 aims to help the reduction of cancer morbidity and mortality in the African Region (WHO Regional Office for Africa, 2008b). That strategy targets both prevention and control of cancers, with reduction in smoking being a major target. Guiding principles and priority interventions are largely informed by those of the regional Strategy on Health promotion (WHO Regional Office for Africa, 2012).

The trajectories of NCDs and related risk factors over time in Africa, characterized by escalating figures, testify that the growing awareness and good will are not yet translating into sufficient concrete action to prevent and control NCDs and risk factors. For instance, a recent survey on the availability of treatment guidelines for major NCD risk factors found that of the 49 countries included in the survey, 69% had guidelines for hypertension, 65% for cardiovascular diseases, 53% for diabetes, and only 10% (five countries) had treatment guidelines for dyslipidemia (Valluri & Gaziano, 2013). Existing guidelines were not always optimally disseminated and made readily available.

There is a relationship between the wealth of countries as measured by the GDP and how much countries spend on health; the larger the per capita income, the larger the expenditure is on health (WHO, 2012c). This trend is also observed in Africa, where the top 10 countries in terms of GDP spent on health appear to be the wealthiest, with the per capita GDP in 2011 ranging from $3,798 in Cape Verde to $2,742 in Equatorial Guinea (World Bank, 2013). Although there is no recommended level of spending on health, it has been shown that increasing expenditures on health are associated with better health outcomes, particularly for low-income countries such as those in Africa (WHO, 2012c). According to this exponential relationship, countries with life expectancy at birth closer to 80 years in 2009 were likely to be those spending more than US$2,000 (per capita) on health. No country in Africa is currently performing at this level of life expectancy, and only 11 sub-Saharan countries would be potentially able to spend up to that level, even assuming that all of their GDP was spent on health. This is very significant in the sense that governments in Africa are already spending less to provide adequate care for the commonest conditions, and yet they have virtually no additional existing capacity to invest further and optimally to improve healthcare in general, including for NCDs (Kengne, June-Rose et al., 2013). This results in heavy reliance on out-of-pocket expenditures for health that may lead to financial barriers for poor people. Paradoxically, the poorer the country is, the higher the share of out-of-pocket spending in total health expenditures. In 2009 this share was only about 13% in high-income countries compared with over 60% across Africa as a whole (WHO, 2012c).

Much Work Still to Do

As the percentage of mortality due to NCDs continues to rise globally, especially as more low- and middle-income countries see the size of their middle class and life expectancy both increase, although many meetings have been held, strategic plans been devised, and treaties been agreed to, outside of North America, Europe, and the developed countries of the Western Pacific region, where rates of NCD incidence and mortality (especially those related to heart disease) have begun to decline, little progress has been made. Table 13.1 shows the percentages of countries in Latin America and the Caribbean (LAC, PAHO countries minus Canada and the United States) and in Africa that have adopted various government policies and practices.

As seen in Table 13.1, African health systems are currently ill equipped and do not have the required capacity to efficiently deliver the prevention and control solutions for NCDs (Abegunde et al., 2007). As such, they will need to undergo significant transformation, with massive investment in health to efficiently address the double burden of communicable and noncommunicable diseases, and the challenge is huge. For instance, the cost of treating diabetes alone in sub-Saharan Africa in 2011 was estimated to be $2.8 billion, and is expected to increase by 61% by 2030, representing the largest relative global increase (International Diabetes Federation, 2011). Furthermore, even the cost of implementing effective diabetes control measures appears to be higher in

Table 13.1 Status of NCD Prevention and Control, and Percentage of Latin American/Caribbean and African Countries Meeting Each Criterion

Indicator	% of LAC Countries	%. of African Countries
Health ministries have a unit or department for NCDs	96%	93%
Funding available for NCD treatment/control, prevention, and surveillance and monitoring	60%	40%
National health reporting system and annual reports include indicators of NCD mortality, morbidity, and risk factors	80%	24%
Maintains national cancer registry	24%	16%
Implementing national policy/plan for prevention/control of CVD	44%	22%
Implementing national policy/plan for prevention/control of cancer	68%	31%
Implementing national policy/plan for prevention/control of respiratory diseases	28%	20%
Implementing national policy/plan for prevention/control of diabetes	44%	31%
Implementing national policy/plan for prevention/control of tobacco	64%	36%
Implementing national policy/plan for prevention/control of alcohol	48%	24%
Implementing national policy/plan for prevention/control of physical inactivity	52%	29%
Implementing national policy/plan for prevention/control of obesity/unhealthy diet	64%	31%
Number with at least one tobacco mPOWER measure implemented at highest level of achievement	52%	10%
Number with at least three tobacco mPOWER measures implemented at highest level of achievement	8%	0%

Africa than Asian countries with similar levels of development. The annual cost per capita for implementing intensive glycemic control augmented with retinopathy screening and photocoagulation in 2005 has been estimated at $3.14 for countries within the WHO African subregion against $2.11 for countries within the WHO Asian subregion (Ortegon et al., 2012).

African governments are grappling with the costs of NCDs on the continent. However, there are promising data (Kengne, Echouffo Tchcugui et al., 2008) suggesting there is some level of readiness on the continent as African governments have empowered themselves to be able to begin facing the global crisis of NCDs. Of all sub-Sahara African countries, as of 2008, 93% have a dedicated unit branch or department within the National Ministry of Health to tackle diseases such as CVD and diabetes. However, only 22% have operational integrated policies dedicated at managing and treating CVDs and only 31% have such a policy/plan for diabetes. For instance, only 13% of the countries have an existing and operational policy/strategy/action plan for tobacco control, with official government tobacco control policy for developing and coordinating the implementation of a plan of action, as well as for building a national infrastructure to carry out the implementation of this plan. More than half of these African countries are implementing fiscal interventions to influence behavior change (e.g., taxation on alcohol, tobacco products, and on high sugar content beverages). There is also hope because almost half of the African countries (40%) have a national surveillance system for NCDs. For instance, 72% of the countries have general availability of diabetes testing at primary care level. Also shown in Table 13.1, only 24% of African countries have a national health reporting system including NCD indicators, only 16% have a national cancer registry, and only 10% have implemented *any* national level tobacco measure recommended in mPOWER recommendations.

Latin America and the Caribbean are doing much better, but still have much work to do. Eighty percent have national reporting systems including indicators of NCDs, and around two-thirds have policies or plans for prevention and/or control of cancer, tobacco, and obesity or unhealthy diet. Around half have policies or plans focused on cardiovascular diseases, diabetes, alcohol, and physical activity. A majority have implemented at least one recommended tobacco control measure, but only 8% have implemented three out of the five recommendations.

NCDs are a huge challenge for human health and undermine development prospects, as they are a cause and effect of poverty. Yet there is a range of population and individual measures that can be combined to reduce the levels and impact of these problems. They require an all-of-society approach given the complexity of NCDs, their risk factors, and determinants such as poverty and lack of education, and lack of access to quality health services. And they require strengthened health systems and services, including, most importantly, the capacity to measure health conditions and risks and use the information for policy planning and evaluation.

The very need for an intersectoral approach is a huge challenge, and the health sector needs to play a leadership role for which it needs to be strengthened. Policy incoherence within government is common, for example, urban and transport developments without provision for biking and walking; state lands being used for tobacco growing; education sector focusing almost wholly on academic achievement and ignoring health promoting aspects such as physical activity; agriculture policy emphasizing meat production and/or export of fruit and vegetables with little or no attention to local populations' consumption. Senior health officials need to be able to engage other sectors and speak their language to accelerate multisector action.

Because NCDs are not perceived as a security threat to the North, the higher burden of NCDs in developing countries has to be addressed almost completely based on local resources, with very low levels of international assistance. Less than 3% of development assistance for health is directed at NCDs and risk factors, despite NCDs being the largest avoidable health and cost burden (Nugent & Feigl, 2010). We hope that the situation will shift as the UNHLM declaration is implemented.

No matter how successful we are at prevention, the demographic shift underway in developing countries will tend to drive increasing levels of NCDs and associated problems like dementia. Healthy aging programs need to be mainstreamed, which largely equates with the same measures to prevent and control NCDs; otherwise the prospect of health costs outstripping pension costs is real.

Childhood obesity and associated problems like Type 2 diabetes in adolescents represents another kind of complex challenge that requires a life course and multilevel approach, from prenatal care and breastfeeding through early childhood nutrition and school feeding programs, and taxes and price measures to favor healthy food.

The region of the Americas and the European region of WHO are the most affected by NCDs of the six WHO regions, and Africa is increasing rapidly in the impact of NCDs, but still least affected of all regions. The problem of NCDs and related risks is rapidly expanding in low- and middle-income countries in these regions and elsewhere in the world, which often have simultaneous burdens of traditional infectious diseases and injuries.

The UNHLM was a historic event in global health with leadership from the Americas and particularly the Caribbean. The challenge is how to maintain the issue of the political agenda nationally and globally. This will necessitate health and the NCD advocacy movement to show the links with and co-benefits of other major development challenges like climate change and poverty reduction. Ongoing leadership is needed from ministries of health and from the World Health Organization and its regional offices (like PAHO and the African Regional Office) and the United Nations, and continued pressure by civil society, academic advocates, and economic development organizations such as the World Bank. The UN system has begun to take the issue on board as a development issue, including in poverty reduction (UNDP), youth programs (UNICEF), and agriculture policy (FAO).

Organizations like PAHO and WHO have leadership roles in global health promotion, developing the evidence and making the case, setting norms and standards, and securing agreement across countries for joint action in public policy, supportive environments, strengthening health systems, community action, setting up networks and partnerships.

Summary

This chapter provides a rich oversight, a panorama, of contemporary uses of health promotion in the prevention and control of noncommunicable diseases in the Americas and in Africa, the major health challenge and avoidable health cost in the former, and a major emerging challenge in the latter.

The narrative brings home the importance of the catalytic role played by WHO and its regional offices, and value of the regional and subregional approach, with the Pan American Health Organization, regional office of WHO for the Western Hemisphere, and the Caribbean countries having played major roles in advancing the issue of NCDs onto the global agenda.

NCDs represent the second time a major health issue came onto the UN Agenda (the first was HIV/AIDS in the 2001 UN General Assembly), with leadership of the Caribbean countries.

The chapter is a rich feast of health promotion strategies being used in the prevention and control of NCDs, beginning with healthy public policy and advocacy, and including collaboration with civil society organizations and networks of professionals across national boundaries. A clear picture emerges of the wide range of actors involved and how political will and mobilization took place at different levels—national, regional, and global—making a historic step forward in 2007 when the Caribbean heads of state declared NCDs a threat to their development; through the UN High Level Meeting on NCDs in 2011, and the subsequent agreement in 2014 on a Global Monitoring Framework with Targets and Indicators, which will be incorporated into the sustainable development goals (SGDs).

For the Americas, a range of initiatives are described, including creation of supportive environments by regional efforts to eliminate trans fatty acids in the diet in the Americas; a SaltSmart consortium to reduce dietary salt consumption; an initiative to reduce marketing of food to children; the promotion of physical activity including innovations such as *Ciclovias,* and the implementation of the WHO Framework on Tobacco Control. Many communications initiatives are overviewed, including one leveraging new social media and mobile phones in an SMS-based GetTheMessage campaign to drive policymakers to attend the UNHLM in New York. Health services reorientation, especially as guided by the chronic disease model, is described. The use of networks and alliances is also described, including regional networks and creation of novel public-private-civil society platforms for taking action.

In Africa, the NCD epidemic is perhaps not as well developed, yet its human and economic impact is blossoming at a time when countries are struggling with debt and other major health and environmental issues. But the response is very dynamic and evolving as governments begin to come to grips with the problem. Most progress has perhaps been made with tobacco, and healthy diets, including salt reduction and tackling obesity, have much potential for action. Africa in many parts faces a double whammy of infectious diseases and NCDs and obesity, which it can ill afford. Lessons learned from other parts of the world can usefully be shared to stimulate increased attention and direction of resources. In turn, lessons on integration of NCDs into primary health care.

It took several decades to arrive at the NCD epidemic now unfolding, driven by demographic changes, widespread risk factors, and determinants in the social, economic, and environmental fabric of societies. It will probably take at least a generation to reverse the trends, and ongoing research and application of evidence and sharing of lessons learned between different parts of the world can only benefit the world.

KEY TERMS

1. **Healthy public policy:** Public policies that determine the present and future of a population's health
2. **Extreme poverty:** Generally considered living on less than $1.25/day
3. **Noncommunicable diseases (NCDs):** Chronic diseases such as cardiovascular diseases, diabetes, obesity, cancer, and chronic respiratory diseases. Internationally, mental illness and substance abuse are sometimes considered NCDs as well
4. **Recommended salt intake:** 5g per day

REVIEW QUESTIONS

1. How is the proportion of mortality due to NCDs changing in some parts of the world?
2. What region of the world has the lowest proportion of mortality due to NCDs?
3. What regions of the world have the highest proportion of mortality due to NCDs?
4. What are some strategies countries can use to reduce trans fat and salt use?
5. What are some strategies countries can use to reduce tobacco use?
6. What are some national policies whose implementation needs to be increased to better monitor and control NCDs?

References

Abegunde, D. O., Shengelia, B., Luyten, A., Cameron, A., Celletti, F., Nishtar, S., … Mendis, S. (2007). Can non-physician health-care workers assess and manage cardiovascular risk in primary care? *Bulletin of the World Health Organization 85*(6), 432–440.

African Union. (2007). *Africa health strategy: 2007–2015*. Johannesburg.

Asaria, P., Chisholm, D., Mathers, C., Ezzati, M., & Beaglehole, R. (2007). Chronic disease prevention: Health effects and financial costs of strategies to reduce salt intake and control tobacco use. *Lancet, 370*, 2044–2053.

Bertram, M. Y., Steyn, K., Wentzel-Viljoen, E., Tollman, S., & Hofman, K. J. (2012). Reducing the sodium content of high-salt foods: Effect on cardiovascular disease in South Africa. *South African Medical Journal, 102*(9), 743–745.

Bibbins-Domingo, K., Chertow, G. M., Coxson, P. G., Moran, A., Lightwood, J. M., Pletcher, M. J., & Goldman, L. (2010). Projected effect of dietary salt reductions on future cardiovascular disease. *New England Journal of Medicine, 362*, 590–599.

Bloom, D. E., Cafiero, E. T., Jané-Llopis, E., Abrahams-Gessel, S., Bloom, L. R., & Fathima, S. (2011). The global economic burden of non-communicable diseases: A report by the World Economic Forum and the Harvard School of Public Health Geneva: World Economic Forum, retrieved from http://www3.weforum.org/docs/WEF_Harvard_HE_GlobalEconomicBurden NonCommunicableDiseases_2011.pdf

Brown, I., Tzoulaki, I., Candeias, V., & Elliott P. (2009). Salt intakes around the world: Implications for public health *International Journal of Epidemiology, 38*(3), 791–813.

CARICOM. (2007). *Uniting to stop the epidemic of NCDs.* Heads of Government Declaration. Retrieved from http://www.caricom.org/jsp/communication/meetings_statements/declaration_port_of_spain_chronic_ncds.jsp?menu-communications

Charlton, K. E., Steyn, K., Levitt, N. S., Zulu, J.V.D., Jonathan, F., Veldman, J., & Nel, J. H. (2005a). Diet and blood pressure in South Africa: Intake of foods containing sodium, potassium, calcium, and magnesium in three ethnic groups. *Nutrition 21*(1), 39–50.

Charlton, K. E., Steyn, K., Levitt, N. S., Zulu, J.V.D., Jonathan, F., Veldman, J., & Nel, J. H. (2005b). Ethnic differences in intake and excretion of sodium, potassium, calcium and magnesium in South Africans. *European Journal of Cardiovascular Prevention and Rehabilitation: Official Journal of the European Society of Cardiology, 12*(4), 355–362.

Charlton, K. E., Steyn, K., Levitt, N. S., Peer, N., Jonathan, D., Gogela, T., … Lombard, C. J. (2008). A food-based dietary strategy lowers blood pressure in a low socio-economic setting: A randomised study in South Africa. *Public Health Nutrition 11*(12), 1397–1406.

Claro, R. M., Linders, H., Ricardo, C. Z., Legetic, B., & Campbell, N.R.C. (2012). Consumer attitudes, knowledge, and behavior related to salt consumption in sentinel countries of the Americas. *Revista Panamericana de Salud Pública, 32*(4), 265–73.

Cobiac, L. J., Vos, T., & Veerman, J. L. (2010). Cost-effectiveness of interventions to reduce dietary salt intake. *Heart, 96*(23), 1920–1925.

Committee on Strategies to Reduce Sodium Intake, Food and Nutrition Board, Institute of Medicine (US); Henny, J. E., Taylor, C. L., & Boon, C. S. (Eds.).

(2010). *Strategies to reduce sodium intake in the United States.* Washington, DC: National Academies Press.

Healthy Caribbean Coalition 2011 GetTheMessage campaign. Retrieved from http://healthycaribbean.org/get-the-message.php

Hofman, K. J., & S. M. Tollman. (2013). Population health in South Africa: A view from the salt mines. *Lancet Global Health 1*(2), e66–e67.

Hospedales, J., & Jane-Llopis, E. (2011). A multi stakeholder platform to promote health and prevent NCDs in the Americas: The Pan American Health Organization Partners Forum for Action. *Journal of Health Communication. 16*(Aug, Suppl. 2), 191–200. Retrieved from http://www.ncbi.nlm.nih.gov/pubmed/21916722

Hublet, A., Kuntsche, E., Nic Gabhainn, S., Godeau, E., Kokkevi, A., HBSC Risk Behaviour Focus Group (2009). Gender specific trends in alcohol use: Cross-cultural comparisons from 1998 to 2006 in 24 countries and regions. *International Journal of Public Health, 54,* 199–208.

International Conference on Diabetes and Associated Diseases. (2009). *The Mauritius call for action.* Mauritius, East Africa: World Health Organization, International Diabetes Federation, Mauritius Ministry of Health and Quality of Life.

International Diabetes Federation. (Ed.). (2011). *Updated diabetes atlas 2011.* Brussels: Author.

Iqbal, R., Anand, S., Ounpuu, S., Islam, S., Zhang, X., Rangarajan, S., … , & Yusuf, S. (2008). Dietary patterns and the risk of acute myocardial infarction in 52 countries: Results of the INTERHEART study. *Circulation 118*(19), 1929–1937.

Kengne, A. P., Echouffo-Tcheugui, J., Sobgnwi, E., & Mbanya, J. C (2013). New insights on diabetes mellitus and obesity in Africa. Part 2: Prevention, screening and economic burden. *Heart 99*(15), 1072–1077.

Kengne, A. P., June-Rose. Z., McHiza, A., Amoah, G., & Mbanya, J. C. (2013). Cardiovascular diseases and diabetes as economic and developmental challenges in Africa. *Progress in Cardiovascular Diseases, 56*(3), 302–313.

Li, X. Y., Cai, X. L., Bian P. D., &. Hu, L. R. (2012). High salt intake and stroke: Meta–analysis of the epidemiologic evidence. *CNS Neuroscience and Therapeutics, 18*(8), 691–701.

Mackey, J., & Erikson, M. (2002). *The tobacco atlas.* Geneva: World Health Organization.

Metta, E., Msambichaka, B., Mwangome, M., Nyato, D. J., Dieleman, M., Haisma, H., … Geubbels, E. (2014). Public policy, health system, and community actions against illness as platforms for response to NCDs in Tanzania: A narrative review. *Global Health Action, 7,* 23439.

Milio, N. (1981). *Promoting health through public policy.* Philadelphia, PA: F. A. Davis.

Milio, N. (1985a). *Promoting health through public policy.* Ottawa: Canadian Public Health Association.

Milio, N. R. (1985b). Healthy nations: Creating a new ecology of public policy for health. *Canadian Journal of Public Health, 76*(Suppl. 1), 79–87.

Milio, N. (1988). Public policy as the cornerstone for a new public health: Local and global beginnings. *Family and Community Health, 11*(2), 57–71.

Mosca, L., Hammond, G., Mochari-Greenberger, H., Towfighi, A., & Albert, M. A. (2013). Fifteen-year trends in awareness of heart disease in women: Results of a 2012 American Heart Association National Survey. *Circulation, 127*, 1254–1263.

NCD Alliance. (2014). *NCD Alliance Report 2013–2014: Putting non-communicable diseases on the global agenda*. London: Author.

Nugent, R., & Feigl, A. (2010). *Where have all the donors gone? Scarce donor funding for non–communicable diseases*. Working Paper No. 228. Washington, DC: Center for Global Development.

Ortegon, M., Lim, S., Chisholm, D., & Mendis, S. (2012). Cost effectiveness of strategies to combat cardiovascular disease, diabetes, and tobacco use in sub–Saharan Africa and South East Asia: Mathematical modelling study. *British Medical Journal, 344*, e607.

Pan American Health Organization. (2007a). *Control of chronic diseases, including diet, physical activity and health*. Washington, DC: Author.

Pan American Health Organization. (2007b). *Regional strategy and plan of action on an integrated approach to the prevention and control of NCDs*. Washington, DC: Author.

Pan American Health Organization. (2008). *Premature mortality due to cerebrovascular disease in the Americas circa 2006*. Washington, DC: Author.

Pan American Health Organization. (2009). *National capacity for the management of chronic diseases in Latin America and the Caribbean*. Washington, DC: Author.

Pan American Health Organization (2011). *Report of a high level regional consultation against NCDs and Obesity*. Retrieved from http://www.paho.org/hq/index.php?option=com_docman&task=doc_view&gid=13836&Itemid=

Pan American Health Organization. (2011). *Recommendations from a Pan American health organization expert consultation*. Washington, DC: Author.

Pan American Health Organization. (2012). *Building a healthier future: Prevention of NCDs*. Washington, DC: Author.

Pan American Health Organization. (2013). *Assessing national capacity for the prevention and control of non-communicable diseases: Report of the Americas Region*. Washington, DC. Author.

Pan American Health Organization/World Health Organization. (2011). *Non-communicable diseases in the Americas: Basic indicators*. Washington, DC: Author.

Pan American Health Organization/World Health Organization Task Force on Trans Fats Free Americas. (2007). *Conclusions and recommendations*. Washington, DC: Author.

Poulter, N. R., Khaw, K. T., Hopwood, M., Mugambi, B. E., Peart, W. S., Rose G., & Sever, P. S. (1990). The Kenyan Luo migration study: Observations on the initiation of a rise in blood pressure. *British Medical Journal, 300*(6730), 967–972.

Rice, M. (2011). *Trends and achievements in promoting health in the Americas: Developments from 2003–2011.* Washington, DC: Pan American Health Organization.

Samuels, T., Kirton, J., & Guebert, J. (2014). Monitoring compliance with high-level commitments in health: The case of the CARICOM Summit on Chronic Non–Communicable Diseases. *Bulletin of the World Health Organization, 92,* 27B0–276B.

Samuels, T. A, & Fraser, H. (2010). Caribbean Wellness Day: Mobilizing a region for chronic noncommunicable disease prevention and control. *Revista Panamericana de Salud Pública, 28*(6), 472–479.

Sarno, F., Claro, R. M., Levy, R. B., Bandoni, D. H., Ferreira, S.R.G., & Monteiro, C. A. (2009). Estimated sodium intake by the Brazilian population, 2002–2003. *Revista de Saúde Pública, 43,* 219–225.

Simons-Morton, B. G., Farhat, T., ter Bogt, T. F. M., Kuntsche, E., Gabhainn, S. N., et al., (2009). Gender specific trends in alcohol use: Cross-cultural comparisons from 1998 to 2006 in 24 countries and regions. *International Journal of Public Health, 54,* S199–S208.

Sodium Working Group. 2010. *Ottawa, Canada: Health Canada.* Retrieved from http://www.hc-sc.gc.ca/fn-an/alt_formats/pdf/nutrition/sodium/strateg/index-eng.pdf

Sookram, C., Munodawafa, D., Phori, P. M., Varenne, B., & Alisalad, A. (2015). WHO's supported interventions on salt intake reduction in the sub–Saharan Africa region. *Cardiovascular Diagnosis and Therapy, 5*(3), 186–190.

Strazzullo, P., D'Elia, L., Kandala, N. B, & Cappuccio, F. P. (2009). Salt intake, stroke, and cardiovascular disease: Meta-analysis of prospective studies. *British Medical Journal, 339,* b4567.

Suhckre, M., Nugent, R., Stuckler, D., & Rocco, L. (2006). *Chronic disease: An economic perspective.* Oxford: Oxford Health Alliance.

Tumwine, J. (2011). Implementation of the framework convention on tobacco control in Africa: Current status of legislation. *International Journal of Environmental Research and Public Health, 8*(11), 4312–4331.

United Nations, 2011. *Political declaration of the high level meeting of the General Assembly on the prevention and control of non-communicable diseases.* A/66/L.1. Retrieved from http://www.un.org/ga/search/view_doc.asp?symbol=A/66/L.1

Valluri, S., & Gaziano, T. A. (2013). Progress in national and regional guidelines development and deployment for the clinical prevention and control of CVD and diabetes in Africa. *Progress in Cardiovascular Diseases, 56*(3), 336–343.

Thorpe, S. (2006). Oral health issues in the African region: Current situation and future perspectives. *Journal of Dental Education, 70*(Suppl. 11), 8–15.

World Bank. (2011). *Chronic emergency: Why NCDs matter.*

World Bank. (2013). *Data–Indicators.* Retrieved from http://data.worldbank.org/indicator

World Economic Forum. (2011). *From burden to best buys. Reducing the impact of noncommunicable diseases in low and middle-income countries.* Retrieved from: http://www.who.int/nmh/publications/best_buys_summary.pdf

World Economic Forum on Latin America/Pan American Health Organization. (2011). *Dietary sodium/salt reduction in the Americas: 2011 statement of Rio de Janeiro.* April 27. Rio de Janeiro, Brazil: Author.

World Health Organization. (1986). *Ottawa charter on health promotion.* Geneva: Author.

World Health Organization. (2000). *Global strategy for the prevention and control of noncommunicable diseases.* Geneva: Author.

World Health Organization. (2001). *Macroeconomics and health: Investing in health for economic development.* Geneva: Author.

World Health Organization. (2003). *Framework convention on tobacco control.* Geneva: Author.

World Health Organization. (2004). *Global strategy on diet, physical activity and health.* Retrieved from http://www.who.int/nmh/wha/59/dpas/en/

World Health Organization. (2006). Sodium *intakes around the world.* Retrieved from http://www.who.int/dietphysicalactivity/Elliot-brown-2007.pdf

World Health Organization. (2010a). *Creating an enabling environment for population–based salt reduction strategies.* Report of a joint technical meeting held by WHO and the Food Standards Agency. United Kingdom, July. Geneva: Author.

World Health Organization. (2010b). *Global strategy to reduce the harmful use of alcohol.* Geneva: Author.

World Health Organization. (2010c). *Set of recommendations on the marketing of foods and non-alcoholic beverages to children.* Geneva: Author.

World Health Organization. (2011a). *Global status report on noncommunicable diseases* 2010. Retrieved from http://www.who.int/nmh/publications/ncd_report_full_en.pdf

World Health Organization. (2011b). *Scaling up action against NCDs: How much will it cost?* Geneva: Author.

World Health Organization. (2011c). *First global ministerial conference on healthy lifestyle and NCD control.* Geneva: Author.

World Health Organization. (2012a). *Comprehensive global monitoring framework including indicators and voluntary targets for the prevention and control of noncommunicable diseases.* Geneva: Author.

World Health Organization. (2012b). *Guideline: Sodium intake for adults and children.* Geneva: Author.

World Health Organization. (2012c). *WHO global health expenditure atlas.* Geneva: Author.

World Health Organization. (2013). *NCD global monitoring framework*. Retrieved from http://www.who.int/nmh/global_monitoring_framework/en/

World Health Organization Regional Office for Africa. (1999). *The Lome declaration on the contribution of parliamentarians to tobacco control in the African Region*. Lome: Author.

World Health Organization Regional Office for Africa. (2000a). *Noncommunicable diseases: A strategy for the African Region*. Brazzaville: Author.

World Health Organization Regional Office for Africa. (2000b). *Regional strategy for mental health 2000–2010*. Brazzaville: WHO.

World Health Organization Regional Office for Africa. (2001). *Health promotion: A strategy for the African Region*. AFR/RC51/18. Brazzaville: WHO.

World Health Organization Regional Office for Africa. (2007a). *Diabetes prevention and control: A strategy for the WHO African Region*. Brazzaville: WHO.

World Health Organization Regional Office for Africa. (2007b). *Technical consultation on the public health problems caused by harmful use of alcohol in the African Region*. Final report. Brazzaville: WHO.

World Health Organization Regional Office for Africa. (2008a). *Cancer prevention and control: A strategy for the WHO African Region*. Yaounde: WHO.

World Health Organization Regional Office for Africa. (2008b). *Implementation of the regional oral health strategy: Updates and the way forward*. Report of the regional director. Yaounde: WHO.

World Health Organization Regional Office for Africa. (2010a). *Reduction of the harmful use of alcohol: A strategy for WHO Africa Region*. AFR/RC60/4. Malabo: WHO.

World Health Organization Regional Office for Africa. (2010b). *A strategy for addressing the key determinants of health in the African Region*. AFR/RC60/3. Malabo: WHO.

World Health Organization Regional Office for Africa. (2011a). *Progress report on the implementation of the regional health promotion strategy*. Yamoussoukro: WHO.

World Health Organization Regional Office for Africa. (2011b). *United Against NCDs: The time to act is now. The Brazzaville Declaration on noncommunicable diseases prevention and control in the WHO African Region*. Brazzaville: WHO.

World Health Organization Regional Office for Africa. (2012). *Health promotion: Strategy for the African Region*. Luanda: WHO.

World Health Organization Regional Office for Africa. (2013). *Multi-stakeholder dialogue on risk factors for non-communicable diseases*. Brazzaville: WHO.

CHAPTER 14

WOMEN'S CANCERS

Silvana Luciani and Irene Agurto

Women are often characterized as the primary caregivers and social agents of change because of their central role in families, communities, and societies. Health promotion and disease prevention programs tend to have a particular emphasis on women, to address their unique health issues, to safeguard their health, and to reach out to women to serve as inherent health promoters within their social sphere of influence.

Much attention and collective international action has been garnered toward women addressing their health needs during their reproductive years, and with a focus on the determinants of health (Box 14.1). The International Conference on Population and Development in 1994, as well as the United Nations Conference on Women (1995), catalyzed much of this global attention on women's health and provided a strategic framework to reduce maternal mortality and increase access to reproductive and sexual health services, including family planning. The Millennium Development Goals (2000), which include targets for maternal mortality, further leveraged the earlier global commitments to women's health. It is as a result of the investments and interventions directed to these significant women's health issues that overall maternal mortality has been decreasing. However, although gains have been made in reducing maternal mortality, now overall more women die of breast and **cervical cancer** each year than in childbirth (Knaul et al., 2012).

As countries progress in their economic development, many are experiencing an epidemiological transition related to changes in lifestyles, reproductive patterns, and longevity. Noncommunicable diseases (NCDs) are now the leading causes of morbidity and mortality in almost all countries around the world (World Health Organization [WHO], 2011). Cancer is the second most common NCD in both men and women, second only to cardiovascular disease. Among women, breast and cervical cancer are the leading cancer types in terms of both incidence and mortality.

LEARNING OBJECTIVES

By the end of this chapter, the reader should be able to:

- **Appreciate the global burden of women's cancers and the inequities associated with breast and cervical cancer**
- **Understand the public health perspectives on the prevention and control of breast and cervical cancer**
- **Know about community-based health promotion strategies that can improve breast and cervical cancer prevention and control**

BOX 14.1 WOMEN'S CANCERS ARE NOT JUST ABOUT HEALTH

Cancer has wide-reaching social, economic, and human rights implications. All people have the right to access proven and effective cancer prevention, early diagnosis, treatment, and palliative care services on equal terms, regardless of income, gender, education, ethnicity, or geographic location, and without suffering hardship as a consequence.

The social impact on women and their families of this high burden of cancer is tremendous, because a diagnosis of cancer associated with reproduction often leads to women's discrimination and stigma. For example, treatment of these types of cancer often involve the removal of a breast, or removal of the cervix and uterus, which make women more vulnerable to social exclusion (Knaul et al., 2012).

Much is known about the risk factors and causes of these two cancer types, though much less is known about **breast cancer** than cervical cancer. Effective public health interventions are available to prevent cervical cancer, detect early stages of breast and cervical cancer, and treat these cancers effectively. Health promotion is a key part of the health care continuum for the prevention and control of these two common types of women's cancers.

In this chapter, we review the prevention and control of breast and cervical cancer and community based health promotion interventions. The objective of this chapter is to improve understanding of the high burden of women's cancers, the inequities associated with these diseases, their preventable nature, and how health promotion strategies can be applied to improve their prevention and control.

Global Burden of Women's Cancers

Worldwide, breast and cervical cancer are the most common cancers; breast cancer is the leading cause of cancer diagnosis in 135 countries, and cervical cancer the leading cause in 45 countries. For cancer deaths, breast cancer is the leading cause in 99 countries, and cervical cancer is the leading cause in 55 countries (Bray et al., 2012).

An estimated 1.64 million women were diagnosed with breast cancer and 454,000 women were diagnosed with cervical cancer in 2010 in the world. The number of breast cancer cases has more than doubled since 1980, increasing at an annual rate of 3.1%. Cervical cancer has increased in that time period at a slower pace, with an annual rate of 0.6% (Forouzanfar et al., 2011).

If no action is taken, the number of new breast and cervical cancer cases is projected to increase to almost 3 million women by 2030, largely because of population growth (Ferlay et al., 2010). This is more than a 50% increase in just 20 years, which will exert a tremendous toll on lives and on economies and health care systems. The bulk of these new cases are estimated to occur in low- and middle-income countries (LMIC) because of increasing life expectancy, but also because of the reductions in infectious diseases and changes in reproductive and lifestyle patterns that affect risk, particularly for breast cancer.

An estimated 425,000 women and 200,000 women worldwide died from breast and cervical cancer respectively in 2010. Since 1980, the number of breast cancer deaths has almost doubled and has increased annually by 1.8%; cervical cancer has increased by 26,000 cases in that period, with an annual increase of 0.46% (Forouzanfar et al., 2011).

Despite the myth that cancer is an illness of the elderly, these diseases affect women in the prime of their lives, when they are contributing to the family income, society, and the care of children. The median age of death from breast cancer is 54 years of age, and for cervical cancer it is 55 years of age (Fourouzanfor et al., 2011). There is a perception that in developing countries, breast cancer affects younger women; however, the rates are not higher in younger women in developed versus developing countries (El Saghir et al., 2011).

These overall trends mask the big problem of cancer in low- and middle-income countries because the majority of these women's cancers occur in women in developing countries, where 76% of cervical cancer cases and 51% of breast cancer cases occur (Ferlay et al., 2010). Furthermore, in LMIC since 1980, breast cancer incidence increased by 60% and mortality increased by 53%; and cervical cancer incidence increased by 24% and deaths by 19%, much larger increases than observed in developed countries (Fourouzanfor et al., 2011). In the Region of the Americas, the disparities in cancer mortality can be observed with cervical cancer mortality, where rates in Central America are up to six times higher than those in the United States or Canada, which may be attributable to the level of development and differences in access to health services (Luciani et al., 2013).

This cancer situation in LMIC is further exacerbated by the fact that women in these countries have poorer outcomes than their developed country counterparts. This is noted by comparing the ratio of mortality to incidence (MIR) for the case-fatality rate, which tend to be higher in developing countries. For example, the cervical cancer MIR in the United States is 0.27, while in developing countries overall it was 0.53. For breast cancer, the MIR in the United States is 0.22, compared to less developed regions, where it was 0.39 (Ferlay et al., 2010).

The poorer outcomes are linked to the late stage of presentation of the disease. For example, more than 70% of women in LMIC present with advanced clinical breast cancer, when cure is less likely (El Saghir et al., 2011). Breast cancer five-year survival remains low in low-income countries, reported as low as 19% in some countries in Africa, as compared to 80% or higher in the United States. This has been attributed to low awareness of community and providers, barriers to access to treatment, and absence of early detection programs.

Preventing and Controlling Women's Cancers

About a third of all cancer cases can be prevented by reducing modifiable risk factors, notably tobacco use, harmful use of alcohol, unhealthy diet, physical inactivity, exposures to environmental carcinogens and infections from human papilloma virus (for cervical cancer), and other infectious agents. Screening asymptomatic populations for cancers detectable at early stage, such as is the case for cervical and breast cancer, can be a very effective public health intervention to reduce the burden of these cancers. Many cancers have a high chance of cure if diagnosed early and treated in a timely and appropriate manner, and all cancer patients can benefit from palliative care and supportive care services. In this section, information is provided on the public health interventions for cervical and breast cancer.

Cervical Cancer

Unlike other cancer types, cervical cancer is highly preventable because of its natural history and because knowledge and tools are available to prevent it. Persistent infection with oncogenic types of **human papillomavirus** (HPV) is the principal cause of cervical cancer. HPV is a very common sexually transmitted virus, and most sexually active people are exposed to HPV in their lifetimes. The majority of HPV infections clear spontaneously as a result of normal immune response, and most women with HPV infection do not develop cervical cancer. In a minority of cases, when the high-risk HPV infection persists, it may evolve into precancer, which, left untreated, can further evolve to invasive cancer. It is estimated that it takes approximately 20 years from initial HPV infection to the development of invasive cervical cancer (WHO, 2009).

Of the more than 100 HPV types, about 14 types are known to be oncogenic; the most common of these are HPV 16 and 18, responsible for approximately 70% of all cervical cancer cases (WHO, 2009). HPV type distribution varies around the world, but the dominant type in all regions is HPV 16. Other common oncogenic HPV types found in cervical cancer include HPV 31, 33, 45, and 58. HPV types 6 and 11 are also common types, not associated with cancer, but they can cause genital warts.

Other risk factors are associated with cervical cancer and can contribute to a woman's increased risk for developing the disease. These include increasing number of sexual partners, early age at first birth, increasing parity, coinfection with HIV or other sexually transmitted infections such as herpes simplex virus 2, chlamydia, or gonorrhea, tobacco smoking, and long-term use of oral contraceptives (WHO, 2006).

Public Health Interventions

Technologies are an important aspect of public health interventions, and a range of cost-effective technologies are available to prevent and control women's cancers, as noted in Box 14.2. For cervical cancer prevention, HPV vaccines are available to prevent genital HPV infections. A bivalent vaccine, licensed in 2007, targets the main oncogenic types HPV16 and 18, and a quadrivalent vaccine, licensed in 2006 targets these same types, in addition to HPV 6 and 11 to prevent genital warts. A 9-valent HPV vaccine was licensed in 2015, and targets five additional HPV types as well as those in the quadrivalent vaccine. These vaccines require two to three doses over a six-month period of

BOX 14.2 TECHNOLOGIES TO PREVENT, DETECT, AND TREAT WOMEN'S CANCERS

Technological advancements have contributed significantly to the improvement of cancer prevention, detection at earlier stages, and treatment outcomes. For cervical cancer, the development of **HPV vaccines** has revolutionized how cervical cancer can be prevented and will lead to significant reductions in mortality. Also, new diagnostic tests such as HPV tests are enabling more accurate detection of early, precancerous cervical lesions. For breast cancer, the development and deployment of **mammography** equipment has enabled disease detection at much earlier stages, although implementing mammography screening in limited-resource settings continues to be a challenge.

time, and are non-infections because they do not contain live viruses. They are designed to be prophylactic and not therapeutic, that is, they are to prevent HPV infection, not clear existing HPV infections.

These vaccines have been proven safe and efficacious in clinical trials. The global policy position on HPV vaccines, issued by WHO in 2009 following an extensive review of evidence and advice from the Strategic Advisory Group of Experts (SAGE) on Immunization, recommends that routine HPV vaccination should be included in national immunization programs if it is programmatically feasible and sustainable. Because the HPV vaccines are most effective in women not exposed to the virus, the primary target population is young adolescent girls, ages 9 to 13. The vaccination of males is not recommended at this time, because the investment should be high vaccination coverage (>70%) in young adolescent girls, which is expected to be more cost-effective in reducing cervical cancer (WHO, 2009). The global recommendation was for a three-dose HPV immunization schedule (WHO, 2009), and based on more recent results from trials evaluating a two-dose schedule, the Pan American Health Organization Technical Advisory Group, as well as the Strategic Advisory Group of Experts on Immunization of the World Health Organization, have now recommended a two dose schedule (Pan American Health Organization [PAHO], 2013; WHO, 2014).

Models predict that vaccination could reduce the lifetime risk of cervical cancer by 35 to 80% if coverage is high (>70%) and if protection lasts for more than 10 years. These models also indicate that HPV vaccination in LMIC may be cost-effective if the cost per vaccinated girl is less than US$10 and produce cost savings if less than US$5 per dose (Goldie et al., 2005).

By late 2015, there were approximately 84 countries implementing HPV vaccines as part of their national public health programs (Cervical Cancer Action, 2015). Many more LMICs, where the burden of cervical cancer is greater, are expected to introduce HPV vaccines in the near future as a result of the decreasing price of the vaccines as well as the growing evidence on their safety, protection, and cost-effectiveness (Jauregui et al., 2011). HPV vaccine prices have been reduced with growing demand and through bulk procurement mechanisms such as the Pan American Health Organization Revolving Fund for the Americas and the Global Alliance for Vaccine and Immunization.

The adolescent population is a unique one for vaccine delivery, and several strategies have been shown to be effective in achieving high coverage of this population. School-based strategies as well as health center-based approaches have been successful in reaching this audience (Ladner et al., 2012; LaMontagne et al., 2011; Lu et al., 2011). Because public knowledge about cervical cancer and HPV can be somewhat limited, public education has increased vaccine acceptance. These strategies have included education about reducing behaviors that increase the risk of acquiring HPV infection, and information about the diagnosis and treatment of precancerous lesions.

Screening women for precancerous cervical lesions, before invasive cancer develops, is another important public health strategy to reduce cervical cancer mortality. HPV induced changes to cervical cells can be detected by cytology, known as the **Papanicolaou (Pap) test**. The Pap test has been implemented mainly in developed countries since the 1960s and has led to an approximately 50% reduction in cervical cancer mortality (Kitchner et al., 2006). But this strategy of Pap testing has proven less effective in developing countries, mainly because of the infrastructure, equipment, and logistical challenges associated with the screening procedures, as well as the test characteristics itself.

As a result, new tools and strategies have been developed for cervical **cancer screening** appropriate for low-resource settings. This includes visual inspection screening with acetic acid (VIA), which has shown in demonstration projects to be safe, feasible, and effective to detect cervical precancer (Sherris et al., 2009). In addition, a cost-effectiveness modeling has demonstrated that VIA screening only once in a lifetime of a 35-year-old woman could reduce the lifetime risk of cervical cancer by 25%; and twice screening, at ages 35 and 40, could reduce the risk by 65% (Goldie et al., 2005).

HPV DNA testing has also emerged as a new cervical cancer screening strategy, although its deployment thus far has been limited mainly to developed countries because of its high cost and infrastructural requirements. A recent large study found that a program strategy based on a single round of HPV testing was associated with reductions of about 50% in cervical cancer incidence and mortality (Sankaranarayanan et al., 2007). A low-cost, simpler HPV test has been developed for low-resource settings and is currently being produced for introduction in China (Qiao et al., 2008).

By late 2015, many countries had begun to take up these new technologies into their programs, with 26 countries using VIA in their national screening programs and 36 countries using VIA in demonstration projects. HPV DNA testing, although more costly than VIA, has not yet had full uptake, with only 6 countries integrating it fully into their programs and about 11 countries evaluating its use as part of pilot projects (Cervical Cancer Action, 2015).

Health education is a critical aspect of increasing awareness of cervical cancer risks, ensuring high vaccination coverage as well as high screening coverage. Men, women, and adolescents need to be aware of the factors associated with the development of cervical cancer and how their risks can be lowered. The use of condoms offers some protection against HPV by reducing risk of infection with HPV as well as other sexually transmitted infections

Table 14.1 Risk Factors for Cervical Cancer

Cervical Cancer Risk Factors	Risk Reduction Strategies
Persistent infection with human papilloma virus (HPV)	Delaying initial sexual activity
Increasing number of sexual partners	Reducing number of sexual partners
Early age at first birth	Receiving an HPV vaccination
Increasing parity	Use of barrier method of birth control (condom or diaphragm)
Coinfection with HIV or other sexually transmitted infections such as herpes simplex virus 2, chlamydia, or gonorrhea	Quitting smoking
Tobacco smoking	
Long-term use of oral contraceptives	

that are cofactors for cervical cancer. Reducing the number of sexual partners, stopping smoking, and delaying first intercourse are also important health education messages to help prevent cervical cancer. Table 14.1 shows the risk factors and risk reduction strategies for cervical cancer.

Breast Cancer

Breast cancer is a disease with likely more than one natural history (International Research on Cancer [IARC], 2002). Breast cancer diagnosed in premenopausal women is likely associated with different risks than for that diagnosed postmenopausally, which is more common. A small proportion, about 5% of breast cancer cases, are genetic and caused by the "breast cancer susceptibility genes" BRCA 1 and 2. Yet, the biological nature of breast development and progression of breast cancer is not fully understood, and much more research is needed to understand what causes it, how to reduce risk, and how to prevent it.

Estrogen, the female hormone, can increase the risk of breast cancer because it stimulates breast cell division. And breast cells are susceptible to bind carcinogens, especially when they are not fully mature, as is the case in girls and women before their first full-term pregnancy. Thus, a woman's risk for breast cancer is increased with events that increase the number of menstrual cycles and therefore increase lifetime exposure to estrogen. This includes low parity, late age at first pregnancy, young age at menarche, and later age at menopause (IARC, 2002). Conversely, life events that protect against breast cancer include late menarche, early pregnancy, bearing children, and early menopause. Lactation is also a protective factor against breast cancer (World Cancer Research Fund, 2010).

The interaction between genes and the environment plays a clear role in breast cancer development, so how women develop in their lifetimes, what they eat, drink, how they stay active, as well as the chemical, microbiological, and physical agents to which she is exposed over her lifetime all have a role to play. Evidence shows increased breast cancer risks for the following environmental factors: use of hormone therapy (estrogen and progestin combined), exposure to ionizing radiation (e.g., with medical procedures such as CT scans), alcohol consumption, and physical inactivity. Tobacco use has been concluded by some studies to be causally related to breast cancer, although other studies show limited evidence (Institute of Medicine, 2011). For premenopausal cancers, obesity (body fatness) is probably a protective factor, whereas for postmenopausal women, body fatness increases the risk of breast cancer. Physical activity is probably a protective factor (World Cancer Research Fund, 2010).

The chemical BPA (bisphenol A) widely used in plastic containers has shown in animal studies to have clear link to breast cancer, but the studies to assess risk in humans are inadequate or lacking. There is no evidence to support that hair dyes or non-ionizing radiation (microwave ovens, electrical devices) increase breast cancer risk (Institute of Medicine, 2012). Table 14.2 shows the risk factors and protective factors for breast cancer.

Public Health Interventions

Breast cancer is much more challenging to prevent than cervical cancer, which has one clear causative agent and for which a vaccine exists to prevent it. Preventive actions that may reduce breast cancer risk relate to healthy living and include avoiding smoking, increasing physical activity, maintaining a healthy weight, limiting or eliminating alcohol consumption, avoiding postmenopausal hormone replacement therapy, and avoiding unnecessary medical radiation (Institute of Medicine, 2012).

The greatest impact on reducing breast cancer incidence and mortality has been from early detection through mammography screening, with appropriate diagnosis and timely treatment. The goal of breast cancer screening is to detect smaller tumors, before signs and symptoms appear (e.g., lump, mass, nipple discharge) and before they advance to clinically evident stages, and when the tumors are amenable to treatment and cure.

Population-based mammography screenings have been introduced in national or sub-national levels in many developed countries, following randomized controlled trials demonstrating effectiveness for early detection. WHO has recommended that screening programs need a population coverage of at least 70% in order to have a significant impact on mortality (WHO, 2011). Maximizing coverage through strategic approaches such as invitation

Table 14.2 Risk and Protective Factors for Breast Cancer

Breast Cancer Risk Factors	Breast Cancer Protective Factors
Low parity	Lactation
Late age at first pregnancy	Physical activity
Young age at menarche	
Later age at menopause	
Use of hormone therapy	
Obesity (postmenopausal)	
Tobacco use	
Alcohol use	
Exposure to ionizing radiation	

letters and call/recall systems must be part of screening program. Opportunistic approaches, such as mobile vans sporadically delivering services to those who show up, are unlikely to have an impact on mortality compared to systematic and active strategies that attain high coverage.

There is a debate over whether or not and by how much mammography screening has an impact in reducing breast cancer mortality. Recent studies indicated a 15% overall reduction in mortality from mammography screening (Bleyer & Welch, 2012). European studies that have used mortality trends to estimate the impact of screening estimate mortality reductions in the range of 1% to 9% annually over 10 years after introduction of mammography screening, and mortality reductions of 28% to 36% from pre-screening to postscreening (Paci et al., 2012). This degree of impact is similar to that experienced in the United States, where breast cancer mortality decreased 28% since the 1990s, probably because of a combination of screening and treatment (Bleyer & Welch, 2012).

Screening, however, raises risk of overdiagnosis and overtreatment, and communicating this weighing of risk and benefit at population and individual levels is a challenge. The harms of mammography screening include false positives, radiation exposure from screening and imaging, invasive procedures, overdiagnosis, and unnecessary treatment anxiety associated with this. In the United States, an estimated 31% of all breast cancers are overdiagnosed (Bleyer & Welch, 2012). The benefits, of course, are deaths averted and life years gained from earlier detection.

Other controversies over screening mammography remain, including age of screening and frequency. Many clinical guidelines call for screening women ages 50 years and older every two years, based on review of evidence and weighing of risks and benefits. Yet many argue that screening should begin at age 40, arguing that a considerable proportion of the overall burden of disease is in this age group of 40–49 years, and the risk of false positive or overdiagnosis ranges from 0% to 50%. Others support beginning at age 50, noting that mammography is less accurate in younger women because of breast biology and low incidence of disease resulting in higher false positives. And still others question whether or not population-based screening mammography is effective at all, claiming that treatment advances have surpassed the benefits of mammography and that harms of screening outweigh benefits (Miller et al., 2014; Smith et al., 2012).

In developing countries, where resources are limited and health systems weaker, mammography screening is not always possible and thus has not been extensively introduced in countries outside the developed world. In these settings, women most commonly present with large, visible, or easily palpable tumors. Thus, the goal of public health interventions in these settings is clinical downstaging, which may be achieved by screening with **clinical breast exams** (CBE) performed by trained medical providers. Current trials in India and other developing countries are exploring the effectiveness of CBE to reduce mortality rates (Sankaranayaran et al., 2007). Breast self examination (BSE) as an early detection method has been questioned because current evidence suggests that BSE does not reduce breast cancer mortality. Nonetheless, its use has been encouraged to promote greater awareness among women of breast symptoms and the need to seek medical attention earlier (Smith et al., 2006).

Public awareness and education is a critical component of breast cancer prevention and early detection, especially in LMIC. Limited public awareness in LMIC has been recognized as a significant barrier to reducing disease burden (Knaul et al., 2012). Women need to understand the utility and benefits of seeking care even without any signs or symptoms and following up on that care to create demand for such services. Health care providers need to meet women's demand and ensure quality of care for women and satisfaction with screening, timely diagnosis, and treatment.

Attention has been called for urgent public health interventions for breast cancer in developing countries, given the high burden, inequities in access to care, and the rise in incidence. The interventions have called for (a) increasing public awareness about breast cancer as a treatable disease and the importance of early detection; (b) improving health system capacity for diagnosis and treatment, including availability of oncological medicines, radiotherapy, and pathology; and (c) increasing health care financing, infrastructure, and human resources for medical oncology (Anderson et al., 2008).

Regardless of the cancer type, radiotherapy services, basic oncological medications, and surgery capacity are important parts of the cancer care continuum. In low- and middle-income countries, this is often the greatest barrier for care for women who show signs and symptoms or suspicion of cancer, and who don't have the access to life-saving treatment technologies. For breast cancer, this includes surgical capacity for radical mastectomy, availability of endocrine therapy with generic tamoxifen, and pathology capacity to detect estrogen receptor status. Although this capacity for treatment exists in much of the developed world, it is unknown at this point what resources are required to build this capacity in the developing world. Telemedicine and collaboration and twinning between institutions in developed and developing countries are the current strategies being used to address some of these gaps in treatment.

Women's Perceptions of Cancer

Social and cultural factors strongly influence how people perceive and understand their risks for cancer as well as the disease itself. With women's cancers, there is much stigma and discrimination, probably because of cancers' association with reproduction (Knaul et al., 2012). The meaning of cancer is often developed through direct experience with the disease. For instance, qualitative studies in women who received a diagnosis of breast cancer indicate that women share their information with other generational family members, and they all reinterpret medical information based on the direct cancer experience of the individual (Tavares & Trad, 2005).

Perceptions and understanding are usually important factors affecting women's willingness to seek preventive services, including HPV vaccination. Understanding these perceptions and how they affect behaviors is thus critical for the development of appropriate health promotion and information, education, and communication strategies.

Associations of cancer with death, fear, and fatality are common among women, particularly those in socially and economically disadvantaged and vulnerable populations. The phrase *breast cancer* itself is associated with inevitable death, terror, suffering, incurability, devastation, powerlessness, and pain and has implications for women's self-image and physical attractiveness (Giraldo-Mora, 2009).

Stigma

Cancer-associated stigma often depends on the degree to which the individual perceives being responsible for the disease and whether the disease leads to disfigurement or disability (Chapple, Ziebland, & McPherson, 2004). The stigma associated with cancer may lead people to hide their condition and not seek or not complete their treatment.

Women's cancers are often associated strongly with blame and self-blame, which serve as psychological barriers to seeking health services. For example, women have cited the causes of breast cancer as personal and emotional problems and certain daily habits, including inadequate nutrition. And the most commonly cited barriers to women seeking breast cancer screening include negligence to take care of themselves, lack of information, anxiety, and fear (Agurto et al., 2006; Giraldo-Mora, 2009).

Social support from partners and families is a key factor affecting women's willingness to seek cervical and breast cancer prevention services. When a woman's cancer is diagnosed, a male partner's behavior can range from full support, to denial, to abandonment, depending on the cultural context (Nigenda, Caballero, & Gonzalez-Robledo, 2009). It appears that women's relationships with their male partners and families are very complex after detecting breast cancer because of the need for deeper psychological and emotional involvement.

Awareness and Sources of Information

Awareness is increasing about cancer prevention screening and early detection, but there is still much misunderstanding and low awareness about the specific preventive nature of breast and cervical cancer.

Women usually receive health messages through mass media, in their communities, and through health services, but the effects on behaviors are different depending on the source. Mass media as well as some public information announcements play a role in understanding cancer. Messages, however, need a balance between motivating healthy behaviors and avoiding developing or increasing self-blame, shame, and stigma. For example, some educational materials add powerful images to messages about the risk for developing cancer to foster self-responsibility, but these same messages can lead to fear and nonresponsiveness in seeking care (Chapple et al., 2004; Giraldo-Mora, 2009).

A global media audit about how cancer was being reported showed that many articles call upon citizens, advocacy organizations, or governments to take actions to improve cancer control across a variety of areas (e.g., increase education, increase funding, improve access to screening, and so on). Each of these calls to action represents a potential motivation for seeking preventive services, but most of the calls for action were nonspecific, such as "More needs to be done" (Livestrong Foundation, 2010). This raises the importance of having specific, directed messages orienting women toward what to do for cancer prevention and screening.

Barriers and Approaches to Screening

In addition, health service related factors such as limited hours of operation, distance to health centers, cost of service, quality of care, including comfort and privacy, and lack of health insurance serve as barriers to seeking care and contribute to late stage diagnosis. Physician-related factors, such as not having a primary care provider or not having a physician recommend screening, are also notable barriers (Binghman, 2003; Schueler, Chu, & Smith-Bindman, 2008).

Patient navigation is a relatively new strategy used to improve access to cancer care by assisting people to go through the complex and often confusing health services for screening, diagnosis, and treatment. A recent review revealed that patient navigation is an effective approach and can improve adherence to breast cancer screening and early diagnosis (Robinson-White et al., 2010).

HPV Vaccine

The HPV vaccine is also affected by similar perceptions, attitudes, and beliefs as those about cervical cancer as well as its acceptability by peers and health providers. Overall there is public acceptance of the HPV vaccines, and most parents are interested in having their preadolescent and adolescent children vaccinated for HPV. This appears to also be influenced by the positive effects attributed to children's vaccination. This occurs despite the fact that there continues to be limited knowledge and misunderstanding about HPV, the HPV vaccine, and cervical cancer screening (Ladner et al., 2012; La Montagne et al., 2011; Zimet, 2005).

There have been public concerns about the HPV vaccine's safety and long-term effectiveness, and some have feared that the vaccine would affect fertility or sexual behavior, which have affected acceptance and intention to be vaccinated (Young, 2010).

There have been sociopolitical issues around HPV vaccine introduction that have affected public acceptance of this vaccine, though not in all countries. For example, in the United States, when HPV vaccines were beginning to be introduced across the country, controversy arose over whether to mandate it for school attendance. Concerns included the need for more safety data, the need for longer-term efficacy data, and concerns that HPV vaccines would increase risky sexual behavior among teens (Luciani, Prieto-Lara, & Vicari, 2011).

Health Promotion Strategies

Health promotion strategies can be used to raise awareness about women's cancers and promote screening among women and HPV vaccination among girls. The specific strategies and messages need to be suitable to the cultural and social context in which they are delivered, and thus developed to meet the needs of identified target populations. It is important to address misinformation and rumors about HPV vaccination and women's cancers that may be present within communities (United Nations Population Fund [UNFPA], 2010).

Health promotion strategies can generally be described according to their overall purposes: (a) awareness raising and providing information to the public; and (b) behavior change strategies to increase uptake of screening and early detection as well as HPV vaccination.

Strategies to Change Behaviors

Interventions that have been successfully applied and appear to increase women's participation in cancer screening programs include client oriented interventions, such as group education, one on one education, provision of informational materials, community mobilization, peer to peer support/ education, traditional and social media; as well as provider-oriented interventions such as client reminders, incentives, and improving satisfaction with care, including comfort, privacy, and accessibility of services (Task Force on Community Preventive Services, 2005). (See Box 14.3.)

Raising Awareness and Providing Information to the Public

Mass media interventions, including public service announcements, can be useful to promote health awareness and provide information to the general public

BOX 14.3 STRATEGIES FOR BEHAVIORAL CHANGE

Health providers, the community, and family members can assist women in changing their behaviors to support cancer prevention and to improve health-seeking behaviors that will support participation in screening programs and adherence to treatment. For instance, health providers may counsel women on healthy lifestyles, including not smoking or quitting smoking, engaging in regular physical activity, and consuming more fruits and vegetables, as well as provide information and support women's decision making regarding cancer screening.

Different theories can be used to affect behavioral skills, among them self- efficacy, social learning and cognitive approaches, reasoned and planned action, stages-of-change models, and health action process. Developing behavioral skills typically include a set of actions such as goal setting and self-monitoring of progress toward those goals, building social support for new behaviors, behavioral reinforcement through self-reward and positive self-talk, structured problem solving to maintain the behavior change, and prevention of relapse behavior. Health behaviors are usually shaped by sociocultural as well as environmental factors and cannot be considered, or changed, solely by interventions targeted at individuals. For example, women can be instructed to seek cancer screening services, but the availability, accessibility, affordability, and quality of these services will affect their health-seeking behavior.

about cancer prevention and screening. Communication channels include print media (newspapers, magazines), broadcast media (radio, television), social media, billboards, and the Internet. Health communication strategies using social marketing and "edutainment," such as embedding messages into soap operas and music videos, are also used to promote acceptance of HPV vaccination and cancer screening.

The effectiveness of mass media campaigns to change behaviors, particularly in increasing cancer screening uptake, however, has proven to have limited evidence (Sabatino et al., 2012). Mass media interventions help create overall awareness about wellness and primary prevention, and when combined with specific behavior change messages are effective in altering lifestyle risk factors (e.g., smoking prevention, physical activity promotion) (Task Force on Community Preventive Services, 2005). Mass media campaigns, however, can be costly interventions and may not be affordable, particularly for developing countries.

Cancer survivors, particularly breast cancer survivors, have been an instrumental group for raising public awareness and advocate for improving services for cancer prevention. Examples of this include the organized survivorship movements being supported and stimulated by nongovernmental organizations such as the American Cancer Society and the Susan G. Komen Foundation in the United States and EuropaDonna in Europe. Fostering and supporting survivor moments for education, awareness, and advocacy has, however, been more limited in developed countries and has yet to evolve in developing countries according to their own cultures and needs.

Reaching women in their communities where they reside and work, rather than relying solely on women to come into contact with health services, is an important outreach strategy. The most active recruitment strategies, such as those that use personalized letters inviting women to screening services, mailed educational materials, phone calls, and directed reminder notices are more effective than spontaneous or opportunistic screening to ensure high coverage of screening (Bonfil et al., 2001; Ferroni et al., 2012). More resource-intensive outreach strategies, such as home visits to personally invite women to screening, are not deemed cost-effective (Ferroni et al., 2012).

Sexual health education for preadolescent and adolescent girls, including condom use and reducing the number of sexual partners, is effective not only to increase HPV vaccine uptake but also to reduce overall risk for HPV infection. Sexual health education, when combined with sexual negotiation skills, which teaches adolescents about reducing sexually risky behaviors, are effective to encourage at least short-term sexual risk reduction behavior (Shepherd et al., 2003).

Health education at schools with parents of preadolescents and adolescents and community outreach have proven to be effective for increasing acceptance of HPV vaccination among girls. Experiences with HPV vaccine implementation have shown that community education is important, especially to reduce the stigma associated with HPV as a sexually transmitted infection, address the misconceptions about HPV and cervical cancer, and reinforce the benefits and positive perceptions of screening and HPV vaccination (La Montagne et al., 2011).

A special focus on health education and outreach needs to be given to those groups of women and girls who are at higher risk of developing cancer and have perhaps more limited access to prevention and care services, for instance, socially and economically vulnerable populations, hard-to-reach groups, and girls who are not attending school. In this regard, community-led and community-based interventions are useful to educate women and girls and increase their participation in prevention programs. These strategies include the involvement and training of lay community health workers or volunteers, engaging community organizations, including faith-based organizations, enlisting the support of local leaders who might have an influence in women's health-seeking decisions, and adapting information and education materials to be more culturally and linguistically relevant to the community.

Information Technology

Communications technology, e-health, and mobile technology are increasingly being used to improve service delivery and to increase women's awareness and participation in screening and girls' uptake of HPV vaccination. For example, an information technology system was used to identify women overdue for mammograms, connect them to primary care providers using a web-based tool, create automatically generated outreach letters for patients specified by providers, monitor for subsequent mammography scheduling and completion, and provide practice delegates with a list of women remaining unscreened for reminder phone calls (Atlas et al., 2012).

Web portals are also a tool for health promotion activities, particularly for providing information tailored to the needs of the users and promoting preventive interventions. Although current scientific evidence suggests that some Internet-based interventions are more effective than others, their effectiveness depends on how accessible, understandable, and relevant the information provided is for the target audience. Interactive and personalized programs can also be effective (D'Addario et al., 2011).

Mobile phones are also increasingly being used to promote knowledge and as reminders. Client reminders, regardless of the modality used, are an effective strategy to promote health-seeking behaviors, increasing attendance and reducing the cost of nonattendance to health centers. For example, an intervention using mobile phone text messages and e-mail in Australia improved knowledge about sexually transmitted infections (STI) and promoting STI testing, but it did not increase condom use (Lim et al., 2012). In another example, text messages to personal mobile phones were used in studies in China and in Brazil to improve attendance rates at health centers; this was more cost-effective than telephone reminders (Chen et al., 2008, da Costa et al., 2010). As the use of mobile phone text messages is evolving, and there are not yet published results of interventions specific for cancer, these examples show the potential of using mobile technology to increase screening and HPV vaccination.

Reducing Health System and Service Barriers

The process of care for women's cancer prevention and control requires community-based and health service–based primary prevention, such as health education, counseling, and HPV vaccination; screening of asymptomatic women and early detection of cervical precancer, including clinical breast examination; diagnosis, through pathology and cytology services; and treatment (surgery, radiotherapy, and systemic therapy or chemotherapy). This level of service delivery requires many public health and medical disciplines, including primary care physicians, nurses, community health workers, working together with pathologists, oncologists, surgeons, and radiologists. Although developed countries may be able to meet these requirements, it is precisely this complex mix of process, need for specialized care providers, and level of resources that can limit the access to prevention and control services in LMIC.

The shortage of specialized health care providers in many LMICs is further exacerbated by migration (brain drain), poor work environments, and poor remuneration. Thus, strategies for health promotion and community education need also to be coupled with provider education, especially of primary care level providers, to train and retain health providers for screening, diagnosis, and treatment. The strategy also must include task shifting, whereby motivated and highly capable health workers are trained to complete specific tasks, relieving physicians to do more complex tasks and treating larger volumes of patients.

Women need to be supported through education and reducing health system barriers to seek preventive health services when there are no signs and symptoms of cancer. Most breast cancers in developing countries are detected by women themselves when a visible lump is felt and other symptoms, such as pain, ulcer, or discharge, appear; and for cervical cancer when symptoms such as pain, discharge, or bleeding appear. Demonstration projects have shown heightening awareness in the community, making preventive clinical services more available to women in primary care settings, and training providers in clinical breast exams can lead to earlier stage diagnosis of breast cancers (El Saghir et al., 2010).

Innovative strategies to reduce breast and cervical cancer morbidity and mortality are being tested, and the focus is on primary level of care so that services are delivered closer to where women and girls reside. Some have advocated for a diagonal approach to woman's cancers through health system strengthening that integrates the delivery of disease specific interventions, not in a vertical isolated program, but addressing the needs of the population and people (Knaul et al., 2012). For example, messages about breast and cervical cancer screening can be integrated as part of sexual and reproductive health and maternal health delivery platforms without missing opportunities to promote education and early detection among women. Breast and cervical cancer prevention for older women can be packaged into NCD interventions, and HPV vaccine into adolescent health programs, but the right package of services is determined by the providers' technical capacity.

Improving the quality of health care can reduce health service barriers and increase women's satisfaction with care, thus increasing their participation in screening and adherence to follow-up treatment. For example, in a study in El Salvador, a model for quality improvement was applied to decrease cervical cancer among hard to reach women. The quality elements, which reduced health service barriers while increasing satisfaction with care, included adapting examination rooms to better accommodate privacy for pelvic exams and overcome shame, reducing the amount of time in which women receive test results and thus limiting the time they experience anxiety or fear of cancer, and improving the quality of test samples to improve accuracy of testing and thus eliminate the need for retesting (Agurto et al., 2006).

Civil society organizations, led by patients, survivors, and women themselves, have contributed to not only provision of supportive care for women, but to health system improvements for better outcomes in developed countries, particularly in the United States. A similar degree of civil society advocacy, activism, and supportive care for women's cancer is evolving in many LMICs to increase access to prevention and treatment (Azenha et al., 2011).

Global Agendas

Although innovations in health service delivery for women's cancer are being developed and tested, there are several global health agendas that will help drive change for increased access to women's cancer services in the future.

Globally, there is a renewal of primary health care and this agenda for strengthening primary care offers an opportunity to improve services at the community level for women in midlife and to incorporate cervical and breast cancer screening as essential, routine health services. Indeed, many countries are going that route, and in a recent survey 57 countries reported having cervical cancer screening services available as primary care services, though the coverage rates were quite low in the developing countries (average of 19% coverage as compared to 63% in the developed world) (Gakidou, Nordhagen, & Obermeyer, 2008).

The United Nations high-level meeting on noncommunicable diseases has initiated a global response to the growing problem of NCDs and is stimulating investments in NCD prevention and control programs and policies. This is creating opportunities for synergy between primary prevention messages about healthy living, healthy eating, physical activity, smoking prevention, and alcohol reduction, which can have some influence on breast cancer because they are risk factors, but it also is creating opportunities to scale up access to screening and treatment for breast and cervical cancer screening. WHO has created a global monitoring framework to guide the NCD agenda and serve as the accountability framework. This includes indicators on cancer incidence, HPV vaccination, and cervical cancer screening, thus spurring investments and service orientation.

Last, the Millennium Development Goals that have driven global investments and collaborations in health over the past decade are being renewed to a post-MDG era. Discussions are ongoing on the priorities, but one thing is clear: NCDs, including women's cancers, will be a top priority for the development community post-2015.

Looking Ahead

Women's cancers, notably breast and cervical cancer, lead to unnecessary deaths among women in the prime of their lives throughout the world. Effective public health interventions are available to reduce death and suffering. For cervical cancer, these include HPV vaccination, HPV screening, Pap testing, visual inspection screening, and treatment for both preinvasive and invasive cervical cancer. For breast cancer, the interventions include clinical breast examination, mammography screening, and treatment (surgery, radiotherapy, chemotherapy). Central to the prevention efforts for women's cancers is health promotion and health education to ensure maximal HPV vaccination coverage, and women's participation in screening and follow-up treatment.

There are many challenges to implementing these health promotion and health service interventions, particularly in limited-resource settings. Yet many countries in the developing world have already established both HPV vaccination and cervical cancer screening programs, and several have begun to initiate population-based breast cancer screening programs.

As the global health community defines its priorities for NCD prevention and control, and establishes a new development agenda for the post-2015 period, women's cancers will certainly feature more prominently on the political agenda. This bodes well for worldwide scale-up and provision of more and better quality services for women and girls in order to save lives. Slowly but surely, capacity and infrastructure will be strengthened, community and individual attitudes and beliefs about cancer will change, and the impact of breast and cervical screening and HPV vaccination, especially in developing countries, will soon be experienced.

Summary

This chapter has provided an overview of the situation of breast and cervical cancer incidence and mortality throughout the world and described the cost-effective strategies and community-based health promotion strategies for their prevention and control.

KEY TERMS

1. **Breast cancer:** An abnormal cell growth in the breast tissue, most commonly in the inner lining of milk ducts or the lobules that supply the ducts with milk, with the potential to spread to other parts of the body
2. **Cancer screening:** A test applied to apparently healthy individuals, on a population-wide basis, to identify disease early when there are no signs or symptoms; enables earlier intervention and treatment to reduce cancer mortality and suffering

3. **Cervical cancer:** An abnormal mass of tissue in the cervix as a result of abnormal cell growth, caused by persistent infection of high-risk HPV types
4. **Clinical breast examination:** A physical examination of the female breasts by a trained health care provider, to feel for lumps or other abnormalities in an attempt to achieve an earlier diagnosis of breast cancer
5. **HPV vaccine:** A vaccine that prevents human papillomavirus (HPV) infection from certain types of HPV associated with the development of some types of cancer, and/or genital warts; three HPV vaccines are currently available on the market: a bivalent HPV vaccine (HPV types 16 and 18) a quadrivalent HPV vaccine (HPV types 6, 11, 16, 18) and a 9-valent HPV vaccine (HPV types 6, 11, 16, 18, 31, 33, 45, 52, and 58)
6. **Human papillomavirus (HPV):** A group of more than 150 related viruses, of which 30–40 HPV types are commonly transmitted through sexual contact and cause infection; most resolve on their own, but some HPV infections may lead to health problems, including genital warts and some types of cancer
7. **Mammography:** A type of radiography used on the breasts for screening of apparently healthy women in an attempt to achieve an earlier diagnosis of breast cancer (*screening mammography*); also used to aid in the diagnosis of a woman who is experiencing symptoms suspicious for breast cancer (*diagnostic mammography*)
8. **Papanicolaou test:** Known as the *Pap test,* or *Pap smear,* a test used for cervical cancer screening; can detect potentially precancerous and cancerous cells in the cervix, and, if warranted, lead to interventions to prevent progression to cervical cancer

REVIEW QUESTIONS

1. How significant a public health problem are women's cancers?
2. What are the attitudes and perceptions of women about breast and cervical cancer?
3. What health promotion strategies are effective to prevent and control these women's cancers?
4. What are the issues and obstacles to improving access and care for women, especially in limited-resource settings, for breast and cervical cancer?
5. What global health opportunities can be garnered to improve women's cancer care?

References

Agurto, I., Sandoval, J., De La Rosa, M., & Guardado, M. E. (2006). Improving cervical cancer prevention in a developing country. *International Journal of Quality in Health Care, 18*(2), 81–86.

Anderson, B. O., Yip, C. H., Smith, R. A., Shyyan, R., Sener, S. F., Eniu, A., ... Harford, J. (2008). Guideline implementation for breast health care in low-income and middle-income countries: Overview of the Breast Health Global Initiative Global Summit 2007. *Cancer, 113*(Suppl. 8), 2221–2243.

Atlas, S. J, Ashburner, J. M, Chang, Y., Lester, W. T, Barry, M. J, & Grant, R. W. (2012). Population-based breast cancer screening in a primary care network. *American Journal of Management and Care, 18*(12), 821–829.

Azenha, G. , Bass, L. P., Caleffi, M., Smith, R., Pretorius, L., Durstine, A., & Perez, C. P. (2011). The role of breast cancer civil society in different resource settings. *Breast, 20*(Suppl. 2), S81–S87.

Bingham, A., Bishop, A., Coffey, P., Winkler, J., Bradley, M., Dzuba, I., & Agurto I. (2003). Factors affecting utilization of cervical cancer prevention services in low-resource settings. *Salud Publica Mexico, 45*(Suppl.), 283–291.

Bleyer, A., & Welch, H. G. (2012). Effect of three decades of screening mammography on breast-cancer incidence. *New England Journal of Medicine, 367*(21), 1998–2005.

Bonfill, X., Marzo, M., Pladevall, M., & Martí, J. (2001). Strategies for increasing women's participation in community breast cancer screening. *Cochrane Database of Systematic Reviews* (*1*), 2943.

Bray, F., Jemal, A., Grey, N., Ferlay, J., & Forman, D. (2012). Global cancer transitions according to the Human Development Index (2008–2030): A population based study. *Lancet Oncology, 13*(8), 790–801.

Cervical Cancer Action. (2015). *Global progress in cervical cancer prevention.* Retrieved from http://www.cervicalcanceraction.org/comments/maps.php

Chapple, A., Ziebland, S., & McPherson, A. (2004). Stigma, shame, and blame experienced by patients with lung cancer: A qualitative study. *British Medical Journal, 328*, 1470.

Chen, Z. W., Fang, L. Z., Chen, L. Y., & Dai, H. L. (2008). Comparison of an SMS text messaging and phone reminder to improve attendance at a health promotion center: A randomized controlled trial. *Journal of Zhejiang University Science B, 9*(1), 34–38.

da Costa, T. M., Salomão, P. L., Martha, A .S., Pisa, I. T., & Sigulem, D. (2010). The impact of short message service text messages sent as appointment reminders to patients' cell phones at outpatient clinics in São Paulo, Brazil. *Journal of Medical Informatics, 79*(1), 65–70.

D'Addario, M., De Vito, C., Marzuillo, C., Vacchio, M. R., Ferroni, E., & Villari, P. (2011). Online communication regarding health promotion and protection: The public health perspective. *Ingeneira Sanita Pubblica, 67*(6), 757–775.

El Saghir, N. S., Adebamowo, C A., Anderson, B. O., Carlson, R. W., Bird, P. A., Corbex, M., ... Cazap, E. (2011). Breast cancer management in low resource countries: Consensus statement from the Breast Health Global Initiative. *Breast, 20*(Suppl. 1), S3–S11.

Ferlay, J., Shin, H. R., Bray, F., Forman, D., Mathers, C., & Parkin, D. M. (2010). GLOBOCAN 2008. v1.2, *Cancer incidence and mortality worldwide: IARC CancerBase no. 10*. Lyon, France: International Agency for Research on Cancer. Retrieved from http://globocan.iarc.fr/Default.aspx

Ferroni, E., Camilloni, E., Jimenez, B., Furnari, G., & Borgia, P. (2012). How to increase uptake in oncologic screening: A systematic review of studies comparing population-based screening programs and spontaneous access. *Preventive Medicine, 55*, 587–596.

Forounzanfar, M. H., Foreman, K. J., Delossantos, A. M., Lozano, R., Lopez, A. D., Murray, C. J., & Naghavi, M. (2011). Breast and cervical cancer in 187 countries between 1980 and 2010: A systematic analysis. *Lancet, 378*(9801), 1461–1484.

Gakidou, E., Nordhagen, S., & Obermeyer, Z. (2008). Coverage of cervical cancer screening in 57 countries: Low average levels and large inequalities. *PLoS Med, 5*(6), e132.

Giraldo-Mora, C. V. (2009). Persistence of social representation regarding breast cancer. *Revista de. salud pública, 11*(4), 514–525.

Goldie, S. J., Gaffikin, L., Goldhaber-Fiebert, J. D., Gordillo-Tobar, A., Levin, C., Mahé, C., Wright, T. C. (2005) Cost-effectiveness of cervical-cancer screening in five developing countries. *New England Journal of Medicine, 353*(20), 2158–2168.

Institute of Medicine. (2011, December). *Breast cancer and the environment: A life course approach*. Retrieved from http://iom.nationalacademies.org/Reports/2011/Breast-Cancer-and-the-Environment-A-Life-Course-Approach.aspx

International Research on Cancer. (2002). *IARC handbooks of cancer prevention: Breast cancer screening*. Lyon, France: IARC Press.

Jauregui, B., Sinha, A., Clark, A. D., Bolanos, B. M., Resch, S., Toscano, C. M., Ruiz Matusa, C., & Andrus, J. K. (2011). Strengthening the technical capacity at country-level to make informed policy decisions on new vaccine introduction: Lessons learned by PAHO's ProVac Initiative. *Vaccine, 29*(5), 1099–1106.

Kitchner, H. C., Castle, P. E., & Cox, J. T. (2006). Achievements and limitations of cervical cytology screening. *Vaccine, 24*(Suppl. 3), S63–S70.

Knaul, F. M., Bhadelia, A., Gralow, J., Arreola-Ornelas, H., Langer, A., & Frenk, J. (2012). Meeting the emerging challenges of breast and cervical cancer in low- and middle-income countries. *International Journal of Gynaecology and Obstetetrics, 119*(Suppl. 1), S85–S88.

Ladner, J., Besson, M. H., Hampshire, R., Tapert, L., Chirenje, M., & Saba, J. (2012). Assessment of eight HPV programs. *BMC Public Health, 12*, 370.

LaMontagne, D. S., Barge, S., Le, N. T., Janmohamed, A., Kumakech, E., Mosqueira, N. R., … Jumaang, A. O. (2011). Human papillomavirus vaccine delivery strategies that achieved high coverage in low- and middle-income countries. *Bulletin of the World Health Organization, 89*(11), 821–830.

Lim, M. S., Hocking, J. S., Aitken, C. K., Fairley, C. K., Jordan, L., Lewis, J. A, & Hellard, M. E. J. (2012). Impact of text and email messaging on the sexual health of young people: A randomised controlled trial. *Epidemiology and Community Health, 66*(1), 69–74.

Livestrong Foundation. (2010). *Cancer stigma and silence around the world: A Livestrong report.* Retrieved from http://livestrong.org/pdfs/3-0/LSGlobalResearchReport]

Lu, B., Kumar, A., Castellsague, X., & Giuliano, A. R. (2011). Efficacy and safety of prophylactic vaccines against cervical HPV infection and diseases among women: A systematic review and meta-analysis. *BMC Infectious Diseases, 12*(11), 13.

Luciani, S., Cabanes, A., Prieto-Lara, E., & Gawryszewski, V. (2013). Cervical and female breast cancers in the Americas: Current situation and opportunities for action. *Bulletin of the World Health Organization, 91*, 640–649.

Luciani, S., Prieto-Lara, E., & Vicari, A. (2011). Providing vaccines against human papillomaviruses to adolescent girls in the Americas: Battling cervical cancer and improving overall health. *Health Affairs, 30*(6), 1–6.

Miller, A. B., Wall, C., Baines, C. J., Sun, P., To, T., & Narod, S. A. (2014). Twenty-five year follow up for breast cancer incidence and mortality of the Canadian National Breast Screening Study: Randomized screening trial. *British Medical Journal, 348*, g366.

Nigenda, G., Caballero, M., & Gonzalez- Robledo, L. M. (2009). Access barriers in early diagnosis of breast cancer in the federal district and Oaxaca. *Salud pública México, 51*(Suppl. 2), S254–S262.

Paci, E., & the Euroscreen Working Group. (2012). Summary of the evidence of breast cancer service screening outcomes in Europe and first estimate of the benefit and harm balance sheet. *Journal of Medical Screening, 19*(Suppl. 1), 5–13.

Pan American Health Organization. (2013, July). *Report of the XXI Technical Advisory Group on Vaccine-Preventable Diseases.* Retrieved from http://www.paho.org/hq/index.php?option=com_content&view=article&id=1862&Itemid=2032&lang=en)

Qiao, Y., Sellors, J., Eder, P. S., Bao, Y. P., Lim, J. M., Zhao, F. H., ... Lorincz, A. T. (2008). A new HPV DNA test for cervical cancer screening in developing regions: A cross sectional study of clinical accuracy in rural China. *Lancet Oncology, 9*(10), 929–936.

Robinson-White, S., Conroy, B., Slavish, K. H., & Rosenzweig, M. (2010). Patient navigation in breast cancer: A systematic review. *Cancer Nursing, 33*(2), 127–140.

Sabatino, S. A., Lawrence, B., Elder, R., Mercer, S. L., Wilson, K. M., DeVinney, B., ... Glanz, K. (2012). Community Preventive Services Task Force. Effectiveness of interventions to increase screening for breast, cervical, and colorectal cancers: Nine updated systematic reviews for the *Guide to Community Preventive Services. American Journal of Preventive Medicine, 43*(1), 765–786.

Sankaranarayanan, R., Esmy, P. O., Rajkumar, R., Muwonge, R., Swaminathan, R., Shanthakumari, S., ... Cherian, J. (2007). Effect of visual screening on cervical cancer incidence and mortality in Tamil Nadu, India: A cluster-randomized trial. *Lancet, 370*(9585), 398–406.

Sankaranarayanan, R., Nessa, A., Esmy, P. O., & Dangou, J. M. (2012). Visual inspection methods for cervical cancer prevention. *Best Practices Research in Clinical Obstetetrics and Gynaecology, 26*(2), 221–232.

Sankaranarayanan, R., Ramadas, K., Thara, S., Muwonge, R., Prabhakar, J., Augustine, P., ... Mathew, B. S. (2011). Clinical breast examination: Preliminary results from a cluster randomized controlled trial in India. *Journal of the National Cancer Institute, 103*(19), 1476–1480.

Schueler, K. M., Chu, P. W., & Smith-Bindman, R. (2008). Factors associated with mammography utilization: A systematic quantitative review of the literature. *Journal of Women's Health, 17*(9), 1477–1498.

Shepherd, J., Weston, R., Peersman, G., & Napuli, I. Z. (2003). Interventions for encouraging sexual lifestyles and behaviours intended to prevent cervical cancer (*Cochrane Review*). The Cochrane Library.

Sherris, J., Wittet, S., Kleine, A., Sellors, J., Luciani, S., Sankaranarayanan, R., & Barone, M. (2009). Evidence-based, alternative cervical cancer screening approaches in low-resource settings. *International Perspectives on Sexual and Reproductive Health, 35*(3), 147–152.

Smith, R. A., Caleffi, M., Albert, U., Chen, T. H. H., Duffy, S. W, & Franceschi, D. (2006). Breast cancer in limited-resource countries: Early detection and access to care. *Breast Journal, 12*(Suppl. 1), S16–S26.

Smith, R. A., Kerlikowske, K., Miglioretti, D. L., & Kalager, M. (2012). Mammography screening for breast cancer. *New England Journal of Medicine, 367*, e31(1)–e31(3).

Task Force on Community Preventive Services. (2005). *The guide to community preventive services: What works to promote health?* New York, NY: Oxford University Press.

Tavares, J. S., & Trad, L. A. (2005 Breast cancer metaphors and meanings from the perspective of five families. [Article in Portuguese]. *Cadernos de Saude Publica, 21*(2), 426–435.

United Nations Population Fund. (2010). *Cervical cancer prevention and control: Guidance for countries.* New York, NY: Author.

Young, A. (2010). HPV vaccine acceptance among women in the Asian Pacific: A systematic review of the literature. *Asian Pacific Journal of Cancer Prevention, 11*, 641–649.

World Cancer Research Fund/American Institute for Cancer Research. (2010). *Food, nutrition, physical activity, and the prevention of breast cancer.* Continuous Update Project Report. Retrieved from http://www.wcrf.org/int/research-we-fund/continuous-update-project-findings-reports/breast-cancer

World Health Organization. (2006). *Comprehensive cervical cancer control: A guide to essential practice.* Geneva: Author.

World Health Organization. (2009). Human papillomavirus vaccines. WHO position paper. *Weekly Epidemiological Record, 15*(84), 118–131.

World Health Organization. (2011). *Global status report on non-communicable diseases.* Geneva: Author.

World Health Organization. (2014). Meeting of the Strategic Advisory Group of Experts on Immunization, April 1–3. Conclusions and recommendations. *Weekly Epidemiological Record, 89,* 221–236.

Zimet, G. D. (2005). Improving adolescent health: Focus on HPV vaccine acceptance. *Journal of Adolescent Health, 37*(Suppl. 6), S17–S23.

CHAPTER 15

HEALTH PROMOTION IN FAMILIES AND COMMUNITIES

An Integrated Approach from Latin America and the Caribbean

Fernando Zacarías, Adrián Díaz, Manuel Peña, Adela Páez Jiménez, Leticia Martínez, and Gina Tambini

The public health approach to **family** and **community** health is based on the values of equity and solidarity and is supported by the argument that health is a basic human right. Its six principles: (1) participation, (2) collaboration, (3) opportunity, (4) integration, (5) interculturalism, and (6) comprehensiveness guide the following four lines of action:

1. health promotion,
2. prevention of disease and risks,
3. intersectoral action in health, and
4. equitable access to quality health services.

LEARNING OBJECTIVES

By the end of this chapter, the reader should be able to:

- **Describe the characteristics of families and communities and their role in achieving better health**
- **Understand the impact of inequities in the health status and social conditions of communities such as indigenous populations**
- **Define the steps necessary to implement an integrated family and community health approach in close collaboration with health services**

Why This Approach?

Healthy families help create healthy communities, and, in turn, healthy communities help create healthy families. Most important, families and communities contribute to the achievement of optimal health and well-being of individuals and populations and thus promote and produce human and social development. Health should be viewed as a continuum that encompasses all **life stages**. The **life course** of people is a dynamic representation of a chronological and biological process made up by the different stages of life (i.e., conception, pregnancy, birth, infancy, childhood, adolescence, adulthood, and old age), each of which is characterized by specific health risks and influenced by specific individual, family, and community determinants, including access to quality health services. This approach to health focuses on the health risks and the social and environmental determinants that are especially associated with age, gender, ethnicity, and culture (Bengston & Allen, 1993).

Also, from a biological standpoint, an increasing body of evidence has pointed out that the future health of a child or adult might not be solely the result of his or her genetic make-up at the time of conception, pregnancy, or the postnatal period (Champagne, 2008). The origins of adult diseases are often found among developmental and biological disruptions occurring during the perinatal period and the early years of life, either as a result of cumulative exposure to stressful experiences or by latent effects of adversity during sensitive developmental periods. **Epigenetic modifications** may be the mechanism linking early life factors to adult onset of risk and disease (Kaati et al., 2007). In practical terms, the evidence suggests that reducing significant social disadvantage early in life may be a powerful strategy for decreasing the burden of chronic morbidity and premature death in the population. Indeed, the life course approach provides a comprehensive vision of health and its determinants, which calls for the development of health services networks that are centered on people's needs at each stage of their lives and address the **social determinants of health**.

Families and Communities

To understand the family and community health approach, it is necessary to recognize the diversity and the changes in the structure of families and communities in the past decades, as well as the increasing public awareness of the role of the social, economic, political, and environmental determinants that affect individual and collective health.

Why Families?

Individuals are born and raised within families. The family provides the basic setting and context in which health knowledge, beliefs, attitudes, practices, and health-seeking behaviors are first formed and established. Notably, the role of the family in health and illness prevention has gained more prominence since the World Health Organization's (WHO) publication of the Statistical Indices of Family Health in 1976 (WHO, 1976).

Traditionally, and in most parts of the world, the concept of the nuclear family—that is, a man and a woman and their children—has been used when defining a family. However, for the purposes of this document, a family is defined as two or more people related by blood, marriage, or affinity, who share a common history, the same household and basic resources (food and shelter), and self-identify as such. In reality, families come in different forms, such as laterally extended families (e.g., uncles, aunts, cousins, in-laws, etc.), transgenerationally extended families (e.g., grandparents, parents, and grandchildren living in the same household), mixed families (e.g., sequential spouses, stepchildren, etc.), families with same-sex partners, and two-member families (e.g., childless couples, single mother with one child, etc.). Consequently, along with these structural differences in the family, the past few decades have seen a dramatic shift in its definition.

Single-parent households, particularly female-headed households, are becoming increasingly common. In Chile, female-headed households increased from 25% in 1992 to 32% in 2002; in Jamaica, female-headed households accounted for 41% of households according to the 2001 census; and in El Salvador, an estimated 37.3% of households were headed by women, with female-headed households making up a larger share of urban households (43.2%) than of rural households (30.7%) (Pan American Health Organization [PAHO], 2007). Additionally, a higher average age for marriage and childbirth has delayed the formation of first families. For example, in Canada in 2004, more than one-third (34.7%) of births to women in their thirties were first births, a trend that is beginning to appear in middle-income countries in Latin America and the Caribbean (LAC) (PAHO, 2007). This delay is tied to the entrance of women into higher education and the labor force in unprecedented numbers, which has changed gender roles and shifted the balance of economic responsibilities in families throughout the Region of the Americas. Furthermore, decreased family and household size (e.g., in Colombia there were 4.1 children per household in 1998 versus 2.6 children in 2002); an increased burden on working-age family members by young and older dependents (e.g., in Argentina, 21% of households have an elderly person who requires supervision and care); and increasing numbers of sequential and simultaneous families as a result of divorce, separation, or multiple liaisons have contributed to the changing concept of the family (PAHO, 2007).

Interactions among family members are the main catalyst of individual and family development, decision making, and adoption of healthy behaviors and practices. Thus, the decision to seek medical care is not always made by an individual itself but by the parents, the husband, or other family member (Christensen, 2004). The foundation for strong families lies in good parenting and the provision of a safe, loving, healthy, and organized environment for children from birth through adolescence (Hoghughi, 1998). The quality of relationships (i.e., cohesion and emotional closeness, degree of privacy, and the ability to solve problems) within a family can have a direct impact on the health of family members. Additionally, the quality of education; prevalence and incidence of disease; health and social problems; availability of resources in the community; and the cultural beliefs, traditions, and societal perspectives on life shape the behavior of families in regard to health and disease (Ferrer, Palmer, & Burger, 2005).

Families have a life course of their own, which starts with the willingness of two people to live together and share their individual resources. In a nuclear family, the couple might decide to have or adopt children, and the family will grow in size while all their individual members continue their passages through different stages of their own life courses. The children become adolescents and young adults and probably leave home to start their own families. The parents mature and age, and the nuclear family dissolves when one of its two original members is no longer alive. This chain of events has implications for the interactions among the family members and for the family role in the community. For this reason, the type of interventions and health promotion approaches required to address individual and family health and welfare throughout their life course need to be adjusted accordingly (Soubhi & Potvin, 2000). It is worth noting that some individuals do not live in a family environment throughout their lives, e.g. children in orphanages, inmates serving long sentences, homeless people, long-term psychiatric patients, abandoned elders, etc. However, *in lieu* of the family, other individuals, social groups, or specific communities can provide, under ideal circumstances, the kind of support necessary for achieving a better life.

Why the Community?

The family is part of an even larger social setting: the community. The complexity of health problems affecting individuals at the family level must be addressed within the context of the community. Commonly, geographical terms are employed to define communities; however, several other characteristics may be used to define a community: (a) sharing common interests, perspectives, and values; (b) joint action, a sense of coherence and identity; (c) social ties; and (d) diversity (the social complexity of a given community) (MacQueen et al., 2001). Moreover, there are communities unified by common characteristics such as language, profession, or race, that transcend geographical boundaries.

Individuals and families live in communities, and this, in turn, may determine their health status and quality of life. Communities can shape individual and collective behavior through a system of exchange and influence. As with healthy and vulnerable families, there are prosperous communities as well as communities that are highly vulnerable to adverse environmental and social factors (Table 15.1); therefore, it is imperative that efforts be centered

Table 15.1 Some Vulnerability Factors in Families and Communities

Families	Communities
Head of household unemployed	Poor leadership and governance
Poor or indigenous	Scarcity of food and basic products
Belonging to a minority group	Geographic, cultural, ethnic, linguistic, political, or economic isolation
Single, working mother	Insecurity and high crime rate
Illiterate parents	Lack of or sufficient infrastructure (roads, communications, electricity, water and sanitation, schools, health services, sport facilities, etc.)
Displaced family	
Lack of access to medical and social services	Uncontrolled physical growth and unplanned development or urbanization
Chronically ill, mentally ill, or incapacitated family member	Rapid demographic changes (massive migration, displaced communities, etc.)
Drug use, alcohol use, violence	Exposure to natural or human-made disasters, including civil or armed conflict
Sexual abuse	Unsafe environment (toxic substances, pollution, erosion, deforestation, desertification)
Suicidal family member	
Family member who is a victim or perpetrator of a serious crime; e.g., homicide, rape	Lack of cohesion or antagonism within the community
Incarcerated parent	
Poor housing	
Indoor pollution	
Death of one or more children	
Migrant and absent parent	

on these at-risk communities and families to ensure that they achieve their health, welfare, and lifestyle goals (Duque, Klevens, & Ramirez, 2003; Frohlich & Potvin, 2008).

Social Determinants of Health and Indigenous Communities

Consideration of socioeconomic determinants of health is essential to the formulation and implementation of an intercultural family and community health approach. According to the World Health Organization (WHO, 2008), the social determinants of health are the conditions in which people are born, grow, live, work, and age and include the health system. These social circumstances are shaped by economic factors such as the distribution of money, power, and resources at local, national, and global levels, which themselves are many times influenced by policy choices. Gwatkin (2007) uses the acronym **PROGRESS** to describe several important social determinants of health: *p*lace of residence, *r*ace, *o*ccupation, *g*ender, *r*eligion, *e*ducation, *s*ocioeconomic status, and *s*ocial capital. These socioeconomic determinants are mostly responsible for the health inequities—that is, the unfair and avoidable differences in health status—seen within and between countries and specific populations.

The Case of Indigenous Communities

Nowhere are the consequences of social determinants more clearly seen than in the indigenous communities of Latin America and the Caribbean. Approximately 40 million indigenous people live in the LAC region. Although they make up about 10% of the total regional population, indigenous people constitute anywhere from 1% to 60% of the total population of each country (Kronik & Verner, 2010). Regionally (and globally), the burden of disease, disability, and premature death is consistently higher among indigenous communities than among the rest of the population. Moreover, indigenous populations still lack opportunities to participate in their own health care, and health care providers and society as a whole have little understanding of the cultural complexities and needs of these communities. Available health indicators for indigenous people demonstrate that urgent action is needed.

The aforementioned socioeconomic and local determinants contribute to vast inequities in indigenous health. Indigenous peoples, and particularly indigenous women, have the worst sociodemographic indicators and the largest inequalities in terms of access to social services in the Latin American region. These communities suffer from high illiteracy, poverty, and unemployment rates, as well as a lack of access to basic health services when compared to their nonindigenous counterparts.

Additionally, high levels of infant and maternal mortality, malnutrition, and infectious diseases have been traditionally commonplace among indigenous populations. In a literature review, Montenegro and Stephens (2006) describe various infant mortality rates that have been reported in specific indigenous communities. In 1994, the national average infant mortality rate in Ecuador was 22 per 1,000 live births, whereas the rate reached 83 and 67 per 1,000 live births in the indigenous communities of Colimbuela and Cumas. Of indigenous children in the Peruvian Amazon, the Campa-Ashaninka had an infant mortality rate of 99 per 1,000 live births and the Machiguenga had a rate of 100 per 1,000. Other studies show that high rates of infant mortality still persist and can be three to four times higher than national averages, despite demographic recovery in some communities. Infant mortality in indigenous communities in Ecuador is as high as 100 per 1,000 live births, compared with a national average of 30 per 1,000.

Maternal mortality is also higher for indigenous communities, particularly in remote areas where maternal mortality rates could be twice or even three times as high as national averages. In Guatemala in 2007, maternal mortality for the indigenous population (163 per 100,000 people) was more than double the rate for the nonindigenous population (77 per 100,000) (Government of Guatemala, 2011).

As these populations become more urbanized and mobile, issues such as drug and alcohol abuse, mental illness, sexually transmitted diseases, and assimilation of traditional medical practices to a more mainstream approach have become prevalent. Issues of inequity and discrimination within the health system and in society have also contributed to the poor health status of the indigenous populations in the LAC region. For example, about 40% of the indigenous population lacks access to conventional health-related services (PAHO, 2006). Persistent issues of poor-quality service provision, such as limited technical or linguistic communication competency and staff noncompliance with evidence-based treatment protocols, medication shortage, and poor staff retention are common in the remote areas that these indigenous populations inhabit. Further complicating matters are cultural barriers, which perhaps pose the most significant challenge to indigenous health. These stem from a lack of understanding of the social and cultural factors deriving from the knowledge, attitudes, and practices in the health of indigenous peoples. About 80% rely on traditional healers as their principal health care providers (PAHO, 2006). Thus, bias toward conventional medicine practices may be construed as inappropriate or even offensive for practitioners of traditional medicine. Finding trained health care providers who speak indigenous languages and understand their cultural practices is difficult. Poor communication that may result from this can seriously compromise access to quality care. Moreover, nonindigenous staff members often discriminate against indigenous people in health centers. This behavior arouses feelings of fear and distrust, which can turn indigenous communities off from seeking the care they need.

Health Promotion in Communities

Knowledge of local determinants affecting the health of community members is an essential tool in planning health interventions in the community. The social, economic, and physical characteristics of neighborhoods are increasingly recognized as having both short- and long-term consequences for residents' quality and years of healthy life (Novilla, et al., 2006). Among the most prevalent local determinants of health is the issue of family housing, specifically the inadequate supply of affordable housing for low-income families and the spatial segregation of households by income, race, ethnicity, or social class into unsafe neighborhoods. When affordable housing is unavailable to low-income households, family resources are diverted to housing costs. Furthermore, the increased concentration of poverty can manifest itself in the physical and social deterioration of neighborhoods. Other important local determinants that must be considered include issues of education, employment, transportation, pollution, crime, sanitation, and sports and leisure activities. Also, access to information regarding employment opportunities and available health resources to promote healthy behaviors and positive life choices can decline. These factors lead to conditions of instability that in turn can lead to a lack of medical care and preventive health services, among other issues.

There are several strategies to promote health in individuals and populations. Two general approaches to health promotion are **health behavior change** (Favin, Naimoli, & Sherburne, 2004) and **empowerment** (Tengland, 2008). Behavior change interventions use various kinds of theories to target people's behavior (Redding et al., 2000), which they do through information, persuasion, pressure and health-oriented control, whereas empowerment focuses on the inclusion of individuals, families, and communities in the decision-making and action processes.

Empowerment

Community empowerment has roots in community psychology, health education and health promotion, the liberation philosophy of Paulo Freire (Minkler & Cox, 1980), community organizing, rural and community development, and social work. Community empowerment is the social action process by which people, organizations, and communities gain mastery over their lives and affairs through changes in their social and political environments.

Strength and self-reliance are central to the idea of community empowerment, with two core aspects based in relationships with others: control over resources (material, human, financial) and control over ideology (values, attitudes, beliefs). Power over others may be exercised through direct or indirect control over peoples' opportunities for education, employment, living conditions, or other political-economic structures that favor certain interests or classes of people over others.

Empowerment strategies therefore mean challenging control and social injustice, through political, social, and psychological processes that uncover the mechanisms of control, the institutional or structural barriers, the cultural norms and social biases, and therefore enable people to challenge internalized helplessness and oppression and to develop new representations of reality (Sadan, 2004).

Two related concepts have been articulated by health professionals: community capacity and **social capital**. **Community capacity** is identified as containing various dimensions, including participation, support networks, sense of community, and access to power, with processes and tools to measure capacity outcomes in development (Chaskin, 1999). Social capital, or the norms and social networks that facilitate coordination for mutual benefit, has captured the imagination of health professionals largely because of epidemiologic studies that have correlated the variables of trust, reciprocity, and civic engagement to morbidity and mortality statistics (Dasgupta & Serageldin, 2001). Both of these have overlapping definitions and may be used interchangeably, though social capital is more an attribute of communities than a strategy.

Tangible evidence of political commitment and support of local and national authorities along with appropriate funding is necessary to establish and sustain the family and community health approach. The values, principles, challenges, and advantages of establishing family and community-oriented health services must be known by decision makers.

Local governments also play a fundamental role in the promotion of healthy practices by coordinating the efforts of different social players in the community, such as health care facilities, schools, community-based organizations, families, churches, and community health agents. Success in carrying out these practices will depend on adequate planning, selecting the appropriate promotional activities, and forming strategic alliances with other social players in the community.

One example of successful collaborative community participation in health initiatives is the Integrated Management of Childhood Illness (IMCI) strategy, designed by WHO and UNICEF in the early 1990s to reduce child mortality and morbidity due to preventable illnesses through interventions focused on not only clinics and health systems but on the community as well (Community IMCI Regional Partnership, 2006a). The IMCI strategy was implemented in the Chao district in Peru from 2002 to 2004 through the utilization of multipartner health committees with representatives from local government (i.e., the mayor's office, police, education sector, and others), the local Red Cross volunteer network, the health centers for the Ministry of Health, and various community-based organizations. This collaboration generated improvements in maternal and child health through the inclusion of parenting classes and maternal and child health curricula in schools (Community IMCI Regional Partnership, 2006b).

Implementation of the Family and Community Health Approach

The family and community health approach seeks to accomplish several goals. First, it seeks to create healthy behaviors and develop strong and resilient communities, families, and individuals. Secondly, this approach aims to reduce risks to health and prevent diseases by decreasing exposure to harmful situations and avoiding the causes of illness and death. Further, by providing equitable access to quality health services, adopting a strategy for the renewal of primary health care, and respecting local culture, it seeks to forge and complement linkages between health services and the community. Further still, the family and community health approach addresses health determinants by conducting intersectoral actions; building alliances, partnerships, and networks; and adopting the "health in all policies" strategy. Last, this approach seeks to promote the development and establishment of organized communities that fully exercise

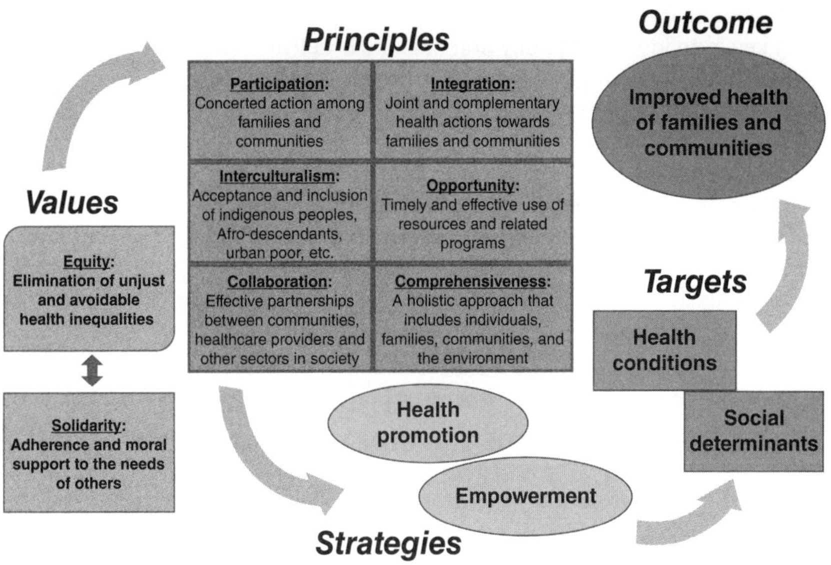

Figure 15.1 Values, Principles, and Strategies of the Family and Community Health Approach

their right to the enjoyment of the highest attainable standard of physical and mental health ("Right to Health") (Figure 15.1).

Six fundamental principles guide the family and community health approach:

1. *Participation:* Involvement of communities and families as active partners sharing responsibility in decision making and management, which is essential for attaining and maintaining their health, based on the identification of their own problems and needs;
2. *Collaboration:* Joint efforts of families, communities, health services, and institutions to produce a synergistic impact on the health of the population. In this sense, the strategy of primary health care (PHC) provides a critical reference point for these efforts (Starfield et al., 2005)
3. *Integration:* Fusion of actions and programs in a continuous, complementary, and synergistic approach to the health of individuals and families
4. *Comprehensiveness:* Recognition of the health disease process as a totality that includes the person throughout the life course and his/her relations with family, community, and the social and physical environment
5. *Interculturalism:* Acceptance and harmonization of the perceptions, interpretations, knowledge, cosmo-vision, and practices of the traditional medicine of indigenous peoples and conventional academic medicine as part of a mutually beneficial relationship
6. *Opportunity:* Advantageous timing and synchronicity with political, social or economic events and structural or policy changes; and/or utilization of already present logistical frameworks, programs, and interactions among individuals, families, communities, and health services to implement simultaneous and timely health interventions

In practical terms, at the core of the family and community approach lies a set of key individual and family practices such as IMCI, including care-seeking behavior and following the advice of health care providers, which in many communities includes members of the community who practice traditional medicine. This approach is intended to strengthen the capacity and efficacy of health systems and service networks to provide integrated and comprehensive care, bringing people closer to the health services and community resources that can improve their quality of care, their health, and their well being. Case Study 15.1 (below) illustrates the real life application of the six principles of the family and community health approach.

CASE STUDY 15.1 REDUCTION OF CHRONIC MALNUTRITION IN CHILDREN THROUGH POLITICAL MOBILIZATION: THE CASE OF PERU

At the beginning of the 2000s, Peru was part of a group of countries in Latin America, including Guatemala, Haiti, Honduras, Ecuador, and Bolivia, with a high prevalence of chronic malnutrition in children five years or younger. Likewise, a global analysis carried out in 2008 placed Peru among the 36 countries in the world that concentrated 90% of the chronically undernourished children five years or younger (Black et al., 2008).

The national average of chronic malnutrition in Peru was 31.3% in 2007, with large gaps between the more developed and the poorest regions of the country, the latter characterized by a predominance of rural and indigenous populations (PAHO, 2012; UNICEF, 2008).

In January 2006, a group of organizations in civil society, bilateral agencies, and agencies of the United Nations agreed to form the Initiative Against Child Malnutrition (IDI) with the goal of reducing the high rates of chronic malnutrition in Peru. This goal was to be accomplished through political advocacy, general and specific information dissemination, and social vigilance and accountability. Members of IDI called upon all the candidates for president in the 2006 elections and asked each one of them to pledge to reduce chronic malnutrition of children five years or younger by 5% in the five years of their future mandate. The newly elected President Alan García made IDI one of the priorities of his government and incorporated this initiative into a major social governmental program, **CRECER** (Government of Peru, 2007).

Thus, there was a turning point in national policy between 2007 and 2012, resulting in a decrease from 31.3% to 18.1% in the national average of chronic malnutrition in children five years and younger (10.5% in urban areas and 31.9% in rural areas). This represented an annual reduction of 1.0 percentage points in urban areas (vs. 0.4 in the 2000–2007 period), 2.8 in rural areas (vs. 0.2 in the 2000–2007 period), and 2.1 at the national level (vs. 0.4 in the 2000–2007 period) (National Institute of Statistics and Informatics, 2014).

These encouraging results were attributed to the following factors:

- *Involvement at all levels of government:* Beyond a narrow sectoral plan, IDI resulted in the active and ongoing involvement of the central, regional, and local governments whose actions were directed to those geographic areas presenting the greatest problems and where the process of local administration with community participation was to take place.

- *Action on the social determinants of health:* IDI and CRECER recognized that the problem of malnutrition in children was mainly due to the socioeconomic context, the level of social participation, housing quality, food security, basic education, access to basic health services, physical and social environment, women empowerment, and labor conditions in the communities.
- *Sectoral interventions with supra sectoral coordination:* The national strategy at the highest political level was structured to address food security, health, education, housing, and social protection. Likewise, the coordination and intersectoral planning facilitated the convergence of social programs in CRECER, toward the most vulnerable regions and those provinces and municipalities with the highest levels of malnutrition.
- *Life course approach:* Recognizing that multiple socioenvironmental factors and risks leading to malnutrition or lack of growth are present throughout the life course, especially at its early stages, actions were specifically directed to newborns and infants as well as pregnant women and mothers.
- *Coordination and alignment of the various cooperation agencies:* The joint and coordinated efforts of all participants, the use of media and other means of communication about the nutritional problems, and the strategies to ameliorate them were instrumental for the success of this program.
- *National monitoring of the process:* National actors and cooperative agencies accompanied and monitored this process periodically underlining the progress and change in the implementation of the national strategy and its execution by the subnational and local governments and communities. The involvement of the media gave visibility and transparency to the process of monitoring and evaluation.

In summary, the *opportunity* presented by the presidential election allowed for the development of a nationwide program with the effective *participation* and *collaboration* of multiple partners and stakeholders at the subnational and community levels.

The *integration* of this initiative into a major governmental social program permitted the implantation and sustainability of actions directed to the most remote and neglected communities of Peru. Also, because of their ethnic diversity this initiative required the implementation of an *intercultural* approach to the indigenous, rural and urban families and communities in the country. Finally, IDI and CRECER addressed the underlining social determinants of malnutrition using a *comprehensive* approach based on the early stages of the life course (preconception, pregnancy, birth, and infancy).

The family and community health approach seeks to ensure that the individual, the family, and the community receive health care that looks not only at a person's health but also at his/her relations with the family and the community. The family and community health approach respects community values, providing a participatory model for the social management of care through the strategy for the renewal of primary health care, which includes the guiding principles of health systems organization.

Several important steps must be taken to ensure a successful approach. First, *identification of community leaders* who legitimately represent the best interests of the community, as well as priority health, socioeconomic, and development issues, is essential. This should be followed by a *diagnosis of the community health situation*. This diagnosis should involve the active participation of key community members to identify and define the most important health problems that are amenable to intervention. Next, a *decision on alternative actions* should be made based on priorities, resources, and known effectiveness of the various possible interventions. Finally, the *implementation and evaluation of selected interventions* should follow. This may include promoting key family and community health practices; training health care workers; linking families, households, and community institutions with the critical components of primary care services and the overall health system. These activities and their impact should be closely monitored and evaluated. It is also sensible to conduct operational research within the community when necessary. Finally, the information attained via these evaluation practices should be disseminated and used to improve the effectiveness and efficiency of current and future interventions (Butterfoss, 2006; Cashman et al., 2008).

Strategically, the necessary measures for designing and implementing these steps for family and community health within the health services include:

1. A *stakeholder analysis* can systematically gather information on each individual party and actors that are affected and can influence the process, and further analyze their strategic positions as drivers, blockers, supporters, bystanders, or abstainers regarding the planned intervention (Hyder et al., 2010).
2. *Advocacy*—the act of supporting a cause or proposal—must be employed with the goal of promoting this approach; for example, the media should be used to engage the necessary parties and stakeholders, ensuring civil society participation.
3. *Development of alliances, partnerships, and networks* among individuals and institutions that can provide technical, political, and financial collaboration and support should be actively pursued.
4. Further, the *formulation of policies, programs, plans, projects, and legislation* when necessary, with a clear and respectful understanding of the needs, rights, and cultural values of individuals, families, and communities,

along with strategies and mechanisms for their execution, monitoring, and evaluation must also be developed.

5. *Social participation* must be stressed. Organized communities will allow for their own empowerment in exercising their right to health.
6. This type of participation will necessitate *the mobilization of human and financial resources* at the local, national, and sometimes, international levels.
7. It will also create the need to *educate and train human resources* at every level to develop multidisciplinary teams whose members can collaborate with and learn from each other.
8. Other actions such as *technical cooperation geared to problem solving;* and *research promotion* (especially applied and participatory research) should be designed to develop new methodologies and knowledge.
9. *Surveillance, monitoring, and evaluation,* to assess the situation, measure progress and results, determine needs, and make adjustments when necessary.
10. *Dissemination of information,* in order to both share findings with society as a whole and to give feedback to decision makers, health services, communities, and families, must be considered.

The success and sustainability of the family and community health approach depend on the development of policies, actions, and tools that aim to empower individuals, families, communities, and health services (Fawcett et al., 1995). Individuals and families are empowered by acquiring health literacy through information and education, by having available options, and by having the right and the ability to choose. Communities are empowered through strong leadership, commitment to health and effective social organization and mobilization in the full exercise of their right to health. Health services are empowered by providing health personnel with ongoing training and economic incentives; access to adequate information, technology, and technical know-how, as well as good managerial practices and logistical, administrative, and financial support for health programs.

Finally, international and multilateral political alliances and financial support for technical interventions at the country level often serve to strengthen governmental and societal resolve to address priority health problems. Box 15.1 describes the Pan American Alliance for Nutrition and Development, an initiative of the United Nations agencies specifically directed to alleviate malnutrition in children in countries of Latin America. We must remember, however, that it is at the family and individual levels that the actions implemented and the success or failure of an intersectoral health and social program will have a critical impact on the health, welfare, development, and future of the community.

BOX 15.1 PAN AMERICAN ALLIANCE FOR NUTRITION AND DEVELOPMENT FOR THE ACHIEVEMENT OF THE MILLENNIUM DEVELOPMENT GOALS

A Social Determinants Approach to Malnutrition and Health in the Americas

The Pan American Alliance for Nutrition and Development (PAND) was conceived for the purpose of implementing comprehensive intersectoral policies and programs that are both sustainable and coordinated. These policies and programs lie within the framework of an intercultural rights-based gender approach, and their purpose is to accelerate achievement of the Millennium Development Goals (MDGs). The alliance is an example of high-level international collaboration in which UN agencies with different mandates have recognized that malnutrition and ill health result from the interaction of many factors, some originated in the individual person, and many others stemming from the social and economic conditions in which individuals are born, grow, work, and age during their life course.

The Centrality of Nutrition in the Creation of the Alliance

Poverty and vulnerability maps overlap with the malnutrition map, especially the chronic malnutrition map. In the targeting of scenarios, as opposed to the targeting of individuals—low height-for-age (stunting) is an optimal tracer of vulnerabilities. The reduction of chronic malnutrition is a sensitive, though nonspecific, indicator of changes in the configuration of its determinants.

Low height-for-age is the result of many factors (e.g., improper child care and child-rearing practices, food insecurity, inadequate health care, lack of access to safe water and basic sanitation, repeated bouts of infection throughout the life course, and low levels of education) that occur simultaneously over extended periods (Black et al., 2008).

Interventions to prevent nutritional problems, especially chronic malnutrition, are effective for a wide range of situations that occur in pregnancy, the first two years of life, and throughout life. These interventions impact health and human development and have transgenerational effects. Although these characteristics are not exclusive to nutrition, low height-for-age has the broadest and most visible horizontal intersection with health and development and their determinants than any other indicator.

The Social Determinants Approach

There is a constellation of known factors operating as social determinants of health that include socioeconomic context, poverty and inequality, social exclusion, socioeconomic status, income, public policies, education, the quality of housing, transportation, the physical and social environment, and social and community support networks. All these factors are clearly found at different levels of a hierarchy. Moreover, the influence of these factors is not summative; some factors behave like underlying causes or intermediate causes, and some modify the effects of other factors in a causative network.

Although providing a child with adequate food and health care is critical, these actions alone are not the most efficient because they do not address the mechanisms that generate food insecurity and greater vulnerability to disease. This fact, which is true for the individual, is even more apparent at the population level. The main objective of the alliance is to reduce malnutrition through a determinants-based approach. However, given the common causality spectrum, addressing the determinants of chronic malnutrition will also have a positive—and paradoxical—impact on the reduction of overweight and obesity, which will help reduce the prevalence of chronic diseases.

Consequently, if it is recognized that health and nutrition are determined by social factors, then the objective of the interventions must focus not only on individuals, but also on the physical and social environments that produces the individual's health, such as the **family and community** environment (Bacallao et al., 2012).

It should be pointed out, however, that the negative aspects of the social determinants—lack of education, and so on—produce and increase health inequalities, not only in society as a whole, but also among specific and vulnerable social groups. Furthermore, these inequalities can be transmitted intergenerationally (i.e., the children of the poor and malnourished are likely to be poor and malnourished), thus impeding social mobility and development and perpetuating the vicious cycle of poverty, ill health, and malnutrition. Malnutrition is a convincing political flagship for advocacy and for enlisting the involvement of those responsible for designing and implementing public policy. However, successfully tackling malnutrition will require the support of all the agencies. The alliance is especially well positioned to crystallize into specific action the spirit of reform in UN organizations and the common goal of "health in all policies" in Latin America and the Caribbean.

Summary

The family and community health approach introduced in this chapter, is one of the health sector strategies to achieve universal health coverage and universal access to health and social services for as many people as possible, especially the most neglected communities and social groups. It is based on the ethical public health values of equity and solidarity, and the practical principles of participation, collaboration, integration, interculturalism, opportunity, and comprehensiveness. Examples of this approach to prevent malnutrition and to improve child health in indigenous communities in Latin America are included in this chapter. For its implementation, the family and community health approach relies on effective leadership and management (individual or shared) as well as the synergistic application of measures such as advocacy, policy, and program formulation; the forging of partnerships and intersectoral alliances; and the mobilization of human and financial resources. In this chapter we posit that the most important factor for the success of this approach is the effective use of health promotion and self reliance strategies to achieve positive behavioral changes and empower individuals, families, and communities to understand, manage, and maintain their own health.

KEY TERMS

1. **Community:** A social setting with a variable number of members (from a few dozen to several thousand) which are connected by a common geography and/or a shared set of characteristics like language, ethnicity, socioeconomic status, identity, etc.
2. **Community capacity:** The combination of participation, support networks, sense of belonging, access to power, and tools to measure outcomes in community health and development (overlaps with definition of social capital)
3. **CRECER:** A national strategy in Peru during the government of Alan García with the purpose of linking either directly or indirectly the diverse sectors, programs, and projects of the national, regional, and local government to the fight against poverty and malnutrition
4. **Empowerment:** The social action process by which people, organizations, and communities gain mastery over their lives and affairs through changes in their social and political environment
5. **Epigenetic modifications:** Externally or environmentally induced changes in gene activity which are not caused by changes in the DNA sequence. These changes can produce cellular and physiological trait variations that can be transmitted from one generation to the next
6. **Family:** The basic social unit consisting of two or more people related by blood, marriage, or affinity, who share a history, the same household and basic resources, and self-identify as such
7. **Health behavior change:** The modification and avoidance of harmful actions and practices, and the adoption and maintenance of beneficial actions and practices related to health
8. **Life course:** A dynamic representation of an individual's passage through the continuum of life, from conception to death
9. **Life stages:** The different biological and chronological phases in an individual's life, from conception, birth, infancy, and childhood to adolescence, adulthood, and old age, with each period being characterized by a distinct set of risks and determinants of health
10. **PROGRESS:** Acronym for social determinants of health (place of residence, race, occupation, gender, religion, education, social economic status, and social capital)

11. **Social capital:** Norms and social networks that facilitate coordination for mutual benefit among community members (overlaps with definition of community capacity)
12. **Social determinants of health:** The economic, social, and political conditions of everyday life that influence the health of individuals, communities, and populations. The conditions in which individuals are born, grow, live, work, and age

REVIEW QUESTIONS

1. Is it possible to reduce health inequities in indigenous populations? How would you approach this problem?
2. What are the various sources of power of individuals, families, and communities? How are people empowered?
3. How would you improve a health program by taking advantage of a political event or a high-priority social or environmental program, for example, education, water and sanitation, change of government, or others?
4. You are a health promotion specialist and a well-known problem solver. How many of the vulnerability factors of families and communities in Table 15.1 are amenable to health promotion interventions? How would you approach those in which health promotion is not effective or warranted?

References

Bacallao, J., Peña, M., & Díaz, A. (2012). Reducción de la desnutrición crónica en las bases biosociales para la promoción de la salud y el desarrollo. *Revista Panamericana de Salud Pública, 32*(2), 145–150.

Bengston, V. L., & Allen, K. R. (1993). Life course perspective. In *Sourcebook of family theories and methods: A contextual approach*. New York, NY: Plenum Press.

Black, R. E., Allen L. H., Bhutta, Z. A., Caulfield L. E., de Onis, M., Ezzati, M., … Rivera, J. (2008). Maternal and child undernutrition: Global and regional exposures and health consequences. *Lancet, 371*(9608), 243–260.

Butterfoss, F.D. (2006). Process evaluation for community participation. *Annual Review of Public Health, 27*, 323–340.

Cashman, S. B., Adeky, S., Allen, A. J. 3rd, Corburn, J., Israel, B. A., Montaño, J., … Eng, E. (2008). The power and the promise: Working with communities to analyze data, interpret findings, and get to outcomes. *American Journal of Public Health, 98*(8), 1407–1417.

Champagne, F.A. (2008) Epigenetic mechanisms and the transgenerational effects of maternal care. *Frontiers in Neuroendocrinology, 29*(3), 386–397.

Chaskin, R.J. (1999). *Defining community capacity: A framework and implications from a comprehensive community initiative.* Chicago: University of Chicago Chapin Hall Center for Children.

Christensen, P. (2004). The health promoting family: A conceptual framework for future research. *Social Science and Medicine, 59*(2), 377–387.

Community IMCI Regional Partnership. (2006a). *Community component of the IMCI strategy: Conceptual framework.* Washington DC: Pan American Health Organization, American Red Cross, and United Nations Foundation.

Community IMCI Regional Partnership. (2006b). Community IMCI: The engendering of social empowerment in Chao, Peru. Washington DC: Pan American Health Organization, American Red Cross, and United Nations Foundation.

Dasgupta, P., & Serageldin, I. (Eds.). (2001). *Social capital: A multifaceted perspective.* Washington, DC: World Bank.

Duque, L.F., Klevens, J., & Ramirez, C. (2003). Cross sectional survey of perpetrators, victims, and witnesses of violence in Bogotá, Colombia. *Journal of Epidemiology and Community Health, 57*(5), 355–360.

Favin, M., Naimoli, G., & Sherburne, L. (2004). *Improving health through behavior change: A process guide on hygiene promotion.* Washington, DC: Environmental Health Project, Pan American Health Organization, Plan, and US Agency for International Development.

Fawcett, S. B., Paine-Andrews, A., Francisco, V. T., Schultz, J. A., Richter, K. P., Lewis, R. K., … Fisher, J. L. (1995). Using empowerment theory in collaborative partnerships for community health and development. *American Journal of Community Psychology, 23*(5), 677–697.

Ferrer, R. I., Palmer, R., & Burger, S. (2005). The family contribution to health status: A population level estimate. *Annals of Family Medicine, 3,* 102–108.

Frohlich, K. L. & Potvin, L. (2008). Transcending the known in public health practice: The inequality paradox: The population approach and vulnerable populations. *American Journal of Public Health, 98* (2), 216–221.

Government of Guatemala. (2011). *National study on maternal mortality: Final report* (in Spanish). Guatemala: Serviprensa.

Government of Peru. (2007). CRECER national strategy: Plan of operations (in Spanish). Retrieved from http://www.apci.gob.pe/marco/atach/PlanDeOperacionesCRECER.pdf

Gwatkin, D.R. (2007). 10 best resources on … health equity. *Health Policy and Planning, 22*(5), 348–351.

Hoghughi, M. (1998). The importance of parenting in child health. *British Medical Journal, 316,* 1545.

Hyder, A., Syed, S., Puvanachandra, P., Bloom, G., Sundaram, S., Mahmood, S., … Peters, D. (2010). Stakeholder analysis for health research: Case studies from low- and middle-income countries. *Public Health, 124*, 159–166.

Kaati, G., Bygren, L.O., Pembrey, M., & Sjöstrom, M. (2007). Transgenerational response to nutrition, early life circumstances and longevity. *European Journal of Human Genetics, 15*, 784–790.

Kronik, J, & Verner, D. (2010). *Indigenous peoples and climate change in Latin America and the Caribbean.* World Bank Publications.

MacQueen, K. M, McLellan, E., Metzger, D. S., Kegeles, S., Strauss, R. P., Scotti, R., … Trotter, R. T. II. (2001). What is community? An evidence-based definition for participatory public health. *American Journal of Public Health, 91*(12), 1929–1937.

Minkler, M., & Cox, K. (1980). Creating critical consciousness in health: Applications of Freire's philosophy and methods to the health care setting. *International Journal of Health Services, 10*(2), 311–322.

Montenegro, R. A., & Stephens, C. (2006). Indigenous health in Latin America and the Caribbean. *Lancet, 367*(9525), 1859–1869.

National Institute of Statistics and Informatics. (2014). *Breastfeeding and nutrition of girls, boys and mothers.* Government of Peru. Retrieved from http://www.inei.gob.pe/media/MenuRecursivo/publicaciones_digitales/Est/Lib1211/pdf/cap010.pdf

Novilla, M .L. B., Barnes, M. D., De la Cruz, N. G., William, P. N., & Rogers, J. (2006). Public health perspectives on the family: An ecological approach to promoting health in the family and community. *Family and Community Health, 29*(1), 28–42.

Pan American Health Organization. (2006). *Health of the indigenous peoples of the Americas.* Washington, DC: Author.

Pan American Health Organization. (2007). *Health in the Americas* (2007 ed.). Washington, DC: Author.

Pan American Health Organization. (2009). *Pan American alliance for nutrition and development. Basic document, conceptual premises and strategic principles.* Washington, DC: Author.

Pan American Health Organization. (2012). *Health in the Americas* (2012 ed.). Washington, DC: Author.

Redding, C. A., Rossi, J. S., Rossi, S. R., Velicer, W. F., & Prochaska, J. O. (2000). Health behavior models. *International Electronic Journal of Health Education, 3*, 180–193.

Sadan, E. (2004). Developing a theory of empowerment. In *Empowerment and community planning*. Tel Aviv: Hakibbutz Hameuchad Publishers. Retrieved from http://www.mpow.org/

Soubhi, H., & Potvin, L. (2000). Homes and families as health promotion settings. In B. D. Poland, L. W. Green, & I. Rootman (Eds.), *Settings for health promotion: Linking theory and practice* (pp. 44–67). Thousand Oaks, CA: Sage.

Starfield, B., Shi, L. et al. (2005). Contribution of primary care to health systems and health. *Milbank Quarterly, 83*(3), 457–502.

Tengland, P. A. (2008). Empowerment: A conceptual discussion. *Health Care Analysis, 16*(2), 77–96.

UNICEF. (2008). *Situation of children in Peru, executive summary.* Lima: UNICEF and INEI. Retrieved from http://www.unicef.org/peru/spanish/Folleto_ing_correc_1.pdf

World Health Organization. (1976). *Statistical indices of family health.* Report of a WHO study group. Geneva. February 17–21, 1975.

World Health Organization. (2008). *Closing the gap in a generation: Health equity through action on the social determinants of health.* Final Report of the Commission on Social Determinants of Health. Geneva: World Health Organization.

CHAPTER 16

ORAL HEALTH PROMOTION

Margaret Scarlett and Gary L. Kreps*

Oral diseases are extremely common, and risks for oral diseases are nearly universal. Although declared a human right and part of overall health by the WHO, oral health remains a relatively neglected public health issue. There is no population-based oral health system, and oral health has not been integrated into the overall health system. These gaps are a major cause for concern.

One important barrier to widespread oral health promotion is the lack of standard measures for assessing the oral health and the risk of oral disease of populations, and common oral diseases and their reversal in individuals. There is an especially acute need for simple, reliable measures that can be used by professionals outside of oral health and understood by policymakers. New technologies such as social media hold promise for assessing and promoting population-wide oral health at relatively low cost, but their promise cannot be fulfilled if the measurement challenges remain unmet.

This chapter begins with an examination of oral health at the biological level, and reviews some simple daily preventive measures an individual can take to care for the mouth and teeth to reduce oral health risks. It goes on to outline major barriers to performing those behaviors, and to emphasize a population-based view of oral health. This perspective entails the recognition that individuals share responsibility for oral health with dentists, other clinicians, public health workers, policymakers (insurers and politicians) who fund health care, schools, and private sector employers. Recent advances and steps that are still needed at the levels of scientific consensus, disease surveillance, health care and health information delivery, policy, and the physical environment are described.

LEARNING OBJECTIVES

By the end of this chapter, the reader should be able to:

- Explain the nature and scope of the oral disease problem
- Provide examples of science-based oral health promotion strategies
- Identify key barriers to implementing oral health promotion
- Describe appropriate measures of success for oral health promotion
- Highlight the common risk factor approach to integrated oral health promotion
- Suggest ways to integrate oral health promotion with other public health efforts
- Outline advances in international policy relevant to oral health promotion

*The authors gratefully acknowledge May Kennedy, PhD, for her inputs for revisions of the chapter, as well as her thoughtful insights. Recognition is also given to Dr. Nigel Pitts of King's College London and Dr. Chris Fox of the International Association of Dental Research for their review.

What Is Oral Health?

Optimal oral health includes sound teeth, free of any kind of restoration or filling, and the absence of oral diseases and conditions in the soft tissues of the oral and perioral areas (Pitts et al., 2014). The most common oral diseases are **tooth decay** (dental **caries**), **gum disease** (**periodontitis**), and **oral cancer** (oral carcinoma). See Box 16.1 for a list of major impacts that oral diseases can have on individuals and populations.

Oral health goes beyond a focus on teeth alone, encompassing the entire oral area and perioral areas (i.e., the mouth and area around the mouth), including the gingiva (gums), oral and perioral soft tissues, chewing muscles, hard and soft palate, tongue, lips, and salivary glands. All of these structures play a part in allowing people to eat, speak, socialize, and express emotions without discomfort or embarrassment (DHHS, 2000). The mouth also provides a snapshot of overall health, as both the beginning of the digestive tract that processes nutrients and an easily accessible body cavity (DHHS, 2000). Conceived even more broadly, optimal oral health means freedom from exposure to (a) infectious disease organisms, (b) chronic diseases like diabetes, (c) excessive forces, such as wear or trauma (see Box 16.2), and (d) damaging environmental agents such as tobacco and excessive alcohol.

Tooth loss has become synonymous with poverty and is one of the most visible and stigmatizing indicators of low socioeconomic status (Watt & Petersen, 2012). Consistent with the 1948 World Health Organization (WHO) definition of optimal health, oral health is an important aspect of overall physical and psychological health and well-being (WHO, 1948). Nevertheless, oral health remains an under studied and under addressed public health issue.

BOX 16.1 THE IMPACT OF COMMON ORAL DISEASE

Tooth decay, gum disease, and oral cancer can:

- cause pain, bleeding, infections, destruction of oral tissues or perioral areas, and even death;
- reduce the ability of oral function, including difficulty speaking or chewing, from loss or misalignment of teeth or by destruction of oral hard and soft tissues by oral cancers;
- damage esthetics, resulting in embarrassment, as well as social and psychological impact, such as avoiding socializing or smiling;
- economic impact, especially to lower socioeconomic groups, for care, as well as lost school and work hours; and
- cause or exacerbate diseases in other parts of the body.

Sources: Petersen & Kwan (2011); US Department of Health and Human Services [DHHS] (2000).

Human Microbiome

The mouth includes the teeth, the gums or **gingiva**, the tongue, cheeks, lips, hard palate, and soft palate. The perioral area includes the area on the face around the mouth, as well as the tonsils, oropharyngeal area, esophagus, Eustachian tube and middle ear, trachea, lungs and nasal passages, and sinuses. All of these structures are populated by micro-organisms; together they are defined as the human oral microbiome. It contains more than 600 identified organisms (Dewhirst et al., 2010), is likely to modulate both health and disease in the oral cavity, and can serve as a port of entry for infectious disease micro-organisms.

Dental Caries

Caries is a disease of both the primary or **deciduous teeth** and permanent teeth, and is nearly universal. Caries starts with transmission of bacteria to infants early in life; it is a process of destruction of tooth structure that, if not reversed at the earliest stages, ends years later with a "hole" or cavitation in a tooth, often called a **cavity** (American Academy of Pediatrics Section on Pediatric Dentistry and Oral Health [AAP] (2014), Keels et al., 2008; American College of Obstetricians and Gynecologists, 2013; Kohler, Andreen, & Jonsson, 1984). A biofilm or "acquired pellicle," commonly called **plaque**, composed originally of salivary proteins on the **enamel** of teeth, combines with bacteria and bacterial by-products to colonize the tooth (Dorian, 2002). High levels of certain colonizing bacteria, most notably *Streptococcus mutans*, *Streptococcus sobrinus*, and some *Lactobaccillus* species, are associated with caries (Corby et al., 2005; Domejean, White, & Featherstone, 2011; Featherstone, 2000). Triggered by ingestion of sugars and fermentable carbohydrates, the biofilm produces acid that attacks the tooth, the hardest material in the body. Over time, this acid can damage the tooth unless it is balanced by protective factors, such as proper salivary flow, routine plaque removal, proper nutrition, and higher pH, as well as replacement of **fluoride**, calcium, and other minerals lost from tooth enamel (Keels et al., 2008; Featherstone, 2000). A balance between these destructive and protective factors is essential to controlling caries, and a point of emphasis for oral health programming.

The best predictors of caries in children at age 3 are high maternal levels of bacteria (>100 **CFUs**) and caries when the children were age one (Chaffee et al., 2014; Corby et al., 2005). Dental treatment with sealants and **fluoride varnish** can protect the deep grooves in primary and permanent teeth; these sealants and varnishes are applied by health professionals.

Periodontitis

Periodontitis is a common, often chronic, bacterially induced inflammatory disease that destroys local bone and connective tissues that support the teeth and raises systemic inflammation (Tonetti & Claffey, 2005). The composition of the oral human microbiome is related to the severity of disease (Yucel-Lindberg & Bage, 2013). Species of bacteria in plaque associated with periodontitis include *Porphyromonas gingivalis, Tannerella Forsythia, Aggregatibacter actinomycetemcomitans,* and hundreds of others. Plaque alone is necessary but insufficient to produce disease because response to plaque is mediated by host factors; in other words, inflammatory and other genetic responses to this bacterial challenge are greater in some individuals over others. For persons prone to inflammation, bacterial plaque can cause destruction of the bony and soft tissues around the tooth (Bartold & Van Dyke, 2013; Giannobile et al., 2013).

In early stage disease, inflammation can be reversed, with resolution of inflammatory markers in the soft and hard tissues around the teeth. This early, reversible stage of caries is called **gingivitis**. Recently identified compounds, called resolvins, lipoxins, and protectins, are host mediators that may play a role in resolution (Bartold & Van Dyke, 2013; Van Dyke, 2011). In the end stage disease process, **attachment loss** of the tooth to the gingiva and/or alveolar bone in the upper and lower jaws occurs, making teeth loose or mobile. Recent evidence indicates that individual, genetically influenced inflammatory responses, environmental and perhaps **epigenetic factors** are likely to affect the severity of disease (Bartold & VanDyke, 2013: Giannobile et al., 2013; Haffajee et al., 2009). Most candidate antibiotic treatments for periodontitis have not been shown to be effective. However, recent evidence suggests that targeting host response with dual action agents, those such as Azithromycin that have both antibiotic and anti-inflammatory effects, may inhibit and even control the destructive cycle of periodontitis (Haffajee, Torresyap & Socransky, 2007).

Major Risk Factors

In general, population-level risk for oral diseases increases with age and poverty. But even within income and age groups in a given context, oral disease is unequally distributed. Personal genetics play a key role in modulating oral diseases, as described in the previous discussion of plaque and periodontal disease. And periodontal diseases are caused by non-plaque as well as plaque conditions; systemic health conditions or diseases (e.g., measles, mumps, diabetes) are likely to impact the severity of periodontal disease. In addition, the oral cavity is not immune to infections (bacterial, fungal or viral), allergic reactions, or dermatologic conditions.

There are also risk factors for oral diseases at the behavioral, cultural, and environmental levels. Some of these are modifiable (see Box 16.2), and may be appropriate foci for health promotion efforts. Petersen and Baehni (2012) have argued that the key modifiable risk factors for periodontal disease are tobacco use, excessive alcohol consumption, poor diet and nutrition, obesity, psychological stress, and insufficient personal and **oral hygiene.** Note that all of these risk factors are shared with other chronic conditions. Other possible foci that should be considered include being vaccinated for preventable infectious diseases and being treated for existing diseases and related secondary inflammatory conditions.

BOX 16.2 POTENTIALLY MODIFIABLE RISK FACTORS FOR ORAL DISEASE

- inconsistent or inadequate personal oral hygiene
- inadequate amounts of fluoride in water supplies, food, and/or toothpaste or **mouth rinse**
- a diet high in fermentable carbohydrates and sugars
- a lack of cultural understanding of oral health risks and/or low overall health literacy
- prolonged oral exposure to harmful substances, such as tobacco, alcohol, and betel nut
- sexual behaviors that can introduce HPV or other sexually transmitted pathogens into the oral cavity
- routine exposure to gastric fluid, such as self-induced vomiting, or to dietary acids, as in sucking lemons
- head trauma or work-related injuries (e.g., holding sewing needles in the mouth, sports-related head injuries)
- use of oral devices (e.g. tongue rings, lip piercings, tongue bars)
- systemic diseases that have been associated with oral conditions (e.g., obesity, diabetes, some cancers or cancer treatments, measles, mumps, and other vaccine preventable diseases)
- more than 600 pharmaceutical products that cause **dry mouth**, which increases risk of oral disease and makes denture wearing more difficult

Sources: Hennequin-Hoenderdos, Slot & Van der Weij (2015); Petersen & Baehni (2012); Sheiham & Watt (2000); Tonetti & Claffey (2005); Yucek-Lindberg and Bage (2013).

Nearly Universal Prevalence of Oral Diseases

Around the globe, almost everyone will suffer at some point from an oral disease, mostly dental caries or periodontitis. The prevalences of oral diseases, along with their relative importance among nearly 300 diseases and injuries, have been assessed periodically in eight global regions since 1990 by the Global Burden of Disease Study. Untreated caries in permanent teeth, severe **periodontal disease,** and/or severe tooth loss were estimated to affect 2.5–4 billion people for the year 2010. This number includes nearly 600 million children, at a cost of 15 million Disability Adjusted Life Years (DALYs) (Marcenes et al., 2013). Compared to 1990, DALYs lost to oral disease increased more than 20% by 2010. Severe, untreated tooth decay in permanent teeth was more frequently reported than any other disease, with a global prevalence of 35% for all ages combined. Untreated decay among children alone ranked as the 10th most prevalent condition or disease. Severe periodontal or gum disease ranked as the 6th most common condition. The average loss of healthy life implied for untreated caries in permanent teeth alone was 224 years per 100,000 population (Marcenes et al., 2013).

Arguably, for such extremely common diseases, what matters most is out come severity, and the severity of oral disease outcomes is strongly associated with social determinants of health such as education and income (Petersen & Kwan, 2011). In fact, from a population perspective, the oral health landscape mirrors access to health care by income level (Kwan & Petersen, 2011). Disadvantaged and poor people suffer stark inequalities in oral disease outcomes because population-level oral health promotion is lacking and preventive oral care is beyond their reach in terms of both accessibility and affordability (Petersen 2005; Petersen & Kwan, 2011).

Oral cancers are a particular concern, although they affect fewer people. The prevalence of oral cancer in developed countries is similar to that of the United States, where lifetime risk has been estimated at 1.1 per 100 (National Cancer Institute [NCI], 2015), but it is higher in some developing countries (Petersen, 2005). Oral cancer rates are rising worldwide, especially in southern Asia, but also in developed countries (Chaturvedi et al., 2013; Petersen, 2005). These diseases can recur and spread throughout the body, and their treatment can be disfiguring or disabling. Even in the United States, only about a third of oral cancers are detected in the earliest stages, when treatment is most effective and least invasive (US DHHS, 2010), and almost 40% of patients fail to survive for five years after diagnosis (NCI, 2015). In many developing countries, early diagnosis and treatment of oral cancers lags even further behind.

Oral health status declines with increasing age, even among children. For example, in a cohort of children followed in Hong Kong, oral health declined from early childhood to late adolescence (Lu et al., 2011). As discussed earlier with regard to the population at large, economic status dictated whether or not a child in Hong Kong received professional oral health services. Other evidence from both developed and developing countries suggests that, throughout the world, children in poorer segments of society are harmed disproportionately (Braveman, Egerter & Mockenhaupt, 2011; Braveman & Gruskin, 2003; Gift, Reisine, & Larach, 1992; Watt & Petersen, 2012). There is a bright spot at the other end of the age spectrum; tooth retention among older adults has increased over the past 13 years worldwide (Petersen & Yamamoto, 2005). This progress underscores the importance of prevention for the aging populations that will make increased demands on the care system in the future. Regardless of age, saliva and adequate saliva production is essential for maintaining good oral health. Xerostomia, from systemic health issues or improperly functioning salivary glands or pharmaceuticals, results in poor oral health status.

Globally, there is little doubt that the increasingly widespread use of tobacco and the overuse of alcohol (WHO, 2005b; Petersen, 2005; Warnakulasuriya, 2009) are central contributors to the development of oral cancers. Population-attributable risks of smoking and alcohol consumption were estimated as 80% for males, 61% for females, and 74% overall (Petersen, 2009). According to the International Agency for Research on Cancer, alcohol use (independent of tobacco) is associated with oral cancers. Frequent use of Quid, Khat, and Maté contribute to oral cancer rates in some parts of the world too. More than a billion people—mostly males in India, but also Indian immigrants in the United States, the Caribbean, and South Africa—use betel nut with tobacco formed into a chewing wad (Quid). In India, this has resulted in the highest rates of oral cancers in the world (Dangi, Kinnunen & Zavras, 2012; Gupta & Ray, 2004; Petersen, 2003a). About 10 million people, mostly males in Djibouti, Somalia, Ethiopia, and Yemen, chew Khat, a mild opiate plant. Khat chewing and oral cancer have been linked, but a recent review of 17 studies concluded that the association was still debatable because of methodological flaws in the research to date (El-Zaemey, Schüz, & Leon, 2015). Maté, used in teas in Central and South America, has been incompletely studied, but one epidemiologic study suggests higher cancer risk for female tea drinkers who also smoke (Loria, Barrios, & Zanetti, 2009).

In developed countries, the primary behavioral risk factor for oral cancer is strikingly different. Patterns of oral sexual behavior have changed in the United States and Europe; their fastest-growing subset of oral cancers is attributed to **human papillomavirus** (HPV) infection by direct contact and from the exchange of fluids during oral sex (Chaturvedi et al., 2011; DeSouza, 2009; Gillison, 2012).

The prevalence of behaviors that effect oral health, and of the theoretical psychological determinants of positive oral health behaviors, should be tracked to guide prevention and promotion activities. One such theoretical determinant is oral health literacy. Unfortunately, exactly how to define oral health literacy and how it is expected to relate to oral health behaviors are matters of current debate. Scant evidence has emerged to support the view that oral health literacy is a strong behavioral determinant, although higher oral health literacy among caregivers has been shown by one research group to translate to better oral health status among children (Divaris et al., 2012; Miller et al., 2010; Lee et al., 2012; Vann, Lee, & Divaris, 2010). Measures of the oral health literacy construct are weak (Institute of Medicine [IOM], 2013). Finally, promoting oral health behavior directly is still more widely understood and endorsed by oral health professionals (IOM, 2012) than is promoting oral health literacy. While researchers explore health literacy, it may be prudent for program designers to attempt to increase levels of more established theoretical predictors of oral health behavior, such as knowledge, attitudes, and perceived norms.

Measuring Oral Health and Disease

Meaningful and consistent measurement of oral health and disease has eluded clinicians and public health professionals alike. For example, there is a lack of consensus on how to evaluate both populations and individual clinic patients for caries and periodontal disease. Across the globe, there are many cross-sectional studies of caries among school aged children, but most countries lack country-wide surveillance systems for tracking caries rates. Furthermore, the best accepted oral health measures are used only by specially trained dental professionals, not the majority of practicing dental professionals and other health professionals, thereby marginalizing personnel who could play central roles in oral health promotion (Frenk, 2010; Frenk et al., 2010; Petersen, 2010). The lack of simple, universally accepted measures of oral health itself has hampered the accumulation of knowledge about the effectiveness of oral health promotion efforts. Moreover, available oral health measures are complex and not readily understood by the general public and policy makers.

Caries Measurement

Caries is generally understood to be destruction of the tooth, resulting in a hole in the tooth. However, even among dental professionals, there is a lack of agreement about the best way to measure caries, and there is no measure that is feasible for other health professionals to use, as of this writing.

Since the 1930s, the most common measure of dental caries has been the **Decayed, Missing, Filled Teeth** index (DMFT). The D(ecayed) component is a binary measure (caries/no caries) of decay in the **dentin**, one of the three parts of a tooth. One disadvantage of the DMFT is that demineralization or early decay in the outer surface of the tooth, called the enamel, is not measured. Another disadvantage is the failure of the DMFT to capture the severe consequences of tooth decay on the inner part of the tooth (or **pulp**) that contains small blood vessels and nerve tissue. Recently released country-wide data on adults and children from Malta and Portugal show that the DMFT underestimates caries by 45% or more, even up to 100% (Pitts N., personal communication, 2015). Early decay in young children under 6 is most often underestimated.

A new approach to caries measurement, the International Caries Disease Assessment System (ICDAS), assesses decay in all three parts of the tooth on a progressive scale ranging from 0-6 (Ismail et al., 2007). The ICDAS includes individual assessments and tracking of early changes. The IDCAS is part of a package of tools called the International Caries Classification and Management System (ICCMS™) (Pitts et al., 2014). (See Figure 16.1.) The ICCMS bridges diagnosis, management of early decay, and minimum interventions to the treatment of moderate and severe decay. Commendably, the ICCMS relies on methods with sound evidence of successful oral health outcomes (Pitts et al., 2014). Combined with a measure of severe decay consequences on the pulp of teeth, the Exposed Pulp, Ulceration, Fistula and Abscess (PUFA) survey, the ICCMS captures most tooth-related decay and could simplify and standardize clinical responses (Monse et al., 2010). A free version of the ICDAS is available for population-based studies of tooth decay (https://www.icdas.org/the-icdas-and-iccms-epidemiology-tool). Use of the ICCMS by non-dental professionals, however, remains a key challenge.

Periodontal Disease Measurement

The most common sign of periodontal disease is **gingival** bleeding, a characteristic of gingivitis. The severity of this disease is measured clinically by dentists in terms of gingival pocket depths and gum attachment around the tooth, but other health professionals do not have easy, consistent ways to measure periodontal disease. Definitions of periodontal disease have varied over time,

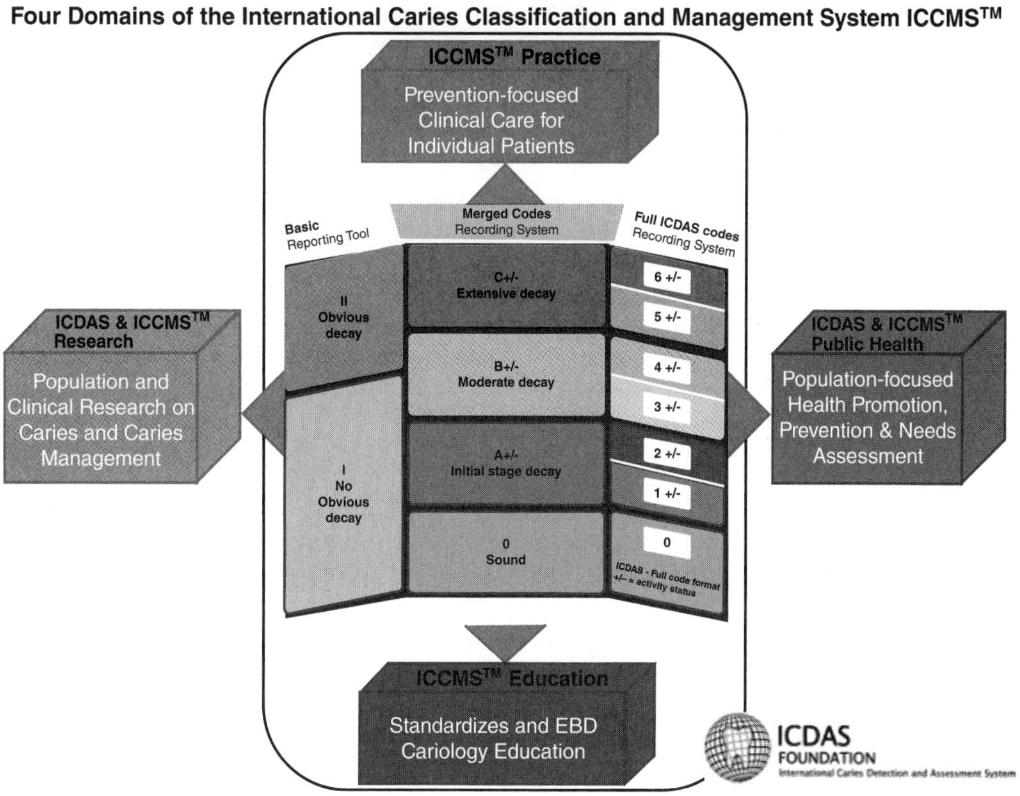

Figure 16.1 Standardized Measurement and Treatment of Tooth Decay with ICCMS
Source: International Caries Classification and Management System™.

both within the dental profession and in population-based periodontal disease surveillance (Page & Eke, 2007). This inconsistency has compromised reporting quality in the epidemiological research on periodontal disease to date. Recently, new standard principles for reporting the prevalence and severity of periodontal diseases were developed for use in epidemiological studies (Eke et al., 2012; Tonetti & Claffey, 2005). They were adopted first in Europe and then in the Americas; by 2017, they are expected to bring about greater consistency in the measurement of gum disease. This European-led refinement and standardization of periodontitis measures is a model for refining definitions of caries and other oral diseases or erosive tooth wear in the United States and other developed nations. For epidemiologic purposes, there has been some progress in standardization of prevalence and severity of periodontal disease (Graetz, Schützhold, Plaumann, Kahl, Springer et al., 2015).

Surveillance of Oral Disease

There is a worldwide dearth of routine, country-specific surveillance of oral health patterns and cases of disease. Incidence and prevalence of oral diseases is not routinely measured. To fill this gap, access to basic oral health services (supplemented by focused regional strategies) sometimes has been used as a surrogate measure of population-based oral health status (Petersen & Baehni, 2012).

Then, in 2014, two or three dentists in each country started sentinel surveillance of caries, in collaboration with the national associations of the Federation Dentaire Internationale (FDI) (daSilva & Eiselé, 2012; Glick & Fisher, 2012). This limited sentinel system measures a single disease in a sample of individual dental patients, but it may contain the seeds of an institutional base for tracking the oral health status of the broader country populations.

In the absence of preferable alternatives, PUFA will remain the standard measure of gross untreated caries (Baginska et al., 2013; Monse et al., 2010). Population-based surveillance would be facilitated by the availability of simple, self-report outcome measures for adults and children; see the description of the OHIP in the section below for a model. The measures should use short scales to assess four parameters: (1) pain, (2) disease, (3) function, and (4) esthetics. Combined with new mobile and other technologies, such streamlined self-report measures hold promise for the rapid advancement of the measurement of oral health (Lee et al., 2013; Lee et al., 2014).

Psychosocial Impact of Oral Health

Psychosocial impact is another promising surrogate for direct disease surveillance—one that can be employed by lay health workers and may be highly salient to policymakers and publics. One sophisticated measure of the psychosocial impact of oral health problems is the Oral Health Impact Profile (OHIP) (Allen, McMillan, & Locker, 2001; Slade, 1997; Slade & Spencer, 1994). The long (49-item) version of the questionnaire provides separate scores for seven domains (e.g., functional limitation, pain, psychological discomfort) based on Likert responses to questions such as "Have you had to interrupt meals because of problems with your teeth, mouth or **dentures**?" A 14-item short version of the OHIP is also available to assess pain, function, psychosocial, and esthetic issues with one score (Slade, 1997).

Measurement Issue Overview

Oral health promotion efforts are hampered because methods to measure tooth decay and gum disease remain inconsistent, lack clinical relevance among dental and other health professionals, and are assessed independently of other health conditions. The lack of precise, consistently used measures of oral health and disease makes it very difficult to evaluate the benefits of oral health promotion. Also, as of this writing, there is still no consensus on how to conduct routine surveillance of the most prevalent oral diseases, and finding measures that are simple enough to be understood by policy makers and the public remains a challenge. However, proxy measures have emerged and additional progress is on the horizon. One very promising development is that WHO has updated its measures of oral health diseases and conditions to be compatible with chronic disease surveillance systems (Petersen & Baez, 2013). Widespread use of such a comprehensive approach to measurement should facilitate interprofessional training and the kinds of common risk factor oral health promotion strategies that are discussed below.

Oral Health Promotion Strategies

Common oral conditions (i.e., tooth decay, gum disease, and some oral cancers) are largely preventable. Reflecting the reality that there are risk factors for oral disease at several system levels, efforts to promote oral health have been undertaken at various levels. Strategies have ranged from instructions from dentistry personnel to patients about how to maintain proper oral hygiene, to multi-issue, community-based interventions and alterations of the physical environment. Interventions at each of these levels are described in the following sections. With adequate resources and political will, interventions from the various levels could be integrated into coordinated programs that approach the scale of the oral health problem and respond to the specific needs of each country.

Promotion to Individuals

Tooth decay and gum disease can be prevented at the earliest stages by removing the gingival plaque that accumulates on teeth after eating. At the individual level, oral health promotion primarily has been teaching patients that removing the plaque is important and showing them how to remove it. Dental professionals (dentists, dental hygienists, dental assistants, dental therapists, dental lab workers, dental industry personnel, and dental education specialists) have served as the primary channel for conveying oral hygiene information to individuals to date; these specialized personnel can tailor their advice closely to a patient's needs and circumstances. However, enthusiasm for oral health promotion at the individual level must be curbed by a severe staffing shortfall; there are far too few dentistry personnel to deliver face-to-face oral health messages to every person who needs to hear these messages (see Figure 16.2).

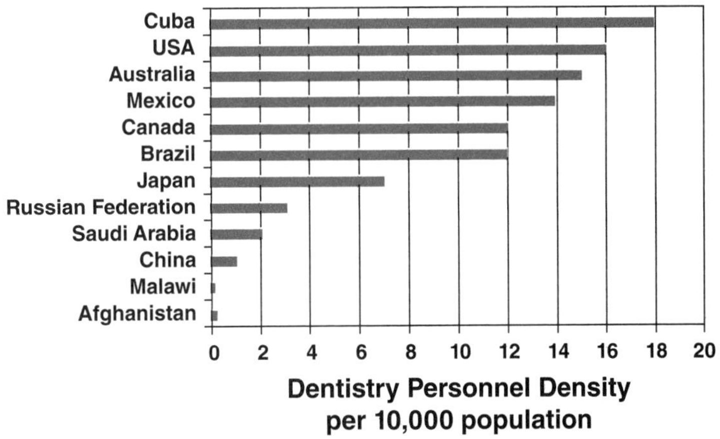

Figure 16.2 Dentistry Personnel Density by Selected Countries

Source: WHO World Health Statistics (2010).

The basic oral hygiene techniques that are normally recommended to individual patients are outlined in the next section of this chapter, but the reader should be cautioned that the finer points of these self-care procedures require a stronger evidence base. In fact, a lack of evidence for many specific self-care and professionally administered prevention practices hampers effective oral health promotion (Twetman, 2015). And even if everyone had sufficient motivation to perform the recommended cleaning behaviors consistently, they would not all have access to the simple manufactured tools recommended for removing dental plaque.

Tooth Brushing

Tooth brushing has been shown to be an effective means of removing dental plaque, and thus is key to preventing periodontal disease and caries (Slot & Van der Weijden, 2015; Van der Weijden & Slot, 2015). There is less agreement about how long and how often tooth brushing should be performed by adults and (or for) children. Wide variations in recommendations about tooth-brushing techniques have been reported among dental professionals, toothpaste companies, and dental associations. Many kinds of toothbrushes and toothpastes are available globally, with no consensus on the best one to use for cleaning teeth and gums, although a Cochrane collaboration review did confirm that fluoride toothpaste was beneficial (Walsh et al., 2010). Brushing at the gumline in a circular motion has been promoted as more effective than other techniques to remove plaque, but, like other oral issues, has been incompletely studied, or studied for only short periods of time (i.e., three or six months) (Wainwright & Sheiham, 2014). Manual toothbrushes have been shown to be less effective than powered toothbrushes with rotational oscillation, but the cost of powered brushes is a barrier to most of the world's population (Marinho et al., 2003, Yaacob et al., 2014). Incorporation of oral care into longer term clinical trials of treatments for non-oral diseases may be useful in answering questions about oral care for healthy and diseased individuals.

Chewing Sticks

In studies among Asians and Africans, Meswak, a chewing stick from the plant *Salvadora persica,* has been shown to be as effective as a toothbrush in removing bacteria associated with caries and periodontal disease (Al-Otaibi et al., 2003; Chaurasia et al., 2013; Sukkarwalla et al., 2013). Meswak contains fluoride, calcium, and phosphorus, which are minerals that are important in reversing early tooth decay. Meswak may be available to refugees, migrants and individuals in isolated areas when toothbrushes and fluoride toothpaste are not; recommending regular use of this low-cost oral hygiene tool is a promising strategy in low-resource settings.

Dental Floss and Interdental Devices

Cleaning between the gums with **floss** can remove dental plaque mechanically. However, a meta-analytical assessment of flossing instruction failed to show benefits on gingival bleeding and inflammation, or on tooth plaque

(Berchier et al., 2008; Sambunjak et al., 2011). There is a need for longitudinal cohort assessments with evaluation points beyond three to six months to confirm the benefits of using floss and interdental picks and brushes at various frequencies, as well as the benefits of instruction in the use of interdental devices.

Antimicrobial Mouth Rinses and Toothpastes

Oral rinsing with antimicrobial mouth rinses may add to the effectiveness of an oral hygiene regimen intended to manage periodontal disease and caries (Boyle, Koechlin, & Autier, 2014; Van Strydonck et al., 2012). Slots (2012) has described povidone-iodine and sodium hypochlorite as first-choice antiseptics in managing periodontal diseases because these are inexpensive and readily available throughout most of the globe. Evaluation of antimicrobial toothpastes and stannous fluoride toothpastes has been hampered by short study durations and measurement issues (Sälzer et al., 2015).

Messages From Dental Care Providers

Individual-level health promotion permits substantial tailoring of oral hygiene instructions to a patient's particular circumstances (e.g., telling a new mother to start wiping the baby's mouth soon after birth with clean, soft cloths, and to brush her child's teeth with fluoride toothpaste beginning after the first tooth erupts at around age one, or advising gum chewers to buy gum containing xylitol rather than sugars) (Boyle et al., 2014; Isokangas et al., 2000). But oral health promotion at the individual level can and should go beyond tailored oral hygiene messages to encourage protective behaviors with multiple health benefits, such as avoiding excessive sugar consumption and tobacco use, and being vaccinated for HPV before sexual initiation (FDI, 2012). The appropriateness of other recommendations would depend on the context (e.g., advice to drink fluoridated tap water if the safety of the municipal water supply were monitored, or to support an initiative to fluoridate a local water supply in an upcoming election).

Motivational Interviewing and Health Coaching

Advice from health professionals is often insufficient to change behavior, and this is a major concern when patients are at high risk of serious negative health outcomes. Two techniques for working with high risk patients require more of a health professional's time than didactic message delivery demands, but they engage the patient more actively, have worked in other health areas, and may hold promise for oral health.

The first technique, *motivational interviewing*, is brief, patient guided, reflective counseling that focuses on the patient's personal reasons for resisting a behavior change. In a systematic review of 16 studies, motivational interviewing was found to be superior to education on at least one oral health outcome, but gains were often short-lived (Gao et al., 2014). More recently, in a Thai study of elderly Type 2 diabetics, several oral hygiene and other protective behaviors were sustained for at least six months after motivational interviews in a dental setting (Saengtipbovorn & Taneepanichskul, 2015).

The second technique, *health coaching*, is an intervention that starts with setting specific goals and creating an action plan, and then continues with encouragement, feedback, and problem-solving geared to goal attainment. There are often a few sessions involved, but some can be distance based. A growing body of evidence underpins claims of the relative effectiveness of coaching compared with simple education; for example, an experiment in Istanbul, Turkey among Type 2 diabetics showed relatively positive effects for coaching on both oral health and blood sugar outcomes (Cinar, Oktay, & Schou, 2014).

Interprofessional Education

The current dentist-based model of care is inadequate to meet global need, as illustrated by the WHO statistic that 30% of people 65 to 74 years old worldwide have no natural teeth (WHO, Fact Sheet 2012, http://www.who.int/mediacentre/factsheets/fs318/en/). Prevailing structures for education in the dental professions and the other health professions are relatively siloed, exacerbating the staffing shortfall in oral health care. One way to begin to address the shortfall is to train other health professionals to perform basic oral health promotion procedures. Such interprofessional education (IPE) brings together practitioners or students from two or more professions to learn from and with each other to improve health outcomes (IPEC, 2011). Regional meetings of an IPE Coalition in the United States already include oral health on their agendas, just as they include medicine, pharmacy, nursing, and other health disciplines. Haber et al. (2015) recommended developing interprofessional curricula for health professional training globally, and oral health content now has been included successfully in training for physician assistants and pediatric nurses (Langelier, Glicken, & Surdu, 2015; Spurr, Bally & Ogenchuk, 2015). In addition, non-dental-health professionals such as oncology nurses are starting to feel comfortable including oral exams in routine head and neck examinations (Perry et al., 2015).

The Common Risk Factor Approach

Another way oral health could extend the reach of its promotional efforts is to leverage parallel resources for addressing common causes of oral diseases (e.g., tobacco use) (Sheiham & Watt, 2000). Because it could extend care and is potentially cost-effective, a common risk factor approach has been endorsed by WHO and the Institute of Medicine (IOM, 2011a; Sheiham & Watt, 2000; Watt & Petersen, 2012). The need for such an approach is especially acute in developing countries that have severe staffing shortages throughout the health professions and a paucity of dental training centers (Hescot, 2013).

Some of the major areas of commonality and intersection between oral health and other health issues and services are presented in Figure 16.3. This is only a rough conceptual road map for common risk factor strategies, but some progress has been made in understanding by fleshing out the particulars of

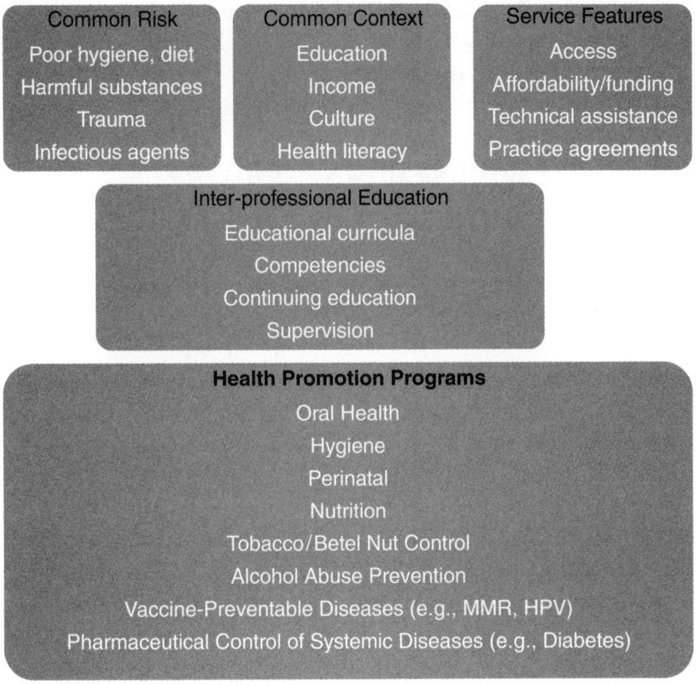

Figure 16.3 Points of Intersection in a Common Risk Factor Approach to Oral Health Promotion

such relationships (US DHHS, 2001). Natural allies for further progress might be health promotion efforts that emphasize common risk factors (e.g., poor diet), and/or promote similar behaviors (e.g., handwashing).

The complexity of interprofessional education should not be underestimated. Health care providers (e.g., dentists, oral hygienists, physicians, nurses, pharmacists, and public health professionals) need to be taught not only what to say, but how to say it, if they are to communicate effectively with at-risk patients about beneficial oral health practices (Kreps & Neuhauser, 2013; Neumann et al., 2010). Simply conveying factual information is not enough when vulnerable groups face socioeconomic challenges, limited levels of education and health literacy, and other cultural and societal barriers to acting on the information (Kreps, 2006). Effective communication rests on audience analysis research that identifies knowledge gaps and the best ways to fill them (Kreps, 2012a). Communication tools such as targeted websites, pamphlets, books, videos, and materials in other media formats are needed to supplement oral interpersonal communication between consumers and providers about oral health (Kreps, 2012a). Finally, interpersonal oral health messages from health providers may be most effective when they are supplemented and reinforced by interventions at the group, institutional, and mass media levels. There is a great need for culturally sensitive, evidence-based interventions that can (a) influence oral health behavior, (b) sustain positive changes, and (c) be implemented within families, religious institutions, schools, businesses, community centers, libraries, and other organizations (Kreps, 2012b). Effective and cost-effective mass media campaigns are also needed.

Promotion to Families and Caregivers

Preschool children around the world suffer from high rates of early childhood caries (ECC). For example, one study found that a quarter of children between three and five years of age in French-speaking Switzerland were burdened with this disease (Baggio et al., 2015). ECC has serious sequelae, ranging from pain and sleep problems to physical and mental growth deficits, but it can be prevented if the child's teeth are brushed with fluoride toothpaste, sugary foods and beverages are avoided (especially late at night), and there are dental visits during early childhood.

Mothers and others who care for young children often face service access barriers to obtaining oral health care for the children. Psychosocial factors also can limit oral health service utilization. For example, a caregiver's oral health beliefs, norms of caregiver responsibility, and personal dental experiences have been shown to predict a child's receipt of oral health care services (Kelly et al., 2005; Trubey, Moore, & Chestnutt, 2015; Zimmerman, 1988). Controlled studies of brief dyadic (mother/child) and small group interventions, some of them explicitly theory-based, have been conducted in Iran (Makvandi et al., 2015), Brazil (Azevedo et al., 2015), and Australia (Gibbs et al., 2015). Gains for treatment group caregivers vs. control group caregivers have been observed on outcomes including dental knowledge, attitudes, and brushing the children's teeth, as well as physiological measures of the children's oral health status.

Reliable self-report outcome measures for young children (Tsakos et al., 2012) and adults, in addition to new mobile and other media technologies for intervention delivery, should speed advancements in family-level interventions (Lee et al., 2013). The new media tools can either stand alone or be active parental components of preschool-based interventions in the form of homework that caregivers complete with children, or games that children and caregivers play (Cooper et al., 2013). See Box 16.3 for some examples of new media tools.

Role of Schools

Schools can educate children and parents about dental hygiene, develop positive habits in children, and serve as points of universal access to children over 5 for screening, product distribution and preventive treatment. The need is clear: Nepalese children ages 5–12 knew about oral hygiene but not about the benefits of fluoride and, as is the case for children around the world, their diet and the type of oral care professionals they visited when experiencing mouth pain were heavily influenced by social determinants of health (Knevel et al., 2008). Many adolescents consume foods with high sugar content, and a study in Ghana showed that urban adolescents were more than twice as likely as

BOX 16.3 NEW MEDIA TOOLS FOR PARENTS AND CAREGIVERS

- MySmileBuddy is a mobile tablet app(lication) for health workers that helps assess risk for early childhood caries and helps clients make healthy food choices. https://mysmilebuddy.ccnmtl.columbia.edu/accounts/login/?next=/
- Attack! of the S. Mutans is a 3-D interactive video game that teaches children over age eight. Users learn how to eliminate acid byproducts of bacteria after they devour sugars and carbohydrates using a Wii-type gun, guided through the mouth by Dentisha, their virtual assistant. http://www.attackofthemutans.com/
- Mouth Healthy Website and Materials offer advice on how to brush and floss teeth and two-minute cartoons and music videos to use during tooth brushing for children of varying ages. http://www.2min2x.org/kids-healthy-mouths
- Brush DJ is a free tooth-brushing app for smartphones and tablets. Approved by the British National Health Service, this free app allows users to customize music from a playlist to use while brushing teeth and sends reminders about daily brushing and dental visits. http://www.brushdj.com/
- Text2Floss is a free brushing and flossing application with daily text reminders for iPhones and iPads. https://itunes.apple.com/us/app/text2floss/id797806327?mt=8
- myCAMBRA is an evidence-based caries management-by-risk-assessment app for dentists and patients who work together to design a customized plan. http://www.mycambra.com/

their rural counterparts to consume sugared cakes or biscuits (Blay, Astrom, & Haugejorden, 2000). Patterns of childhood risk must be studied within countries in order to inform school-based and other interventions mounted in particular cultural contexts.

There have been successful attempts to intervene at the school level in many places. In Thailand, an experimental program that involved supervised tooth brushing with fluoride toothpaste during school hours resulted in significantly less caries than was observed in control schools (Petersen et al., 2015). In Sweden, placing dental hygienists in secondary schools part time for two years resulted in greater knowledge about oral health and fewer enamel caries in teens, although their attitudes toward tobacco were unaffected (Hedman, Gabre, & Birkhed, 2015).

It appears that school-based programs that combine education with services have the greatest impact on dental outcomes, as well as on other medical outcomes. As a case in point, a successful tooth brushing/hand washing/deworming program in schools in the Philippines shows great promise for replication in other countries (Monse et al., 2013). Successful programs are also likely to require the cooperation of governments and families, in addition to cooperation from school personnel, who may themselves need instruction in such topics as how to deal with traumatic dental injuries in children (Bayrak, Tunc & Sari, 2012).

Promotion of Oral Health in the Workplace

Workplace oral health promotion programs are few, but companies are well positioned to encourage workers to brush, floss, and rinse at work and at home, and job sites can require use of procedures and devices that minimize risk of oral trauma. Some large workplaces (e.g., a BMW plant in the United States) have begun to offer dental services on site to reduce absenteeism. A six-week workplace-based oral health awareness campaign in England showed improvements in two clinical measures of periodontal disease (gingival bleeding and pocket probing depth) in intervention workers compared with wait-list controls (Fishwick, Ashley, & Wilson, 1998). Workplace clinics are also good locations for studying associations between risk factors and dental outcomes among generally healthy adults. The cost-effectiveness of workplace oral health promotion has been studied, but mainly with a focus on insurance costs, not oral health status impact. However, one worksite in Japan that offered brief dental exams, minor scaling, and hygiene instruction found the program cost-effective for workers who used the facility a moderate amount (Ichihashi, Muto, & Shibuya, 2007). In the future, workplaces may present an opportunity to assess and address common risk factors for oral health problems and conditions such as obesity.

Use of Mass Media

To promote good oral health, concerted efforts are needed to educate the public at large about identifying and avoiding oral health risks. Through mass media, preferably in combination with interpersonal communication, members of the public can be encouraged to engage in behaviors that promote good oral health. Media campaigns can target not only behaviors but also their presumed cognitive prerequisites, several of which could be considered aspects of oral health literacy (see Table 16.1).

Some mass media campaigns that were designed to promote oral health have been evaluated and reported in the scientific literature; see Table 16.1 for examples. Again, as is likely with interventions at other system levels, mass media campaigns that are consciously and explicitly based in formal behavior change theory may be most likely to bring about behavior change among members of their intended audiences. Table 16.1 omits "Mouth Healthy," a major recent effort to encourage low income children in the United States to brush their teeth twice a day for two minutes, because its outcome evaluation is still underway. Regardless of the findings of the evaluation, however, the campaign is noteworthy for forging a collaboration between the US Advertising Council, the Dental Trade Alliance, the American Dental Association, and over 30 business and corporate entities, all of whom contributed substantial in-kind campaign resources.

Table 16.1 Mass Media Campaigns Promoting Oral Health

Author (date published)	Audience(s)	Component(s)	Outcome(s)
Friel et al. (2002)	Children 7–12 in Ireland	Messages in a TV show, Smile of the Year contest, dental nurse visiting schools	Use of recommended amount of toothpaste and brushing for three minutes among those exposed to TV, more gains from exposure to nurse
Gholami et al. (2014)	Adults 18–50 in Iran	TV	Significant increases in periodontal knowledge among those recalling campaign exposure
Jedele & Ismail (2010) Ismail et al. (2012)	African American adults in urban Detroit, Michigan, USA	Radio, billboards, newspaper ads, education sessions, a toll-free hotline, mailings to physicians and dentists	Providers reported higher patient campaign exposure and requests for oral cancer screening in intervention area; most hotline callers prompted by radio ad; campaign cost considered "relatively low"
Logan et al. (2013)	African American adults in four rural counties, Florida, USA	Posters, handheld fans, brochures, large car magnets	Compared to those in three control counties, intervention county participants had greater campaign exposure, oral cancer concern, and oral cancer screening intentions
Rise & Sogaard (1988)	Adults in Norway	Booklet with five simple rules, radio, TV, illustrated newspaper articles	Knowledge about tooth brushing to prevent periodontal disease increased
Saleh et al. (2012)	Adults in Malaysia	TV	Awareness of oral cancer increased, effects were uneven across ethnicities
Schou (1987)	Mothers and five- to seven-year-old children in Scotland	TV, radio, magazine ads, brochures with active aspects sent home from school	Brochures remembered best, magazine ads remembered least

As discussed in previous sections of this chapter, oral health attitudes and behaviors can be difficult to influence, in part because they are culturally ingrained and/or habitual. In addition, those individuals at greatest risk for serious oral health problems often have limited access to relevant, timely, accurate health information (Dutta & Kreps, 2013), and they may face educational and economic barriers that make it difficult for them to understand and/or respond to health messages in the media (Kreps, 2006). Achieving the adoption and maintenance of health behaviors among at-risk populations demands highly strategic behavioral change communication (Neuhauser & Kreps, 2010). Oral health campaigns should be tailored for specific audiences; to be culturally sensitive and appropriate, the communication must be informed by pre-campaign audience research that identifies the best communication channels, messages, and sources to use (Kreps, 2012a, 2012b; Kreps & Sparks, 2008). Campaigns should also involve community stakeholders from the earliest planning stages (see Box 16.4).

BOX 16.4 CASE STUDY: A U.S. TOOTHBRUSHING CAMPAIGN FOR LOW LITERACY MOTHERS OF CHILDREN UNDER SIX

In 2007, following the death of a 12 year old African-American child from untreated tooth decay that spread to his brain, the U.S. state of Maryland (MD) created a dental action committee, convened by the governor. It created a bold action plan to address oral health literacy and education, prevention of injuries and oral infectious diseases, and other policy issues that affect the oral health of the state's children. Much of the plan was carried out, but compared to their white and more affluent counterparts, children from racial and ethnic minority groups and low-income families continued to have poorer oral health. A 2012 MD study on oral health literacy found that parents from low income and minority groups were not aware that oral health is important to overall health, and did not know how to prevent dental disease. Another telephone survey of oral health literacy among 400 low-income individuals identified knowledge gaps regarding toothbrushing.

The MD Oral Health Learning Alliance (MOHLA) was formed to plan a toothbrushing campaign. MOHLA was composed of key state partners, such as the library association, Head Start and the Women Infants and Children's nutrition supplementation program, Medicaid, an online repository of clinical treatment records, the pediatric and medical associations, the University of MD (UMD) dental hygiene and dentist training programs, and other advocates.

With $800,000 of state grant funding from the CDC, MOHLA worked with the dental office of the state health department in a strategic alliance to develop an oral health literacy campaign. Message testing was conducted with focus groups of pregnant and parenting minority women, the intended campaign audience, and gatekeepers. The *Healthy Teeth, Healthy Kids* campaign was launched in March 2012. It stressed the safety and importance of daily use of fluoridated toothpaste to prevent decay for children under 6, and receipt of clinical oral health services by pregnant women. Components of the campaign included a website, www.HealthyTeethHealthyKids.org, TV and radio spots, bus shelter ads, brochures, posters, and a hotline. Nine million paid media media impressions were estimated, and dozens of news media stories resulted in added campaign exposure. Over 20,000 kits of toothbrushes and 54,000 brochures were distributed. Public libraries hosted oral health story times that reached more than 4,000 low-income children and caregivers. Supported largely by additional funding from the UMD's Horowitz Center for Health Literacy, a Spanish language version of the campaign was launched via radio and with community outreach, generating several million additional estimated impressions.

The campaign evaluation had very limited funding, and was forced to rely on Google Analytics and other free measures of usage of online campaign materials. There were no data available to tie campaign exposure to rates of caries progression or dental visits. A follow-up oral health literacy survey did show a modest increase in oral health knowledge over the 6-month campaign period. However, a simultaneous media campaign developed by the national Ad Council also promoted toothbrushing, so knowledge gains could not be attributed to Healthy Teeth, Healthy Kids with confidence. The Spanish language version of the campaign had no funding for evaluation.

But knowledge and awareness of important oral health recommendations did increase among community and nurse outreach workers, and campaign planners believe that a number of important lessons were learned about this kind of campaign:

1. Small group reinforcement of campaign messages was important.
2. Good small group leaders knew when to get out of the way to permit collective action.
3. Using volunteers brings in new partners, creating opportunities to improve and expand existing programs.
4. Mentorship is needed to nurture the development of oral health champions and leaders.
5. Partners from racially and ethnically diverse groups can help develop materials that are culturally appropriate for diverse groups and more likely to bring about behavior change in such groups.

Mass media messaging becomes very complicated and may not be suitable when the intended audience is persons with co-morbidities, such as patients with cardiovascular disease and stroke. And even in the United States, there is still no clear consensus on effective oral health messages for the elderly (McGrath, Zhang, & Lo, 2009). However, the promotion of good oral hygiene is part of the general guidelines for patient care following stroke. (British Society of Gerodontology, 2010). The elderly, and those patients after stroke, or other co-morbidities that may limit toothbrushing ability, are unlikely to be harmed by effective oral hygiene promotion. (Marinho et al., 2003).

Limiting the advertising of harmful substances such as tobacco products, especially ads aimed at adolescents and other vulnerable populations, could be thought of as the other side of the mass media coin. Serious consideration should be given to ad regulation as a prevention strategy, given the impact of tobacco on overall health and oral health. In South Africa, Panama, and Mongolia, having seen more than two sources of tobacco advertisements was associated with significantly increased odds of cigarette smoking among adolescents (Agaku et al., 2013). Similarly, advertising of e-cigarettes has been shown to affect curiosity and trial of e-cigarettes in the United States (Villanti et al., 2015). However, the extent of nicotine product advertising varies widely around the world. Furthermore, in low and middle income countries, a regulator's task is complicated by the likelihood that tobacco products are positively depicted or actively promoted in videos that were produced abroad and then distributed in-country through unauthorized channels.

Community Environment

Concrete aspects of the environment can (a) be beyond the control of individual audience members, (b) limit an individual's ability to respond to health messages, and/or (c) increase the risk of oral health problems. Laws and treaties have a central role to play in ensuring that the environment is conducive to oral health.

Adequate fluoride intake guards against caries, and water fluoridation advocacy has been the most visible environmental-level activity in oral health promotion by far. Delivering fluoride through a water or food supply delivers benefits evenly throughout the population, regardless of social determinants, helping to ensure health equity.

Furthermore, like many environmental interventions, municipal fluoridation avoids the need for voluntary message compliance, which entails near-inevitable lapses. China and Korea have instituted school-based fluoride rinse programs, but in Beijing, a lack of knowledge of the benefits of fluoridated self-care products on the parts of schools and parents was a barrier to program effectiveness (Liu et al., 2007). Continuous, costly messages about the benefits of fluoridated self-care products were required to sustain their use.

It should be noted, however, that overexposure to fluoride carries its own risks. Fluoride is now added to many dental products and is also found in foods (e.g., farmed fish or irrigated produce from areas that fluoridate water). The amount of fluoride that should be added to a water supply will vary by locale, and should reflect intake of fluoride from other sources. Total fluoride intake from non-local food sources has not yet been adequately assessed for populations.

A safe supply of potable water is a prerequisite for fluoridation, making the strategy irrelevant in many places in the world. That said, the personnel, equipment, and supply costs for keeping fluoride levels in water at or below 0.7 parts per million are reasonably affordable. Malaysia, Singpore, Hong Kong, Ho Chi Minh City in Vietnam, and Brunei have all fluoridated their municipal water supplies. Alternative strategies can work where central water supplies are limited; salt fluoridation has been used in Laos and Cambodia, and milk fluoridation in Thailand. Finally, new technologies that allow users to test community water virtually should allow for expansion of water fluoridation methods to smaller water systems.

Direct political action has been undertaken to convince policymakers and voters to support fluoridation policies. For water fluoridation advocacy to be effective, it is critically important to understand the governance structures that have local jurisdiction in the matter. In the state of New South Wales, Australia, for example, the decision to fluoridate water rests with local government councils, not a state body. Advocates in New South Wales localities distributed fluoridation information packets with data on oral health disparities between fluoridated and unfluoridated communities. They also conducted outreach to local policymakers, arranged to have public health leaders make presentations in local public forums, and built rapport with local media spokespeople who could help build citizen support; consequently, they won the local votes required for fluoridation (Sivaneswaran, 2012). In Calgary, Canada (population 820,000), an expert panel reviewed water fluoridation as a public policy. Although four of the five members agreed that there was insufficient evidence to warrant substantial changes to the existing policy to fluoridate, the city's Standing Policy Committee on Operations and Environment recommended a vote on water fluoridation in the next election. The ballot addition was endorsed by the city council. Local oral health advocates formed a fluoride education committee with three strategies: building partnerships, educating health professionals, and educating the public. Despite anti-fluoridation activities, the eventual vote was 55% in favor of continuing fluoridation (Pryce and Smorang, 1999). In Pinellas County, Florida in the United States, an anti-fluoridation threat was countered by electing new officials who understood the benefits of community water fluoridation (Easley, 1985; Easley, 2013). However, Portland Oregon defeated fluoridation efforts by 60%. (http://www.huffingtonpost.com/2013/05/22/portland-oregon-fluoridation_n_3320388.html accessed 11/30/15).

Protecting the environment from contamination by the materials used in dental supplies and appliances is also a policy matter. Environmental concerns about dental amalgam, which sometimes contains mercury, are being raised in the negotiation of an international treaty to limit environmental sources of mercury (Minamata Convention on Mercury, http://www.mercuryconvention.org/). There is also ongoing consideration of limiting compounds used in some dental **sealants** and tooth-colored tooth restoration filling materials (e.g., Bis-As and Bis-Phenol GMAs by the European Food Safety Authority (http://www.efsa.europa.eu/).

Oral Health Promotion Policy

Since the early 2000s, WHO, regional health policy groups, professional associations, and industry councils have published policy documents that address oral health issues (see Table 16.2). Key among these is the 60th World Health Assembly's Call to Action for Oral Health Promotion (WHO, 2007), which covered health topics comprehensively and situated oral health within a larger public health context. Some of the other documents addressed oral health only by implication; these documents called for healthy public policies, intersectoral action for health, and health in all policies (Collins & Koplan, 2009; WHO, 1986; WHO/HiAP, 2014). Still other documents dealt with particular oral health topics in detail; examples include the Crete Declaration from the 10th Congress on Oral Cancer (2005) that was endorsed by representatives from 57

Table 16.2 Oral Health Policy Milestones

Date	Sponsor	Document
2007	WHO	Call to Action for Oral Health Promotion
2009	WHO	Global Conference on Health Promotion—toward integration of oral health Nairobi, Kenya—Call to Action
2010	WHO	Framework for action on interprofessional education and collaborative practice
2011	United Nations	Political Declaration on the Prevention and Control of Noncommunicable Diseases

countries, and the WHO paper on oral health measurement (Petersen & Baez, 2013). Policy analysts typically have treated oral health as a noncommunicable disease (UN, 2011), although some common oral diseases can be communicable (Caufield & Griffen, 2000; Kohler, Andreen, & Jonsson, 1984). The potential impact of oral health on issues such as immigration or global security has not been explored from a policy perspective.

Overall, this body of policy literature has raised the visibility of the burden of disease attributable to oral diseases and conditions. The documents have condemned the disparities in oral health; identified needs for local capacity building, early intervention, risk assessment, disease monitoring, and service integration; and provided guidance on best practices in surveillance, care, and prevention.

The International Association for Dental Research (IADR) organizes the World Congress on Preventive Dentistry (WCPD) in collaboration with the WHO every four years with a focus on community interventions to promote oral health. The 2005, 2009 and 2013 WCPD's resulted in the Liverpool, Phuket and Budapest Declarations, respectively (Clarkson et al., 2010; WHO, y, 2005a; Mossey & Petersen, 2014). Unfortunately, resource constraints, both fiscal and human, continue to block implementation of the policies at the scale of the global oral health problem.

Shared Risk Factors

Oral health has risk factors in common with a number of other aspects of health. Thus, integrating oral health into efforts to promote health in areas with shared risk factors has been strongly endorsed in policy documents. However, in practice, the systematic incorporation of oral health into other health promotion activities can be overwhelming. One simplifying framework lists sample steps that health educators and policy-makers can take to help reach shared objectives; Table 16.3 illustrates the use of this framework as it pertains to tobacco content.

In addition to a list of activities, integrated health promotion also requires a time-consuming process of building coalitions and partnerships prior to launching collaborative activities. Trust must be established, a shared understanding of the problems being addressed must be developed, roles and responsibilities must be negotiated, and the commitment of stakeholders and frontline staff must be gained (IOM, 2011b; Rosenberg et al., 2010; Rosenthal et al., 2006). Policymakers should allocate resources to this coalition-building process; early attention to group dynamics will help build success into coordinated clinical, educational, and environmental change activities (Frenk et al., 2010).

Within the ranks of public health, consensus and coordination may be facilitated by including oral health into public health core competencies. The new competencies (which should focus more on prevention than treatment) should lead, in turn, to more support for oral health in intraprofessional education curricula (Gilbert, Yan, & Hoffman, 2010).

More inclusive partnerships across multiple sectors, both public and private, will be necessary if the common risk factor approach is to be

Table 16.3 Tobacco Control Strategies for Educators and Policymakers

WHO-Recommended Objectives	Sample Activities for Educators	Sample Activities for Policymakers
Use of the most updated state-of-the-science and knowledge	Collate available literature and surveys Use and distribute WHO Basic Oral Health Methods	Communicate tobacco-related deaths and tobacco use Develop policy briefing sessions
Assistance to countries in risk behavior analysis and surveillance	Conduct population-based and individual risk assessments Conduct risk surveillance	Develop policies and laws to foster reductions in behavioral risks
Translation of knowledge into action programs in countries and communities	Promote oral health in schools and workplaces	Restrict tobacco advertising on television, radio & public facilities by laws/regulations Provide incentives for having health insurance (developed countries) Ban sale of tobacco to minors
Use of evaluation, monitoring, and surveillance	Develop goals for educational programs Develop common surveillance with tobacco-control programs	Assure common funding to include oral health promotion in tobacco-control activities

Source: Adapted from Petersen (2003b).

employed at the full scale of the oral health problem. There have been calls for patient-centered partnerships (Scarlett, 2007; Rosenman, 2013). Others have encouraged corporate partnerships (Riggs et al., 2008), novel community/academic partnerships (Dugdill & Pine, 2011; Pine & Dugdill, 2011; Yamalik, 2011), or partnerships around relatively rare, but compelling oral diseases, such as Noma, a devastating, facially disfiguring disease that affects malnourished children (Barmes, 1999).

The FDI World Dental Federation, the international professional organization for the dental profession, has permitted use of its global infrastructure of regional and country dental associations to support and advocate for oral health integration efforts (FDI, 2012). Country-wide advocacy is necessary to spur the adoption and implementation of integrated service policies; individual private practitioners may have little incentive to broaden their topical portfolios or spend time planning service integration. Partnerships on oral diseases may also be extended to tropical diseases (Liese et al., 2010).

Building the Knowledge Base

There is a real dearth of monitoring of rates of oral health diseases and conditions, individual oral hygiene and risk behaviors, and the receipt of dental services. Policymakers should provide support for addressing these information gaps, so that health promotion strategies can be prioritized, tracked and evaluated. While dedicated data collection systems evolve, the Health Impact Assessment process (endorsed by Collins & Koplan, 2009) may help to guide policy. The aim of this process is to use multiple existing data sources, including stakeholder input, and a variety of analytical methods to anticipate the effects of a proposed policy, plan, program, or project on the health of a population or group. Health Impact Assessments are being initiated in several places around the world, and the state of California in the United States has already used the process to inform decisions about incorporating oral health into other health programs. Finally, multisector impact assessments are needed to predict the utility and cost-effectiveness of including oral health-relevant components in policies about food, public water supplies, soft drinks, concessions in schools and sports venues and tobacco point-of-sale purchases (IOM, 2011a and b).

An ambitious Global Oral Health Inequalities Research Agenda has been generated by the IADR (Challacombe et al., 2011; Marmot & Bell, 2011; Sgan-Cohen et al., 2013). It prioritizes the social determinants of health, prevention over treatment, developing better oral health measures, and the delivery of preventive services in cultural context.

Preventing Oral Health Problems in Children Avoids Deferred Costs

Based on United Nations Development Program estimates, health care costs attributable to oral health care are significant, ranging from 3.5% in the United States and several other developed nations to 12.5% in Israel in 2012. Controlling these costs over the long term is much more feasible if strategies focus more on children than on adults. Schools are the natural place to reach children with oral health promotion programs.

Southern Asia has been at the forefront of school-based oral health promotion. Three regional documents, the Toyko, Ayutthaya, and Bangalore declarations (first Asian conference, 2001; second Asian conference, 2003; Commonwealth Association for Mentally Handicapped and Developmental Disabilities [CAMHADD], 2005), have led to community support for working together to promote oral health in schools, and have sped information sharing about model services.

Rights to Oral and Reproductive Health

The Nairobi Call to Action (Kwan & Petersen, 2010) framed oral health as a human right, just as reproductive/sexual health had been framed 15 years earlier (UN International Conference on Population and Development, 1994), but policy analysis has yet to trace the complex web of linkages between these two rights domains. There is a sound empirical link between HPV infection and oral cancer (Gillison et al., 2008; Gillison et al., 2012; DeSouza G et al., 2007; DeSouza et al., 2009; Chaturvedi et al., 2011), but HPV vaccines have not been approved for the prevention of this kind of cancer. Intimate oral contact can transmit HPV and is a known transmission vector for a variety of other STDS including HIV. Integrating rights-based perspectives on reproductive/sexual health and oral health could increase advocacy, research attention, and resources for these interrelated health concerns.

Summary

Oral disease is ubiquitous. Stigmatizing oral disease, along with accompanying pain and inability to smile, chew or speak, ensures that oral needs are not met among populations and individuals around the globe. Like many other health conditions, poverty and other social determinants of health pose greater risks for oral diseases among all populations. Because the oral health workforce is inadequate to address the problems of oral diseases, health and community workers, including public health nurses, are beginning to be trained in oral health to address this problem. However, a shift is needed in the cultural context of oral health so that potential workers can find and maintain employment and students learning about health understand their roles in reversibility of early oral disease. Culturally, oral health may be viewed as an individual responsibility, but when oral health needs go unmet, the consequences escalate and the costs are shifted onto the health system and society. The responsibility for oral health should be shared among individuals, dentists, other clinicians, policymakers (insurers and politicians) who fund health care, schools, public health workers, and private sector employers.

The risk factors for common oral diseases are present months to years before disease onset, and much oral disease can be prevented. Common oral disease like tooth decay and gingivitis can be reversed at early stages by medical management. Risk reduction should start early in life, and health promotion efforts should skew resource allocation towards young children and pregnant women.

Because of the severe worldwide shortage of dental professionals, population-based communication efforts and environmental interventions are more likely than individual-level efforts to have a substantial impact on global oral health. Communication strategies should be theory-based and culturally competent, and they should offer specific information about how to reduce risks. Messages about the overconsumption of fermentable carbohydrates, especially processed sugar (e.g., in the form of sugary beverages) are badly needed because of the great risk these foods pose for tooth decay. Messages warning about the risks of tobacco and betel nut use, heavy consumption of alcohol, and oral sex are also very important because of the risks these behaviors pose for mouth and throat cancers and for other diseases. Future health promotion efforts should evaluate effectiveness of oral health promotion based on outcomes measures for oral health and health over a longer period of time than 3 or 6 months. Scientific consensus among health professionals is needed for measuring common oral diseases and successful reversal of oral diseases at the earliest stages with the same intensity currently reserved for treatment.

Screening can detect oral cancers at an early and often treatable stage, but oral cancer screening is underutilized. Screening does not have to remain the sole purview of dentistry professionals—interprofessional education should include this aspect of oral health promotion in its curricula.

Finally, the science on the connection between general health and oral health is still emerging, but increasingly it shows that oral diseases can adversely affect other parts of the body and vice versa. There is a strong argument for including oral health promotion in other health promotion activities.

KEY TERMS

1. **Attachment loss:** The gum or gingival attachment around a tooth is lost and is a key indicator of gum disease
2. **Caries:** Tooth decay that can cause a hole in the tooth from by-products of a biofilm comprised of various bacteria, including *S. mutan*, *S. sobrinus*, and *Lactobacillus*
3. **Cavity:** A hole in the tooth caused by caries
4. **CFUs:** Colony-forming units, a measurement of the number of bacteria in a sample size
5. **DMFT:** Developed as a dental epidemiologic screening tool in the 1930s, this outmoded measure has been used by dental epidemiologists for calculating tooth decay in individuals and populations. This is a measure for D (decayed), M (missing), Filled (F), teeth (T). DMFT is a crude measure because it lacks sensitivity and specificity to determine the cause of M (missing). Teeth may be missing due to caries, natural exfoliation or removal because of trauma or orthodontic reasons. It is difficult to use with mixed dentition of adolescents. Inconsistent with the biology of caries, DMFT is not used to measure and track reversal of early enamel decay.
6. **Decay:** Another word for dental caries or cavities that cause a hole in the tooth
7. **Deciduous teeth:** The 20 teeth that erupt in young children, generally before age 3; also called primary teeth and are usually exfoliated by age 12
8. **Dentin:** The middle layer of a tooth
9. **Dentures:** False teeth that replace natural teeth
10. **Dry mouth:** See **Xerostomia**
11. **Enamel:** The hard calcified outer portion of the tooth, covered by dentin on the top part or crown of a tooth
12. **Epigenetic factors:** External, environmental factors that switch genes on and off
13. **Esthetics:** Appearance
14. **Floss:** A tape or tiny ribbon that removes trapped food and bacteria from between teeth that cannot be removed by tooth brushing alone.
15. **Fluoride:** One of the minerals, along with calcium and acidulated phosphate, that strengthens the crystalline structure of the outer portion of teeth or the enamel
16. **Fluoride varnish:** Fluoride liquid painted onto the teeth to harden teeth, usually primary teeth before the age of 3
17. **Gingiva:** The gums in the area around the teeth. Also **Gingival:** refer to the gum or pocket of soft tissue around a tooth.

18. **Gingivitis:** An inflammatory condition related to gum tissue that can cause redness or bleeding
19. **Gum disease:** Also called periodontal disease
20. **Human Immunodeficiency Virus** (HIV)**:** A type of virus that weakens the immune system
21. **Human Papillomavirus** (HPV)**:** A type of virus; certain HPVs such as 16, 18, 19 are linked to both cervical and oral cancers
22. **ICCMS-International Caries Classification and Management System:** A system of clinical, epidemiologic and treatment classification for managing tooth decay based on the biology of tooth decay and evidence for managing tooth decay. This also includes medical management of tooth decay, that is without use of surgical interventions, to preserve tooth structure. See also Figure 16.1 and reference Pitts et al. (2014).
23. **Mouth rinse:** Oral rinse to reduce the bacterial by-products or change the pH to reduce susceptibility to caries and gingivitis
24. **Oral Cancer or Oral Carcinoma:** Cancer of the mouth, perioral areas, including oropharyngeal cancers. Also referred to as **Carcinoma, a common form of cancer which is often not detected early**. This type of cancer is rapidly increasing due to oral sexual transmission of HPV in many Western countries. See also Human Papillomavirus. In Asia, use of betel nut and tobacco has resulted in the highest oral cancer rates in the world
25. **Oral hygiene:** Cleaning of the teeth that includes brushing of the teeth, tongue, and dentures
26. **Periodontal disease:** A term used to describe various types of gum disease that affect gingival health and the attachment of the tooth to bone
27. **Periodontitis:** A severe form of gum disease that can lead to tooth loss
28. **Permanent teeth:** Teeth that begin to erupt at about age 6 or 7, replacing the primary teeth; total up to 32 teeth for adults
29. **Plaque:** The accumulation of bacteria and by-products into a soft film that is often visible on the teeth
30. **Pulp:** Blood supply and nerves for the tooth
31. **Sealant:** A plastic coating for the crevices on molar teeth
32. **Tooth decay:** A hole in the tooth caused by the acid in plaque; more common name—cavity
33. **Xerostomia:** Dry mouth caused by decreased salivary secretions

REVIEW QUESTIONS

1. What is the key problem related to oral health?
2. What are three barriers to implementation of oral health promotion?
3. What risk factors do oral diseases have in common with other public health issues, such as vaccine-preventable diseases, diabetes management, or cardiovascular disease?
4. What are some strategies for population-based prevention of oral disease?
5. How can population-based oral health promotion activities be translated to and engage influential individuals outside of the oral health professions?
6. What key translation strategies for implementing population-based oral health promotion activities are promoted to engage peers and the public?

References

Agaku, I. T., Adisa, A. O., Akinyamoju, A. O., & Agboola, S. O. (2013). A cross-country comparison of the prevalence of exposure to tobacco advertisements among adolescents aged 13–15 years in 20 low and middle income countries. *Tobacco Induced Diseases, 11*(1), 11.

Alexander, D., Clarkson, J., Buchanan, R., Chadwick, G., Chesters, R., Drisko, C. L., ... & Warren, P. (2008). Exploring opportunities for collaboration between the corporate sector and the dental education community. *European Journal of Dental Education, 12*(Suppl 1), 64–73.

Allen, P. F., McMillan, A. S., & Locker, D. (2001). An assessment of sensitivity to change of the Oral Health Impact Profile in a clinical trial. *Community Dentistry and Oral Epidemiology, 29*(3), 175–182.

Al-Otaibi, M., Al-Harthy, M., Söder, B., Gustafsson, A., & Angmar-Månsson, B. (2003). Comparative effect of chewing sticks and toothbrushing on plaque removal and gingival health. *Oral Health and Preventative Dentistry, 1,* 301–307.

American Academy of Pediatrics Section on Pediatric Dentistry and Oral Health. (2014). Maintaining and Improving the Oral Health of Young Children. *Pediatrics, 134*(6), 1224–1229. doi: 10.1542/peds.2014-2984

American College of Obstetricians and Gynecologists. (2013). Oral health care during pregnancy and through the lifespan. Committee Opinion No. 569. *Obstetrics and Gynecology, 122,* 417–422.

Azevedo, M. S., Romano, A. R., Correa, M. B., Santos Ida, S., & Cenci. M. S. (2015). Evaluation of a feasible educational intervention in preventing early childhood caries. *Brazilian Oral Research, 29,* 1–8. Epub July 3. doi: 10.1590/1807-3107BOR-2015.vol29.0089

Baggio, S., Abarca, M., Bodenmann, P., Gehri, M., & Madrid, C. (2015). Early childhood caries in Switzerland: A marker of social inequalities. *BioMedCentral Oral Health, 22*(15), 82.

Baginska, J., Rodakowska, E., Wilczynska-Borawska, M., & Jamiolkowski, J. (2013). Index of clinical consequences of untreated dental caries (PUFA) in primary dentition of children from north-east Poland. *Advances in Medical Sciences, 21*, 1–6.

Barmes, D. E. (1999). A global view of oral diseases: Today and tomorrow. *Community Dentistry and Oral Epidemiology, 27*(1), 2–7.

Bartold, P. M., & Van Dyke, T. E. (2013). Periodontitis: A host-mediated disruption of microbial homeostasis. Unlearning learned concepts. *Periodontology 2000, 62*(1), 203–217.

Bayrak, S., Tunc, E.S., & Sari, E. (2012). Evaluation of elementary school teachers' knowledge and attitudes about immediate emergency management of traumatic dental injuries. *Oral Health & Preventive Dentistry, 10*(3), 253–258.

Berchier, C. E., Slot, D. E., Haps, S. & Van der Weijden, G. A. (2008). The efficacy of dental floss in addition to a toothbrush on plaque and parameters of gingival inflammation: A systematic review. *International Journal of Dental Hygiene, 6*(4), 265–279.

Blay, D., Åstrøm, A., & Haugejorden, O. (2000). Oral hygiene and sugar consumption among urban and rural adolescents in Ghana. *Community Dentistry and Oral Epidemiology, 28*(6), 443–450.

Boyle, P., Koechlin, A. & Autier, P. (2014). Mouthwash use and the prevention of plaque, gingivitis and caries. *Oral Diseases, 20*(Suppl. 1), 1–68.

Braveman, P. Gruskin, S. (2003). Poverty, equity, human rights and health. *Bulletin of the World Health Organization. 81* (7): 539–45.

Braveman, P. A., Egerter, S. A., & Mockenhaupt, R. E. (2011). Broadening the focus: The need to address the social determinants of health. *American Journal of Preventive Medicine. 40*(1S1): S4–S18.

British Society of Gerodontology. (2010). Guidelines for the Oral Healthcare of Stroke Survivors. Accessed http://www.gerodontology.com/content/uploads/2014/10/stroke_guidelines.pdf. on 3/1/15.

Caufield, P. W., & Griffen, A. L. (2000). Dental caries: An infectious and transmissible disease. *Pediatric Clinics of North America, 47*(5), 1001–1019.

Chaffee, B. W., Gansky, S. A., Weintraub, J. A., Featherstone, J. D. B., & Ramos-Gomez, F. J. (2014). Maternal oral bacterial levels predict early childhood caries development. *Journal of Dental Research, 93*(3), 238–244.

Challacombe, S. J., Chidzonga, M., Glick, M., Hodgson, T., Magalhães, M., Shiboski, C., … Naidoo, S. (2011). Global oral health inequalities: Oral infections—challenges and approaches. *Advances in Dental Research 23*, 227–236.

Chaturvedi, A. K., Anderson, W. F, Lortet-Tieulent, J., Curado, M. P., Ferlay, J., Franceschi, S., … Gillison, M. L. (2013). Worldwide trends in incidence rates for oral cavity and oropharyngeal cancers. *Journal of Clinical Oncology, 31*(36), 4550–4559.

Chaturvedi, A. K, Engels, E. A, Pfeiffer, R. M, Hernandez, B. Y., Xiao, W., Kim, E., … Gillison, M. L. (2011). HPV and rising oropharyngeal cancer incidence in the United States. *Journal of Clinical Oncology, 29*(32), 4294–4301.

Chaurasia, A., Patil, R., & Nagar, A. (2013). Miswak in oral cavity: An update. *Journal of Oral Biology and Craniofacial Research, 3*(2), 98–101.

Cinar, A. B., Oktay, I., & Schou, L. (2014). "Smile healthy to your diabetes": Health coaching-based intervention for oral health and diabetes management. *Clinical Oral Investigations, 18*(7):1793–801.

Clarkson, J., Watt, R. J., Rugg-Gunn, A. J., Pitiphat, W., Ettinger, R. L., Horowitz, A. M., … Shin, S. C. (2010). Proceedings: 9th World Congress on Preventive Dentistry (WCPD): Community participation and global alliances for lifelong oral health for all. Phuket, Thailand, September 7–10, 2009. *Advances in Dental Research, 22,* 2. Online version. doi: 101177/00203451 0368736.

Collins, J., & Koplan, J.P. (2009). Health impact assessment: A step toward health in all policies. *Journal of American Medical Association, 302*(3), 315–317. Erratum in: (2009). *Journal of American Medical Association, 302*(9), 946.

Cooper, A. M., O'Malley, L. A., Elison, S. N., Armstrong, R., Burnside, G., Adair, P., … Pine, C. (2013). Primary school-based behavioural interventions for preventing caries. *Cochrane Database Systematic Review, 5,* CD009378.

Corby, P. M., Lyons-Weiler, L., Bretz, B. A., Hart, T. C., Aas, J. A., Boumenna, T., … Paster, B. J. (2005). Microbial risk indicators of early childhood caries. *Journal of Clinical Microbiology, 43*(11), 5753–5759.

Dangi, J., Kinnunen, T. H., & Zavras, A. I. (2012). Challenges in global improvement of oral cancer outcomes: Findings from rural northern India. *Tobacco Induced Diseases, 10*(1), 5. doi:10.1186/1617-9625-10-5

da Silva, O.M., & Eiselé, J. L. (2012). FDI Global Caries Initiative phase 2: Preparing the profession for change. *International Dental Journal, 62*(4), 167–168.

DeSouza, G., et al. (2007). Case control study of human papillomavirus and oropharyngeal cancer. *New England Journal of Medicine, 356,* 1944–1956.

DeSouza, G., Agrawal, Y., Halpern, J., Bodison, S., Gillison, M. L. (2009). Oral sexual behaviors associated with prevalent oral human papillomavirus infection. *Journal of Infectious Diseases, 199*(9), 1263–1269.

Dewhirst, F. E., Chen, T., Izard, J., Paster, B. J., Tanner, A. C R., Yu, W-H., … Wade, W. G. (2010). The human oral microbiome. *Journal of Bacteriology, 192*(19), 5002–5017.

Divaris, K. J., Lee, Y., Baker, A. D., & Vann, W. F. (2012). Caregivers' oral health literacy and their young children's oral health-related quality of life. *Acta Odontologia Scandanavia, 70*(5), 390–397.

Domejean, S., White, J. M., & Featherstone, J. D. B. (2011). Validation of the CDA CAMBRA Caries Risk Assessment: A six year retrospective study. *Journal of the California Dental Association, 30*(10), 709–715.

Dorian, R. M. (2002). Biofilms: Microbial life on surfaces. *Emerging Infectious Diseases, 8*(9), 881–890.

Dugdill, L., & Pine, C. M. (2011). Evaluation of international case studies within "Live.Learn.Laugh": A unique global public–private partnership to promote oral health. *International Dental Journal, 61*(Suppl. 2), 22–29.

Dutta, M. J., & Kreps, G. L. (Eds). (2013). *Reducing health disparities: Communication interventions.* New York, NY: Peter Lang Publishers.

Easley, M. W. (1985). The new antifluoridationists: Who are they and how do they operate? *Journal of Public Health Dentistry, 45*(3), 133–141.

Easley, M. W. (2013). Dental Public Health Practice: Political Science Meets Health Science—A Case Study in Successful Technology Transfer, *Journal of Theory and Practice in Dental Public Health, 1*(1), 15–18.

Eke, P. I., Page, R. C., Wei, L., Thornton-Evans, G., & Genco, R.J. (2012). Update of the case definitions for population-based surveillance of periodontitis. *Journal of Periodontology, 83,* 1449–1454.

El-Zaemey, S., Schüz, J., & Leon, M. E. (2015). Qat chewing and risk of potentially malignant and malignant oral disorders: A systematic review. *International Journal of Occupational and Environmental Medicine, 6*(3), 129–143.

European Food Safety Authority. (2015). Retrieved from http://www.efsa.europa.eu/

Featherstone, J. (2000). The science and practice of caries prevention. *Journal of the American Dental Association, 31*(7), 887–899.

Federation Dentaire International (FDI). (2012). *Oral health and the United Nations Political Declaration on Non-Communicable Diseases: A guide to advocacy.* Geneva: World Health Organization.

Fishwick, M. R., Ashley, F. P., & Wilson, R. F. (1998). Can a workplace preventive programme affect periodontal health? *British Dental Journal, 184*(6), 290–293.

Frenk, J., Chen, L., Bhutta, Z. A., Cohen J., Crisp N., Evans T., … Zurayk, H. (2010). The Interprofessional Education Collaborative, an Independent Commission of the Lancet. Health professionals for a new century: Transforming education to strengthen health systems in an interdependent world. *Lancet, 376*(9756), 1923–1958.

Frenk, J. (2010) The global health system: Strengthening national health systems as the next step for global progress. *PLoS Med. 7*(1), e1000089.

Friel, S., Hope, A., Kelleher, C., Comer, S., & Sadlier, D. (2002). Impact evaluation of an oral health intervention amongst primary school children in Ireland. *Health Promotion International, 17*(2), 119–126.

Gao, X., Lo, E. C., Kot, S. C., & Chan, K. C. (2014). Motivational interviewing in improving oral health: A systematic review of randomized controlled trials. *Journal of Periodontology, 85*(3), 426–437.

Gholami, M., Pakdaman, A., Montazeri, A., Jafari, A., & Virtanen, J. I. (2014). Assessment of periodontal knowledge following a mass media oral health promotion campaign: A population-based study. *BioMedCentral Oral Health, 5*(14), 31.

Giannobile, W. V., Braun, T. M., Caplis, A. K., Doucette-Stamm, L., Duff, G. W., & Kornman, K. S. (2013). A personalized medicine approach combining gene biomarkers with conventional risk factors to stratify populations may be useful in resource allocation for preventive dentistry. *Journal of Dental Research, 92*(8), 694–701.

Gibbs, L., Waters, E., Christian, B., Gold, L., Young, D., de Silva, A., ... Moore, L. (2015). Teeth Tales: A community-based child oral health promotion trial with migrant families in Australia. *British Medical Journal Open, 5*(6), e007321. doi: 10.1136/bmjopen-2014-007321

Gift, H. C., Reisine, S. T., & Larach, D. C. (1992). The social impact of dental problems and visits. *American Journal of Public Health 82*(12), 1663–1668.

Gilbert, J. H., Yan, J., & Hoffman, S. J. (2010). A WHO report: Framework for action on interprofessional education and collaborative practice. *Journal of Allied Health, 39*(Suppl. 1), 196–197.

Gillison, M. L., Gypsyamber, D., Westra, W., Sugar, E., Xiao, W., Begum, S., & Viscidi, R. (2008). Distinct risk factors HPV-16 positive and HPV-negative head and neck cancers. *Journal of the National Cancer Institute, 100*(6), 402–420.

Gillison, M.L, Broutian, T., Pickard, R.K., Tong, Z.Y., Xiao, W., Kahle, L., ... Chaturvedi, A. K. (2012). Prevalence of oral HPV infection in the United States, 2009–2010. *Journal of the American Medical Association, 307*(7), 693–703.

Glick, M., & Fisher, J. (2012). A new model for caries classification and management. FDI World Dental Federation Caries management. *Journal of the American Dental Association, 143*, 546–551.

Graetz, C., Schützhold, S., Plaumann, A., Kahl, M., Springer, C., Sälzer, S., ... Schwendicke, F. (2015). Prognostic factors for the loss of molars–an 18-years retrospective cohort study. *Journal of Clinical Periodontology, 42*(10), 942–950.

Gupta, P. C., & Ray, C. S. (2004). Epidemiology of betel quid usage. *Annals of the Academy of Medicine, Singapore, 33*(Suppl.), 31S–36S.

Haber, J., Hartnett, E., Allen, K., Hallas, D., Dorsen, C., Lange-Kessler, J., ... Wholihan, D. (2015). Putting the mouth back in the head: HEENT to HEENOT. *American Journal of Public Health, 105*(3), 437–441.

Haffajee, A. D., Roberts, C., Murray, L., Veiga, N., Martin, L., Teles, R. P., ... Socransky, S. S. (2009). Effect of herbal, essential oil, and chlorhexidine mouthrinses on the composition of the subgingival microbiota and clinical periodontal parameters. *Journal of Clinical Dentistry, 20*(7), 211–217.

Haffajee, A. D., Torresyap, G., & Socransky, S. S. (2007). Clinical changes following four different periodontal therapies for the treatment of chronic periodontitis: One-year results. *Journal of Clinical Periodontology, 34*, 243–253.

Hedman, E., Gabre, P., & Birkhed, D. (2015). Dental hygienists working in schools: A two-year oral health intervention programme in Swedish secondary schools. *Oral Health and Preventive Dentistry, 13*(2), 177–188.

Hennequin-Hoenderdos, N., Slot, D. E., & Van der Weijden, G. A. (2015). The incidence of complications associated with lip and/or tongue piercings: A systematic review. *International Journal of Dental Hygiene*. [Epub ahead of print]. doi: 10.1111/idh.12118

Hescot, P. (2013). FDI: From research representation to action. *Indian Journal of Dental Research, 24*(5), 525–526.

Ichihashi, T., Muto, T., & Shibuya, K. (2007). Cost-benefit analysis of a worksite oral-health promotion program. *Industrial Health, 45*(1), 32–36.

Institute of Medicine (IOM) and National Research Council. (2009). *Local government actions to prevent childhood obesity*. Washington, DC: National Academies Press.

Institute of Medicine. (2011a). *Advancing oral health in America*. Washington, DC: National Academies Press.

Institute of Medicine. (2011b). *For the public's health: Revitalizing law and policy to meet new challenges*. Washington, DC: National Academies Press.

Institute of Medicine. (2012). *Improving access to oral health for vulnerable and disadvantaged populations*. Washington, DC: National Academies Press.

Institute of Medicine. (2013). *Oral health literacy*. Workshop summary. Washington, DC: National Academies Press.

Interprofessional Education Collaborative Expert Panel (IPEC). (2011). *Core competencies for interprofessional collaborative practice: Report of an expert panel*. Washington, DC: Author. Retrieved from https://ipecollaborative.org/

Ismail, A. I., Jedele, J. M., Lim, S., & Tellez, M. (2012). A Marketing Campaign to Promote Screening for Oral Cancer. *Journal of American Dental Association, 143*(9), e57–66.

Ismail, A. I., Sohn, W., Tellez, M., Amaya, A., Sen, A., Hasson, H., & Pitts, N.B. (2007). The International Caries Detection and Assessment System (ICDAS): An integrated system for measuring dental caries. *Community Dentistry and Oral Epidemiology, 35*(3), 170–178.

Isokangas, P., Söderling, E., Pienihakkinen, K., & Alanen, P. (2000). Occurrence of dental decay in children after maternal consumption of xylitol chewing gum, a follow-up from 0 to 5 years of age. *Journal of Dental Research, 79*(11), 1885–1889.

Jedele, J. M., & Ismail, A. I. (2010). Evaluation of a multifaceted social marketing campaign to increase awareness of and screening for oral cancer in African Americans. *Community Dentistry and Oral Epidemiology, 38*(4), 371–382.

Keels, M. A., Hale, K. J., Thomas, H. F., Davis, M. J., Czerepak, C. S., & Weiss, P. A. (2008). Preventive oral health intervention for pediatricians. *Pediatrics, 122*(6), 1387–1394.

Kelly, S .E., Binkley, C. J., Neace, W. P., & Gale, B. S.(2005). Barriers to care-seeking for children's oral health among low-income caregivers. *American Journal of Public Health, 95*(8), 1345–1351.

Knevel, R. J., Neupane, S., Shressta, B., & de Mey, L. (2008). Buddhi Bangara project on oral health promotion: A 3- to 5-year collaborative programme combining support, education and research in Nepal. *International Journal of Dental Hygiene, 6*(4), 337–346.

Kohler, B., Andreen, I., & Jonsson, B. (1984). The effect of caries-preventive measures in mothers on dental caries and the oral presence of the bacteria

Streptococcus mutans and *lactobacilli* in their children. *Archives of Oral Biology, 29,* 879–883.

Kreps, G. L. (2006). Communication and racial inequities in health care. *American Behavioral Scientist, 49*(6), 760–774.

Kreps, G. L. (2012a). Strategic communication for cancer prevention and control: Reaching and influencing vulnerable audiences. In A. Georgakilas (Ed.), *Cancer prevention* (pp. 375–388). Intech Publishers, available at: http://www.intechopen.com/books/cancer-prevention-from-mechanisms-to-translational-benefits/strategic-communication-for-cancer-prevention-and-control-reaching-and-influencing-vulnerable-audiences.

Kreps, G. L. (2012b). Translating health communication research into practice: The importance of implementing and sustaining evidence-based health communication interventions. *Atlantic Communication Journal, 20,* 5–15.

Kreps, G. L., & Neuhauser, L. (2013). Artificial intelligence and immediacy: Designing health communication to personally engage consumers and providers. *Patient Education and Counseling, 92,* 205–210.

Kreps, G. L., & Sparks, L. (2008). Meeting the health literacy needs of vulnerable populations. *Patient Education and Counseling, 71*(3), 328–332.

Kwan, S., & Petersen P. (2010). Oral health: Equity and social determinants. In E. Blas & A. S. Kurup (Eds.), *Equity, social determinants and public health programmes* (pp. 159–175). Geneva: World Health Organization.

Langelier, M. H., Glicken, A. D., & Surdu, S. (2015). Adoption of oral health curriculum by physician assistant education programs in 2014. *Journal of Physician Assisted Education, 26*(2), 60–69.

Lee, J. Y., Divaris, K., Baker, A. D., Rozier, G., & Vann, W. F. (2012). The relationship of oral health literacy and self-efficacy with oral health status and dental neglect. *American Journal of Public Health, 102*(5), 923–929.

Lee, P. H., McGrath, C. P., Kong, A. Y., & Lam, T. H. (2013). Self-report poor oral health and chronic diseases: The Hong Kong FAMILY Project. *Community Dentistry and Oral Epidemiology, 41*(5), 451–458.

Lee, P. H., McGrath, C. P., Kong, A. Y, & Lam, T. H. (2014). Self-reported oral health and quality of life: A latent growth curve analysis. *International Journal of Behavioral Medicine, 21*(2), 358–363.

Liese, B., Rosenberg, M., & Schratz, A. (2010). Programmes, partnerships, and governance for elimination and control of neglected tropical diseases. *Lancet, 375*(9708), 67–76.

Liu, M., Zhu, L., Zhang, B., & Petersen, P. E. (2007). Changing use and knowledge of fluoride toothpaste by schoolchildren, parents and schoolteachers in Beijing, China. *International Dental Journal, 57*(3), 187–194.

Logan, H. L., Shepperd, J. A., Pomery, E., Guo, Y., Muller, K. E., Dodd, V. J., Riley, J. L. III. (2013). Increasing screening intentions for oral and pharyngeal cancer. *Annals of Behavioral Medicine, 46*(1), 96–106.

Loria, D., Barrios, E., & Zanetti, R. (2009). Cancer and yerba mate consumption: A review of possible associations. *Revista Panamericana de Salud Pública, 25*(6), 530–539.

Lu, H. X., Wong, M. C., Lo, E. C., & McGrath, C. (2011). Trends in oral health from childhood to early adulthood: A life course approach. *Community Dentistry and Oral Epidemioliology, 239*(4), 352–360.

Makvandi, Z., Karimi-Shahanjarini, A., Faradmal, J., & Bashirian, S. (2015). Evaluation of an oral health intervention among mothers of young children: A clustered randomized trial. *Journal of Research in Health Sciences, 5*(2), 88–93.

Marcenes, W., Kassebaum, N. J., Bernabe, E., Flaxman, A., Naghavi, M., Lopez, A., Murray C. J. (2013).Global burden of oral conditions in 1990–2010: A systematic analysis. *Journal of Dental Research, 92*, 592–597.

Marinho, V. C. C., Higgins, J. P. T., Logan, S., & Sheiham, A. (2003). Fluoride toothpastes for preventing dental caries in children and adolescents. *Cochrane Database of Systematic Reviews, 1*, CD002278. doi: 10.1002/14651858.CD00227

Marmot, M., & Bell, R. (2011). Social determinants and dental health. *Advances in Dental Research, 23*(2), 201–206.

McGrath, C., Zhang, W., & Lo, E. C. (2009). A review of the effectiveness of oral health promotion activities among elderly people. *Gerodontology, 26*(2), 85–96.

Miller, E., Lee, J. Y., DeWalt, D. A., & Vann, W. F. (2010). Impact of caregiver literacy on children's oral health outcomes. *Pediatrics, 126*, 107–114.

Minamata Convention on Mercury. (2013). Retrieved from http://www.mercuryconvention.org/

Monse, B., Benzian, H., Naliponguit, E., Belizario, V., Schratz, A., & van Palenstein Helderman, W. (2013). The Fit for School Health Outcome Study: A longitudinal survey to assess health impacts of an integrated school health programme in the Philippines. *BioMedCentral Public Health, 21*(13), 256.

Monse, B., Naliponguit, E., Belizario, V., Benzian, H., & van Helderman, W. P. (2010). Essential health care package for children: The "Fit for School" program in the Philippines. *International Dental Journal, 60*, 85–93.

Mossey, P. A., & Petersen, P. E. (2014). Budapest Declaration. *Journal of Dental Research Clinical Research Supplement, July, 2014*. DOI: 10.1177/0022034514527972.

National Cancer Institute, National Institutes of Health, National Program of Cancer Registries (NPCR), CDC/NCCDPHP; Surveillance, Epidemiology, and End Results Program (SEER). (2015). *Oral cancer fact sheet*. Retrieved from http://seer.cancer.gov/statfacts/html/oralcav.html. Accessed 10/3/2015

Neuhauser, L., & Kreps, G. L. (2010). E-health communication and behavior change: Promise and performance. *Social Semiotics, 20*(1), 7–24.

Neumann, M., Edelhäuser, F., Kreps, G. L., Scheffer, C., Lutz, G., Tauschel, D., & Visser, A. (2010). Can patient–provider interaction increase the effectiveness of medical treatments or even substitute them? A methodological reflection of the specific effect of the provider. *Patient Education and Counseling, 80*, 307–314.

Page, R. C., & Eke, P. I. (2007). Case definitions for use in population-based surveillance of periodontitis. *Journal of Periodontology, 78*(Suppl. 7), 1387–1399.

Perry, A. D., Iida, H., Patton, L. L., & Wilder, R. S. (2015). Knowledge, perceived ability and practice behaviors regarding oral health among pediatric hematology and oncology nurses. *Journal of Dental Hygiene, 89*(4), 219–28.

Petersen, P. E. (2003a). Global framework convention on tobacco control: The implications for oral health. *Community Dental Health, 20,* 137–138.

Petersen, P. E. (2003b). Tobacco and oral health: The role of the World Health Organization. *Oral Health and Preventive Dentistry, 1,* 309–315.

Petersen, P. E. (2005). Strengthening the prevention of oral cancer: The WHO perspective. *Community Dentistry and Oral Epidemiology, 33,* 397–399.

Petersen, P. E. (2009). Oral cancer prevention and control: The approach of WHO. *Oral Oncology, 45,* 454–460.

Petersen, P. E. (2010). Improvement of global oral health: The leadership role of the World Health Organization. *Community Dental Health, 27,* 194–198.

Petersen, P. E., & Baehni, P. C. (2012). Periodontal health and global public health. *Periodontology 2000, 60*(1), 7–14.

Petersen, P.E. & Baez, R.J. (2013). *Oral health surveys: Basic Methods.* Geneva: World Health Organization.

Petersen, P. E., Hunsrisakhun, J., Thearmontree, A., Pithpornchaiyakul, S., Hintao, J., Jurgensen, N., & Ellwood, R. P. (2015). School-based intervention for improving the oral health of children in southern Thailand. *Community Dental Health, 32*(1), 44–50.

Petersen, P. E., & Kwan, S. (2011). Equity, social determinants and public health programmes: The case of oral health. *Community Dentistry and Oral Epidemiology, 39*(6), 481–487.

Petersen, P. E., & Yamamoto, T. (2005). Improving the oral health of older people: The approach of the WHO Global Oral Health Programme. *Community Dentistry and Oral Epidemiology, 33*(2), 81–92.

Pine, C. M., & Dugdill, L. (2011). Analysis of a unique global public–private partnership to promote oral health. *International Dental Journal, 61*(Suppl. 2), 11–21.

Pitts, N. G., Ismail, A. I., Martignon, S., Ekstrand, K., Douglas, G. V. A., Longbottom, C., and 49 participating authors. (2014). *ICCMS Guide for Practitioners and Educators.* London: Kings College.

Pryce, C., & Smorang, J. (1999). Continuing water fluoridation in the city of Calgary, Alberta, 1997–1998. *Journal of the Canadian Dental Association, 65*(2), 101–104.

Rise, J., & Sögaard, A. J. (1988). Effect of a mass media periodontal campaign upon preventive knowledge and behavior in Norway. *Community Dentistry and Oral Epidemiology, 16*(1), 1–4.

Roseman, D., Osborne-Stafsnes, J., Amy, C. H., Boslaugh, S., Slate-Miller, K. (2013). Early lessons from four 'aligning forces for quality' communities bolster the case for patient-centered care. *Health Affairs* (Millwood), *32*(2), 232–241. doi: 10.1377/hlthaff.2012.1085

Rosenberg, M. L., Hayes, E., McIntyre, M., & Neill, M. W. (2010). *Real collaboration: What it takes for global health to succeed*. Berkeley: California/Milbank Books on Health and the Public.

Rosenthal, M. P., Butterfoss, F. D., Doctor, L. J., Gilmore, L. A., Krieger, J. W., Meurer, J. R., Vega, I. (2006) The coalition process at work: Building care coordination models to control chronic disease. *Health Promotion Practice, 7*(Suppl. 2), 117S–126S.

Saengtipbovorn, S., & Taneepanichskul, S. (2015). Effectiveness of lifestyle change plus dental care program in improving glycemic and periodontal status in aging patients with diabetes: A cluster, randomized, controlled trial. *Journal of Periodontology, 86*(4), 507–515.

Saleh A., Yang Y. H., Wan Abd Ghani, W. M., Abdullah, N., Doss, J. G., Navonil, R., ... Cheong, S. C. (2012). Promoting oral cancer awareness and early detection using a mass media approach. *Asian Pacific Journal of Cancer Prevention, 13*(4), 1217–1224.

Sälzer, S., Slot, D. E., Dörfer, C. E., &Van der Weijden, G. A. (2015). Comparison of Triclosan and Stannous Fluoride. *International Journal of Dental Hygiene, 13*(1):1–17. doi: 10.1111/idh.12072. Epub June 19, 2014.

Sambunjak, D., Nickerson, J. W., Poklepovic, T., Johnson, T. M., Imai, P., Tugwell, P., & Worthington, H. V. (2011). Flossing for the management of periodontal diseases and dental caries in adults [CD-ROM]. *Cochrane Database of Systematic Reviews, 12*, CD008829.

Scarlett, M. (2007). A clarion call for partnership and communication for better patient health. *Cranio, 25*(1), 1.

Schou, L. (1987). Use of mass-media and active involvement in a national dental health campaign in Scotland. *Community Dentistry and Oral Epidemiology, 15*(1), 14–18.

Sgan-Cohen, H. D., Evans, R. W., Whelton, H., Villena, R. S., MacDougall, M., Williams, D. M. (2013). IADR-GOHIRA Steering and Task Groups. IADR Global Oral Health Inequalities Research Agenda (IADR-GOHIRA(R)): a call to action. *Journal of Dental Research, 92*(3), 209–211. doi: 10.1177/0022034512475214. Epub 2013 Jan 24.

Sheiham, A., & Watt, R. (2000). The common risk factor approach: A rational basis for promoting oral health. *Community Dentistry and Oral Epidemiology, 28*, 399–406.

Sivaneswaran, S. (2012). The revival of water fluoridation in the state of New South Wales, Australia, in the 21st century. *Community Dentistry and Oral Epidemiology, 40*(Suppl. 2), 65–70.

Slade, G. D. (1997). Derivation and validation of a short-form oral health impact profile. *Community Dentistry and Oral Epidemiology, 25*(4), 284–290.

Slade, G.D., & Spencer, A. J. (1994). Development and evaluation of the Oral Health Impact Profile. *Community Dental Health, 11*(3), 437–441.

Slot, D. E., & Van der Weijden, F. A. (2015). Group A Initiator Paper Plaque control: Home remedies practiced in developing countries. *Journal of the International Academy of Periodontology, 17*(Suppl. 1), 4–15.

Slots, J. (2012). Low-cost periodontal therapy. *Periodontology 2000, 60*(1), 110–137.

Spurr, S., Bally, J., & Ogenchuk, M. (2015). Integrating oral health into pediatric nursing practice: Caring for kids where they live. *Journal for Specialists in Pediatric Nursing, 20*(2), 105–114.

Sukkarwalla, A., Ali, S. M., Lundberg, P., & Tanwir, F. (2013). Efficacy of miswak on oral pathogens. *Dental Research Journal (Isfahan), 10*, 314–320.

Tonetti, M. S., & Claffey, N. (2005). Advances in the progression of periodontitis and proposal of definitions of a periodontitis case and disease progression for use in risk factor research. Group C consensus report of the Fifth European Workshop in Periodontology. *Journal of Clinical Periodontology, 32*(Suppl. 6), 210–213.

Trubey, R. J., Moore, S. C., & Chestnutt, I. G. (2015). The association between parents' perceived social norms for toothbrushing and the frequency with which they report brushing their child's teeth. *Community Dental Health, 32*(2), 98–103.

Tsakos, G., Blair, Y. I., Yusuf, H., Wright, W., Watt, R. G., & Macpherson, L. M. (2012). Developing a new self-reported scale of oral health outcomes for 5-year-old children (SOHO-5). *Health Quality of Life Outcomes, 10*. doi: 10.1186/1477-7525-10-62. PubMed PMID: 22676710; PubMed Central PMCID: PMC3413607

Twetman, S. The evidence base for professional and self-care prevention. (2015). *BioMedCentral Oral Health*, (Suppl. 1), S4.

United Nations. (2011). *Political declaration on the prevention and control of non-communicable diseases*. General Assembly, 66th session. New York, accessed at: http://www.un.org/en/ga/president/65/issues/ncdiseases.shtml

United Nations (UN) International Conference on Population and Development. (1994). UN Programme of Action of the International Conference on Population and Development. Cairo, Egypt: adopted September 5–13, 1994.

US Department of Health and Human Services. (2000). *Oral Health in America: A report of the Surgeon General*. Rockville, MD: US Department of Health and Human Services, National Institute of Dental and Craniofacial Research, National Institutes of Health.

US Department of Health and Human Services, Healthy People 2020. (2010). *Oral health indicators, oropharyngeal cancer*. Washington, DC: Author. Retrieved from https://www.healthypeople.gov/2020/topics-objectives/topic/oral-health/objectives

Van der Weijden, F. A., & Slot, D. E. (2015). Efficacy of homecare regimens for mechanical plaque removal in managing gingivitis: A meta review. *Journal of Clinical Periodontology, 42*(Suppl. 16), S77–S91.

Van Dyke, T. E. (2011). Proresolving lipid mediators: Potential for prevention and treatment of periodontitis. *Journal of Clinical Periodontology, 38*(Suppl. 11), 119–125.

Vann, W. F., Lee, J. Y., & Devaris, K. J. (2010). Oral health literacy among female caregivers: Impact on oral health outcomes. *Journal of Dental Research, 89*(12), 1495–1500.

Van Strydonck, D. A., Slot, D. E., Van der Velden, U., & Van der Weijden, F. (2012). Effect of a chlorhexidine mouthrinse on plaque, gingival inflammation and staining in gingivitis patients: A systematic review. *Journal of Clinical Periodontology, 39*(11), 1042–1055.

Villanti, A. C, Rath, J. M, Williams, V. F, Pearson, J. L, Richardson, A., Abrams, D. B., ... Vallone, D. M. (2015). Impact of exposure to electronic cigarette advertising on susceptibility and trial of electronic cigarettes and cigarettes in US young adults: A randomized controlled trial. *Nicotine Tobacco Research*. [Epub ahead of print] doi: 10.1093/ntr/ntv235

Wainwright J, & Sheiham, A. (2014). An analysis of methods of toothbrushing recommended by dental associations, toothpaste and toothbrush companies and in dental texts. *British Dental Journal, 217*(3). doi:10.1038/sj.bdj.2014.651

Walsh, T., Worthington, H. V., Glenny, A. M., Appelbe, P., Marinho, V. C. & Shi, X. (2010). Fluoride toothpastes of different concentrations for preventing dental caries in children and adolescents [CD-ROM]. *Cochrane Database of Systematic Reviews, 1*, CD007868.

Warnakulasuriya, S. (2009). Causes of oral cancer: An appraisal of controversies. *British Dental Journal* [Online], *207*, 471–475. doi:10.1038/sj.bdj.2009.1009

Watt, R. G. & Petersen, R. G. (2012). Periodontal health through public health: The case for oral health promotion. *Periodontology 2000*, 60, 1147–1551.

World Health Organization. (1948). *Constitution of the World Health Organization*. Geneva: WHO Basic Documents.

World Health Organization. (1986). *The Ottawa Charter for Health Promotion*. First International Conference on Health Promotion, Ottawa, November 21.

World Health Organization. (2005a). *The Liverpool Declaration: Promoting oral health in the 21st century: A call for action*. Geneva: WHO.

World Health Organization. (2005b). *The Crete Declaration on Oral Cancer Prevention 2005: A commitment to action*. 10th International Congress on Oral Cancer. Island (Crete), Greece: World Health Organization. Retrieved from http://www.who.int/oral_health/media/orh_crete_declaration_april05.pdf?ua=117284871

World Health Organization. (2007). *Oral health: Action plan for promotion and integrated disease prevention*. Report by the Secretariat. Sixtieth World Health Assembly A 60/16. March 22.Provisional agenda item 12.9.

World Health Organization. (2009). The Seventh WHO Global Conference on Health Promotion: Towards integration of oral health (Nairobi, Kenya 2009). *Community Dental Health, 27*(Suppl. 1), 129–136.

World Health Organization. (2013). *Oral health surveys: Basic methods* (5th ed.). Geneva: Author.

World Health Organization. (2014). Health in all policies (HiAP) framework for country action. *Health Promotion International, 29*(Suppl. 1), 19–28.

World Health Organization. Oral Health. (2012). Fact Sheet Geneva: April 2012. Available at http://www.who.int.mediacentre/factsheets/fs318/en/). Accessed 12/7/15.

Yaacob, M., Worthington, H. V., Deacon, S. A., Deery, C., Walmsley, A. D., Robinson, P. G., Glenny A.-M.. (2014). Powered versus manual toothbrushing for oral health. *Cochrane Database of Systemic Reviews*. Oral Health Group. Issue 6, Art. No. CD002281. doi: 10.1002/14651858. CD 002281. pub3.

Yamalik, N., Mersel, A., Cavalle, E., & Margvelashvili, V. (2011). Collaboration between dental faculties and National Dental Associations (NDAs) within the World Dental Federation-European Regional Organization zone: An NDAs perspective. *International Dental Journal*, *61*(6), 307–313.

Yucek-Lindberg, T., & Bage, T. (2013). Inflammatory mediators in the pathogenesis of periodontitis. *Expert Reviews in Molecular Medicine*, *5*(15), e7. doi: 10.1017/erm.2013.8

Zimmerman, R. S. (1988). The dental appointment and patient behavior: Differences in patient and practitioner preferences, patient satisfaction, and adherence. *Medical Care*, *26*(4), 403–14.

CHAPTER 17

ADAPTATION AND IMPLEMENTATION OF PUBLIC HEALTH INNOVATIONS IN DEVELOPING COUNTRIES

Bonita Stanton, Xiaoming Li, and Linda Kaljee

Over the past decade, public health and health research institutions across the globe have focused resources at an unparalleled level on translating scientific breakthroughs into practice. This effort serves as the foundation for the National Institutes of Health (NIH) Roadmap Initiative (Zerhouni, 2006a and b), which seeks to move science through an ordered process of experimentation in a laboratory to a controlled clinical setting, to clinical and community practice. The Center for Disease Control's Prevention Synthesis Program (CDC, 2015a) seeks to identify effective behavioral interventions and its counterpart, the "Dissemination of Effective Behavioral Interventions (DEBI) program" selects certain "best evidence programs" and packages them to enable communities to implement them in a fashion most likely to retain their effectiveness (Collins, Harshbarger, Sawyer, & Hamdallah, 2006; Dworkin et al., 2008; Lyles et al., 2007; CDC, 2015b).

Earlier chapters in this book have discussed the many effective programs designed to reduce maternal and infant mortality (Murthy, 2016); to effectively reduce transmission of multiple diseases (Rice et al., 2016), including malaria (Farooq & Bergman-Leitner, 2016) and HIV and other sexually transmitted diseases (DiClemente, Seth, & Mehrotra, 2016); to prevent and diminish the severity of chronic diseases (Hospedales et al., 2016), including cancer (Luciani & Agurto, 2016); and to promote health-sustaining community-based activities including good nutrition (Zacarías et al., 2016). Some of these interventions have been developed in low- and middle-income countries, although the majority have been developed and evaluated in higher-income settings, with a relative paucity of interventions developed in and for low-income settings (Bhutta et al., 2005; Haws et al., 2007; Opiyo & English, 2010). Regardless

LEARNING OBJECTIVES

By the end of this chapter, the reader should be able to:

- **Understand the importance of and difference between the aspects of and steps in "implementation" of effective interventions**
- **Recognize the state of our understanding about the aspects of a program that are critical to its effectiveness**
- **Understand the importance of the field of implementation science to advances in domestic and global public health**

of the site of their origin and evaluation, the process of intervention design and effectiveness trials are labor intensive, time consuming, and expensive. Likewise, substantial revisions of previously effective interventions for new settings are resource intensive, including the need for reassessment of intervention effectiveness. Resource constraints, especially in lower-income settings, therefore argue against redesigns and reevaluations of effective prevention and treatment programs as they are transported from one setting to another. However, different cultural, behavioral, epidemiologic, economic, and geographic backgrounds of new settings argue in favor of repeated modification and evaluation of interventions before bringing them to practice in a new setting.

This desire to address substantial public health needs in a timely fashion with apparently effective approaches is tempered by the concern that action without guidance from research-based **adaptation** is not new. Moreover, communities may be skeptical about an intervention's reputed effectiveness; having been shown once or twice to be effective under study conditions does not necessarily translate into effectiveness in a "real-world" situation (Collins et al., 2006; Cronbach, 1982). Certainly there are many examples of interventions that were effective in one setting that were less effective in a different setting. For example, in-service neonatal emergency care training has been effective for hospital-based personnel in industrialized settings, but results are less encouraging for similar training administered to community-based workers in developing countries (Opiyo & English, 2010). Approaches such as demonstration projects (Warren & Liamba, 2004), rapid ethnographic assessments (Bentley et al., 1988), and "process research" (M. M. Rogers, 1995) were all born out of the uncertainty as to when and how to apply interventions that had been effective in other settings.

Along with and emerging from these varied but related adaptation approaches has been growing awareness and interest in the science of innovation (including interventions) utilization or application (Kilbourne et al., 2007). Broad elements or phases that have been identified as critical to innovation application include **diffusion** of new innovations, including ideas, technology, and practices (defined as "the uncontrolled or natural spread of innovations"), **dissemination** (defined as "purposeful or deliberate efforts to move an innovation"), and the final step, **implementation** (defined as "adoption or utilization of the innovation") (Dearing, 2008, 2009; Green et al., 2009).

Implementation

Several decades of rich literature focuses on readiness of the community to embrace a new intervention (Green & Glasgow, 2006; Rubenstein et al., 2000; Sales et al., 2006). This literature, often following the outlines of diffusion theory (Rogers, 2003) and stages of change theory (Prochaska, et al., 1994; Zimmerman, Olsen, & Bosworth, 2003), emphasizes the need for the organization or community to be "ready for change," explicates phases in this readiness, identification of individuals who are amenable to acceptance of change, characteristics of the innovation that might increase its acceptance, and/or the ability to facilitate the acceptance of innovation among individuals. These issues are critical to utilization of innovation—and have received much attention in the research and public health literature. By contrast, until recently, the fourth phase of innovation application, **implementation,** had typically not been the primary focus of the research or field activity (Dearing, 2008; Green et al., 2009; Rotheram-Borus, Swendeman, & Chovnick, 2009). Therefore, although all of these processes are critical (and interrelated) to utilization of innovations, this chapter focuses primarily on implementation.

Critical Issues

Although much of the remainder of this chapter may apply to innovations in general, we focus on issues relevant to the utilization of interventions, both behavioral and a combination of behavioral and biomedical, that have been demonstrated through randomized, controlled trials to improve one or more health outcomes in at least one population or target audience. Public health implementation of such an intervention include both or either use in a wider setting but in a similar population (e.g., the intervention may have been conducted in a limited number of schools in a city or state and now will be implemented in all schools through the city or state), or in a new population (whether geographic, cultural, socioeconomic, or demographic) or a different public health use (e.g., a different disease, secondary versus primary prevention, etc.).

A wide range of issues affect the ability to implement an intervention in a real-world setting in a manner that retains the effectiveness achieved in the research setting. The science of evidence-based interventions is rapidly evolving. We first discuss each of the issues that have been found or are hypothesized to be of importance in intervention implementation, providing examples from the literature to illustrate approaches, findings, and remaining questions. We conclude the chapter with a summary of implications for the field of intervention utilization.

Elements of an Effective Intervention

In developing an intervention designed to alter or sustain a specific behavior or behaviors, behavioral researchers rarely rely on a single item or approach. For example, an investigator may rely on one theory of behavioral change or may integrate two or more (e.g., a social cognitive theory [Bandura, 1986] or stages of change theory [Prochaska et al., 1994] or motivational interviewing [Naar-King & Suarez, 2010)]). Likewise, the investigator may incorporate several different activities or approaches to illustrate and support the point that he or she is trying to make. For example, in our adolescent sexual risk reduction intervention, Focus on Youth and Informed Parents Together (FOY and ImPACT (https://effectiveinterventions.cdc.gov/en/highimpactprevention/Interventions/FOY.aspx), we utilized multiple approaches to teaching and reinforcing condom use: a movie discussing reproductive health followed by a discussion; a condom demonstration; a condom "race"; team games regarding facts about reproductive health; a "condom hunt," in which youths must obtain condoms in the community and bring them back to the next class; and a role play convincing a partner to use a condom.

We do not know which of these activities and approaches is critical; we suspect that all may be important because each one supports an important aspect of appropriate condom use. Clearly knowing why a condom should be used is as important as the correct steps in condom use. Without having handled a condom, a youth would not know whether or not he could apply it correctly. By applying it during a time of tension (e.g., the condom race), she is required to use it correctly when she is excited or there is some "pressure." Even if a youth knows how to use it, if he is not able to obtain a condom and likewise if she cannot convince her partner to use a condom (or be able to refuse sex if the partner will not use it), knowledge about correct use will not be helpful. But do we know that each of these activities is necessary or sufficient? No, really we do not. We do not know which of the component parts were necessary for the original success of the program in one setting—and we certainly do not "know" which ones would be necessary in a new setting.

This is a problem with significant public health implications. The Centers for Disease Control has advocated for a practical approach, striking "a balance between adaptation to fit local needs and maintaining the **core elements** that made the original intervention effective" (Harshbarger et al., 2006, p. 185). This approach has a compelling practical logic to it—but still begs the question as to what is a "core element." The CDC is well aware of this conundrum and thus has developed a guide for researchers and organizations interested in adapting an intervention and remaining "true" to the core elements. The authors of the guide argue that the core elements are those aspects of the intervention that are critical to the "internal logic" of the intervention (Harshbarger et al., 2006; Kelly, Heckman et al., 2000; Kelly, Somlai et al., 2000). Internal logic is the mapping of risk determinants and behaviors with intervention activities—such as what we described for condom use. The internal logic argument suggests that it would be necessary to include activities or approaches to underscore each of the determinants of condom use in any adaptation of Focus on Youth—but the specific activities (called **key characteristics** by the CDC, Harshbarger et al., 2006) could be changed. So, for example, rather than a teacher demonstrating proper use of a condom, this could be done by a nurse or physician or a movie. Rather than a role play of a discussion as to the use of a condom, clips of movies illustrating discussions could be shown, followed by a live discussion. Uncertain still—but possible—is the use of condom cards (in which correct cards must be identified and placed in proper order) if it is not permissible for youth to handle condoms (Stanton et al., 2009). See Box 17.1 for more detailed definitions of core elements, adaptation, key characteristics, and internal logic (McKleroy et al., 2006).

Alteration of activities that appear to be "key characteristics" can be hazardous in the absence of technical training (Gandelman & Reitmeijer, 2004). For example, we found that in removing the "most offensive" condom activities (typically those in which teachers and/or youth touched condoms) without thoughtfully replacing them with other activities that underscored the specific learning objectives even though other condom-use exercises were retained, undermined the effectiveness of the intervention (Stanton et al., 2005).

BOX 17.1 DEFINITIONS OF IMPLEMENTATION TERMS

- *Core elements* are required elements that reflect the underlying theory and internal logic of the intervention. It is presumed that these are the intervention components producing the intervention's main effects. Core elements are identified through research and program evaluation. Because core elements define an intervention, they must be preserved with fidelity during adaptation and implementation.
- *Adaptation* is the process of modifying an intervention while preserving the core elements and internal logic. An intervention should be modified to be consistent with the cultural context in which it will be implemented, including new or altered determinants of risk and protective behaviors of the target population, and other local variables.
- *Key characteristics* are important, but not essential, to an intervention's success. They may be modified and substituted to be culturally appropriate and fit the risk and/or protective factors and behaviors, behavioral determinants, and other unique circumstances of the new setting. Changes to the key characteristics should not conflict the core elements, theory, and internal logic of the intervention.
- *Internal logic* of an intervention is the theory describing the relationships among intervention that activates behavioral determinants and the intended outcome of the intervention.

Source: Adapted from McElroy (2006).

To guide groups who wish to implement effective interventions in new settings but plan to change some of the activities, the CDC has developed the DEBI program. By packaging interventions in such a fashion as to explicitly identify the core elements of the intervention and the key characteristics, and by providing specific examples of changes in the key characteristics that would not alter the internal logic of the intervention, the DEBI program seeks to facilitate implementation in new settings (Harshbarger et al., 2006; Dworkin et al., 2008; Lyles et al., 2007) in a manner that retains the effectiveness of the original intervention. Accordingly, in the process of transforming an "effective program" into a DEBI program, the researchers, adapters, and CDC work to identify the core elements or critical characteristics of the original (effective) intervention without which it is questionable that the intervention would retain its effectiveness (CDC, 2015b). Core elements can be considered to be in two categories: *implementation-pedagogy* (characteristics relating to the logistics of establishing a positive learning environment and the teaching process used); and *content* (the information, skills, values, etc., that are being taught). Each of these components is considered critical in diffusion and adaptation of interventions. (See Figure 17.1 for an example of how the use of core elements can facilitate appropriate adaptation of an existing effective intervention into a new setting.)

Focus on Youth Core Elements
Implementation–pedagogy Core

1. Delivering intervention to youth in community-based settings:
   Modification: Delivered in community-set elementary school
2. Using two skilled facilitators to implement the youth group sessions:
   Modification: Used one trained teacher
3. Using "friendship groups" to strengthen peer support
   Modification: Used classroom of local neighborhood children

Content Core

4. Using culturally appropriate interactive activities proven as effective learning strategies to help youth capture the important constructs in the theory
5. Including a "family tree" to contextualize and personalize concepts such as decision making and risk assessment
6. Enabling participants to learn and practice a decision making model
7. Training participants in assertive communication and refusal skills specifically related to negotiation of abstinence or safer sex behaviors
8. Teaching youth proper condom use skills

ImPACT Core Element
Implementation–pedagogy Core

1. Deliver the intervention to individual parent-youth dyads in their home or a convenient community-based setting (e.g., CBO, church, recreation center, or school) at a time that fits the schedule of the parent/guardian.
   Modification: Delivered to groups of parents without youth
2. Use of health educators whom parents and adolescents find credible and are skilled at building rapport with parents and youths at the beginning of the session.
3. Ideally, ImPACT should be delivered prior to the child beginning the Focus on Youth intervention or before completion of Session 3.
4. Use of documentary that shows the challenges and importance of parents monitoring and talking to their children ages 12-15 about sex, abstinence, STDs, HIV, and condoms.
5. The health educator, parent, and child should watch the video together.

Content Core

6. The intervention allows parents an opportunity to practice and improve their monitoring skills and parents and children an opportunity to improve and practice communication skills.
7. Teach parent and child proper condom use skills.
8. All parents receive a pamphlet on good communication, how to talk to your kids; importance of parental monitoring; facts on STIs and HIV, including prevalence data among young African Americans.

Figure 17.1 Adaptation of an Effective Intervention into a New Setting Using Core Elements

We believe that the field has been substantially advanced by the concept of core elements. Core elements cannot be changed. Key characteristics can be modified—as long as they do not alter a core element and thereby disrupt the internal logic of the intervention.

Fidelity of Implementation

Fidelity of implementation (henceforth referred to only as "fidelity") refers to the degree to which program trainers implement programs as intended by the program developer—and as reflected in adherence to the core elements of the program and its internal logic. Given that there is a danger that core elements might be disrupted unintentionally, wouldn't it be better not to alter the intervention at all when applying it to new populations? That is, shouldn't we strive to maintain fidelity to the original intervention as much as possible?

The simple answer is probably not, for at least two reasons. First, in new communities some change will be needed. Frameworks have been provided to identify when and how cultural adaptation might be needed. Lau has suggested that such modification is needed when there are clear indicators that populations differ, especially if there is reason to believe that these differences may affect the local propensity to engage in risk or protective behaviors or interventions (DePue et al., 2010; Lau, 2006). This is particularly true when moving behavioral interventions from a setting with a different racial, religious, ethnic, and cultural background than the new one, as is typically seen between high- and low-income countries. Resnicow et al. (2005) have described these differences as "deep structures" that may require substantial changes to an intervention. By contrast, "surface structures" include cosmetic changes such as places, familiar names, songs, and so on, that can be changed to make potential participants more comfortable with an intervention. Second, a long history of implementation assessment resoundingly confirms that, as a practical matter, implementation of interventions in new settings *is* associated with change. Dating back at least to the mid-1970s with the Rand report "Implementation of Educational Innovation," concerns have been raised regarding the fidelity of implementation; the consensus of multiple evaluations of implementation of education and behavioral interventions is that some degree of adaptation is unavoidable (Bell et al., 2007; Berman & McLaughlin, 1976; Dusenbury et al., 2003; Galbraith et al., 2008; Halfors & Godette, 2002; Ringwalt et al., 2004). Ringwalt et al. (2004) reported that among a representative sample of US teachers, 79.8% reported adapting their curricula for prevention of disease. Other investigators have noted that there are ways to increase fidelity to an original intervention. For example, Perrin et al. (2006) reported that employment of consistent implementation procedures and program materials increases fidelity of implementation.

Related to concerns about overzealous adaptation is the problem of low-quality implementation. For example, in their assessment of delinquency-prevention programs in US schools, Gottfredson et al. (2000) concluded that about one-half of school-based activities were of very low quality and thus could not be expected to achieve the intended outcome. Reacting to this observation, Chris Melde concluded, "With such concerns about the degree and quality of program implementation, it becomes necessary to question the extent to which program failure is an artifact of poor programs as opposed to poorly implemented programs" (Melde, Esbensen, & Tusinski, 2006, p. 716).

In response to concerns regarding unguided adaptation and/or poor implementation of interventions in new settings, researchers have noted the importance of providing early, structured technical assistance to communities as a way of guiding the adaptation without discouraging it (Collins et al., 2006; Kelly, Heckman, et al., 2000; Kelly, Somlai, et al., 2000; O'Donnell et al., 2000). Thus the DEBI program approach should increase fidelity to the adapted program. It recognizes and embraces the inevitability of adaptation but both define acceptable limits *and* establish support structures to decrease further adaptation.

Optimal Balance Between Fidelity and Adaptation

For many years, researchers, public health experts, communities, research institutions, and public health institutions have identified the need for moving research findings into the community (Durlak, 1998; Institute of Medicine [IOM], 2003; Kelly, Spielberg, & McAuliffe, 2008). Much progress has been made as individuals and groups from disparate backgrounds have come together to identify and package effective programs and to delineate frameworks for the transfer of these former research projects into communities and classrooms (CDC, 2009; Cottrell et al., 2008; DiClemente et al., 2008; Lyles et al., 2004; McKleroy, 2006; Wingood & DiClemente, 2008). Much has been written regarding the balance between scientific rigor and community needs and realities (Dworkin et al., 2008). Some studies have replicated evidence-based programs in community or clinic settings, in a few cases even assessing some measures of fidelity of implementation (e.g., Cornman et al., 2008). Some investigators have conducted the primary effectiveness trials in large-scale community and school settings (e.g., Coyle et al., 2004; Kirby et al., 1991). Still missing have been large-scale implementation studies of evidence-based interventions "taken to scale," in which both the fidelity of implementation and outcomes are assessed. Studies exploring the fidelity outcomes issue from related fields (substance abuse and delinquency prevention, for example) provide suggestive, but inconclusive, evidence supporting this relationship.

For example, in a study of the relationship of fidelity and outcomes in evaluations of family and youth competence training regarding substance abuse refusal, Spoth et al. (2002) defined "higher adherence schools" as those achieving adherence to more than 80% of the components in the intervention. Using this definition, 23 of the 35 schools in the studies were categorized as "higher adhering." The authors concluded that high levels of implementation fidelity can be achieved, but the relationship between adherence and outcomes was less clear: "In relatively lower-adherence schools there was only limited evidence of adverse effects on outcomes" (Spoth et al., 2002, p. 512). The coding scheme employed in this study for adherence was "yes/no" and appeared to address all curricular contents equally—for example, there was no specification of "core elements."

Although conducted a quarter-century ago, one of the most comprehensive examinations of fidelity and effectiveness to date was conducted by Blakely et al. (1987), assessing seven nationally disseminated education and criminal justice projects. The researchers measured program fidelity as the proportion of finite program components that were implemented; they developed detailed process measures that allowed observation of specific program components to measure adoption or implementation by each site to determine fidelity. Multiple methods, including extensive interviews and in-person observations, were utilized. Validity was analyzed by comparing data across the various measures obtained. Multiple sources of data were available for 75% of items at each site. The investigators found an exact-agreement convergence rating of .96 for the between-source comparison strategy summed across all 70 sites. They found that high-fidelity adopters tended to be more effective than implementers with low fidelity, local additions to the model tended to enhance effectiveness, and modifications not distracting from fidelity were unrelated to effectiveness.

As significant as this research is there are several reasons why additional research on the relationship between fidelity of intervention delivery and outcomes is still critically important. First, as the researchers themselves describe, the outcomes data were left up to the sites to describe and provide and thus were inconsistent in nature and of variable quality. The procedure to examine any relationship was limited to a ranking procedure, and the relationship itself was suggestive rather than definitive. Further, conceptualization of fidelity has progressed since Blakely and his colleagues (1987) conducted their study. Finally, and arguably of less importance, it is possible that in different audiences with different types of interventions (e.g., a health rather than a criminal justice focus) the results may differ.

There is a strong suggestion that fidelity of implementation is important to outcomes, but that fidelity cannot be the only "driver". It appears then, that much uncertainty remains with regard to the tension between "fidelity" and "adaptation". Both clearly defined fidelity data and outcomes data are critical to understand the relationship between fidelity and sustained effectiveness of evidence-based interventions and to confirm the hypothesis that underlies so much of current public health replication efforts: that is, that fidelity of implementation is critical to program effectiveness.

Determining Fidelity

The NIH Behavior Change Consortium has identified five areas to consider in conceptualizing treatment fidelity in conducting research: study design; training providers; delivery of treatment; receipt of treatment; and enactment of treatment skills (Bellg et al., 2004; Domitrovich & Greenberg, 2000). To illustrate the importance of each of these actions, Bellg et al. (2004), on behalf of the NIH Behavior Change Consortium, draws upon an example employed by Lichstein, Riedl, and Grieve (1994):

> Assessment of whether a physician wrote a prescription (delivery) is inadequate for ensuring that the treatment has been implemented as intended. To receive an active dose of a treatment, the patient must then fill the prescription (receipt) and take the medicine as prescribed (enactment). (Bellg et al., 2004, p. 444)

Although there are many ways in which these factors could be grouped, we categorize them according to those that could potentially be affected during the training and adoption process, those that may be affected by fixed characteristics of the trainers (teachers) or the respondents, and those associated with the intervention itself.

Factors That Could Be Modified During Training and Adoption

Characteristics that may be alterable through targeted training or other approaches that have been identified as associated with increased fidelity include those that potentially increase (a) trainer confidence; (b) perceived relevance; (c) sense of ownership; and (d) relative benefit. Those factors that could be altered and might result in increased trainer *confidence* include (a) intensive in-service training that follows a set curriculum itself (compared to no training, training that is ad hoc or variable in nature, nonparticipatory training, and/or brief training); (b) less curricular discretion (e.g., a more detailed script or lesson plan); and (c) practice in their ability to teach the curriculum and to use interactive methods. Those factors that potentially result in increased *relevance* include a perception that the situation being addressed in the intervention applies to the community in which the intervention is being adopted. The extent to which relevance is more local (as opposed to a global or national relevance), may be a stronger motivator of fidelity. *Ownership* appears to be important—that is, a sense on the part of the trainees that the intervention addresses a local issue *and* that they or their community had significant input into the development of the intervention. The importance of incorporating community contextual factors has been repeatedly stressed in the literature. Support for the importance of the intervention being adopted by local authorities (e.g., in the case of a school-based intervention, the school principal and guidance counselors) serves to indicate the relative *benefit* to be derived from teaching this curriculum as opposed to more time spent on another subject (such as math or reading). Also relevant to the question of benefit is the perception of the effectiveness of currently available curricula; if the existing curriculum is perceived as adequate, substitution with a new one is likely to be more difficult. Finally, given the significance of testing in many educational systems, it is likely that a decision by the teacher or the school authorities to test and grade children on the curriculum may reinforce the perceived benefit of the material to the student and to the teacher (Backer, 2002; Berman et al., 1976; Dworkin et al., 2008; Dusenbury et al., 2003; Dusenbury et al., 2005; Elliot & Mihalic, 2004; Fors & Doster, 1983; Kelly, Somlai, et al., 2000; Mihalic, Fagan, & Argamaso, 2008; Parcel et al., 1991; Perry, Murray, & Griffin, 1990; Ringwalt et al., 2004; Rohrbach, Graham, & Hansen, 1993).

Factors Affected by Characteristics of the Teachers and Respondents

Characteristics of the teachers and teaching environment that may or may not be affected by training have also been shown to increase fidelity. Examples include shorter duration of time as a teacher, initial feelings about the existing curriculum (in this case the existing HIV prevention in the schools), and an overall positive attitude toward prevention in general. Likewise organizational characteristics including receptivity to innovation and decreased turmoil have been associated with increased fidelity (Bauman, Stein, & Ireys, 1991; Dusenbury et al., 2003; Kelly, Heckman, et al., 2000; Kelly, Somlai, et al., 2000; Parcel et al., 1995; Rohrbach et al., 1993; Wandersman et al., 1988).

Factors Associated With the Intervention

Complex programs are less likely to be successfully implemented; as a corollary, programs that are packaged and present the materials in a straightforward manner are more faithfully executed. Detailed instruction manuals for the trainers increase fidelity. As part of the DEBI process, the selected effective interventions are packaged to fulfill these criteria. Because there were relatively few changes in the U.S. version of the HIV prevention program Focus on Youth when it was adapted in The Bahamas (Focus on Youth Caribbean–FOYC) and in the parent component ImPACT when it was converted to CaribbeanImPACT (CImPACT), in the same training manuals with only minor modifications can (and have been) used in teacher training (Bauman et al., 1991; http://www.effectiveinterventions.org; Dusenbury, 2003; Gottfredson, 1984; Luborsky & DeRubeis, 1984).

Assessing Fidelity and Adaptation

It is important to be able to assess fidelity and adaptation of intervention implementation. Unfortunately, to date, standardized measures of fidelity and adaptation are lacking. In a review of the issues surrounding fidelity, Song et al. (2010) note that frequently trial integrity and intervention fidelity are conflated. Likewise they note that following the steps proposed as likely to increase treatment fidelity does not mean that fidelity has in fact been achieved. Further, in behavioral interventions, it is not just whether and how many elements of an intervention are delivered, but how they are delivered (Dumas et al., 2001; Hawe, Shiell, & Riley, 2004). As a corollary, when customization occurs, it must be described.

Song, Happ, and Sandelowski (2010) describe the need for fidelity instruments that will (a) assess the theoretical basis of the intervention as well as the specific tasks of the intervention; (b) describe and otherwise address delivery of unplanned additions to the intervention; (c) describe and otherwise address modifications made in response to a subject interaction (e.g., Were these modifications part of or outside of the script for the intervention?); and, (d) note the sequencing and delivery pace of an intervention (e.g., delivery of an intervention over eight hours in eight weekly sessions may or may not have the same impact as eight hours in one day).

Sustainability

Given the current early stage of efforts and theoretic guidelines to describe, document, and monitor implementation of effective interventions in public health settings, it is perhaps not surprising that intervention sustainability has received relatively little attention in the literature (Stirman et al., 2012). There is little reason to assume that the factors leading to implementation will necessarily be the same as those resulting in sustainability (Bowman et al., 2008; Massatti et al., 2008); accordingly, extrapolation of findings from implementation research should be accompanied with a high degree of caution. So, for example, "early adapters" (Rogers, 2003) are unlikely to champion sustainability. Likewise, although adaptation may occur within or outside of the established infrastructure, sustainability of an intervention will require either the incorporation of the intervention into the existing environment or change of the existing environment that houses the "new" intervention—or both. This in turn may affect how "fidelity" is measured and regarded. If the intervention replaces the existing infrastructure in large measure, "fidelity" of the new intervention may be high; by contrast, if the intervention needs to be incorporated into an existing program, fidelity is likely to be lower (Scherer & Dearing, 2011; Stirman et al., 2012).

A recent review of 25 papers examining sustainability found that "partial sustainability," in which some but not all elements were retained, was generally thought to be high (Stirman et al., 2012). However, few studies included in the review reported an operational definition of sustainability and/or independent assessments of sustainability. The authors further noted that the absence of a working framework of "sustainability" was an important limitation of the published studies in this area. Most of the studies did not identify the "core elements" of the intervention, further limiting interpretation as to what exactly was sustained.

Summary

In this chapter, we focus on the application and implementation of health interventions in low- and middle-income countries as one important phase in the translation process from scientific breakthroughs to practice. With a focus on examples of health interventions which have undergone rigorous scientific evaluations, we discuss issues which have been identified as integral to effectively transitioning from research to "real world" public health settings. Issues discussed include: 1) identifying "core elements" of interventions, 2) program fidelity and implications for programmatic adaptation and change, 3) utilization of technical assistance to guide adaptation to increase likelihood of retaining program effectiveness throughout the implementation process, 4) the need for continuing research which incorporates both program fidelity and outcomes data particularly in large-scale implementation settings, and 5) standardization of measurements for fidelity and adaptation. While implementation science has made substantial in-roads to identify and address these issues, an outstanding need remains to define and assess program sustainability.

KEY TERMS

1. **Adaptation:** The process of modifying an intervention so that it is appropriate for the new audience while preserving the core elements
2. **Core elements:** Required elements that reflect the underlying theory and internal logic of the intervention; Core elements define an intervention and must be preserved with fidelity during adaptation and implementation
3. **Diffusion:** The uncontrolled or natural spread of a new idea, program, or innovation

4. **Dissemination:** The purposeful or deliberate attempt to introduce a new idea, program or innovation
5. **Implementation:** The adoption, utilization and/or administration of a new idea, program, or innovation
6. **Key characteristics:** Important but not essential aspects of an intervention; as such they may be modified and substituted during the process of adaptation of an intervention to a new audience

REVIEW QUESTIONS

1. What differentiates "implementation" from "dissemination" and/or "diffusion" of an intervention?
2. What is the current understanding of the relationship between fidelity of implementation of an intervention and intervention impact?
3. What factors appear to influence whether or not a trainer delivers an intervention with fidelity?

References

Backer, T. E. (2002). *Finding the balance: Program fidelity and adaptation in substance abuse prevention: A state-of-the-art review.* Rockville MD: Center for Substance Abuse Prevention. Retrieved from http://www.samhsa.gov/cents/csap/modelprograms/pdfs/Findingbalance/pdf

Bandura, A. (1986). *Social foundations of thought and action: A social cognitive theory.* Englewood Cliffs, NJ: Prentice-Hall.

Bauman, L. J., Stein, R.E.K., & Ireys, H. T. (1991). Reinventing fidelity: The transfer of social technology among settings. *American Journal of Community Psychology, 19,* 619–639.

Bell, S. G., Newcomer, S. F., Bachrach, C., Borawski, E., Jemmott, J. B. III, Morrison, D., … Zimmerman, R. (2007). Challenges in replicating interventions. *Journal of Adolescent Health, 40,* 514–520.

Bellg, A. J., Borrelli, B., Resnick, B., Hecht, J., Minicucci, D. S., Ory, M., … Czajkowski, S. Treatment Fidelity Workgroup of the NIH Behavior Change Consortium. (2004). Enhancing treatment fidelity in health behavior change studies: Best practices and recommendations from the NIH Behavior Change Consortium. *Health Psychology, 23,* 443–451.

Bentley, M. E., Pelto, G. H., Straus, W. L., Schumann, D. A., Adegbola, C., de la Pena, E., ... Huffman, S. L. (1988). Rapid ethnographic assessment: Applications in a diarrhea management program. *Social Science and Medicine, 27*(1), 107–116.

Berman, P., & McLaughlin, M. (1976). Implementation of educational innovation. *Education Forum, 40*, 345–370.

Bhutta, Z. A., Darmstadt, G. L., Hasan, B. S., & Haws, R. A. (2005). Community-based interventions for improving perinatal and neonatal health outcomes in developing countries: A review of the evidence. *Pediatrics, 115*, S19–S102.

Blakely, C. H., Mayer, J. P., Gottschalk, R. G., Schmitt, N., Davidson, W. S., Roitman, D. B., Emshoff, J. G. (1987). The fidelity-adaptation debate: Implications for the implementation of public sector social programs. *American Journal of Community Psychology, 15*, 253–268.

Bowman, C. C., Sobo, E. J., Asch, S. M., Gifford, A. L., & HIV/Hepatitis Quality Enhancement Research Initiative. (2008). Measuring persistence of implementation: QUERI Series. *Implementation Science, 3*(1), 21.

Centers for Disease Control (2015a). *Prevention Synthesis Project.* Retrieved from http://www.cdc.gov/hiv/dhap/prb/prs/. Last updated March 18, 2015.

Centers for Disease Control (2015b). *Diffusion of Effective Behavioral Interventions (DEBI).* Retrieved from https://effectiveinterventions.cdc.gov/en/AboutDebi.aspx

Collins, C., Harshbarger, C., Sawyer, R., & Hamdallah, M. (2006). The Diffusion of Effective Behavioral Interventions project: Development, implementation, and lessons learned. *AIDS Education and Prevention, 18*(Suppl. A), 5–20.

Cornman, D. H., Kiene, S. M., Christie, S., Fisher, W. A., Shuper, P. A., Pillay, S., ... Fisher J. D. (2008). Clinic-based intervention reduces unprotected sexual behavior among HIV-infected patients in KwaZulu-Natal, South Africa: Results of a pilot study. *Journal of Acquired Immune Deficiency Syndrome*; *48*, 553–560.

Cottrell, L., Rishel, C., Cottrell, S., & Branstetter, S. (2008). Program sustainability in a changing world. In B. S. Stanton, J. S. Galbraith, & L. Kaljee (Eds.), *The uncharted path from clinic-based to community-based research* (237–254). New York, NY: NovaScience Publishers.

Coyle, K., Kirby, D., Marin, B., Gomez, C., & Gregorich, S. (2004). Research and practice: Draw the line/respect the line: A randomized trial of a middle school intervention to reduce sexual risk behaviors. *American Journal of Public Health*, 843–851.

Cronbach, L. J. (1982). *Designing evaluations of educational and social programs.* San Francisco, CA: Jossey-Bass.

Dearing, J. W. (2008). Evolution of diffusion and dissemination theory. *Journal of Public Health Management Practice, 14*(2), 99–108.

Dearing, J. W. (2009). Applying diffusion of innovation theory to intervention development. *Research on Social Work Practice, 19*(5), 503–518.

DePue, J. D., Rosen, R. K., Batts-Turner, M., Bereolos, N., House, M., Forster, R., ... McGarvey, S. T. (2010). Cultural translation of interventions: Diabetes care in American Samoa. *American Journal of Public Health, 100*(11), 2085–2093.

DiClemente, R. J., Seth, P., & Mehrotra, P. (2016). The Evolving Global HIV Pandemic: Epidemiology, Prevention, and Future Priorities. In R. S. Zimmerman (Ed.), R. J. DiClemente (Ed.), J. K. Andrus (Ed.), E. N. Hosein (Ed.), Society for Public Health Education (SOPHE). *Introduction to Global Health Promotion.* Somerset, NJ: Jossey-Bass.

DiClemente, R. J., Wingood, G. W., Crittenden, C. P., & Rose, E. S. (2008). Translational research: Adapting evidence-based HIV interventions in diverse environment. In S. Stanton, J. S. Galbraith, & L. Kaljee (Eds.), *The uncharted path from clinic-based to community-based research* (pp. 201–218). New York, NY: NovaScience Publishers.

Domitrovich, C. E, & Greenberg, M. T. (2000). The study of implementation: Current findings from effective programs that prevent mental disorders in school-aged children. *Journal of Educational Psychology Consulting, 11,* 193–221.

Dumas, J. E., Lynch, A. M., Laughlin, J. E., Phillips, S. E., & Prinz, R. J. (2001). Promoting intervention fidelity: Conceptual issues, methods, and preliminary results from the EARLY ALLIANCE prevention trial. *American Journal of Preventive Medicine, 20*(Suppl.), 38–47.

Durlak, J. A. (1998). Why program implementation is important. *Journal of Prevention and Intervention in the Community, 17,* 5–18.

Dusenbury, L., Brannigan, R., Falco, M., & Hansen, W. B. (2003). A review of research on fidelity of implementation: Implications for drug abuse prevention in school settings. *Health Education Research, 18,* 237–256.

Dusenbury, L., Brannigan, R., Hansen, W. B., Walsh, J., & Falco, M. (2005). Quality of implementation: Developing measures crucial to understanding the diffusion of prevention interventions. *Health Education Research, 20,* 308–313.

Dworkin, S. L., Pinto, R. M., Hunter, J., Rapkin, B., & Remien, R. H. (2008). Keeping the spirit of community partnerships alive in the scale up of HIV/AIDS prevention: Critical reflections on the roll out of DEBI (Diffusion of Effective Behavioral Interventions). *American Journal of Community Psychology, 42,* 51–59.

Elliot, D., & Mihalic, S. (2004). Issues in disseminating and replicating effective prevention programs. *Prevention Science, 5,* 47–53.

Farooq, F., & Bergman-Leitner, E. S. (2016). Malaria Prevention and Control. In R. S. Zimmerman (Ed.), R. J. DiClemente (Ed.), J. K. Andrus (Ed.), E. N. Hosein (Ed.), Society for Public Health Education (SOPHE). *Introduction to Global Health Promotion.* Somerset, NJ: Jossey-Bass.

Fors, S. W., & Doster, M. E. (1983). Implication of results: Factors for success. *Journal of School Health, 55,* 332–334.

Galbraith, J., Stanton, B., Boekeloo, B., King, W., Desmond, S., Howard, D., Black, M. (2008). Exploring implementation and fidelity of evidence-based behavioral interventions for HIV prevention: Lessons learned from the Focus on Kids diffusion case study. *Health Education and Behavior,* April 29, 1–18.

Gandelman, A., & Reitmeijer, C. A. (2004). Translation, adaptation, and synthesis of interventions for persons living with HIV: Lessons from previous HIV prevention interventions. *Journal of Acquired Immunodeficiency Syndrome, 37,* S126–S129.

Gottfredson, G. D. (1984). A theory-ridden approach to program evaluation: A method for stimulating researcher–implementer collaboration. *American Psychologist, 39,* 1101–1112.

Gottfredson, G. D., Gottfredson, D. C., Czeh, E., Cantor, D., Crosse, S., & Hantman, I. (2000). A national study of delinquency prevention in school. Final report. Ellicot City, MD: Gottfredson Associates, Inc. Retrieved from http://files.eric.ed.gov/fulltext/ED459409.pdf.

Green, L. W., Ottoson, J. M., Garcia, C., & Hiatt, R. A. (2009). Diffusion theory and knowledge dissemination, utilization, and integration in public health. *Annual Review of Public Health, 30,* 151–74.

Green, L. W., & Glasgow, R. E. (2006). Evaluating the relevance, generalization, and applicability of research: Issues in extended validation and translation methodology. *Evaluation and the Health Professions, 29,* 1–3.

Halfors, D., & Godette, D. (2002). Will the "principles of effectiveness" improve prevention practice? Early findings from a diffusion study. *Health Education Research, 17,* 461–470.

Harshbarger, C., Simmons, G., Coelho, H., Sloop, K., & Collins, C. (2006). An empirical assessment of implementation, adaptation, and tailoring: The evaluation of CDC's National Diffusion of VOICES/VOCES. *AIDS Education and Prevention, 18*(Suppl. A), 184–197.

Hawe, P., Shiell, A., & Riley, T. (2004). Complex interventions: How "out of control" can a randomized controlled trial be? *British Medical Journal, 328*(7455), 1561–1563.

Haws, R. A., Thomas, A. L., Bhutta, Z. A., & Darnstadt, G. H. (2007). Impact of packaged interventions on neonatal health: A review of the evidence. *Health Policy and Planning, 22,* 193–215.

Hospedales, C J., Kengne, A. P., Legetic, B., & Marquizo, A. B. (2016). Non-Communicable Diseases (NCDs): Moving toward Health Promotion. In R. S. Zimmerman (Ed.), R. J. DiClemente (Ed.), J. K. Andrus (Ed.), E. N. Hosein (Ed.), Society for Public Health Education (SOPHE). *Introduction to Global Health Promotion.* Somerset, NJ: Jossey-Bass.

Institute of Medicine. (2003). *The future of the public's health in the 21st century.* Washington, DC: National Academies Press.

Kelly, J. A., Heckman, T. G., Stevenson, L. Y., Williams, P. N., Ertl, T., Hays, R. B., … Neumann, M. S. (2000). Transfer of research-based HIV prevention interventions to community service providers: Fidelity and adaptation. *AIDS Education and Prevention, 12*(Suppl. A), 87–98.

Kelly, J. A., Somlai, A. M., DiFranceisco, W. J., Otto-Salaj, L .L., McAuliffe, T. L., Hackl, K. L., … Rompa, D. (2000). Bridging the gap between the science and service of HIV prevention: Transferring effective research-based HIV prevention interventions to community AIDS service providers. *American Journal of Public Health*.

Kelly, J. A., Spielberg, F., & McAuliffe, T. L. (2008). Defining, designing, implementing and evaluating Phase 4: Prevention effectiveness trials for vulnerable populations. *Journal of Acquired Immune Deficiency Syndrome, 47*, S28–S33.

Kilbourne, A. M., Neumann, M. S., Pincus, H. A., Bauer, M. S., & Stall, R. (2007). Implementing evidence-based interventions in health care: Application of the replicating effective programs framework. *Implementation Science, 2*, 42.

Kirby, D., Barth, R., Leland, N., & Fetro, J. (1991). Reducing the risk: Impact of a new curriculum on sexual risk-taking. *Family Planning Perspectives* (November–December), 253–263.

Lau, A. S. (2006). Making the case for selective and directed cultural adaptation of evidence-based treatments: Examples from parent training. *Clinical Psychology: Science and Practice, 13*(4), 295–310.

Lichstein, K. L., Riedl, B. W., & Grieve, R. (1994). Fair tests of clinical trials: A treatment implementation model. *Advances in Behavior Research and Therapy, 16*, 1–29.

Luborsky, L., & DeRubeis, R. J. (1984). The use of psychotherapy treatment manuals: A small revolution in psychotherapy research style. *Clinical Psychology Review, 4*, 5–14.

Luciani, S., & Agurto, I. (2016). Women's Cancers. In R. S. Zimmerman (Ed.), R. J. DiClemente (Ed.), J. K. Andrus (Ed.), E. N. Hosein (Ed.), Society for Public Health Education (SOPHE). *Introduction to Global Health Promotion*. Somerset, NJ: Jossey-Bass.

Lyles, C. M., Kay, L. S., Crepaz, N., Herbst, J. H., Passin, W. F., Kim, A. S., ... Mullins, M. M.; & HIV/AIDS Prevention Research Synthesis Team. (2007). Best-evidence interventions: Findings from a systematic review of HIV behavioral interventions for US populations at high risk, 2000–2004. *American Journal of Public Health, 9*,133–143.

Massatti, R. R., Sweeney, H. A., Panzano, P. C., & Roth, D. (2008). The de-adoption of innovation of mental health practices (IMPH): Why organizations choose not to sustain an IMPH. *Administration and Policy in Mental Health and Mental Health Policy Research, 35*, 50–65.

McKleroy, V. S., Galbraith, J. S., Cummings, B., Jones, P., Harshbarger, C., Collin, C., ... Carey, J. W.; & ADAPT Team. (2006). Adapting evidence-based behavioral interventions for new settings and target populations. *AIDS Education and Prevention, 18*, 59–74.

Melde, C., Esbensen, F. A., & Tusinski, K. (2006). Addressing program fidelity using onsite observations and program provider descriptions of program delivery. *Evaluation Review, 30*, 714–740.

Mihalic, S. F., Fagan, A. A., & Argamaso, S. (2008). Implementing the LifeSkills training drug prevention program: Factors related to implementation fidelity. *Implementation Science*, 3. Retrieved from http://www.implementationscience.com/content/3/1/5

Murthy, P. (2016). Reducing Maternal and Infant Mortality: Meeting a Global Challenge. In R. S. Zimmerman (Ed.), R. J. DiClemente (Ed.), J. K. Andrus (Ed.), E. N. Hosein (Ed.), Society for Public Health Education (SOPHE). *Introduction to Global Health Promotion*. Somerset, NJ: Jossey-Bass.

Naar-King, S., & Suarez, M. (2010). Motivational interviewing with adolescents and young adults. *Application of motivational interviewing*. New York, NY: Guilford.

O'Donnell, L., Scattergood, P., Adler, M., Doval, A. S., Barker, M., Kelly, J. A., ... Neumann, M. S. (2000). The role of technical assistance in the replication of effective HIV interventions. *AIDS Education and Prevention, 12*(Suppl.), 99–114.

Opiyo, N., & English, M. (2010). In-service training for health professionals to improve care of the seriously ill newborn or child in low- and middle-income countries (Review). *Cochrane Database Systematic Reviews, 4,* CD007071.

Parcel, G. S., O'Hara-Tompkins, N. M., Harrist, R. B., Basen-Engquist, K. M., McCormick, L. K., Gottlieb, N. H., & Eriksen, M. P. (1995). Diffusion of an effective tobacco prevention program: II. Evaluation of the adoption phase. *Health Education Research, 10,* 297–307.

Parcel, G. S., Ross, J. G., Lavin, A. T., Portnoy, B., Nelson, G. D., & Winters, F. (1991). Enhancing implementation of the teenage health teaching modules. *Journal of School Health, 61,* 35–38.

Perrin, K. M., Burke, S. G., O'Connor, D., Walby, G., Shippey, C., Pitt, S., ... Forthofer, M. S. (2006). Factors contributing to intervention fidelity in a multi-site chronic disease self-management program. *Implement Science, 1,* 26.

Perry, C. L., Murray, D. M., & Griffin, G. (1990). Evaluating the statewide dissemination of smoking prevention curricula: Factors in teacher compliance. *Journal of School Health, 60,* 501–504.

Prochaska, J. O., Velicer, W. F., Rossi, J. S., Goldstein, M. G., Marcus, B. H., Rakowski, W. (1994). Stages of change and decisional balance for 12 problem behaviors. *Health Psychology, 13,* 39–46.

Resnicow K, Jackson A, Blissett D, Wang T, McCarty F, Rahotep S, Periasamy S. (2005). Results of the Healthy Body Healthy Spirit trial. *Health Psychology, 24*(4), 339–348.

Rice, M. E., Andrus, J. K., Swezy, V. & Zimmerman, R. S. (2016). Global Immunization Initiatives from a Health Promotion Perspective. In R. S. Zimmerman (Ed.), R. J. DiClemente (Ed.), J. K. Andrus (Ed.), E. N. Hosein (Ed.), Society for Public Health Education (SOPHE). *Introduction to Global Health Promotion*. Somerset, NJ: Jossey-Bass.

Ringwalt, C., Vincus, A., Ennett, S., Johnson, R., & Rohrbach, A. (2004). Reasons for teachers' adaptation of substance use prevention curricula in schools with non-white student populations. *Prevention Science, 5,* 61–67.

Rogers, M. M., Peoples-Sheps, M. D., & Sorenson, J. R. (1995). Translating research into MCH service: Comparison of a pilot project and a large-scale resource mothers program. *Public Health Reports, 110*(5), 563–569; discussion 562.

Rogers, E. M. (1995). *Diffusion of innovations* (4th ed.). New York, NY: Free Press.

Rogers, E. M. (2003). *Diffusion of innovations* (5th ed.). New York, NY: Free Press.

Rohrbach, L. A., Graham, J. W., Hansen, & W. B. (1993). Diffusion of a school-based substance abuse prevention program: Predictors of program implementation. *Preventive Medicine, 22*, 237–260.

Rotheram-Borus, M. J., Swendeman, D., & Chovnick, G. (2009). The past, present, and future of HIV prevention: Integrating behavioral, biomedical, and structural intervention strategies for the next generation of HIV prevention. *Annual Review of Clinical Psychology, 5*, 143–167.

Rubenstein, L. V., Mittman, B. S., Yano, E. M., & Mulrow, C. D. (2000). From understanding health care provider behavior to improving health care: The QUERI framework for quality improvement. Quality Enhancement Research Initiative. *Medical Care, 38*(6, Suppl. 1), 1129–1141.

Sales, A., Smith, J., Curran, G., & Kochevar, L. 2006). Models, strategies, and tools: Theory in implementing evidence-based findings into health care practice. *Journal of General Internal Medicine, 21*(Suppl. 2), S43–S59.

Scheirer, M. A., & Dearing, J. W. (2011). An agenda for research on the sustainability of public health programs. *American Journal of Public Health, 101*, 2059–2067.

Song, M. K., Happ, M. B., & Sandelowski, M. (2010). Development of a tool to assess fidelity to a psycho-educational intervention. *Journal of Advanced Nursing, 66*(3), 673–682.

Spoth, R., Guyll, M., Trudeau, L., & Goldberg-Lillehoj, C. (2002). Two studies of proximal outcomes and implementation quality of universal preventive interventions in a community-university collaboration context. *Journal of Community Psychology, 30*, 499–518.

Stanton, B., Deveaux, L., Lunn, S., Yu, S., Brathwaite, N., Li, X., ... Marshall, S. (2009). The Condom Use Skills Checklist (CUSC): A proxy for assessing condom use skills when direct observation is not possible. *Journal of Health, Population and Nutrition, 27*, 406–13.

Stanton, B., Guo, J, Cottrell, L., Galbraith, J., Li, X., Gibson, C., ... Harris, C. (2005). The complex business of adapting effective interventions to new populations: An urban to rural transfer. *Journal of Adolescent Health, 37*(163), e17–163.e26.

Stirman, S. W., Kimberly, J., Cook, N., Calloway, A., Castro, F., & Charns, M. (2012). The sustainability of new programs and innovations: A review of the empirical literature and recommendations for future research. *Implementation Science, 7*, 17.

Wandersman, A., Morrissey, E., Davino, K., Seybolt, D., Crusto, C., Nation, M., ... Imm, P. (1988). Comprehensive quality programming and accountability: Eight essential strategies for implementing successful prevention programs. *Journal of Primary Prevention, 19*, 3–30.

Warren, C., & Liamba, W. (2004). *Safe motherhood demonstration, Western Province: Approaches to providing quality maternal care in Kenya*. Nairobi: Population Council.

Wingood, G. M., & DiClemente, R. J. (2008). The ADAPT-ITT model: A novel method of adapting evidence-based HIV interventions. *Journal of Acquired Immune Deficiency Syndromes, 47*(Suppl. 1), S40–S46.

Zacarías, F., Díaz, A., Peña, M., Jiménez, A. P., Martínez, L. & Tambini, G. (2016). Health Promotion in Families and Communities: An Integrated Approach from Latin America and the Caribbean. In R. S. Zimmerman (Ed.), R. J. DiClemente (Ed.), J. K. Andrus (Ed.), E. N. Hosein (Ed.), Society for Public Health Education (SOPHE). *Introduction to Global Health Promotion.* Somerset, NJ: Jossey-Bass.

Zerhouni, E. (2006a). Clinical research at a crossroads: The NIH roadmap. *Journal of Investigative Medicine, 54*(4), 171–173.

Zerhouni, E. (2006b). Translational research moving discovery to practice. *Clinical Pharmacology & Therapeutics, 81,* 126–128.

Zimmerman, G. L., Olsen, C. G., & Bosworth, M. F. (2000). A "stages of change" approach to helping patients change behavior. *American Family Physician, 61,* 1409–1416.

CHAPTER 18

HEALTH PROMOTION IN THE GLOBAL SETTING

The Role of International Organizations and Governments

John (Jack) Bryant and F. Curtiss Swezy

As we enter the 21st century the nature of global health threats is changing. At the end of World War II the preponderance of morbidity and mortality in less developed areas of the world were still largely attributable to diarrhea, pneumonia, and vaccine-preventable diseases. Vector-borne malaria was a significant cause of death, as was tuberculosis, which responded poorly to the vaccine BCG.

There are countries that continue to have high death rates and low **life expectancy at birth** (LEB). Many countries have seen measures such as child mortality drop below 65 and LEB rise above 60 years of age. However, the magic bullets of oral rehydration therapy (ORT), expanded programs in immunization (EPI), and antibiotics for such diseases as acute respiratory infection (ARI) no longer protect from the new assaults on human health, specifically noncommunicable diseases (NCDs). Increased client participation is now required to address such an issue as obesity. Poverty is clearly a factor in overcalorie malnutrition, including physical and financial access to healthy foods. But so is knowledge and personal action. There is a growing recognition that injury has always been a health problem in both developed and developing countries. But there is no immunization to prevent child drowning, and it will take a great deal more than spooning some ORS into an infant to slow and reverse injuries and deaths from drowning or adults from road traffic injuries (RTIs).

With common vector-borne diseases such as malaria and dengue fever, mosquitoes are becoming more resistant to insecticides and the infectious agents are adjusting to drug therapies. Therefore, clients themselves will have to become much more engaged, including proper use of bednets and careful, selective spraying of house walls against mosquitoes. Infected individuals will have to use antimalarial therapies correctly and persistently.

LEARNING OBJECTIVES

By the end of this chapter, the reader should be able to:

- Understand the history of global health organizations in the evolution of global health and their key contributions to health promotion
- Appreciate how health promotion has moved from passive to active client participation
- Explain the shift after World War II to improving the status of health in resource-poor nations around the world
- Understand the key role of global health organizations in the post–World War II period on the evolution of health promotion

A large number of preventive health interventions initially required **passive health behaviors**, that is, the intervention was done for recipient individuals and populations requiring little or no behavior change. As more complex health conditions have been addressed, there has been an increasing need for **active health behaviors** on the part of individuals and communities to promote and improve their health. Active behavior change is always more difficult to achieve.

Huge gains in the reduction of disease and improvement in the status of health have been accomplished by institutional changes. One of the first and perhaps most famous was John Snow's successful petition to have the handle removed from the Bank Street well pump and the London cholera epidemic of 1854 was stopped (Aschengrau & Seage, 2008).

Joseph Goldberger initiated research that led to the discovery that the "infectious" disease pellagra is caused by a deficiency of niacin in the diet. In the United States niacin is added to flour by law, and pellagra is nonexistent. In each of these instances, participation by the clients is passive. Individuals need do nothing, nor even fully appreciate that the water has been cleaned and the niacin added to the bread for them.

The growing health issues we face on a global scale are going to require the active participation of the beneficiaries. This makes imperative an effective new approach to health promotion. Cessation of smoking is one of the single biggest health promotion actions we can take. Nicotine is addictive. There is some research that implies that sugar may be similarly addictive. Although changes in the law could raise the price of cigarettes and lower the content of sugar, once brain changes have occurred in the individual there is no pill to stop the cravings.

Proactive participation in health is not limited to individuals. History is replete with examples of health failures due to lack of political will. This runs the gamut from addressing outbreaks of cholera to providing comprehensive reproductive health services so that couples can have the number of children they want when they want them, creating a world free of unwanted pregnancies.

Collective and proactive participation will be required to protect the environment, including eliminating water and air pollution, and to address anthropogenic (human-caused) changes in climate. As developing countries move up the economic ladder, individual citizens will want to drive cars, as their role models in developed countries have been doing for a century. But cars fueled by hydrocarbons pollute the air. A current initiative is to harvest "clean" hydrocarbons in the form of methane through a process of hydrofracturing (fracking). This mining technique clearly fouls adjacent water sources. Similarly, megadams are viewed as an alternative to burning hydrocarbons for fuel. But the physical alterations to the topography and impact on human and wildlife populations mean these sources of clean energy come at a higher price than advertised.

Health promotion will be effective in the 21st century only if it is implemented proactively. And this participation must take place at the individual, community, national, and international levels. This chapter adds a roadmap for this new, proactive health promotion to our continuing quest to improve health around the world by governments and international health organizations.

Early Vestiges of Health Promotion

Health promotion in the international setting began as a defensive mechanism by wealthy trader nations during the earliest colonial periods. Health protection was needed for the Western adventurers and soldiers who traveled to remote areas of the world. Specifically, there was great concern about importing cholera from the Indian subcontinent into Europe and yellow fever into the United States. Eventually, this protection for Western travelers slowed the transmission of communicable diseases to Europe and North America from the less developed regions of the world.

International health (**global health** as we know it today) began as a component of the expansion of wealthy European nations into the technologically and economically less developed areas of the globe from the 15th to the 20th centuries. This expansion was fueled by the United Kingdom, Spain, Portugal, the Netherlands, and France. By the 19th century Russia had gotten in on the action, and the expansion extended as far as what is now the West Coast of the United States. Less ambitious initiatives were also undertaken by Germany, Italy, and Belgium, to name a few.

The three main players of colonialist expeditions were soldiers, bureaucrats, and clergy. Some entourages included adventurers, soldiers of fortune, and indentured servants. The initial forays were to stake out territory for the European host country. In most instances, Christianity, favored by the European powers, was integrally a part of the mission. These expeditions were expected to take territory, by force if necessary, convert the local populations to Christianity, and return wealth—preferably gold—to the home country. Medical practitioners on these expeditions were included to take care of the European members of the expeditionary force.

East–West trade from the Indian subcontinent was frequently accompanied by the importation of cholera to Europe. The science of the day could not explain why some infectious diseases seemingly spread between groups of people. In the 19th century there were thought to be two categories of disease: the **contagionists,** diseases that spread when people were in proximity to each other, and the **noncontagionists,** diseases that were linked to the environment. The former are now known as infectious diseases, and the latter environmental health. (Malaria was literally "bad air," because intuitively the natural scientists of the day could correlate "bad night air" with malaria.)

Many ships from India arrived with the majority of their crews stricken with cholera. When large numbers of pilgrims traveled from India to Arabia for the annual *hajj,* cholera accompanied these travelers.

In 1854 the Italian physician and researcher, Filippo Pacini, published an article on the vibrio cholera. Pacini was one of the first to subscribe to germ theory. In the same year, John Snow, through his brilliant epidemiological investigation, drew a correlation between cholera and water in the London epidemic of that year. Neither was aware of the other's work for a number of years.

International Sanitary Conferences

While these trading nations were aggressively independent, they clearly recognized that disease is not stopped by international boundaries. This gave rise to the recognition that collective action by multiple nations was needed to address the problems. Thus was born the idea of having multinational conferences to address international health issues.

Europe

The political and commercial leadership of Europe decided that something had to be done about the importation of contagionist diseases onto the continent, particularly from India. At the urging primarily of the French, the first international sanitary conference was convened among the principle trading nations of Europe in Paris in 1851.

The participants agreed that diseases cross international boundaries. But attempts to implement quarantine regulations were lost in debates about contagonist and noncontagionist transmission of disease. Britain, which had a large investment in shipping from India to Europe, was opposed to quarantines.

The fourth sanitary conference convened in Vienna was called for by Russia, which was concerned about quarantines interfering with its trade in the Bospherous. Out of this meeting came one durable precedent: in matters of international health, each country had an equal voice: "One country, one vote."

The Americas

In parallel a series of international health conferences were held in South America to address cross-border disease transmission. The United States became involved in 1881 when it hosted an international sanitary conference in Washington, D.C., the first that included representatives from both Europe and the Americas. The intent was to persuade European countries to agree that US Foreign Service officers could inspect ships in their home ports before departing for the United States. The European countries were not about to agree to this. A committee was formed to study the "American" disease of yellow fever, waves of which had periodically swept into the United States from South America. (Yellow fever probably originated in Africa and may well have been transmitted to the Americas during the early slave trade. There continue to be outbreaks of the disease on both continents.)

The Pan American Sanitary Bureau

An international health meeting of American states was convened in Mexico City in 1901–1902. This led to an Inter-American Sanitary Conference in Washington later in 1902. These two meetings launched the first multinational health secretariat, the Pan American Sanitary Bureau. The United States wanted to control the organization and agreed to fund the secretariat in Washington. For a number of years the US Surgeon General was simultaneously the director general of the Sanitary Bureau (the name later changed to the **Pan American Health Organization** [PAHO]).

It was the first time that a group of nations had come together to address the transnational nature of disease transmission.

> While a permanent international health office had been proposed not only at the Washington conference of 1881, but also at the fourth International Sanitary Conference in Vienna in 1874, it was the American States that had independently taken the initiative of creating such an agency, if on a regional rather than a universal basis. *World Health Reports,* December 1972. (Howard-Jones, 1972)

Paris: Office International d'Hygiene Publique

In Europe, the succession of international health meetings led to the establishment of the ***Office International d'Hygiene Publique*** (OHIP, or simply the Paris office) in Paris in 1907. Although two multinational secretariats were established at the beginning of the 20th century, neither was global in its mandate or reached the concept of working universally on international health problems.

The establishment of these two secretariats, the Paris Office and the Pan American Sanitary Bureau, were not primarily focused on improving health in the very poor areas of the world with high incidence rates of infectious disease. The offices had been established in Paris and Washington primarily to keep infectious diseases out of Europe and the United States. As germ theory became more established, quarantine became the first line of defense. But these were defensive mechanisms on the part of the wealthy nations of the world; improving health in the poor nations of the world was not the focus.

Geneva

At the conclusion of World War I under the leadership of US President Woodrow Wilson, the framework for an idealistic world organization, the **League of Nations**, was drawn up. A specific provision was included to address international health issues. Agreement was reached to headquarter the new health organization in Geneva. The intent was to absorb the Paris office into this new health structure. Ironically, a conservative US Senate refused to ratify the agreement, and the United States was left out of the League of Nations and the Geneva office of international health. France protested having the Paris office subsumed by the new Geneva office. Faced with not being able to participate in international health on the European continent, the United States switched positions and supported keeping the Paris office in parallel with the Geneva office. As a result, in the years between World War I and World War II there were three international health offices, the Paris office, the Geneva office, and the Pan American Sanitary Bureau in Washington. On an informal basis, the health professionals of the three agencies cooperated and coordinated their efforts to understand and combat transnational disease transmission. But the focus continued to be on keeping communicable disease out of Europe and the United States, not aggressively addressing health issues in the poorest, predominantly tropical countries of the world.

Post–World War II Evolution

At the conclusion of World War II, international health was again recognized as an important international issue with implications for promoting peace. Under the auspices of the UN, an independent agency was created: the **World Health Organization** (WHO) to address international health.

World Health Organization

When the end of World War II was in sight, representatives of the Allied Powers, the coalition that ultimately won the war, began planning for another multilateral agency, the **United Nations**. Curiously, in the run-up to creating this new world organization no provision was made to address international health. At a planning meeting in San Francisco in 1945, this oversight was recognized and a meeting was planned for New York to address health only.

In New York there emerged a plan for the new World Health Organization (WHO). It was to be headquartered in Geneva and administratively would evolve from the Geneva office. The structure was based upon the Pan American Sanitary Bureau, with every member country belonging to the overall health assembly, the World Health Assembly, an executive committee that provided direct governance and oversight to operations, and a secretariat that implemented the policies of the World Health Assembly. As initiated by PAHO, members would be assessed to provide funds to operate the new secretariat. Harking back to the early international sanitary conferences, the precedent was continued of "one country, one vote" irrespective of a nation's population size or financial contribution.

An interesting procedure was instituted that although WHO was an entity under the United Nations, any country could join; a country did not have to be a member of the United Nations first to join WHO. The result was in the years following World War II, as country after country gained independence from former colonial regimes, they often joined WHO before applying for UN membership. This gave them a couple of years of experience working with a large, multilateral agency before joining the UN proper.

A delicate issue was what to do with the Pan American Sanitary Bureau, which preceded WHO and provided much of the organizational model for the new entity. After much discussion it was agreed that PAHO would be integrated, not merged into WHO. This meant they simultaneously retained their identity and also became the Regional Office for the Americas of WHO: AMRO. Because PAHO retained its funding mechanism of assessments, it is not dependent upon Geneva for an operating budget, and they have retained a degree of autonomy not enjoyed by any other regional office of WHO.

In fact, member countries of PAHO are double assessed, both for PAHO and WHO. But much of the money that is sent to Geneva is returned for program activities in the Americas. This arrangement continues to work satisfactorily to the present day.

The New York meeting also produced the iconic WHO statement of principles of health, a remarkably forward-looking declaration: "Health is a state of complete physical, mental and social well-being and not merely the absence of disease or infirmity."

The Run-Up to Community-Based Primary Health Care

More and more medical practitioners recognized that they were not reaching their potential public or maximizing health outcomes. Increasingly they recognized that treatment could not be top-down clinical services, but must include clients in their own health and address many preventable health maladies.

Medical Missionaries

From the earliest voyages of the colonialists from Europe to the economically underdeveloped continents of the world, clergy were an integral part of most every excursion. Converting indigenous populations to Christianity was often an overt goal. This was the case of the British in India, the French in Indochina, and the Spanish and Portuguese in South America. A melding of medical care and proselytizing grew where indigenous populations were encouraged to adopt "modern" ways and ideologies by providing them health care.

As medical science improved, particularly before the onset of World War I and accelerated between World War I and World War II, this gave rise to what could be termed the Albert Schweitzer Syndrome; medical missionaries who traveled to these undeveloped areas with the specific goal to treat local residents and improve their status of health. Sometimes the clerical role was stressed; in other instances it was less overt and under the mantle of "demonstrating (Christianity) by doing."

The model for these medical missionaries was fairly standard and reflected the worldview of the predominantly European practitioners. A medical facility was built and patients were encouraged to come and avail themselves of the usually free services. Higher-order staff, physicians, nurses, and other specialists were European. Host nationals were employed to provide support services for these facilities. Sick and injured patients were treated and then released back into the community. This conformed to the European model in which churches (and hospitals) were built and parishioners in the catchment areas were expected to attend.

At the conclusion of World War II, a group of largely Protestant medical missionaries gave a hard look at this Western model (McGilvray, 1965). Two meetings were convened at the German Institute for Health and Wellness in Tübingen, Germany, the first in 1964 and the follow-up meeting in 1967. The initial question was what to do with these Christian missionary hospitals in the newly emerging nations around the world. Although initiated with the best of intentions, the international staff of these hospitals were often condescending to the patients; a "good" patient was one who was completely subservient. Also, the costs of operating these facilities were a burden. Initially subsidized by home-country churches, more and more of the operating expenses were being transferred to the host country communities and governments, which they simply could not afford.

At the time of the Tübingen conferences, the Europeans and Americans estimated that the fixed-faculties model was capturing only about 20% of the population in the designated catchment areas. This meant that 80% of the target population was not served. And the figure of 20% served was probably an overestimate. Even with the best of intentions and the most optimistic assumptions, these church leaders concluded the existing model was not working.

In 1968 the Protestant **World Council of Churches** (WCC) created the **Christian Medical Commission** (CMC), headquartered in Geneva, to determine how to make the best use of Christian facilities around the developing world. In their estimation, "by 1910 there were 2100 hospitals and twice that many clinics operated by mission agencies of the Protestant Church alone" (McGilvray, 1965). The role was further complicated by the frequent resentment in newly emerging countries of the missionary–colonial nexus that had created these facilities.

By this time the World Health Organization, also in Geneva, had become operational around the world. Although the wealthy nations of primarily Europe and the United States funded most of the operations, under the policy of one country, one vote, the focus of the World Health Assembly shifted to improving health in the poorest countries of the world with the highest rates of morbidity and mortality. They wanted practical models that worked in poor countries.

In discussions between WHO and the WCC in Geneva, the then-director general of WHO, Dr. Halftan Mahler, charged WCC with providing examples of health programs in poor countries with demonstrable impact on the status of health. WCC came up with three model working programs from the more than 1,000-plus medical missionary programs around the world.

Three Model Programs

The World Council of Churches identified three prototype programs that implemented their field programs in the manner of the new primary health care paradigm. They operated in three geographic regions of the developing world.

Central Java

Dr. Gunawan Nugroho and his wife started a health program in 1963 in Indonesia. Because poverty limited patient access to the program's services, they created a "health fund" so that everyone could receive treatment, and worked to increase family income by expanding chicken and goat farming.

Jamkhed, India

Another husband-and-wife team, Rajanikant and Mabelle Arole, developed a health program in the early 1970s based upon community decision making. They established a viable and effective health care system that involved the community, was planned at the grassroots, used local resources to solve local health problems, and provided total health care, not fragmented services.

Chimaltenango, Guatemala

Dr. Carroll Behrhorst, an American, trained community health promoters and included such activities as literacy, family planning, and agricultural extension in his broad-based program.

These programs all had some characteristics in common.

- They were community-client centered, not facility-provider oriented.
- Services went well beyond traditional health care. This included "non-health" activities to raise income.
- Emphasis was placed on prevention, not just treating disease once people became sick.
- Outreach was implemented into the community and even the individual home.

The change in focus that was occurring in WHO led to a seismic change in international health. No longer a captive of wealthy trading nations, WHO shifted its focus to the efficient improvement of the status of health in developing countries: "health for all by the year 2000." The launch of this new initiative was officially proclaimed at the WHO 1978 **Alma Ata Conference on Primary Health Care**.

Community-Based Primary Health Care

Some of the same WCC leaders worked with WHO to put together the first conference on **primary health care** sponsored by the WHO in the Central Asia provincial capital of Alma Ata. (Alma Ata was the Russian name for *Almaty,* the largest city in what is now the independent republic of Kazakhstan.) The concept of community-based primary health care has expanded and continues to be the guiding approach to global health (Perry, Freeman, Gupta, and Rassekh, 2009). This includes programs that are:

- community based;
- perhaps facilities based, but not facilities-centric: services reach out to and interface with the community;
- emphasize prevention, treatment, and education;
- respond to the perceived needs of the client, not the provider;
- minimize or eliminate barriers to care;
- maintain women/girl-children focus: women are the primary bearers of children and providers of family health care;

- focus on factors that directly and indirectly shape health:
  - sustained sufficient income;
  - education, including girl-children;
  - security;
  - protection from external stresses to health: air, water, natural disasters, and so on;
- provide service at the lowest level of technical competence;
- utilize community-based outreach workers, paid or unpaid, interfacing between the health system and the community.

Global Health Organizations

Many organizations, government, multigovernment (multilateral), and nongovernmental organizations (NGOs) have become engaged in global health. They have played very important roles in the evolution of health behaviors over the past half century.

Multilateral Organizations

World Health Organization Ottawa Conference, 1986

The first international health promotion conference was convened in Ottawa in 1986 (WHO, 1983). The meeting was a follow-up to the iconic WHO primary health care meeting in Almaty, Kazakhstan, in 1978. The result of the 1978 meeting was to promote "health for all by the year 2000." The Ottawa conference was intended to pursue specific activities toward accomplishing that goal.

Supported by WHO, Health and Welfare Canada, and the Canadian Public Health Association, representatives of 38 countries formulated a charter on promoting health throughout the world. Although it was based upon the evolution of health care in the economically developed world, it was envisioned as a roadmap for resource-poor countries as well. The components of health promotion were identified to include:

- building healthy public policy;
- creating supportive environments;
- strengthening community action;
- developing personal skills;
- reorienting health services toward prevention.

WHO ProLead

As WHO continued to advocate for health promotion, it focused on rallying community leadership in support of such efforts. Health programs have long been stymied by lack of political leadership within a given community or in nations as a whole. WHO evolved the **ProLead** program: **Health Promotion LEADership and Management Development**. This has led to community-wide health promotion activities in countries around the world. One example is ProLead in the city of Hue in central Vietnam, presented as Case Study 18.1 (Fawkes, Lin, and Chong, 2012).

CASE STUDY 18.1 PROLEAD HUE: VIETNAM

Civic and political leaders in the city of Hue in central Vietnam recognized that there was little involvement on the part of many health stakeholders within the greater Hue community. In a survey of city leaders, relevant agencies, and NGOs it was learned that only 3 of an identified 18 key stakeholders had a role in health promotion. Key reasons for this low involvement included a lack of knowledge about health or their involvement in health, low priority assigned to health among myriad responsibilities, gatekeepers who did not perceive their agency as a health stakeholder, and finally the lack of perceived opportunities to work together even when they were motivated to do so.

The program began with cooperating-country training for the Vietnamese. In the spring of 2006 a group of civic leaders from Hue made a site visit to Kuching City, Malaysia, where the municipal leadership had a model civic health promotion plan in operation. The guests met with members of the Kuching City Healthy City program and made site visits to the waste treatment plant, a "healthy market," a medical clinic, and a township housing project.

A delegation from Kuching City then made a reciprocal visit to Hue to meet with identified stakeholders in that city. This precipitated the creation of a Hue Healthy City Steering Committee under the direction of the senior vice chairman of the Hue City People's Committee, the equivalent of the deputy mayor. The steering committee developed and has continued to implement the Healthy City Action Plan. This case example serves as a model for developing broad recognition and involvement of stakeholders in resource-poor nations to improve political support, develop specific program actions, and efficiently coordinate across a wide range of governmental and community organizations to maximize the impact of health activities within the community. ProLead as a model has been disseminated to many other developing nations around the world.

Bilateral Programs

Every "Western" nation has a bilateral foreign aid program, and health is a prominent component of almost all of these. These national programs have wrestled with the tension of doing good for the people of the world who need it and leveraging political advantage for the donor country. A second tension is donor countries that are very self-conscious about "inventory shrinkage" of funds turned over directly to underdeveloped countries. Some countries maintain rigorous oversight and control over their donated funds; others are more open-ended in allowing host agencies to use the money within broad guidelines. There are some governments and donor organizations that maintain corruption indexes on recipient developing countries around the world.

Many bilateral programs fund both programs with individual countries (bilaterally), as well as contribute to multilateral efforts such as WHO. In the past two decades there have been some interesting trends. Some governments have elevated their foreign assistance programs within their overall government operations. The United Kingdom has moved to elevate the **Department for International Development** (DFID) to cabinet rank, in parallel with the foreign ministry. The **Japan International Cooperation Agency** (JICA) appears to be moving in the same direction, although it is not completely separate from the Ministry of Foreign Affairs at this writing. Since the 1960s the US government has had the **United States Agency for International Development** (USAID) as a semiautonomous agency separate from the Department of State. Recent changes hint at USAID being absorbed more directly into the State Department, with more focus on political leverage for programs they conduct in the field, including a vigorous global health program.

Under President Barack Obama, a Global Health Initiative is being implemented according to the principles of community-based primary health care. As an example, the funds that were originally targeted for **antiretroviral drugs** (ARVs) in the HIV/AIDS program initiated by President George W. Bush, the **President's Emergency Plan for AIDS Relief** (PEPFAR), now are being utilized for capacity building within host country ministries of health, including complementary maternal and child health interventions.

Foundations

A number of foundations have made important contributions to global health. This support ranges from sponsoring graduate education of health professionals to research, service delivery, and program strengthening. Funding can be simply within the foundation, for programs in the field, or financial support to host country programs.

Early in the 20th century, before the wealthy Western nations began to assist developing countries in any meaningful way, private nonprofit foundations began to work in international health. Very wealthy industrialists provided funds for these organizations, and the precedents for supporting global health were begun. Much of the rationale for the shift from defensive international health to proactive global health evolved within these foundations.

The Rockefeller Foundation

One of the earliest to become involved in global health was the Rockefeller Foundation.

In the period after World War II, a number of former colonial territories became independent nations and faced the necessity of providing their populations with the social, economic, and educational advantages enjoyed by the affluent nations. Many of these nations embarked on the development of full-scale medical and nursing schools patterned after Western institutions. With their limited financial and educational resources, such schools could expect at best only a trickle of fully qualified physicians and nurses over the ensuing few decades to serve the needs of millions of sick people. In another approach, reliance was placed on the training and use of a variety of subprofessional personnel, without a clear definition of their capabilities or of the responsibilities that their training equipped them to assume on the medical team.

Understandably, the emerging nations turned to the more technically advanced countries for guidance and support. These countries, unfortunately, were better prepared to tell how they managed at home than to explain how a new country, within a given budget, could best prepare medical personnel in significant numbers in a reasonable period of time to serve the major needs of its people. Indeed, the affluent nations are currently facing the same problem on a larger scale. There clearly was a need for a study to provide guidelines for the architects of medical systems for the developing countries and to serve as a reference, at least, for their political leaders to use in making judgments of how best to spend their limited resources.

The Rockefeller Foundation, in cooperation with the USAID, in the spring of 1964 convened a distinguished advisory committee from several countries and agencies to plan and guide such a study. This committee sought out a team of experts who would visit a sample of developing countries and describe the health problems, the systems for meeting the problems, and the type and effectiveness of the training programs for medical personnel. The result was published in a book entitled *Health and the Developing World* (1960), with John Bryant, MD, a team member, as the author.

The Ford Foundation

The Ford Foundation of the United States funds some of its own staff and programs in developing countries. But they also support host country initiatives and such things as jointly conducted research. Case Study 18.2 presents an example of the foundation's health promotion.

CASE STUDY 18.2 FORD FOUNDATION HEALTH PROMOTION: HO CHI MINH CITY

The Ford Foundation both implements projects in resource-poor countries and funds other organizations to do development work. The foundation was one of the pioneer organizations to support reproductive health programs in the emerging nations of the world after World War II.

Following that tradition, at the turn of the millennium they supported an operations research program in Vietnam to address the spread of HIV/AIDS in that country (Bao et al., 2003). Health promotion to change behavior and risk reduction related to this disease is always a challenge. The Ford Foundation focused on approaching employees in the workplace. They elicited good cooperation from employers. Ford selected a particularly challenging group of transient construction workers, primarily men, in the largest city in that country, Ho Chi Minh City (HCMC) to be the health promoters. These were mobile workers who moved from site to site as each construction project was completed. The majority of the workers were single or living away from their wives. A common practice was on Saturday night to work "the second shift," a visit to a Karaoke bar to drink, sing, and interact with sex workers.

In the best tradition of primary health care, two groups of health promoters were selected and trained for this project. The first group, health communicators (HCs), consisted of university students who were studying social work and were highly motivated to have a positive impact on the community. The second group, peer educators (PEs), was composed of construction workers themselves. Both groups of health promoters were trained in the technical aspects of HIV/AIDS, how to discuss these topics with construction workers, and provided supplies of condoms to distribute to anyone who wanted to accept them.

The project documented that behavior change was possible among this mobile, predominantly male group of workers. The biggest changes occurred at sites where fellow construction workers, PEs, did the health promotion. Some interesting observations were made. At first the university HCs were more knowledgeable about HIV/AIDS than were the construction worker PEs. But by the end of six months this distinction disappeared. Only about 15% of the construction workers were female, while almost half of the HCs were women. The female HCs did not relate well to the male construction workers and were regularly embarrassed by the subject matter. Turnover among this group was high.

The male PEs had better responses from their peers. This was due to such factors as student HCs not being allowed on construction sites because of safety concerns and that men speaking with their peers could be more open in their discussions. An interesting result was as PEs moved to new sites they continued to provide peer education and motivation at their new sites. As the numbers of their fellow workers they interacted with expanded, there was a need to train additional construction PEs to meet the additional target audiences.

Behavior did change. Increasing numbers of construction workers reported using condoms when consorting with non-wives. Overall, the cost of using PEs was cheaper than the university HCs. In the highly sensitive area of sexual behavior and risk avoidance, this peer-to-peer health promotion works even when requiring dramatic active behavior change on the part of the target audience.

The Gates Foundation

One of the most active players in global health is the Bill & Melinda Gates Foundation. They have brought unprecedented resources to programs in developing countries with annual grant payments in excess of $3 billion, more than some donor country's bilateral programs.

In an effort to stimulate innovative health promotion, the Gates Foundation has developed funding streams that encourage higher-risk programs, recognizing that some of these will fail. Their Grand Challenges Explorations encourages bold new approaches by groups and individuals who have not participated in global health before. This should encourage thinking of new ways to implement health promotion in the future.

Nongovernmental Organizations

Nonprofit organizations established in wealthy countries have long promoted health in the developing world. Initially, many of these could be categorized as FBOs, **faith-based organizations**. Albert Schweitzer went to Africa as a representative of the Society of the Evangelist Missions of Paris. In the period after World War II, secular NGOs burgeoned and greatly expanded health programs around the world. Initially, these organizations raised their own funds to support their overseas activities. In an interesting evolution, bilateral government programs now fund many of these NGOs, calling into question how distinct their programs are and can be from sponsoring government agency policies.

An interesting expansion of US government funding of FBOs occurred during the George W. Bush administration, when a large number of FBOs were financed to expand service programs related to HIV/AIDS, particularly in sub-Saharan Africa. PEPFAR is credited with providing antiretroviral drugs to almost 10 million people, with much of this distribution provided by FBOs.

NGOs have further advanced the primary health care methodology to global health, frequently working in individual communities or smaller regional programs within developing countries. Typically, these programs have a small number of expatriates on site to plan and manage the programs. Host country nationals in the employ of the NGO provide many of the services. Critics have pointed out that these programs tend to be expensive; salary and support for expatriates is high. And frequently these programs make high-end expenditures on support costs such as housing and four-wheel-drive vehicles, which appear ostentatious compared to common modes of housing and transportation in developing countries. A repeated complaint of NGOs is that host country government and counterpart organizations regularly attempt to leverage funds for nonessential activities and fees.

Nonetheless, the bottom line is that NGOs, supported by fundraising or government contracts, have made a very large impact in raising the level of services, supplies, professional training, and community awareness and participation in internationally funded global health programs. Case Study 18.3 provides an example from Bangladesh.

CASE STUDY 18.3 TASC INJURY RESEARCH: BANGLADESH

The Alliance for Safe Children (TASC) is a nonsectarian NGO created by the former US ambassador to Vietnam, Douglas "Pete" Peterson. He became focused on the issue of child injury while serving in Vietnam. His foundation has done research documenting the breadth of morbidity and mortality from injury in several countries of Southeast Asia (Linnan et al., 2007).

In Bangladesh TASC has worked with the Institute of Child and Mother Health (ICMH; 2003), Director General of Health Services (DGHS) of Bangladesh to assess what children (under-fives) die from. They have done this by conducting large-scale community surveys. Faculty and students from Bangladesh institutions traveled to the research areas and conducted community surveys. Survivors of child deaths, usually caretakers and close relatives, were interviewed to provide verbal autopsies. Bangla field researchers were facile in languages and even regional dialects when gathering this information. The Institute of Child and Mother Health processed and analyzed the data. This furthered the movement over the past few decades to involve host country organizations in the operational aspects of survey research, assessment, and policy recommendations.

The conclusions are that

- drowning is the single largest cause of child death in Bangladesh;
- most occur in the monsoon season;
- the largest number are children ages one to two;
- the deaths occur mostly between 9:00 am and noon; and
- they occur when the mother is busy with housework.

Health promotion recommendations include:

- creating community crèches, where two or more adults watch a group of children
- erect fences around bodies of water (fish ponds), and teach children survival swimming as young as possible.

These results are now being shared with a wide swath of countries around the world.

Private Sector

For-profit companies are involved in global health in many ways. In straightforward business terms, many pharmaceutical companies manufacture and sell drugs to treat diseases in developing countries. ARVs are used both prophylactically and as an inhibitor to HIV/AIDS death. More recently, governments have teamed with private sector firms in a number of ways. This has included subsidized research for drugs to treat diseases prominent in poor, often tropical countries. These "orphan drugs" are generally not commercially viable.

Other partnerships have used commercial distribution systems (e.g., for soft drinks) to distribute health commodities such as condoms and contraceptive pills.

Information technology is being incorporated into global health programs by host governments, NGOs, and commercial firms. This includes leapfrogging landline telephones and going directly to mobile phones. It is much easier and cheaper for developing countries to install towers than to hard-wire entire nations. Health program directors are using the technology for things like reminding clients to take daily pharmaceuticals, setting schedules for immunizations, and in-service training of community health workers. Each month a new message can be sent in patient care, service delivery, and clinical techniques. These small bites of information constitute an ongoing in-service training for medical staff (Campbell et al., 2014). Additional research is needed to verify which forms of telephonic and instant messaging communication are the most efficacious for various health promotion needs, but movement to adopt this technology in resource-poor countries is very clear.

Universities

The Education of the Physician

The story is told with depressing frequency of the young physician, trained in excellence in the university hospital, who is virtually inadequate in the rural setting. She fails to see the greater challenge of the surrounding communities waiting for her insight, skill, and leadership. What is missing from this style of medical education that has been developed in the more affluent nations? What is the young physician not learning that is essential to the work her host country needs done?

First, the system of health care in which the physician works may require areas of competence that are radically different from those he has learned in the university hospital. For example, he may have to evaluate the health needs of a community and lead a team in the development of a comprehensive health program.

Perhaps his greatest deficiency is in handling the quantity of problems of health care: the large number of people scattered over many miles in many communities, the great variety of problems and obstacles, and the limited resources. Dealing with these issues involves responsibilities, skills, concepts, decisions, and even ethical and moral problems that are vastly different from those exercised in the university hospital. At the center of those differences is the physician's responsibility for all the people of an area rather than for individual patients. Indeed, his primary job is to improve the health of the entire population rather than taking care of people one at a time. He will still have individuals to care for, but it will be against the backdrop of his concern for the larger number. He must continually choose among the many things that need to be done, guided by a sense of cost and benefit in order to use his scarce resources well. His effectiveness will depend largely on how well he works through others who have less training and less understanding of health processes. And program results must often be measured in terms of statistical rather than individual change.

The role of the physician in the university-style hospital and that of the physician in the rural setting are both essential in the spectrum of health care, but we must not underestimate the distance between the two. Neither can we assume that a good education for one is an adequate education for the other. For a recently graduated physician, the transition from one to the other can be shattering. It is in not recognizing the magnitude of the transition and in not approaching its importance that the basis for the failure of universities to provide an adequate education for health personnel largely lies.

Relevance Versus Rigorous Scholarship

There are some who see an involvement of the university in questions of national need as a distraction from the mainstream of academic medicine, from the high standard of patient care and the clinical and laboratory research that can be pursued in the medical school and the university hospital. They see in it a danger of overextending academic resources that are already too thin.

The central question is, "Can a university develop a strong academic setting in which there is a premium on scholarship, creativity, and high standards of performance and at the same time develop programs directed toward understanding and meeting national need?" Which leads us to ask, "What are the purposes of a university and what does it prize as the objects of scholarship and teaching?" Here we argue that the problems of providing health care to large numbers of people on limited resources is a legitimate object of academic concern and that finding solutions to those problems will require sophisticated and rigorous research. For those concerned about having the university and its students involved in a low standard of medical care, we argue that the quality of the enterprise should be judged more by what is accomplished considering the limitations of resources than by using the university hospital as a standard. There is a need to look again at the concept of excellence and the meaning universities attach to it. We see a dilemma. If, on the one hand, the university turns away from an involvement in the community in favor of pursuing scholarship within its own walls, its scholarly successes will only distantly benefit the nation and its people. If, on the other hand, the university forsakes scholarship in favor of a frontal attack on the surface problems of the community, it risks losing the intellectual strength and creativity needed to untie the deeply complex knots of community need. Here we suggest that the rising challenge to universities, indeed the future course of universities, lies in resolving this dilemma, not by choosing one course over the other, but by finding how to couple the two in a philosophy of university action.

Summary

Health promotion has always been important in the global setting. From the days of the earliest explorers traveling to exotic areas, such as East Asia and Africa, concern for disease has always been a paramount priority. As the science of disease improved, the response to health and health promotion adjusted accordingly.

In the mid-19th century concern for diseases coming into Europe and the United States precipitated a series of international health conferences to address these problems. Sovereign countries recognized that diseases do not respect international boundaries and were compelled to find trans-border—international—solutions. This resulted in the creation of a secretariat for health, the Pan American Sanitary Bureau in Washington, D.C., at the start of the 20th century, followed shortly by the Paris office for the Nations of Europe.

At the end of World War II global health expanded exponentially through the establishment of the World Health Organization. This led to four health promotion shifts: curative services changing their focus to preventive health, service in fixed facilities shifting to community outreach, "passive" to "active" health promotion and behavior change, and the addition of "non-health" interventions.

KEY TERMS

1. **Active health behaviors:** Activities that require behavior change on the part of the individual: exercise, smoking cessation, getting enough sleep
2. **Alma Ata International Conference on Primary Health Care:** WHO conference to promote primary health care, particularly in resource poor areas of the world; provided the iconic challenge, "Health for all by the year 2000"
3. **Antiretroviral drugs (ARVs):** Drugs used most prominently in the treatment of patients who are HIV/AIDS-positive
4. **Christian Medical Commission:** A collective of Christian denominations created in 1968 by the World Council of Churches to promote global health
5. **Contagionists:** Scientists who believed diseases spread when people were in proximity to each other; now understood to be infectious diseases
6. **Department for International Development (DFID):** The bilateral foreign aid agency of the United Kingdom; health, including water and sanitation, are priority programs
7. **Faith-based organizations (FBOs):** A subset of NGOs, some of the first Western organizations to provide health care in resource-poor regions of the world
8. **Global health:** A synonym for *international health,* expanded to include health in both developing and developed nations, depending upon the individual author
9. **Health Promotion LEADership and Management Development (WHO ProLead):** A World Health Organization program that rallies political support of and community participation in health promotion
10. **International health:** Health programs focused on improving health in developing regions of the world now generally referred to as Global Health
11. **International sanitary conferences:** A series of meetings held in parallel in Europe and the Americas to address diseases that were crossing international boundaries
12. **Japan International Cooperation Agency (JICA):** The bilateral foreign aid agency of Japan, with emphasis on maternal and child health, infectious disease control, and strengthening health systems
13. **League of Nations:** Intergovernmental organization formed at the end of World War I with the goal of promoting world peace; the United States did not join

14. **League of Nations Health Organization:** International health secretariat established in Geneva in 1920
15. **Life expectancy at birth (LEB):** The number of years a newborn infant would live if prevailing patterns of mortality at the time of its birth were to stay the same throughout its life
16. **Noncontagionists:** Scientists who believed diseases were thought to be linked to the environment; now known as environmental health
17. **Nongovernmental organizations (NGOs):** Nonprofit organizations that have played a pivotal role in expanding health services to developing countries, often predating government-sponsored bilateral programs
18. ***Office International d'Hygiene Publique*:** The first international health office for Europe, established in Paris in 1907
19. **Pan American Health Organization (PAHO):** Originally the Pan American Sanitary Bureau, the first multinational health agency focused on the Americas, established in Washington, D.C., in 1903
20. **Passive health behaviors:** Activities that require no behavior change by individuals; clean water provided by the municipality, niacin added to flour, air bags installed in autos
21. **President's Emergency Plan for AIDS Relief (PEPFAR):** A program initiated by President George W. Bush to provide antiretroviral drugs to HIV-positive clients, particularly in sub-Saharan Africa
22. **Primary health care:** Sometimes referred to as *community-based primary health care*, health care focused on the patient, rather than the provider with emphasis on prevention
23. **The Alliance for Safe Children (TASC):** A nongovernmental organization that focuses on child injury; has conducted research and implemented program interventions in several South and Southeast Asian countries
24. **United Nations (UN):** Successor to the League of Nations, created at the conclusion of World War II
25. **United States Agency for International Development (USAID):** The bilateral foreign aid agency for the United States; a semiautonomous agency under the Department of State
26. **World Council of Churches (WCC):** An international collective of Protestant denominations interested in fostering ecumenism formed in 1948; in 1968 created the World Medical Commission headquartered in Geneva specifically to promote global health by Christian missionaries
27. **World Health Assembly:** The policy-setting body of the World Health Organization; members represented on the premise of "one country, one vote"

28. **World Health Organization (WHO):** The preeminent multinational organization in global health; a specialized agency of the United Nations headquartered in Geneva; successor to the League of Nations Health Organization
29. **World Health Organization Ottawa Conference, 1986:** The first international conference to address health promotion, particularly in resource poor nations

REVIEW QUESTIONS

1. In the 19th century, what infectious (contagionist) disease concerned the political and business leadership of Europe?
2. In the 19th century, what infectious (contagionist) disease concerned the US government?
3. In the 18th and 19th centuries, was international health designed to primarily improve health in poor areas of the world or protect wealthy nations?
4. What is the worldwide global health organization? In what city is the headquarters located?
5. Do member countries of WHO have proportionate representation based upon the amount of money they contribute to the global health organization?
6. In what city was the inaugural WHO conference on health behaviors? In what year?
7. What are passive and active health behaviors?
8. For most noncommunicable diseases, are active or passive health behaviors generally required to address the issue?
9. What are four types of organizations that are currently engaged in global health promotion?

References

Aschengrau, A. and Seage, G.R. (2008). *Essentials of epidemiology in public health.* Boston, MA: Jones and Bartlett.

Bao, Y. V., Guest, P., Pulerwitz, J., Thuy, J. Thao, L., Dinh, D. X., ... Levin, A. (2003). *Expanding workplace HIV prevention programs for a highly mobile population in Ho Chi Minh City.* Horizons Research Summary. Washington, DC: Population Council.

Bryant, J. (1960). *Health in the developing world.* Ithaca, NY: Cornell University Press.

Campbell, N., Schiffer, E., Buxbaum, A., McLean, E., Perry, C., & Sullivan, T. M. (2014). Taking knowledge for health the extra mile: Participating evaluation of a mobile phone intervention for community health workers in Malawi. *Global Health Science and Practice, 2*(1), 1–2. Retrieved from http://dx.doi.org/10.9745/GHSP-D-14–00007

Fawkes, S., Lin, V., & Chong, S. (2012). *Evaluation of medium term outcomes of WHO ProLEAD program: Preliminary overview of results.* Melbourne: LaTrobe University.

Howard-Jones, N. (1972, December). Three score years and ten. *World Health Reports,* 3–7.

Institute of Child and Mother Health, Director General of Health Services, UNICEF Bangladesh, The Alliance for Safe Children, and the Centers for Disease Control. (2003). *Bangladesh Health and Injury Survey: Key findings on child injury.* Dhaka: UNICEF.

Linnan, M., Giersing, M., Cox, R., Linnan, H., Williams, M., Voumard, C. (2007). *Child mortality and injury in Asia: An overview.* Florence: UNICEF Innocenti Research Centre (No 2007-04).

McGilvray, J. C. (1965). *The quest for health and wholeness.* Tübingen: German Institute for Health and Wellness.

Perry, H., Freeman, P., Gupta, S., & Rassekh, B. M. (2009). *How effective is community-based primary health care in improving the health of children? A review of the evidence.* Retrieved from: http://www.comminit.com/early-child/content/how-effective-community-based-primary-health-care-improving-health-children

United States Agency for International Development. (2013). *USAID forward progress report.* Washington, DC: Author.

World Health Organization. (1983). *New approaches to health education in primary health care: Report of a WHO expert committee.* World Health Organization Technical Report Series 690. Geneva: Author.

CHAPTER 19

THE FUTURE OF GLOBAL HEALTH PROMOTION

Rick S. Zimmerman, Jon K. Andrus, and C. James Hospedales

For the first time in history, more people live in urban areas than in rural, and more people are overweight than underweight. For the first time, chronic diseases are killing more people than are infectious diseases. Of the 56 million global deaths in 2012, 38 million (68%) were due to chronic diseases (World Health Organization [WHO], 2014d). This is occurring while the world continues to suffer from the still substantial burden of infectious diseases like HIV, TB, malaria, vaccine-preventable diseases, and tropical neglected diseases.

The challenge for health promotion efforts is to recognize the multiple causes of poor health and integrate health promotion initiatives to mount a more coordinated, systematic, and effective public health response while going well beyond the health sector.

The purpose of this chapter is twofold: (1) to present data demonstrating the extent of progress that has been made as a result of global health promotion in the past 25 years and (2) to examine some of the key challenges that remain. Efforts to strengthen health promotion in the future must account for the rising epidemic of chronic disease driven by aging, economic development, and widespread risk factors while simultaneously tackling the unfinished agenda that infectious diseases impose on the health and well-being of people living in poverty, and at the same time maintaining the gains such as prevention and control of vaccine-preventable diseases. It should be noted that although not specifically discussed in this chapter, health promotion efforts will also be critically needed for substantially strengthening health systems that will allow for progress in all areas of health (see chapter 18 for a more detailed discussion of this area).

In this chapter, we review progress in global health promotion across the six WHO regions of the world and summarize some of the work that still needs to be done.

LEARNING OBJECTIVES

By the end of this chapter, the reader should be able to:

- **Know how successful public health has been in meeting the health-related millennial development goals globally and regionally**
- **Understand trends in risk factors for chronic diseases globally and regionally**
- **Identify parts of the world in which social determinants of health and illness, including poverty, female literacy, human rights, and corruption, still need the most work**
- **Identify two infectious diseases that continue to be a serious concern in the Americas**
- **Identify two neglected tropical diseases**
- **Explain the "all of society" approach to health**

Then we examine a number of broad issues relating to new global approaches to health promotion and large global challenges that will require progress not only in the health sector but throughout societies around the world to reducing morbidity and mortality.

Global and Regional Progress in Addressing Global Health Issues

In this section of the chapter we review the status of global health and the role of health promotion, and use one figure and two tables to summarize key data. Figure 19.1 presents brief labels and pictures corresponding to the eight millennial development goals. Table 19.1 presents progress toward the health-related **Millennium Development Goals** (MDGs) globally and in each of the six World Health Organization regions (United Nations, 2014). Table 19.2 presents progress in a variety of other areas, including social determinants of health, noncommunicable diseases and risk factors, oral health, mental health and substance abuse, and air pollution.

Progress in Meeting Health-Related Millennial Development Goals

As shown in Figure 19.1, the eight MDGs are related to (1) extreme hunger and poverty, (2) universal primary education, (3) gender equity, (4) child mortality, (5) maternal health, (6) HIV, malaria, and other diseases, (7) environmental sustainability, and (8) global partnership for development.

Table 19.1, using primarily 2012 World Health Organization data, presents the status of attainment for the four most health-related MDGs: child mortality; maternal health; HIV, malaria, and other diseases; and environmental

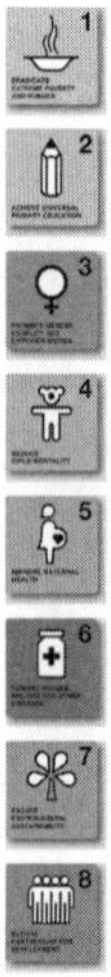

Goal 1: Eradicate Extreme Hunger and Poverty

Goal 2: Achieve Universal Primary Education

Goal 3: Promote Gender Equality and Empower Women

Goal 4: Reduce Child Mortality

Goal 5: Improve Maternal Health

Goal 6: Combat HIV/AIDS, Malaria, and Other Diseases

Goal 7: Ensure Environmental Sustainability

Goal 8: Develop a Global Partnership for Development

Figure 19.1 MDGs

sustainability. The under-five mortality rate has decreased by almost half (from 90 to 48 per 1,000 live births) between 1990 and 2012—though impressive, it does not quite meet the two-thirds reduction targeted as part of MGD goal number 4 (United Nations [UN], 2014). Developed regions almost met their target (reduction from 15 to 6 deaths per 1,000 live births), eastern Asia met its target (reduction from 53 to 14), Latin American and the Caribbean almost met its target (reduction from 54 to 19), and Northern Africa met its goal (reduction from 54 to 19). Sub-Saharan Africa, Southern Asia, Oceania, the Caucasus and Central Asia, Southeastern Asia, and Western Asia have not met or nearly met their goals. Enough success has been achieved throughout the six WHO regions that all regions are considered either on track or insufficient progress, but none "off track." Most of these deaths were from infectious diseases such as pneumonia, diarrhea, and malaria. Measles is another significant cause of death. (See chapter 8 to read more about progress in reducing maternal and infant mortality.) As shown in Table 19.1, significant improvements have been made in measles immunization, improving from 72% to 84% from 2000 to 2009, but stagnating since. Sub-Saharan Africa coverage has increased from 52% to 73% and in Southeast Asia from 61% to 78%, but additional work is needed to access children outside the reach of existing health services in those parts of the world. (See chapter 10 to learn more about vaccination campaigns.) Malnutrition is a significant risk factor for **neonatal deaths**, especially for those with infectious diseases in low-income countries. The best way to reduce neonatal mortality is through better maternal care during the first 24 hours after birth (see MDG 5 discussion, later in the chapter).

Three outcomes related to MDG goal number 5—maternal health—are presented next in Table 19.1. The ambitious goal of reducing the maternal mortality rate by 75% has not been met globally or in any region of the world. Globally the rate has decreased from 380 in 1990 to 210 maternal deaths/100,000 live births in 2013, a 45% reduction. Most regions and subregions have seen similar proportionate decreases, with reductions greater than 50% in Southern Asia, Oceania, Southeastern Asia, Northern Africa, and Eastern Asia. Access to health care solutions for complications (e.g., uterotonic commodities and magnesium sulphate to manage common complications such as bleeding during childbirth and pregnancy-related hypertension) need to be provided especially in vulnerable populations. Skilled birth attendants and contraceptive use and access to family planning are also important, and are the next two sets of data presented in Table 19.1. All areas of the world have increased the percentage of births attended by skilled health personnel from 57% to 72% globally, though Southeast Asia just barely meets the two-thirds target and the Africa and Eastern Mediterranean regions do not. Similarly, although the use of any method of contraception has increased from 52% to 63% between 1990 and 2012, the Africa and Eastern Mediterranean regions are far from meeting the goal of universal use or access (UN, 2014).

Health outcomes related to key infectious diseases are reflected in MDG goal 6. HIV incidence has declined by around 50% in developing regions of the world since 2001, largely due to the widespread introduction of antiretrovirals and continuing behavioral interventions in Africa and the Caribbean. The incidence rate in Southern Africa is still around 1,020 per 100,000 and 290 per

Table 19.1 Health MDGs scorecard for WHO regions

Health MDGs Scorecard for WHO Regions

MDG	Indicator	World	Africa	Americas	Eastern Mediterranean	Europe	Southeast Asia	Western Pacific
4	Under-five mortality rate *per 1,000 live births (2012)*	48	95	15	57	12	50	16
4	Measles immunization *percentage coverage (2012)*	84	73	94	83	94	78	97
5	Maternal mortality ratio *per 100, 000 live births (2013)*	210	500	68	170	17*	190	45
5	Skilled birth attendant *percentage births (2006–2013)*	72	48	94	58	98	67	93
5	Contraceptive use *percentage married women ages 15–49 (2006–2012)*	63	27	74	46	69	59	80
6	HIV incidence *per 100, 000 population (2012)*	33	176	15	9.9	18	12	5.9
6	Malaria mortality rate *per 100, 000 population (2012)*	11	63	0.02**	0.5**	0**	0.07**	0.03**
6	TB treatment *percentage success rate (2011)*	87	82	78	88	66	89	94
7	Water *percentage using improved drinking water sources (2012)*	90 2015 Target: 88	66 2015 Target: 75	96 2015 Target: 95	87 2015 Target: 93	98 2015 Target: 98	91 2015 Target: 85	93 2015 Target: 86
7	Sanitation *percentage using improved sanitation facilities (2012)*	64 2015 Target: 75	33 2015 Target: 64	88 2015 Target: 90	68 2015 Target: 77	93 2015 Target: 96	45 2015 Target: 63	70 2015 Target: 68

On track | Insufficient progress | Off track

* Region with MMR<100 in 1990 is not categorized; **Rates based on reported malaria deaths

2

100,000 in Central Africa, still higher than optimum. The rate is also above the target for the Eastern Mediterranean, at 9.9 per 100,000 population. Only 30% of people living with HIV are currently living in areas where medications are universally available. (See chapter 11 to learn more about global strategies for reducing HIV.) The malaria mortality rate per 100,000 population has declined by 42% globally between 2000 and 2012, from 19 to 11. Africa has made significant progress, but there are still 63 deaths per 100,000 population, most among children under age five (UN, 2014). Two countries, the Democratic Republic of the Congo and Nigeria, account for 40% of malaria mortality worldwide. Although more than 700 million **insecticide-treated nets** (ITNs) were delivered to sub-Saharan Africa countries between 2004 and 2013, still only 36% of the population living in malaria-affected areas in sub-Saharan Africa were sleeping under ITNs in 2013. (See chapter 9 to learn more about global malaria prevention and control.) Globally, for the fourth year in a row, 85% of newly diagnosed tuberculosis (TB) cases have been treated successfully. The relatively low success rate in Europe (66%) appears to be attributable, in large part, to the high prevalence of drug-resistance TB cases in Eastern Europe, many in marginalized groups (e.g., the homeless and injecting drug users, Carvalho, Migliori, & Cirillo, 2010).

The final two sets of data included in the "Health MDGs Scorecard for WHO Regions," Table 19.1, are the percentage of the population that used "improved drinking water sources" and "improved sanitation facilities" in 2012, both related to MDG goal 7. The global percentage increased from 76% to 90% between 1990 to 2012, with the target of cutting in half the proportion of people without access to an improved source (UN, 2014). Asia was the region with the largest increase of having access to an improved source—an increase of around 20% to 91%. Increases in Africa and the Eastern Mediterranean regions have not yet achieved their targets, as shown in Table 19.1. Improved sanitation facilities are now available to 64% of the world's population, as compared to 49% in 1990; the world did not achieve the 75% target by the end of 2015. Africa, the Eastern Mediterranean, and Southeast Asia are also unlikely to meet their 2015 targets and the Americas and Europe may not quite meet theirs. The vast majority (82%) of people currently using open defecation practices now live in middle-income, populous countries such as Nigeria and India. In addition, 70% of people without access to improved sanitation facilities now live in rural areas around the world. (See chapter 3 to read more about social determinants of health.)

Status of Other Health Outcomes and Social Determinants of Health

Table 19.2 presents additional information relating to global health and global health promotion, including global and regional assessments of a variety of social determinants of health. One additional set of data is presented related to MDG 4. Whereas under-five mortality rate was presented in Table 19.1, here we present the infant mortality rate (up to age one) per 1,000 live births. The global rate has declined from 63 in 1990 to 34 in 2013, about the same 45% decrease as in the under-five mortality rate during that time described above (UN, 2014). When comparing the infant mortality rates to the under-five mortality rates presented earlier, it becomes clear that almost all deaths under age five are infant deaths in the Americas, Europe, and the Western Pacific. One-quarter to one-third of the under-five mortality rates are due to ages one to five mortality, more significantly related to immunization rates, childhood diseases, and malnutrition, all significantly more problematic in Africa, Southeast Asia, and the Eastern Mediterranean.

We next present seven sets of data related to noncommunicable diseases (NCDs). We have presented some background epidemiological data in chapter 13 on NCDs, as well as much more information about global strategies to reduce NCDs, but we summarize some of it here as background. Of the 56 million deaths that occurred worldwide in 2012, about 38 million (68%) were due to noncommunicable diseases, principally cardiovascular diseases (48%), cancer (21%), chronic respiratory diseases (12%), and diabetes (4%) (WHO, 2014d). Unfortunately, more than 9 million of these deaths occurred before the age of 60 and could have largely been prevented (WHO, 2011). Low- and middle-income countries were the location for 80% of theses NCDs. In addition, more than 40% of NCD-related deaths in low-income countries occurred in people under age 60, nearly three times the proportion in high-income countries (13%). If the trend cannot be reversed, NCD deaths could reach 44 million deaths by 2020. During the next decade, the greatest increases are expected to occur in the WHO regions of Africa, Southeast Asia, and the Eastern Mediterranean (increases over 20%, compared to a global increase of 15%). "Most non-communicable diseases have globalization, urbanization and aging as underlying determinants; and unhealthy diet, physical inactivity and tobacco/alcohol as common risk factors. They also share intermediate risks like high blood sugar, raised blood pressure, overweight/obesity and abnormal blood lipids. The two major inextricably related issues, aging and chronic disease, create challenges for public health and clinical care in settings already faced with scarce recourses" (Boutayeb, Boutayeb, & Boutayeb, 2013).

In the most recent year for which data are available (2012), 68% of all deaths worldwide were caused by noncommunicable diseases (WHO, 2014d). (Unfortunately regional level data for 2012 have not been reported; the regional-level percentages of deaths due to mortality use 2008 data.) Percentages were highest for regions with the most upper- and upper-middle-income countries, Europe (87%), Western Pacific (80%), the Americas (79%), and the Eastern Mediterranean (79%). Percentages were lowest for Africa (28%) and Southeast Asia (55%). In addition, a higher proportion of NCD-related mortality occurs for individuals younger than 60 in lower- and middle-income than in high-income countries. Though percentages of mortality due to NCDs are lowest in Africa and Southeast Asia because of the generally higher mortality rates as well as the large populations (especially India in Southeast Asia and China in the Western Pacific region), in these parts of the world, the percentage of all global NCD deaths in low- and middle-income countries has now risen to 78%, up from 40% in 1990. This proportion is expected to reach 90% of all NCD global mortality by 2030. Thus it is increasingly important to look at data related to NCDs and risk factors for NCDs globally and regionally in planning global health promotion strategies for the next decades. Shown in Table 19.2 are total deaths due to NCDs by region.

Table 19.2 Health, Wellness, Mortality, and Social Determinants Data by Region

	North America	Latin America/ Caribbean	Western Europe	Eastern Europe	Africa	Eastern Mediterranean	Southeast Asia	Western Pacific*
Infant mortality rate/1,000 live births	15		13		61	43	38	15
Annual mortality due to NCDs	4.9M		8.0M		2.9M	2.2M	7.9M	10.2M
Breast cancer incidence (women)@	78	43	90	46	34	33	36	85/27*
Cervical cancer incidence (women)@	7	22	8	17	34	7	17	6/8
Lung cancer incidence (men)@	49	19	40	54	12	16	17	35/50*
Diabetes prevalence (percentage)	11		8		9	12	10	8
High blood pressure prevalence (percentage)	36		41		47	41	37	38
Percentage of adult smokers	18		29		13	20	18	26
Age-standardized prevalence (%) of obesity in adults ages 20 and up	27%		22%		8%	19%	3%	7%
Decayed, missing, and filled teeth index (percentage of countries averaging moderate to high)	0%	44%	0%	88%	13%	75%	0%	10%
Depression prevalence in sampled countries^	19%	13%	14%	15%+	10%+	10%	9%	18%+/7%*
Alcohol abuse prevalence	6.0%		7.5%		3.3%	0.3%	2.2%	4.6%
Percentage of tested cities exceed IT-2 for air pollution	40	60	40	100	80	100	100	20/100*
Percentage living in extreme poverty (< $1.25 US/day)	3#	5	0.5		47	2	25	8
Females 15+ literacy rate (percentage)	—	92	—	98	50	69	52	—
Human Rights Risk Index (percentage of countries at high or extreme risk)	0	75	0	68	94	90	88	0/80*
Corruption Perception Index (median world rank of countries)	17	94	31	110	119	80	117	16/83*

Note: Shaded cells are most problematic regions in each row of the table.
*Where two numbers are presented, they represent high-income and middle/low-income countries in that region, respectively.
+Only one country, which may not be representative of the region, was studied.
^Only 18 countries were studied, with a total sample size of approximately 50,000.
#Used less than $2/day definition.
@ per 100,000 population.

Next within the category of NCDs, we present incidence data on some key cancers found primarily in men and women globally (Ahmedin et al., 2011). Breast cancer appears to still be an illness found at higher rates in high-income countries of North America, Western Europe, and high-income countries of the Western Pacific. Lung cancer patterns are similar, though in parts of the world where smoking is quite high (e.g., Eastern Europe and China in the Western Pacific), lung cancer prevalence is also relatively high. Cervical cancer, on the other hand, is highly prevalent in low- and middle-income countries where health system infrastructures are less well developed and annual Pap smears are by and large not available, with the highest Eastern Europe, incidence rates in Central and South America, the Caribbean, sub-Saharan Africa, and Southern Asia. (See more about cancers in women in chapter14 and more about human papilloma virus in chapter 10 in vaccination campaigns.) Diabetes prevalence is increasing in both low- and middle-income and high-income countries, with rates in the double digits in most of the regions of the world, with slightly lower rates in Europe, Africa, and the Western Pacific (WHO, 2011). Obesity (presented later in this paragraph) is an increasing risk factor globally for diabetes. The prevalence of high blood pressure is moderately high (between 35% and 50%) in all regions of the world. Data are also presented for two risk factors for NCDs, percentage of adults who smoke and the percentage of adults ages 20 or older who are obese. Smoking is especially prevalent in Europe (and higher in Eastern Europe, not shown in the table) and the Western Pacific (and higher in China than elsewhere in this region). Obesity still appears to be largely a risk factor found in high-income countries of the Americas, Europe, and the Eastern Mediterranean (Ng et al., 2014; WHO, 2011).

Data related to oral and dental health are poorer and collected less often and in fewer countries than any of the other data presented here (Moreira, 2012; Peterson, 2003). We rely on a 2003 map reporting country-level average numbers of decayed, missing, and filled teeth (the DMFT index, widely used as a measure of oral health), in children age 12. Unfortunately, this confounds several factors, including oral health and access to and use of dental health care, because the number of filled teeth requires having seen a dental professional. Countries were classified into quartiles: the lowest quartile were those averaging less than 1.2 DMFT, next quartile 1.2–2.6 DMFT, and the two highest quartiles (classified as "moderate" and "high" and added to arrive at a percentage of countries in each region falling into either of these categories) were 2.7–4.4 DMFT, and finally, greater than 4.4 DMFT. As seen in Table 19.2, high-income regions had the lowest percentages of 12-year-olds with 2.7 or more DMFT (0% to 10%), though Southeast Asia also included no countries with an average of 2.7 or more DMFT. Africa, presumably at least in part because of little availability or use of dental care, had a low percentage of countries with a moderate or high average number of DMFT in 12-year-olds as well. Latin America and the Caribbean had a relatively high level of children with 2.7 or more DMFT (44%), and the Eastern Mediterranean (75%) and Eastern Europe (88%) had the highest proportion of 12-year-olds with 2.7 or more decayed, missing, or filled teeth. (See chapter 16 to learn more about global strategies for improving oral health.)

The next two sets of data presented in Table 19.2 relate to behavioral health, prevalence of depression and alcohol abuse, also considered NCDs in the developing world. The strongest global data concerning the prevalence of diagnosis-level depression were collected in a study of 18 countries with a total sample size of approximately 50,000, including one country only in high-income countries of the Western Pacific, Eastern Europe, and Africa, and so should be considered very cautiously (Kessler & Bromet, 2013). Rates of depression were highest in North America and the one high-income country of the Western Pacific (New Zealand). They were lowest in Southeast Asia, the Eastern Mediterranean, and the one country studied in Africa. Estimates of the prevalence of alcohol abuse are based on significantly more surveys across many more countries. The data suggest the highest rates of alcohol abuse are in the high-income countries of North America and Europe (WHO, 2014a).

We also present in Table 19.2 one kind of data related to global air pollution, an environmental risk factor especially for asthma and other respiratory diseases. This is also related to MDG goal number 7, environmental sustainability. To present the data on air quality, we first need to define some terms. Particulate matter (PM), comprised of solid or liquid material suspended in the atmosphere, is one sort of air pollution that is subjected to WHO compliance testing. $\mathbf{PM_{10}}$ is one regularly used measure of concentration of PM which assesses the percentage of particles $10\mu m$ in diameter ($1\mu m = 1$ millionth of a meter, with $100\mu m = 0.1$ mm) which pass through a size-selective filter. PM_{10} is important because it is also considered the "thoracic fraction," because particles larger than $10\mu m$ generally have a low probability of being carried past the larynx into the lungs. (WHO, 2005, pp. 9–28). The use of the proposed WHO air quality guidelines (AQG) for air quality for particulate matter, IT-5 (Interim Target-2), resulted in just about all of the cities around the world that were sampled not complying with the standard (WHO, 2014c). Thus we chose IT-2 (Interim Target-2) as a somewhat but not extremely high aspirational target in which the annual mean for PM_{10} is 50%. Results indicated that all sampled cities in Eastern Europe, the Eastern Mediterranean, Southeast Asia, and low-income countries of the Western Pacific (including China) exceeded this quality standard, and 80% of African cities did so as well. Western European and North American cities did best (only 40% exceeded the quality standard), and Latin American and Caribbean cities did moderately well (60% exceeded the quality standard).

Finally, and also shown in Table 19.2, we present data for four issues related to human rights and social determinants of health: the percentage of the population living in extreme poverty (Olinto, Beegle, Sobrado, & Uematsu, 2013), the percentage of females 15 and older who are literate (Population Reference Bureau, 2015), the percentage of countries in each region that score at high or extreme risk on the Human Rights Risk Index (Maplecroft, 2013), and the median world rank on the Corruption Perception Index of the countries in each region (Transparency International, 2014). Africa (47%) and Southeast Asia (25%) had by far the highest percentages of their population living in extreme poverty, the lowest percentage of females over age 15 who are literate (both around 50%), the highest percentages of countries in their region scoring at high or extreme risk on the Human Rights Risk Index (around 90%) along with the Eastern Mediterranean, and the highest median rank on the Corruption Perception Index (117 and 119), with countries in Eastern Europe, Latin America and the Caribbean, and the Eastern Mediterranean also scoring high on this last measure (median global country ranks of 110, 94, and 80, respectively).

In short, we found that

- Marked improvements have been made in infant and under-five mortality rates, childhood immunizations, and maternal mortality rates. More work is needed to achieve higher levels of immunization in rural areas and more contraceptive use and antenatal and skilled birth attendant care.
- HIV, malaria, and TB rates are significantly reduced from 15 years ago. More availability of HIV medication and use of insecticide-treated bednets are both needed, as is better diagnosis and treatment of resistant TB in Eastern Europe.
- Improvements in water and sanitation have lagged way behind MDG targets in much of the developing world. Much more financial commitment is required to accelerate health gains related to water and sanitation.
- Risk factors for NCDs are high in high-income countries and increasing in low- and middle-income countries. Obesity, smoking, diet, physical activity, and screening or vaccination for cervical cancer and screening for breast cancer all require greater targeted campaigns.
- Oral health data are so poor that it is difficult to know exactly where to target dental care. It is likely greatly lacking throughout the world, and because of the relationship between oral health and many other diseases, focus on dental health should be increased.
- Depression and alcohol abuse are very significant problems, especially in high-income regions of the world.
- Air pollution is a serious health threat in Eastern Europe, Africa, the Eastern Mediterranean, Southeast Asia, and the low- and middle-income countries of the Western Pacific. Political will is required to change this situation.

Extreme poverty is a pervasive health challenge, but especially in Africa and Southeast Asia. More girls need to be educated in Africa and Southeast Asia, and political work on human rights and corruption is required in Latin America and the Caribbean, Africa, the Eastern Mediterranean, Southeast Asia, and low-income countries of the Western Pacific region.

Key Challenges Ahead

Having described the current state of health outcomes and social determinants of health regionally and globally, in this section of the chapter we describe several key challenges that still remain. These include chronic illnesses (noncommunicable diseases), remaining and emerging infectious diseases, and social determinants and their role in new kinds of explanatory models.

Chronic Disease: Call to Action

The top four chronic disease killers are cardiovascular disease, diabetes, cancer, and chronic respiratory disease (WHO, 2014d). The level of associated disability and avoidable costs are staggering without significant work in global health promotion. Amazingly, the vast suffering that these killer diseases inflict is largely preventable. Perhaps more alarming, we could be the first generation not to live as long as our parents. We face this situation as a direct result of demographic change and profound changes in the way we live, work, and play. This is compounded by our own apathy and neglect on how best to turn back the rising tide of the epidemic of chronic disease, especially because there are cost-effective solutions for countries at every level of development. What is at stake, aside from the loss of life and quality of life?

Recent research at Harvard University estimated that if we maintain the status quo in terms of our investment in the required interventions—that is, do nothing more than what we are already doing—over the next two decades the estimated global cost of chronic disease will be approximately $30 trillion for cardiovascular disease, diabetes, cancer, and respiratory disease (Hunter & Reddy, 2013). If mental illness is included, which is a cross-cutting co-morbidity that is associated with chronic disease, as well as being a possible consequence of chronic disease, the cost is estimated to be an astounding $47 trillion over the next two decades! The regional and national implications are astronomical. To that end, we have run out of time; the time for action is now. Aside from the many humanitarian and human rights reasons, the hard reality is that the cost will be clearly unsustainable for national health systems, particularly in economically vulnerable countries. Senior policymakers must understand the significance of this impending health threat and accelerate efforts for prevention and promotion or we will drown in the costs.

Health promotion efforts often target citizens of the community to change individual behaviors leading to ill health. Equally, if not more important, such efforts must target policymakers who have enormous potential for making living conditions equitable and sustainable. Health policy decisions can lead to healthy foods being more accessible, as well as parks and recreational services and smoke-free environments. The two approaches must be inextricably linked. Educated citizens living in poverty in communities where health food choices or safe and recreational facilities are not available will be at risk for the poor health outcomes that we as health promoters are trying to prevent. The social determinants of health, including education, socioeconomic status, race, gender, ethnicity, and cultural background emerge as critically important factors to be addressed if we are going to avert the economic crisis of health costs that chronic disease will inevitably impose on society if the status quo is maintained. In this context, the factors that influence health go well beyond the health sector. Simply put, any positive impact on health will require an **"all of society" approach**.

A major driver is that the proportion of the population that is aging has also substantially grown and, if projections are accurate, will continue to grow. Folks are living longer lives, thereby acquiring multiple chronic diseases.

This phenomenon is ubiquitous in both developed and developing countries. Investment in policies and programs that promote healthy aging are therefore essential to avoid health costs outstripping pension costs. The good news is that the necessary measures are largely the same as those needed to prevent and control chronic NCDs.

In reality, chronic disease in many countries is both a cause and an effect of poverty. Chronic disease is a consequence of the social determinants of health. It is ironically also an effect of people living longer in countries developing economically with growth in their middle classes. One consequence is that the Americas are the fattest region in the world, a clear precursor to many of the chronic diseases that will lead to morbidity and premature mortality. In the United States, it is not surprising that our nation's poorest states are also our fattest (Ogden et al., 2010).

Childhood obesity—a precursor (early life version of) to the precursor (of chronic illness)—is also increasing. The social determinants prevent access. And, here lies the crux of the problem. To prevent childhood obesity we need a life span and multi-level approach that will ultimately help us mitigate the upcoming economic costs. Approximately 80% of our population lives in rapidly expanding urban environments, many of which are poorly planned, with few adequate transportation and recreational park services (Rydin et al., 2012). Poor urban planning and development ultimately contributes to families having no access to healthy foods, largely compounded by a detrimental national agricultural economic policy that produces poorly nutritious, unsafe foods. No matter how educated that family, a high-fructose, highly refined carbohydrate, poor omega-3 diet, in addition to an already unsafe neighborhood for sustaining a healthy lifestyle, all pave the way for premature suffering and death. Here again, we must acknowledge that the solution goes beyond health, and will require a broader, multilevel, "all of society" approach.

Despite the enormous challenges, highly cost-effective solutions exist that will save lives more quickly (WHO, 2011). But, these solutions will require everyone working together. Scaling up preventive measures to prevent or curb tobacco use is an example of an immediate action point. An additional trigger for action is that with increasing empowerment for girls and women around the world, smoking prevalence is rising faster in girls than in boys in many countries (Pan American Health Organization [PAHO], 2011). So rapid tax increases, smoke-free environments in work and public places, health information and warnings, and bans on tobacco advertising, particularly those targeting our children are required. And tobacco control is one of the clear **"best buys" in global health promotion**.

Good governance, including strong government ownership to implement such actions, is also critical and should be on the agenda of leading promoters of health. Government buy-in to reduce smoking prevalence by 20%, reduce average daily salt intake by 15%, and reach 60% of those folks who already have chronic disease with essential medicines like hydrochlorothiazide for high blood pressure, could avert millions of deaths over the next 10 years in low- and middle-income countries around the world (Gaziano, Galea, & Reddy, 2007).

Those folks would eventually die, but they would lead longer, more productive, happier, and healthier lives. Just those three things: reductions in tobacco and salt use, and better access to care for those who already have these chronic diseases can make an immediate impact. Using such best practices could greatly reduce that 47 trillion dollars in global costs over the next two decades, and is estimated to only cost about $11 billion per year for a basic package of similar best buys.

Toward achieving the needed "all of society" action, WHO and its regional offices, with support from key partners, can be the honest brokers. Engaging the private sector is absolutely essential. But, corporate responsibility is fundamental if such engagement will have sustainable benefit. Health promoters have the opportunity to engage the private sector with corporate responsibility being a key guiding principle. Corporate interests should not dictate the health agenda but be involved in the implementation of policy developed by public health authorities. Food and beverage companies, for example, can demonstrate that responsibility, including product reformulation to reduce salt, fat, and sugar; providing more information to consumers; restricting marketing to children of foods high in fat, salt, and sugar; and promoting physical activity. The story of the scale-up and use of concentrated fructose corn syrup in the United States is an excellent example of the road we do NOT want to take. Many experts now believe that after tobacco the next battle in public health will be curtailing the use of fructose corn syrup and sugar in general (Morenga, Simonette, & Mann, 2013). Fructose is clearly linked to premature mortality through a pathway of fatty liver disease, with the subsequent adverse consequences of diabetes, heart disease, and cancer.

Excellent, highly committed entities in the private sector exist who want to work on these issues in a most constructive manner, including NBA Cares, Merck Foundation, the Bill & Melinda Gates Foundation, and the Carter Center, as well as many other foundations that have emerged as a result of privately accumulated wealth. Many of these private entities only need a platform from which to bridge their philanthropic work. To that end, using the Americas as an example, PAHO has created the Pan American Forum on Chronic Disease Prevention in the Americas (PAHO, 2013). The forum meets yearly to discuss issues and mechanisms of collaboration going forward. Partners report back on actions taken. Additionally, PAHO has a regional plan of action for tackling chronic disease that is replicated at the national and local levels in every country of the region (PAHO, 2007). This plan of action provides mechanisms for member countries to implement four basic objectives. These objectives are to (1) rapidly enhance their policies and partnerships at the local and national levels of government, (2) reduce risk factors and strengthen protective factors, (3) strengthen the health system response, including increasing the capacity of the work force, access to essential medicines and supplies, and also coverage with multi-drug therapies; and finally (4) enhance national surveillance, monitoring and evaluation, and research activities. To sum up, this action plan addresses policy, risk factor prevention, health system capacity to respond, as well as monitoring and research, and is supported by the

CARMEN network of national NCD coordinators, and the aforementioned Pan American Forum. Similar plans have been constructed in other regions of the world. (See chapter 13 for more details about the PAHO plan and for details of the African region's response.)

Infectious Disease Prevention and Control

Any discussion of the unfinished agenda should avoid pitting infectious disease prevention and control against the chronic disease interventions discussed above, and vice versa. This is a trap public health experts often fall into. Make no mistake, from a global health perspective, chronic disease deserves our attention and commitment. For reasons expressed above, the chronic disease pandemic needs urgent attention, but not at the risk of the unfinished agenda. The road ahead must avoid the "tyranny of sequential thinking." Looking through the lens of vaccine-preventable diseases, such diseases, even when once controlled, have a way of rebounding with the deadliest of consequences, respecting no national borders or boundaries, especially if we drop our guard (Andre et al., 2008).

From a humanitarian public health perspective, but also from national, regional, and global security perspectives, the challenges of preventing and controlling disease spread that certainly respects no borders and are only a plane ride away, are daunting. The recent Ebola epidemic, which as of the end of August 30, 2015 has left 11,305 dead (WHO, 2015), is another prime example. To frame the discussion we have two stories from the Americas to share, one that occurred previously in 2006 and the other story continues to evolve.

The first story is about yellow fever. The case fatality ratio of yellow fever is 40%; it is a serious disease that kills (Tomori, 2004). Infected individuals, who die, experience a very painful death of systemic hemorrhage and multi-organ system failure. At one time, yellow fever was the scourge of the Americas. In fact, PAHO, the oldest international organization in the world, was largely founded as a result of Teddy Roosevelt's efforts to thwart the yellow fever threat of the late 1800s and early 1900s (PAHO, 2014).

There are two forms of yellow fever, the jungle or sylvatic form, and the urban or epidemic form. The jungle form is maintained by the animal reservoir of the monkeys in the jungle. A particular mosquito, the *Haemogogus* mosquito, can pass the virus to an unsuspecting human who ventures into the jungle. Jungle yellow fever does not spread from human to human. Jungle yellow fever can only be spread from monkeys to humans via this particular mosquito living in the jungle. As a result, the epidemiology of jungle yellow fever is characterized by a relatively few sporadic cases a year, usually among healthy, young men who go to the jungle to hunt, mine gold, or tend their crops (Barnett, 2007).

With regards to the urban epidemic form of the disease, the vector associated with this form of the disease, the *Aedes aeqypti* mosquito, lives in urban areas throughout Latin America and the Caribbean (Gubler, 2011). It is the same mosquito that leads to the spread of dengue virus, which causes what people often refer to as "break-bone fever," another killer disease in our region. Both jungle and urban yellow fever are equally dangerous to the infected human individual. The key difference between jungle and urban yellow fever is that once the yellow fever virus enters the urban setting where the *Aedes aegypti* mosquito resides, the virus develops the ability to spread from person to person through the mosquito vector, and thus has the high potential to cause large, urban outbreaks in populations of immune-naïve individuals who have not been exposed to yellow fever virus infection for decades.

Until the urban outbreak of yellow fever in Asuncion, Paraguay in 2008, the last urban yellow fever outbreak to occur in our hemisphere was more than 45 years ago (Andrus et al., 2011). Successful public health practices of vector control, and judicious use of vaccination strategies, had prevented ongoing outbreaks. When the outbreak started, the Paraguayan Ministry of Health was ill prepared for such an unexpected calamity. Doses of vaccine available were few. Those early days of the outbreak with shortages of vaccine directly contributed to widespread civil unrest in the nation's capital, Asuncion, that many felt almost toppled the elected government. The world responded to the 2006 outbreak, which acutely caused some 10 deaths in the peri-urban setting of Asuncion over a matter of a couple of weeks, in the following manner:

- The global stockpile maintained in Geneva by WHO and partners had been nearly depleted from the demand caused by the annual outbreaks in the yellow fever belt of Africa. A global call for action was put in place. Supplies from Geneva were freed up, but did not cover the 3.5 million doses needed for a country with a total population of approximately 9 million people.
- PAHO mobilized vaccine donations from neighboring countries of Brazil, Bolivia, Peru, Venezuela, and others.
- Experts were mobilized to assist the country in rapidly vaccinating one-third of the nation's population <1 month after the start of the outbreak.

These actions averted government collapse and civil unrest. The region acted collectively to dodge a bullet, save lives, and maintain national and regional security against a deadly killer thought to be no longer a risk. The International Health Regulations and PAHO's role in overseeing these regulations certainly contributed to the rapid response (Andrus et al., 2010).

In lieu of the social determinants of health and factors leading to climate change, the evidence is pretty overwhelming that we cannot drop our guard against the threats of neglected tropical diseases, leading to our second story (Andrus et al., 2013). **Neglected tropical diseases** are found in tropical or subtropical areas of the world that the United States has been free of for decades, examples include Chagas disease or the American form of trypanosomiasis, a parasitic infection which causes chronic heart problems often indistinguishable from cardiovascular heart disease; and other parasitic infections such as cutaneous leishmaniasis and cysticercosis. But, the list also includes dengue, West Nile virus, typhus, and tuberculosis in diabetic patients, diseases many of which already have a firm foothold in our own backyard of the southern United States. The challenge in countries like the United States will be to define the extent of the problem and the critical need for research. Developing countries already understand the severity of the problem; the challenge is galvanizing the resources to tackle these diseases properly. Diagnostic tests or simple drug therapies may not be available, or are too toxic to administer for some patients, and not necessarily considered economical for development by the pharmaceutical industry.

There are other issues at hand besides the traditional public health response to disease threats. Again, we must keep in mind the social determinants of health. An estimated 46 million Americans live below the poverty line, including 20 million who live in extreme poverty. Roughly, in Texas 1 out of every 5 people live in poverty (Andrus et al., 2013). Neglected tropical diseases clearly disproportionately affect people who live in conditions of poverty.

Chagas disease, the American form of trypanosomiasis, has been targeted for elimination from the Western Hemisphere by 2015 (Andrus et al., 2013). Chagas disease is the leading cause of dilated cardiomyopathy (Andrus et al., 2013). In 2006, some 8 million cases were reported. In 2010, some 6 million cases were still being reported. There has been progress but so much more needs to be done. The kissing bug, which serves as the vector for Chagas disease transmission, is highly prevalent in southern Texas. It is one thing for an adult to contract a disease like syphilis from another adult, but it is much more alarming to have mother to child in utero transmission. The unprotected fetus suffers life-long adverse consequences. The same goes for Chagas. The CDC estimates that some 300,000 cases of Chagas occur in the U.S. annually. But, in reality we really do not know the extent of the problem. We have only passive disease reporting mechanisms in place. We are still at the "tip of the iceberg" in terms of our understanding, or simply put by Peter Hotez, the best metaphor is "the ears of the Armadillo" (Andrus et al., 2013).

With regards to other causes of neglected tropical diseases, in 2012 outbreaks of dengue, or "break bone" fever, have occurred in Houston and parts of Florida (Andrus et al., 2013). Even the US capital is confronted with periodic outbreaks of West Nile virus, not to mention other bacterial threats such as multidrug resistant tuberculosis, and particularly the rapidly growing prevalence of this infection among our diabetic patients.

Tragically the dearth of surveillance data, especially for Chagas disease, only raises more questions, rather than provides answers. To that end in the United States, we urgently need to identify the critical public health gaps and address the specific needs of the southern states along the border with Mexico, especially in Texas. Several studies are required, from just understanding the extent of the disease burden, to defining the best public health interventions or best practices for cost-effective prevention and control, to developing new, more accurate diagnostic tests, to the development of new vaccines, like the vaccines on Chagas and hookworm.

On the part of PAHO and WHO, we are partnering with the best researchers and colleagues in the Ministries of Health of Latin America.

PAHO and WHO provide support to countries primarily through the development of national plans of action, strengthening of the institutional and human resource capacity to respond, strengthening national surveillance and laboratory systems, as well as overseeing the implementation of the International Health Regulations (Andrus et al., 2010).

In Latin America and the Caribbean our most vulnerable communities are indigenous communities, who are at greatest risk for neglected tropical diseases. These vulnerable communities include the Yanomami people along the Venezuela/Brazil border, those folks living in the Chaco region of Bolivia, Argentina, and Brazil, and also the communities of the Amazon Basin, the Chiapas region of Mexico, the highlands of Guatemala, and the Andes mountain range, and certainly the shantytowns of Recife, Port-au-Prince, and Kingston (Cassidy-Seyoum, 2014). And it is among these very communities that women and children carry the greatest risk for suffering caused by the burden of NTDs.

The accelerated fight against the NTDs in the Americas began decades ago. Any progress has been a result of key government leadership with support of key partners. No one entity can make a difference alone. The Americas have been fortunate to have eradicated polio, measles, rubella, and congenital rubella syndrome, all achieved with strong partnerships. For example, polio eradication would likely not have happened without the critical support of partners like the Rotary International (de Quadros et al., 1992). We also have been extraordinarily fortunate to have been supplied with effective donated medicines from Merck to combat onchocerciasis, also known as river blindness, with the ultimate goal of elimination in our region and also globally. With the donation of key drugs like ivermectin and the benznidazoles, and the creation of critical global partnerships between WHO, Ministries of Health, and key players, we have been able to treat millions and millions of people living in the Americas, ranging from entire countries to large populations and the "hotspots" of transmission. Understandably, the *p* in promotion actually underscores the guiding principle of any work going forward, the critical need for effective "partnership."

Consequently, countries have greatly suppressed or interrupted the transmission of onchocerciasis, the cause of river blindness, in all but 2 of 13 originally identified foci. On July 29, 2013 Colombia received the visit of an international team led by WHO/PAHO to verify the elimination of onchocerciasis (Global Network Neglected Tropical Diseases, 2013); Ecuador was declared free of the disease on September 29, 2014 (WHO, 2014b).

Promoting health through partnership has the great potential to achieve equity, access, and better health for all, particularly of the marginalized and the underserved communities. (See chapter 18 for more about collaborations among governments and international organizations and NGOs). In 2008, the partnership of PAHO, WHO, the Global Network for Neglected Tropical Disease, a program of the Sabin Vaccine Institute, and the Inter-American Development Bank pledged to work together to help countries scale up and coordinate integrated NTD programs (Inter-American Development Bank,

Pan American Health Organization, Sabin Vaccine Institute, 2011). Supporting national country leadership, this partnership is working to rapidly accelerate the development of National Plans of Action to eliminate and control the NTDs in Latin America and the Caribbean.

The fact remains that the neglected tropical diseases continue to be "forgotten diseases of forgotten people." If we continue to neglect what should be a legacy for our future generations of children, we will have failed as a global community.

The Hard Part: Social Determinants, Multilevel Models, and the Radical Agenda

One of the themes that has woven throughout this book is that global health promotion, to achieve many of its goals, must include much more than health care. Prevention will require collaboration among all of the public sectors, including education, health, transportation, urban planning and housing, and social services. As David McQueen has reminded us in chapter 2, this will necessitate an increasing use of language that broadens the biomedical public health model to a broader public health discourse that includes social, economic, and behavioral sciences. And as James Hospedales told us in chapter 13 and we have already said here, an "all of society" approach will be required. In order to persuade those in government bureaucracies and political leaders in countries that may have conservative policies that may prefer only the narrowest government approaches to problems, data will be required to show that structural changes, such as economic, educational, and housing programs (rather than specifically health programs) are needed to move the needle as far as it needs to go. Models and theories do not generate as much passion and energy as calls to action to stop neglecting chronic diseases now! Figure 19.2 shows a picture of various levels of variables from individual to structural that we and our colleagues (Kaufman et al., 2014) have proposed all need to be taken into account in both understanding and intervening to reduce HIV transmission. Similarly complex sets of variables will need to be measured and intervened upon with regard to the various health conditions, diseases, and problems that have been discussed in this book. Unfortunately, while lots of pictures have been drawn about groups of variables (like Figure 19.2), much hard theoretical and methodological work is also required to determine how to test such complex, **multilevel models** and show the impact of variables at all of the different levels and the interactions among the levels. But as organizations and research and public health groups increasingly look to cost-effective, evidence-based approaches for global health promotion, we urge that multilevel models be designed to test these interventions related to social determinants of health so government leaders will have no choice but to follow the data and support the big changes needed to arrive at a healthy population.

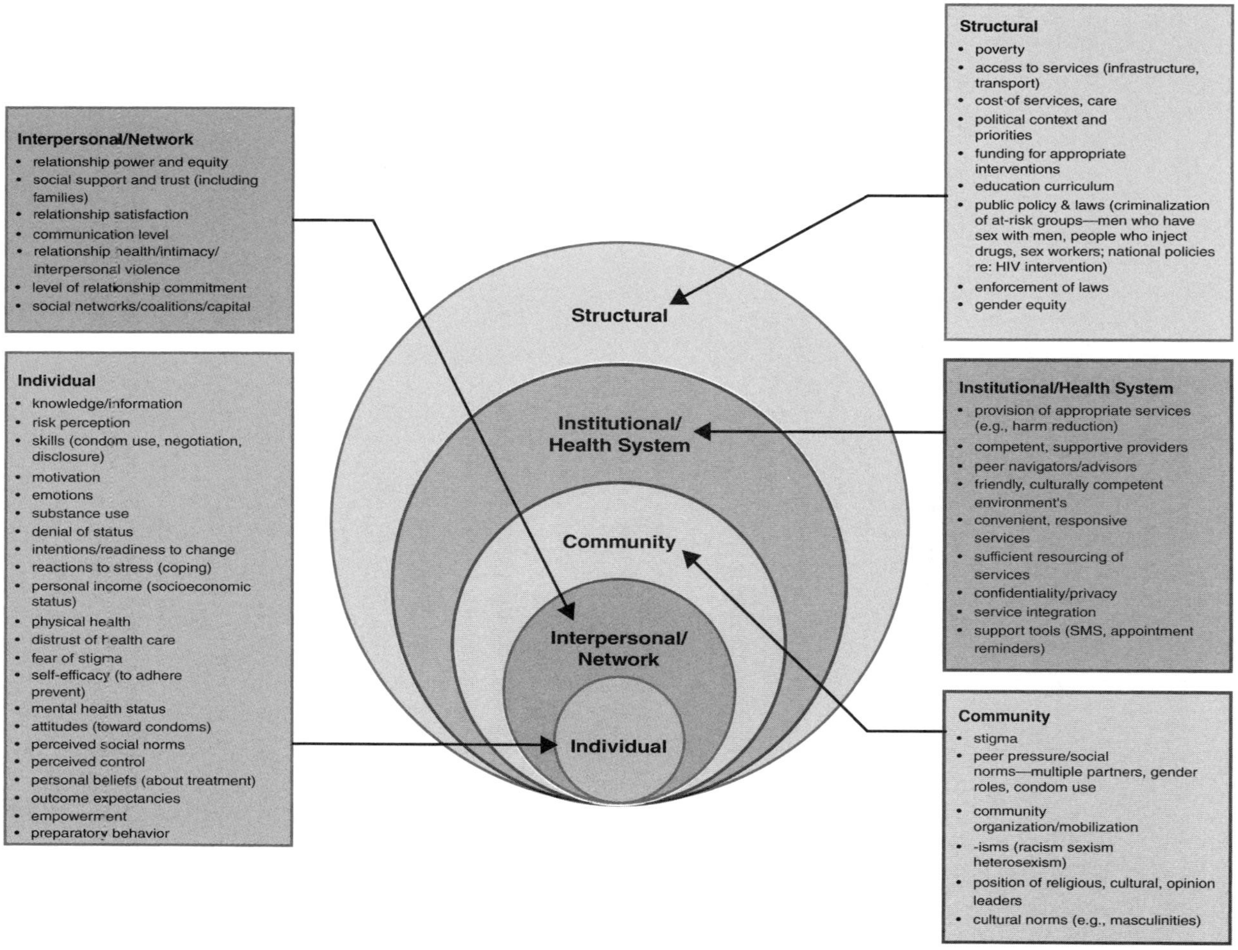

Figure 19.2 Factors Influencing Behavior Change at Each Level of the Socioecological Model, for the Example of HIV

Summary

In the first part of this chapter, we reviewed some data to assess where global health promotion has brought us and what work still needs to be done. In short, we found that marked improvements have been made in infant and under-five mortality, HIV, malaria, and TB rates, though improvements in water and sanitation have lagged behind millennial development goal targets. Risk factors for NCDs are prevalent throughout the world and in many cases are on the increase.

In the second part of the chapter, we presented several key challenges we believe remain for global health promotion. For the first time in recorded history, chronic non-communicable diseases are killing more people than infectious diseases. Maintaining the status quo in the response to prevention and control of chronic diseases will result in unsustainable health care costs for countries over the next two decades. There is still work to be done in reducing infectious diseases, including persistent neglected tropical diseases and other infectious diseases (like Ebola) that emerge and re-emerge over time. Finally, controversial but very important work still remains in reducing serious social determinants of disease and mortality, including poverty and food insecurity. New models also need to be constructed that include concepts at a variety of levels including the social-structural level.

KEY TERMS

1. **All of society approach:** An approach to health in which policies across sectors (education, transportation, banking, etc.) consider the health-related outcomes of the policy, rather than only the health sector focusing on health outcomes
2. **Best buys in global health promotion:** Health promotion approaches that yield significant improvements in mortality or morbidity per dollar spent; tobacco control is one of the best buys in GHP
3. **Decayed, missing, and filled teeth (DMFT):** A measure of oral health that adds the numbers of each of these type of teeth
4. **Insecticide-treated nets (ITNs):** Also called bednets, a primary prevention strategy for malaria
5. **Millennium Development Goals (MDGs):** The eight goals for international development established as a result of the Millennium Summit of the United Nations in 2000, following the adoption of the United Nations Millennium Declaration

6. **Multilevel models:** Models that include variables at multiple levels (e.g., individual, family, neighborhood, system, society) to predict and explain health-related behaviors and outcomes as more complex than the result of primarily or only individual-level factors
7. **Neglected tropical diseases (NTDs):** Diseases in tropical or subtropical parts of the world that the United States has been free of for decades,
8. **Neonatal deaths:** Deaths in the first 28 days of life
9. **PM_{10}:** A regularly used measure of concentration of particulate matter (PM) in which 50% of particles $10\mu m$ in diameter pass through a size-selective filter

REVIEW QUESTIONS

1. What are examples of health or social determinant outcomes that have shown so much progress that they met Millennial Development Goals around the world; examples that have met MDGs only in high-income countries; and examples that have not met MDGs in any regions of the world?
2. What chronic diseases are on the increase in low- and middle-income countries?
3. Why does good governance matter for good health outcomes?
4. Summarize two examples of neglected tropical diseases around the world.
5. Why are new multilevel models needed to help us understand and explain health-related behaviors and outcomes?

References

Ahmedin, J., Bray, F. C., Center, M. M., Ferlay, J., Ward, E., & Forman, D. (2011). Global cancer statistics. *Cancer Journal for Clinicians, 61*, 69–90.

Andre, F. E., Booy, R., Bock, H. L., Clemens, J., Datta, S. K., John, T. J., ... Schmitt, H. J. (2008). Vaccination greatly reduces disease, disability, death and inequity worldwide. *Bulletin of the World Health Organization, 86*, 140–146.

Andrus J. K., Aguilera, X., Oliva, O., & Aldighier, I. S. (2010). Global health security and the International Health Regulations. *Biomedcentral Public Health, 10* (Suppl.), S2.

Andrus, J., Bottazzi, M. E., Chow, J., Goraleski, K. A., Fisher-Hoch, S. P., Lambuth, J. K., … Hotez, P. J. (2013). Ears of the armadillo: Global health research and neglected diseases in Texas. *PloS Neglected Tropical Diseases, 7*(6), e2021, 1–6.

Andrus J. K., de Quadros, C. A., Castillo-Solorzano, C., Roses Periago, M., & Henderson, D.A. (2011). Measles and rubella eradication in the Americas. *Vaccine, 29S*, D91–D96.

Barnett, E. (2007). Yellow fever: Epidemiology and prevention. *Clinical Infectious Diseases, 44 (6)*, 850–566.

Boutayeb, A., Boutayeb, S., & Boutayeb, W. (2013). Multi-morbidity of noncommunicable diseases and equity in WHO Eastern Mediterranean countries. *International Journal of Equity and Health, 12*, 60.

Carvalho, A. C., Migliori, G. B., & Cirillo, D. M. (2010). Tuberculosis in Europe: A problem of drug resistance or much more? *Expert Review of Respiratory Medicine, 4*(2), 189–200.

Cassidy-Seyoum, S. (2014). *Neglected tropical diseases: Latin America and the Caribbean's silent killer*. Council on Hemispheric Affairs. Retrieved from http://www.coha.org/tropical-diseases-latin-america-and-the-caribbeans-silent-killer/

de Quadros, C. A., Andrus, J. K., Olive, J.-M., de Macedo, C. G., & Henderson, D. A. (1992). Polio eradication from the Western Hemisphere. *Annual Review of Public Health, 13*, 239–252.

Gaziano T., Galea, G., & Reddy, K. S. (2007). Scaling-up interventions for chronic disease prevention: The evidence. *Lancet, 370*, 1939–1946.

Global Network Neglected Tropical Diseases. (2013). *Felicidades, Colombia! Colombia Eliminates Onchocerciasis*. Retrieved from http://endtheneglect.org/2013/07/felicidades-colombia-colombia-eliminates-onchocerciasis/#sthash.XSQjHWjT.dpuf

Gubler, D. (2011). Prevention and control of *Aedes aegypti*-borne diseases: Lessons learned from past successes and failures. *Asian Pacific Journal of Molecular Biology and Biotechnology, 19* (3), 111–114.

Hunter, D. J., & Reddy, K. S. (2013). Noncommunicable diseases. *New England Journal of Medicine, 369*, 1336–1343.

Inter-American Development Bank, Pan American Health Organization, Sabin Vaccine Institute. (2011). *A call to action: Addressing soil-transmitted helminths in Latin America and the Caribbean*. Retrieved from http://www.globalnetwork.org/call-action-deworming-needs-latin-america-and-caribbean

Kaufman, M. R., Cornish, F., Zimmerman, R. S., & Johnson, B. T. (2014). Health behavior change models for HIV prevention and AIDS care: Practical recommendations for a multi-level approach. *Journal of Acquired Immune Deficiency Syndrome, 66*(Suppl. 3), S250–S278.

Kessler, R. C., & Bromet, E. J. (2013). The epidemiology of depression across cultures. *Annual Review of Public Health, 34*, 119–138.

Maplecroft (2013). *World Human Rights Index 2014.* Retrieved from http://reliefweb.int/map/world/world-human-rights-risk-index-2014

Moreira, R. da Silveira. (2012). Epidemiology of dental caries in the world. In *Oral health care: Pediatric, research, epidemiology and clinical practices.* V. Mandeep (Ed.), *InTech, OpenScience.* Retrieved from http://www.intechopen.com/books/oral-health-care-pediatric-research-epidemiology-and-clinical-practices/epidemiology-of-dental-caries-in-the-world

Morenga, L., Simonette, M., & Mann, J. (2013). Dietary sugars and body weight: Systematic review and meta-analyses of randomised controlled trials and cohort studies. *British Medical Journal, 346,* e7492.

Ng, M., Fleming, T., Robinson, M., Thomson, B., Graetz, N., Margono, C., … Gakidou, E. (2014). Global, regional, and national prevalence of overweight and obesity in children and adults during 1980–2013: A systematic analysis for the Global Burden of Disease Study 2013. *Lancet, 384*(9945), 766–81.

Ogden, C. L., Lamb, M. M., Carrol, M. D., & Flegal, K. M. (2010). *Obesity and socioeconomic status in adults: United States 1988–1994 and 2005–2008.* NCHS data brief no 50. Hyattsville, MD: National Center for Health Statistics.

Olinto, P., Beegle, K., Sobrado, C., & Uematsu, H. (2013). The state of the poor: Where are the poor, where is extreme poverty harder to end, and what is the current profile of the world's poor? *Economic Premise, October, 2013, number 125.* Washington, DC: Poverty Reduction and Economic Management Network Vice-Presidency of the World Bank. Retrieved from: http://www-wds.worldbank.org/external/default/WDSContentServer/WDSP/IB/2013/10/11/000333037_20131011145101/Rendered/PDF/818010BRI0EP120Box0379844B00PUBLIC0.pdf

Pan American Health Organization. (2007). *Strategy and plan of action for an integrated approach to the prevention and control of chronic diseases, including diet, physical activity and health.* Retrieved from http://www.paho.org/english/ad/dpc/nc/reg-strat-cncds.pdf

Pan American Health Organization. (2011). *Tobacco control report for the region of the Americas.* Retrieved from http://new.paho.org/hq/index.php?option=com_docman&task=doc_view&gid=16836&Itemid=

Pan American Health Organization. (2013). *Pan American forum for action on NCD.* Retrieved from http://new.paho.org/panamericanforum/

Pan American Health Organization. (2014). *PAHO celebrates 112 Years.* PAHO Web bulletin. Retrieved from http://www.paho.org/hq/index.php?option=com_content&view=article&id=10244&Itemid=135&lang=en

Petersen, P. E. (2003). *The world oral health report.* Geneva: World Health Organization.

Population Reference Bureau. (2015). *2015 World population data sheet with a special focus on women's empowerment.* Retrieved from http://www.prb.org/pdf15/2015-world-population-data-sheet_eng.pdf

Rydin, Y., Bleahu, A., Davies, M., Dávila, J. D., Friel, S., De Grandis, G., ... Lai, K. M. (2012). Shaping cities for health: Complexity and the planning of urban environments in the 21st century. *Lancet, 379*(9831), 2079–2108.

Tomori, O. (2004). Yellow fever: The recurring plague. *Critical Review of Clinical Laboratory Science 41*(4), 391–427.

Transparency International. (2014). *Corruption perceptions index.* Retrieved from http://www.transparency.org/cpi2014.

United Nations. (2014). *The Millennium Development Goals report, 2014.* New York, NY: Author.

World Health Organization. (2005). *WHO air quality guidelines for particulate matter, ozone, nitrogen dioxide and sulfur dioxide: Global update 2005, summary of risk assessment.* Geneva: Author.

World Health Organization. (2011). *From burden to best buys: Reducing the economic impact of noncommunicable diseases in low and middle income countries.* Retrieved from http://www.who.int/nmh/publications/best_buys_summary.pdf

World Health Organization. (2014a). *Global status report on alcohol and health.* Geneva: Author.

World Health Organization. (2014b). *WHO declares Ecuador free of onchocerciasis (river blindness).* Retrieved from http://www.who.int/neglected_diseases/ecuador_free_from_onchocerciasis/en/

World Health Organization. (2014c). *WHO's ambient air pollution database: Update 2014.* Retrieved from http://www.who.int/phe/health_topics/outdoorair/databases/AAP_database_results_2014.pdf

World Health Organization (2014d). *Global status report on noncommunicable diseases, 2014.* Geneva, Switzerland: WHO Press.

World Health Organization. (2015). *Ebola situation report 2 Sept. 2015.* Retrieved from http://apps.who.int/ebola/ebola-situation-reports

AUTHOR INDEX

Page references followed by *t* indicate a table and *b* indicate a box.

SUBJECT INDEX

Page references followed by *fig* indicate an illustrated figure; followed by *t* indicate a table and *b* indicate a box.

D

E

N

O

T

Y